Foundation Studies for Caring

How to use this book

Foundation Studies for Caring is a feature-rich textbook that has been developed with you, the student, in mind.

Each chapter begins with outcomes and concepts to help you plan your workload, and ends with a conclusion and reference section to support further learning. Throughout the rest of the book you'll find a wide range of innovative tools, all designed to help you become a capable and confident practitioner.

S **Scenarios**
Case studies which provide real-life situations for you to investigate

a **Learning activities**
Ideas to help you explore key issues, either individually or within your interprofessional learning group

e **Evidence-based practice boxes**
Examples of how best practice has been based on research

c **Professional conversations**
Practitioner perspectives to help you understand the roles of different professionals

t☆ **Practice tips**
Advice to help you provide exceptional care

! **Professional alerts**
Warnings about potential pitfalls, to ensure you work safely and effectively

 Links to *Foundation Studies for Caring*
Cross-references to help you navigate between chapters in this book

 Links to *Foundation Skills for Caring*
Cross-references to help you find relevant chapters in our sister skills volume

<u>W</u> **Web options**
Markers flagging up information that can be sourced online

W **On the websites**
Markers flagging up relevant material on our companion site

Foundation Studies for Caring

Using Student-Centred Learning

edited by Alan Glasper,

Gill McEwing and

Jim Richardson

palgrave
macmillan

First published 2009 by
PALGRAVE MACMILLAN

Palgrave Macmillan in the UK is an imprint of Macmillan Publishers Limited,
registered in England, company number 785998, of Houndmills, Basingstoke,
Hampshire RG21 6XS.

Palgrave Macmillan in the US is a division of St Martin's Press LLC,
175 Fifth Avenue, New York, NY 10010.

Palgrave Macmillan is the global academic imprint of the above companies
and has companies and representatives throughout the world.

Palgrave® and Macmillan® are registered trademarks in the United States,
the United Kingdom, Europe and other countries.

ISBN-13: 987-0-230-55268-5
ISBN-10: 0-230-55268-4

This book is printed on paper suitable for recycling and made from fully
managed and sustained forest sources. Logging, pulping and manufacturing
processes are expected to conform to the environmental regulations of the
country of origin.

A catalogue record for this book is available from the British Library.

10 9 8 7 6 5 4 3 2 1
18 17 16 15 14 13 12 11 10 09

Printed in the UK by
CPI William Clowes Beccles NR34 7TL

Contents

Chapter 28   **Rehabilitation**   573
               Stephen O'Connor

        29   **Loss, grief, bereavement and palliative care**   595
               Lynda Rogers and Pauline Turner

        30   **Emergency care and interventions**   610
               Jessica Knight and Rachel Palmer

        31   **Child emergency care and resuscitation**   635
               Janet Kelsey and Gill McEwing

        32   **Adult emergency care and resuscitation**   648
               Jan Heath

        33   **HIV and infectious disease management**   660
               Vidar Melby

        34   **Primary care**   683
               Sian Maslin-Prothero, Sue Ashby and Sarah Taylor

        35   **Complementary and alternative medicine**   704
               Alistair McConnon

        Names index   721

        Subject index   727

List of figures

List of tables

Acronyms and abbreviations

A&E	Accident and Emergency
AC	Aromatherapy Council
ADH	antidiuretic hormone
ADL	activity of daily living;
AGA	appropriate for gestational age
APHO	Association of Public Health Observatories
ART	antiretroviral therapy
ARS	acute retroviral syndrome
ASC	Action for Sick Children
ASH	Action on Smoking and Health
AVPU	alert, responds to voice, pain or unresponsive
BAPEN	British Association for Parenteral and Enteral Nutrition
BBB	blood brain barrier
BMA	British Medical Association
BMI	body mass index
BNF	British National Formulary
BOS	base of support
BP	blood pressure
bpm	beats per minute
CAIPE	Centre for the Advancement of Interprofessional Education
CBT	cognitive behavioural therapy
CD	controlled drugs
CDI	clostridium difficile infection
CMHN	community mental health nurse
CMV	cytomegalovirus
CNS	central nervous system
COG	centre of gravity
CPAP	Continuous positive airway pressure
CPD	continuing professional development
CPPIH	Commission for Patient and Public Involvement in Health
CPR	cardiopulmonary resuscitation
CSF	cerebrospinal fluid
CT	computed tomography
CVA	cerebrovascular accident
CVD	cardiovascular disease
D&V	diarrhoea and vomiting
DNS	diabetic specialist nurse
DH	UK Department of Health
DVT	deep vein thrombosis
EAR	estimated average [nutrition] requirements
EBL	enquiry-based learning
EBP	evidence-based practice
EFM	electronic fetal monitoring
ESR	erythrocyte sedimentation rate
EU	European Union
EWS	early warning score
FAED	food avoidance emotional disorder
FI	fusion inhibitors
GCS	Glasgow Coma Scale
GINA	Globe Initiative for Asthma
GP	general practitioner
GUM	genito-urinary medicine
HAART	highly active anti-retroviral therapy
HCAI	healthcare associated infections
HCP	healthcare providers
HCV	hepatitis C virus
HI	head injury
HIV	human immunodeficiency virus
HR	heart rate
HSE	Health and Safety Executive
HSV	herpes simplex virus
ICM	International Confederation of Midwives
ICN	International Council of Nurses
ICN	infection control nurse
ICP	intracranial pressure
ICU	intensive care unit
IDU	intravenous drug usage
IID	infectious intestinal disease
ILAE	International League Against Epilepsy

IM	intramuscular
IQ	intelligence quotient
IRB	Institutional Review Board (USA)
IUGD	intra-uterine growth deficit
IV	intravenous
IVI	intravenous infusion
IWL	insensible water loss
LGA	large for gestational age
LINKs	local involvement networks
LOC	level of consciousness
MAR	medicines administration record
MAU	medical assessment unit
MC	Medical Council
M, C&S	microscopy, culture and sensitivity
MDI	metered dose inhaler
MHO	Manual Handling Operations
MHRA	Medicines and Healthcare products Regulatory Agency
mmHg	millimetres of mercury
MMR	measles, mumps and rubella vaccine
MRI	magnetic resonance imaging
MSM	men having sex with men
NAWCH	National Association for the Welfare of Children in Hospital
NCCWCH	National Collaborating Centre for Womens and Children's Health
NCPC	National Council for Palliative Care
NCT	National Childbirth Trust
NELHS	National Electronic Database for Health
NG	nasogastric
NHS	UK National Health Service
NHSLA	NHS Litigation Authority
NICE	National Institute of Clinical Excellence
NICU	neonatal intensive care unit
NMC	Nursing and Midwifery Council
NNRTIs	non-nucleoside reverse transcriptase inhibitors
NPIS	National Poisons Information Service
NPSA	National Patient Safety Agency
NRTI	nucleoside/nucleotide reverse transcriptase inhibitors
NSCLC	non-small cell lung cancer
NSF	National Service Framework
NTE	neutral thermal environment
NU	neonatal unit
OM	omission
ORS	oral replacement solution
PAC	pre-admission clinic
PADSS	post-anaesthesia discharge scoring system
PALS	Patient Advice Liaison Services
PBL	problem-based learning
PCA	patient-controlled analgesia
PCP	pneumocystis carinii pneumonia

PCT	primary care trust
PEA	pulseless electrical activity
PEF	peak expiratory flow
PEG	percutaneous endoscopic gastrostomy
PGD	patient group direction
PHO	public health observatory
PI	protease inhibitor
PLH	people living with the human immunodeficiency virus
PN	practice nurse
PNS	peripheral nervous system
PPE	personal protective equipment
PPROM	premature prolonged rupture of membranes
prn	whenever necessary or needed
PSD	patient specific direction
QOF	Quality and Outcomes Framework
RCM	Royal College of Midwives
RCN	Royal College of Nursing
RCOG	Royal College of Obstetricians and Gynaecologists
RCP	Royal College of Physicians
RDS	respiratory distress syndrome
REC	Research Ethics Committee
RF	reticular formation
RNA	ribonucleic acid
RSCN	Registered Sick Children's Nurse
RSV	respiratory syncytial virus
RTA	road traffic accident
SAP	single assessment process
SARS	severe acute respiratory distress syndrome
SBL	student-based learning
SC	self-caring
SCLC	small cell lung cancer
SfBH	Standards for Better Health
SGA	small for gestational age
SHA	strategic health authority
SRN	State Registered Nurse
STI	sexually transmitted infection
TBI	traumatic brain injury
TBSA	total body surface area
TBW	total body water
TED	thrombo-embolic deterrent
TIA	transient ischaemic attack
TPN	total parenteral nutrition
U&E	urea and electrolyte
VCS	voluntary and community sector
VE	vaginal examination
VL	viral load
WHO	World Health Organization
WRVS	Women's Royal Voluntary Service

Notes on contributors

Sue Ashby, Lecturer in Nursing and Midwifery, School of Nursing and Midwifery, Keele University

Marion Aylott, Lecturer in Children's and Young People's Nursing, School of Health Sciences, University of Southampton

John Bastin, Lecturer in Biology, School of Nursing and Community Studies, School of Nursing and Community Studies, University of Plymouth

Maria Bennallick, Module Lead in Infection Prevention and Control Theory, School of Nursing and Community Studies, University of Plymouth

Margaret Chambers, Lecturer in Nursing (Subject Advisor Paediatrics), School of Nursing and Community Studies, University of Plymouth

Geraldine Clay, Lecturer in Health Studies (Adult Community Nursing), School of Nursing and Community Studies, University of Plymouth

Alison Cochrane, Senior Lecturer, Adult Nursing (Post-Reg) and Course Leader for BSC Professional Practice (Older People), School of Nursing and Caring Sciences, University of Central Lancashire

Michael Cooper, Lecturer in Adolescent Mental Health, School of Health Sciences, University of Southampton

Jenny Dedmen, Lecturer in Stroke Rehabilitation, School of Healthcare, University of Leeds

Rory Farrelly, Director of Nursing, NHS Greater Glasgow & Clyde Acute Services Division & National Advisor CNO (Scotland) for Children and Young People's Nursing

Anne Francis, Lecturer and Practitioner, Burns and Plastic Surgery, Senior Nurse Plastic and Oral Maxillo-Facial Surgery Out Patients Department, Salisbury NHS Foundation Trust

Carolyn Gibbon, Principal Lecturer for Learning and Teaching, School of Nursing and Caring Sciences, University of Central Lancashire

Anthony Gilbert, Deputy Head, School of Applied Psychosocial Studies, University of Plymouth

Alan Glasper (ed), Professor of Nursing, School of Health Sciences, University of Southampton

Kevin Hambridge, Lecturer in Adult Nursing, Faculty of Health and Social Work, University of Plymouth

Jan Heath, Skills for Practice Lead, Southampton University Hospitals NHS Trust

Kevin Humphrys, Lecturer, School of Health Sciences, University of Southampton

Katie Jackson, Lecturer in Applied Psychosocial Studies, School of Nursing and Community Studies, University of Plymouth

Pam Jackson, Head of Acute Care, School of Health Sciences, University of Southampton

Neil Jackson, Lecturer in Learning Disability, School of Health Sciences, University of Southampton

Adele Kane, Lecturer, School of Nursing and Community Studies, University of Plymouth

Janet Kelsey, Senior Lecturer in Health Studies (Paediatric), Academic Lead for Child Health and Programme Lead for BSc Child Health Nursing, Faculty of Health and Social Work, University of Plymouth

Jessica Knight, Lecturer in Nursing, School of Health Sciences, University of Southampton

Vanessa Lockyer-Stevens, Senior Lecturer and Programme Leader for Child Health, School of Health and Social Care, Bournemouth University

Eileen Mann, Nurse Consultant in Pain Management, Poole Hospital NHS Trust, and Lecturer-Practitioner, School of Health and Social Care, Bournemouth University

Sian Maslin-Prothero, Dean of the Graduate School and Professor of Nursing, Clos Moser Research Centre, Keele University

Vidar Melby, Senior Lecturer, School of Nursing, University of Ulster

Hilary McCluskey, Nurse Educator: Public Health Nursing, Waitakere Hospital, New Zealand

Alistair McConnon, Lecturer, School of Nursing and Community Studies, University of Plymouth

Gill McEwing (ed) Senior Lecturer, Faculty of Health and Social Work, University of Plymouth

Jane Morgan, formerly eLearning Co-ordinator, School of Health Sciences, University of Southampton

Stephen O'Connor, Consultant Nurse, School of Health Sciences, University of Southampton

Rachel Palmer, Academic Practitioner, School of Health Sciences, University of Southampton

Theresa Pengelly, Senior Lecturer in Child Health, Institute of Health, Social Care and Psychology, University of Worcester

Jennie Quiddington formerly lecturer, School of Health Sciences, University of Southampton

John Rawlinson, Academic Lead in Mental Health, School of Applied Psychosocial Studies, University of Plymouth

Brenda Rees, Head of Midwifery and Gynaecology Nursing, Cardiff and Vale NHS Trust

Colin Rees, Lecturer and Programme Manager, School of Nursing and Midwifery Studies, University of Cardiff

Jim Richardson (ed), Head of Division, School of Health, Sport and Science, University of Glamorgan

Melanie Robbins, Programme Manager BSc (Hons) Nursing Child, School of Healthcare, University of Leeds

Lynda Rogers, Senior Lecturer, Academic Lead for High Dependency Group, Academic Coordinator for Foundation Degree, School of Nursing and Midwifery, University of Southampton

Chris Taylor, Nurse Specialist, Southampton University Hospital Trust

Sarah Taylor, Diabetes Specialist Nurse, University Hospital of North Staffordshire

Kathryn Tattersall , Staff Nurse, Thoracic Surgery, Glenfield General Hospital, Leicester

Pauline Turner, Lecturer in Nursing, School of Health Sciences, University of Southampton

Acknowledgements

Every effort has been made to trace the copyright holders of third party material in this book. However, if any have been inadvertently overlooked, Palgrave Macmillan will be pleased to make the necessary arrangements at the first opportunity.

The publishers and authors wish to acknowledge the following for their kind permission to use copyright material:

Nursing and Midwifery Council for permission to reproduce Table I.1: NMC outcomes for entry to the branch programme

Wiley-Blackwell for permission to reproduce Figure 7.11 The ethical grid

NHS Clinical Governance Support Team for permission to reproduce Figure 8.2 The seven pillars of clinical governance

NHS Litigation Authority for permission to reproduce Table 8.1 Overview of NHSLA risk areas

Controller of HMSO and Queens' Printer for Scotland for permission to reproduce Figure 10.1 The Eatwell Plate; Table 19.2 Survival and disability rates

Bapen (British Association for Parenteral and Enteral Nutrition) for permission to reproduce Figure 10.2 Malnutrition Universal Screening Tool ('MUST'). Please note that for further information on MUST you should visit www.bapen.org

Nursing Times for permission to reproduce Figure 13.2 Frequently Missed Areas when Washing Hands

World Health Organisation for permission to reproduce Figure 13.3 Five Moments for Hand Hygiene

BMC Pediatrics for permission to reproduce Figure 19.3 Newborn classification by weight, length, head circumference against gestational age. The article from which this figure came is available at http://www.biomedcentral.com/1471-2431/3/13

Clement Clarke International www.clementclarke.com for permission to reproduce Table 21.6 Peak flow normal values

Peter Gardiner of Clinical Skills Ltd for Figure 28.1 Sleep positions following stroke

Resuscitation Council (UK) for permission to reproduce Figure 31.10 Paediatric foreign airway obstruction; Figure 31.18 Paediatric basic life support; Figure 32.3 Anaphylaxis algorithm; Figure 32.4 Adult basic life support

Dawn Johnson for permission to reproduce Figure 34.1 Care in the community

Photographs: Cover image: girl at whiteboard © Tim Wheeler; Chapter 19 Care of the Neonate © Marion Aylott; Chapter 20 Care of the Child and Young Person © Gill McEwing; Chapter 21 Care of the Acutely Ill Child © Gill McEwing; Chapter 30 Emergency Care and Interventions © Jessica Knight & Rachel Palmer; Chapter 31 Child Emergency Care and Resuscitation © Gill McEwing; Chapter 32 Adult Emergency Care and Resuscitation © Jan Heath

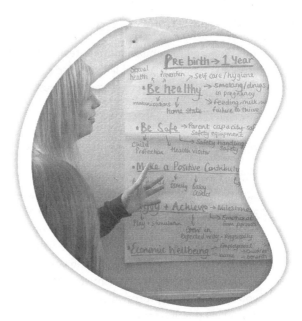

Introduction

Alan Glasper, Gill McEwing
and Jim Richardson

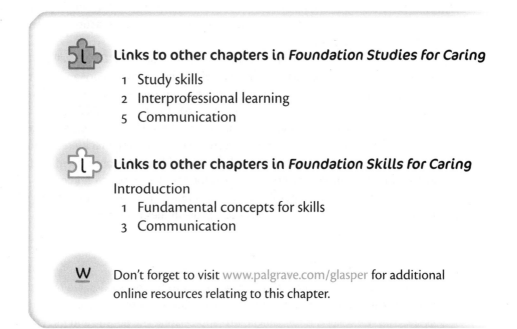

Links to other chapters in _Foundation Studies for Caring_

1 Study skills
2 Interprofessional learning
5 Communication

Links to other chapters in _Foundation Skills for Caring_

Introduction
1 Fundamental concepts for skills
3 Communication

W Don't forget to visit www.palgrave.com/glasper for additional online resources relating to this chapter.

Foundation Studies for Caring: Using student-centred learning

This book and its companion website are just two of the many resources that will help you to acquire the knowledge and skills needed over the foundation component of your programme. They will help you meet the required outcomes and to make the transition towards your chosen healthcare career.

Exploring the patient's experiences to help you learn

Throughout this book scenarios involving actual patient experiences and other clinical situations are visited – in other words, we take a client-focused approach. This is done from an interprofessional perspective so that the scenarios and clinical situations can be explored within the context of any of the fields of nursing and by other healthcare professionals. Therefore, whichever path you choose to follow, this learning will have direct relevance for you and you will be able to apply it in your own practice setting.

The book also takes a student-centred learning (SCL) approach. This means that it involves you in the learning process at every step, rather than simply listing facts. It is characterised by:

- working through activities and seeking out and responding to questions and dilemmas, many of which you are encouraged to pose for yourself.
- active learning – you will be invited to explore issues and gain further insights through local practice observations.
- studying individually and in groups – debating issues with colleagues enriches and diversifies your understanding.

The aim of this book is to help you to embark on the road to becoming a professional nurse or other healthcare practitioner. For this reason the questions and activities that guide your learning will frequently place you in the role of the qualified practitioner, rather than as a student or care assistant.

This book and the companion volume *Foundation Skills for Caring* will introduce you to a new and refreshing approach to learning about healthcare theory and practice. They use real client experiences as the focus for learning about caring. They are therefore more about learning how to think about healthcare and how to approach challenging situations than about providing all the answers. It is the ability of the healthcare professional to seek out solutions and provide the best possible care that separates the registered practitioner from nonprofessional colleagues. Nurses and other health professionals need to be constantly aware of practice developments, often brought about by research findings, so knowledge is ever-evolving and having the skill to access current information is key to professional practice. It is these skills of enquiry that we hope to explore in the chapters in this book.

Learning through enquiry

By taking a client-focused approach we want you to be able to visualise the bigger picture – that is, the full healthcare environment – before being tempted to examine each piece of the jigsaw. This, we believe, is fundamental to appreciating the holistic and integrative nature of contemporary healthcare practice, which crosses professional boundaries in order to provide the best possible patient care. This places learning in context; it gives you the opportunity to experience the excitement and challenge of professional practice from a position of safety, while also acknowledging the frustrations that some days can bring. This reality, together with your own experiences drawn from practice, will enable you to seek out and understand the background and detail behind each event.

Being reflective, being inquisitive and solving problems

Using enquiry as the basis of your learning often means starting with something unfamiliar or confusing and then seeking out the information that helps to explain or make sense of the situation or problem. This is a bit like looking for clues to solve a puzzle, and is something that healthcare professionals such as nurses have to do all the time. Seeking out and making sense of difficult issues and dealing with the uncertainties of life are essential skills for practice, equally as important as learning about hard facts.

This process of investigation is often called being 'reflective' and described as a sequence of events known as the reflective cycle. There are several examples that have been developed (Gibbs, 1988; Schon, 1983).

Figure I.1 is an adaptation from Gibbs (1988):

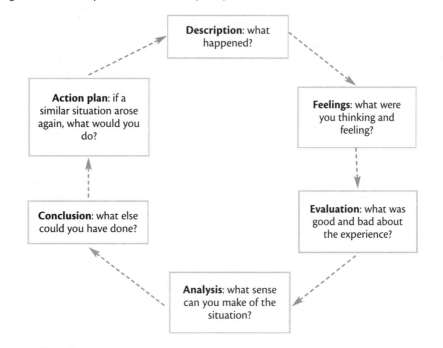

Figure I.1 The reflective cycle

There is a further example of the reflective cycle included in Chapter 14, which illustrates how it can be used in practice.

It will be helpful to keep these reflective stages in your mind as you explore and make sense of the different scenarios, and the complex world of healthcare which unfolds in the chapters of this book. Being reflective means getting in touch and keeping in touch with the way you and others practise.

a Learning activity

Think about a situation that you have recently experienced, perhaps one that did not quite go according to plan. Now work through each of the stages of the reflective cycle exploring your personal experience, looking at what you did and how you might do it differently next time.

Reflection provides a systematic approach to learning and to practising care delivery. You will also hear about problem-based approaches to assessing, planning, implementing and evaluating care.

Like reflection, problem solving can also be seen as a cycle, and makes use of some of the principles that have already been introduced in the reflective cycle. In reality you will use both approaches, depending on the situation you are exploring. For instance, sometimes you will explore a problem and find that there is a definite solution, a right or wrong answer, often proven through past research. On other occasions there is no problem to be solved, just something that appears confusing, that needs to be explored and understood. Such is the world of nursing and the other caring professions.

SCL is an umbrella term which incorporates these approaches we have been describing along with some other similar approaches:

- problem-based learning (PBL)
- enquiry-based learning (EBL)
- case studying
- action learning.

So what are these approaches to learning?

The modern history of the SCL movement began at the medical school at McMaster University in Hamilton, Canada. EBL/PBL found favour there as it was perceived by teachers to be an ideal medium for exploring the real world of patient care, where students could learn how to 'solve problems' and think critically. It is, however, important to understand that the term 'problem' encompasses 'enquiry', or the asking of questions about a particular subject. The enquiry may or may not be directly related to a patient problem as such (for example their illness or disease), but rather the learning issues to be explored.

This is particularly pertinent in higher education, where the emphasis has moved away from direct teaching to a more holistic use of the term 'learning'. Hence strategies to enhance learning opportunities, such as the use of EBL/PBL, have been adopted by many disciplines, including nursing and the other health professions. Additionally many traditional boundaries between the healthcare professions are becoming increasingly blurred in response to changes in healthcare delivery (Humphris and Masterson, 2000), and students are expected to work flexibly across these interprofessional boundaries. This changing workplace environment now requires an innovative approach to healthcare education, which facilitates greater understanding of the roles of different members of the interdisciplinary healthcare team. SCL is an innovative learning method which is suited to interprofessional healthcare education as it challenges students to identify the ideas and skills they will need to tackle the complexities of healthcare delivery (Duch, Groch and Allen, 2001).

All of the learning approaches mentioned here are enquiry based. Whichever approach your particular university favours, all will invite you to explore and learn through practice. They will not give you all the answers, but don't worry – they are not intended to.

EBL has similar principles to PBL, and for the purposes of this book it is not necessary for you to distinguish between the two. The case studying approach similarly uses the principles of EBL/PBL to explore real but anonymised patient case studies. Action learning takes place in a learning group, and is characterised by individuals learning with and from each other by analysing real issues from the world of healthcare. McGill and Brockbank (2004) believe that learning occurs when an individual or groups of individuals learn from reflection, and that this reflective learning in turn facilitates new learning from effective action.

Some reasons for adopting a model of SCL

Since the publication of *Fitness for Practice* (UKCC, 1999), many preregistration nursing curricula have embraced the principles of SCL as a method of educating students. SCL based on enquiry uses genuine real-life client scenarios, which provide the students with an opportunity to explore a range of issues directly pertaining to client care in a variety of contemporary nursing settings (Long, Grandis and Glasper, 1999). Exploration follows a systematic approach to enquiry, reflection and evaluation (Long and Grandis, 2000).

Learning is often undertaken as a group, with individual students taking on specific responsibilities within that group for researching and gathering evidence to bring back to the team. This contributes to the group's overall collective understanding of the issue or problem being explored.

In a Canadian study of second-year nursing students, Morales-Mann and Kaitell (2001) demonstrated that the factors that most influenced the levels of learning within the group were positive attitudes and group effort. Rhem (1998) believes that the reason this method is prevailing within higher education institutions is that it orientates students towards strategies of 'meaning making' over simple fact collecting.

In this way the product of the group is greater than the sum of the parts, resulting in higher levels of attainment in which prior learning is valued and built upon. Additionally, this type of cooperative learning brings with it enhanced social skills (Connolly and Seneque, 1999), which are highly valued in the healthcare professions.

Perhaps more importantly, the linking of clinical skills (prized by practitioners) and theoretical knowledge (prized by academics) through the medium of SCL (O'Neil, Morris and Baxter, 2000) might bridge the theory–practice gap which has bedevilled the profession for so long. Morales-Mann and Kaitell (2001) have described this type of learning strategy as liberating the academic from the traditional roles associated with teaching. This is good news for you and your lecturers, as you will both enjoy the process!

Acknowledging some challenges

Not all students find the approach easy. Indeed some prefer a more structured didactic approach, while others thrive on the freedom to explore, share and learn in a way that they feel reflects the way in which they will practise as professionals. A study by Glasper (2001) looked at a UK cohort of 15 children's nurses on completion of their three-year preregistration programme. Using a nominal group technique, he identified five areas that students liked most about SCL and five that they liked least. Students valued the friendships and support generated by working as a group, and believed that SCL enabled them to share experiences, exchange views and gain confidence. They saw SCL as having made the group work 'exceptionally well'. Conversely, students also voiced their frustrations about a lack of structure, having to rely on others to pull their weight and then being provided with poor-quality feedback by their peers on what they had researched.

Groups are usually led by tutors but can be led by students. Steele, Medder and Turner (2000), in a comparison of student-led versus tutor-led group work, demonstrated a preference for student facilitators. In this study of second-year medical students, peer facilitators were given slightly higher ratings than academics, but it was noted by the investigators that peer-facilitated groups often took short cuts in the SCL process.

You will need to use your skills in reflection to assess your own views on SCL, and take steps to address any problems.

Getting the most from this book

Because this is a different kind of textbook from many others, it is not encyclopaedic. We have selected aspects that we believe you are most likely to want to explore, and which will help you to address each of the Nursing and Midwifery Council (NMC) and other regulatory body outcomes (for entry to a particular field of practice programme). See page xxvi at the end of this chapter for more on the outcome). This book provides you with the opportunity to identify what you need to learn and to equip yourself with the necessary foundations on which to build your own professional practice. It will help you explore and experience new ways of learning and seek out pathways, while pointing you towards resources that will help you to make sense of complex issues. This is SCL, and we hope you enjoy the challenge. We think you will.

There are a number of steps that characterise the approach to learning used in this book. These steps draw on some of the principles of reflection and problem solving outlined earlier in this chapter. There are several examples of process steps. The steps illustrated here have been adapted from McMaster's handbook for tutors (1996) and Woods (1994).

SCL when working in groups

Before you begin there are some basic rules pertinent to SCL groups.

Election of chairperson and scribe

The group facilitator, who will normally be one of your lecturers, will prompt the learning group to elect a chairperson and sometimes a scribe who may summarise on flipchart paper the focus of your discussions. This makes it easier for the group to agree a work schedule. In some universities SCL groups meet weekly, others less often. The chairperson and the scribe might only act in the role for one meeting, or take those roles for a whole scenario often over a period of many weeks. As each group member will act as a chairperson at some point during the semester, everybody can learn the skills of chairing and those of summarising group contributions as scribe.

Setting SCL ground rules

This is important to allow the group to function optimally. Learning groups may consider some of the following:

- Mobile phones should be switched off.
- Everybody must pull their weight by fulfilling what they said they would do for the following SCL meeting (this might be a PowerPoint presentation, a student handout or a poster presentation, for example). There is nothing more embarrassing than not turning up to your SCL group or not having fulfilled your commitment. Note that attendance at SCL groups is usually mandatory in most universities and registers are kept.
- Respect – during SCL meetings whatever an individual person says should be respected even if you disagree. That is all part of SCL, and the freedom to say what you feel must not be compromised.
- Punctuality and other ground rules may be agreed.
- Keep rules to a minimum!

SCL when working as an individual

Working as an individual you may find it useful to consider your own way of learning and to reflect on your learning strategies, study methods and skills of communication to enable you to create and capitalise on a variety of learning opportunities.

The process steps

The enquiry phase

1 Explore the scenario (often an action learning group – also known as a learning set – will develop their own scenario)
   - Do you understand the context of the scenario?
   - Are there words that you need to define?
2 What are the main issues?
   - Analyse the situation, challenges and problems.
3 Identify what you do not know and need to know (because your lack of knowledge is impeding understanding and action).
4 Decide the exact questions on which you need to work, and prioritise them.
5 Plan your use of resources; for example, plan your time to make the best use of learning opportunities.

The reflective phase

6 Share experiences, new knowledge and learning with others whenever you can create the

opportunity. Reflect on the adequacy of the answers to your original questions and identify what remains to be achieved.

When working in a group the seventh stage is:

7 Reflect on the group process (considering what enhances and what inhibits learning within the group learning environment).

Your learning group facilitator, who will understand what you need to achieve over the foundation year of your programme, will steer you away from areas of investigation that are beyond your level, and advise you of when you might explore these areas in future years of the programme.

> **(a) Learning activity**
>
> Just as you did earlier, try taking a patient situation or problem or area of knowledge deficit and by using the process steps explore ways in which you can find an acceptable way forward, or indeed an answer to your problem.

Getting started

In order to maximise and enjoy your learning and make the best use of your study time, read the next section carefully.

Each chapter in this book has expected learning outcomes; however, as an enquiring student, it is likely that you already have many questions about healthcare practice and how this relates to the practice of colleagues from other disciplines. When you start to read each chapter, you may identify with particular clinical or personal experiences which prompt you to question why you thought or reacted in a particular way, so make sure you note these. You may be exploring some topics for the first time with little or no previous experience, so you don't know what you don't know! For many students in healthcare this can initially raise some anxieties, but you are not alone! This is usual and part of the learning process.

There are prompts for learning in the form of questions and activities at regular points in each chapter. Some of these are best attempted before you read on, as they will help you to identify how much you currently know, as well as the level and accuracy of existing knowledge. Sometimes we do not appreciate what we have previously taken for granted until it is clearly brought to our attention – better in a book than in the clinical environment! The companion textbook to this volume, *Foundation Skills for Caring*, has been written to let you see the relationship between theory and practice, and by dipping into each you will begin to build up a picture of your world of healthcare. Additionally there is a companion website that allows you to further explore each chapter topic. The chapter writers have placed kite-marked websites on the online pages to allow you access to other types of material which you will find extremely helpful in your learning groups or action learning sets.

Your most important role as a healthcare student is to constantly question, to gain knowledge and to identify the evidence base that underpins accepted professional practice. Sometimes, you might discover that care is based more on 'custom and practice' than evidence, and there is a need to seek out the most informed sources, rather than follow tradition.

This book helps you to identify the areas of knowledge that you may need to explore, and the kinds of questions that you might choose to ask. Developing the confidence to ask questions is a very important part of being a healthcare professional, since you will need to be able to seek out information from patients and their relatives, often about sensitive or potentially embarrassing topics. All healthcare professionals need also to possess assertiveness and interpersonal skills to be able to appropriately question, and sometimes challenge, colleagues from either the same or other disciplines. Clearly, effective communication is immensely important both now as a student and in your future career (see Chapter 5 on Communication).

Deciding what to focus on

It is also acknowledged that knowledge is constantly changing. This can be a troublesome idea when starting a new career with a vast amount to learn. However, once the overall picture is grasped and the foundations are laid, more complex issues can be tackled. This comes through reading, accessing other resources and also from being an active observer and participant in clinical practice. Soon you will feel more comfortable questioning accepted practice. As a student you are privileged to experience a wide range of practice environments, and you will observe that care might differ between practitioners. Questioning the rationale for those differences will add to your repertoire of knowledge and skill, rather than accepting that it is just the way something is done. The manner in which questions are asked is likely to influence the response you receive!

Key points you may like to consider are:

- Is this the appropriate time?
- Is this person likely to have the correct information or appropriate experience?
- Do I need permission to ask this person?
- How do I phrase the question; for example, to avoid offence or to ensure the question elicits a relevant answer?

Throughout the book you will be invited to seek the opinions of friends, relatives, patients and others, finding out their views related to different health issues. Getting into the habit of seeking others' opinions will help to develop the skills you will need throughout your professional career. Working in healthcare is a lifelong learning experience, which requires you to remain open to others' views and opinions.

Most textbooks are studied in isolation. However, it is well established that learning with others can contribute very positively to the learning experience, not only in making it more interesting and satisfying, but also in extending ideas. Spending time thinking about practice is useful, but it is likely to be yet more productive if you can engage with others. They might identify aspects which you haven't thought about. Your views might be questioned and this may prompt you to think more laterally – to think the unthinkable!

As discussed, your university centre will normally provide you with opportunities for small group learning in the form of a learning group or action learning set, and there might also be an interprofessional group of which you are a member. Perhaps you are also a member of an online learning group facilitated through one of the virtual learning platforms such as Blackboard or WebCT. You will certainly have access to email , and much of your collaborative leaning will be facilitated through this medium. Various chapters in the books examine study methods and optimum methods of using information technology, such as PowerPoint presentations. You may have friends in other healthcare educational institutions with similar learning needs.

Each chapter also presents a set of concepts. This list is not definitive. Again, as you approach the topic area in each chapter, you may have your own concepts to add to the list. When reviewing the concepts embodied within the chapters, view them as broadly as possible as this will enhance your understanding. For example, the concept of 'care' will be viewed differently depending on whether you are a patient, client, husband/wife, child, parent, friend, nurse, manager, doctor, physiotherapist, chaplain, undertaker or employer. Accessing the literature will also broaden and deepen your current understanding of each concept. Continually reflect on your personal experience, your current understanding and how new knowledge can change practice. It is through this process that improvements in practice are made.

Working with scenarios

Most clients/patients first access healthcare in a community setting, with many attending the local health centre, the occupational health facility at work, or being cared for in their own homes. With changes to out-of-hours general practitioner services many now seek health advice from NHS Direct or its equivalents, or NHS walk-in centres. Some patients seek advice over the internet using for example NHS Direct online or accessing digital television health advice programmes. 'E-health' care is becoming a reality. Because of the increasing array of portals for healthcare through which a client can access information, some of the scenarios in this book are set in the community and some are located in a hospital or other residential settings. All however emphasise the importance of providing integrated services, so that wherever people are attended to there is continuity of care.

Central to most chapters is a named individual or a family. They may have health problems which have resulted from disease, injury or handicap, or have been exacerbated by social circumstances resulting in distress. Each is equally important to the student of healthcare. The study of health will enable the student to raise health awareness, promote health, and where possible, reduce the likelihood of disease or recurrence of illness. The skills of healthcare practitioners such as nurses are also directed towards those who are already ill, are disabled or having difficulty coping, in either the short or long term. Much is about enabling people to maximise their level of independence, to live fulfilling lives. Healthcare is not so much about cure, but providing quality of life, providing comfort, and where needed, supporting the whole family through a period of death and bereavement. This philosophy is reflected in the chapters of this book, and the principles are relevant to all healthcare professions, including the fields of practice of nursing.

Practising in a changing world of healthcare

The ways in which new healthcare practitioners are prepared for their unique role within health services have changed radically over the last few years. Different health professions now often learn together. There is now more flexible access as well as opportunities to 'step on' and 'step off' courses, as your individual student needs dictate. This book hopes to introduce you to a way of learning that reflects and complements the diversity of this approach. Whether you embark on your studies in a college of further education or at university, we intend that this book will act as an effective resource as you begin a career in healthcare.

Although the fundamental principles upon which healthcare is founded remain unaltered, the ways in which professionals practise, the roles they occupy with others and the public's expectation are constantly changing. In this century more than ever before, healthcare practitioners will have to adapt their practice to meet the needs of the increasing number of people who are living longer, well into old age. Nurses among others must find ways of providing the best care possible, yet be constrained by tighter costs and account for their every action.

While research and new technologies will enable more and more dreams to be realised, lives to be saved and health to be optimised, some of the longer-established treatments will, as now, be found wanting. We have already entered the arena of the 'superbug'. There are new challenges; old diseases over which we had previous control are increasing again (for example tuberculosis), and the full impact on health from environmental change is yet to be realised. Smoking has increased dramatically among young women and we are yet to see the full impact of the rising tide of obesity in children and adults. The expectations and demands of modern living are leading to increased levels of stress, mental illness and suicide in all age groups. Conversely, for example many people who develop cancer are living much longer after treatment than they previously did and there is improved use of transplants and organ donation. No wonder public expectation constantly rises as the media proclaims that more and more is possible!

Aside from all this, new ways of caring for people within the community aim to support independence more effectively. This brings with it the challenge of taking acceptable risks when public protection must always be paramount. Healthcare professionals have to be able to make such difficult decisions daily. When things go wrong, more people then ever before will know their rights and will have the confidence to seek redress, but because the gap between wealth and poverty continues to widen, the professional's role in safeguarding the interests of the more vulnerable becomes ever more important.

As the boundaries of practice change, nurses and others will choose to extend their skills into new areas. Some will overlap with the skills of other professionals, and yet all will continue to use those skills that the public recognise and know as 'nursing', 'occupational therapy', 'physiotherapy' and so on. It is this mix of essential skills, knowledge and attitudes that is woven into the fabric of the healthcare professional and which is is central to lifelong professional practice. It is these fundamental principles that will be introduced during the initial period of this book, and the way you understand them will influence the way you will practise in the future.

Working towards competence

The Nursing and Midwifery Council (NMC), the regulatory body for nursing, and the other healthcare regulators set out a number of common outcomes that all students, irrespective of where they are studying in the United Kingdom, are required to achieve. For example if you are commencing a nursing course, meeting these first-year outcomes will enable you to proceed to one of four fields of practice programmes: adult, children's, mental health or learning disability nursing. The NMC outcomes to be achieved at the end of the first year are set out in Table I.1.

For examples of other healthcare professional learning outcomes visit the pages on the companion website that accompany this chapter.

Table I.1 NMC outcomes for entry to the branch programme

Domain 1 Professional and ethical practice
Discuss in an informed manner the implications of professional regulation for nursing practice. ➜ Demonstrate a basic knowledge of professional regulation and self-regulation. ➜ Recognise and acknowledge the limitations of one's own abilities. ➜ Recognise situations which require referral to a registered practitioner.
Demonstrate an awareness of the NMC code of professional conduct ➜ Commit to the principle that the primary purpose of the registered nurse is to protect and serve society. ➜ Accept responsibility for one's own actions and decisions.
Demonstrate an awareness of, and apply ethical principles to, nursing practice ➜ Demonstrate respect for patient and client confidentiality. ➜ Identify ethical issues in day-to-day practice.

Demonstrate an awareness of legislation relevant to nursing practice ➜ Identify key issues in relevant legislation relating to mental health, children, data protection, manual handling, and health and safety, etc. ➜ Demonstrate the importance of promoting equity in patient and client care by contributing to nursing care in a fair and anti-discriminatory way. ➜ Demonstrate fairness and sensitivity when responding to patients, clients and groups from diverse circumstances. ➜ Recognise the needs of patients and clients whose lives are affected by disability, however manifest.
Domain 2 Care delivery
Discuss methods of, barriers to and the boundaries of effective communication and interpersonal relationships ➜ Recognise the effect of one's own values on interactions with patients and clients and their carers, families and friends. ➜ Utilise appropriate communication skills with patients and clients. ➜ Acknowledge the boundaries of a professional caring relationship.

Demonstrate sensitivity when interacting with and providing information to patients and clients

Contribute to enhancing the health and social well being of patients and clients by understanding how, under the supervision of a registered practitioner, to:
→ Contribute to the assessment of health needs.
→ Identify opportunities for health promotion.
→ Identify networks of health and social care services.

Contribute to the development and documentation of nursing assessments by participating in comprehensive and systematic nursing assessment of the physical, psychological, social and spiritual needs of patients and clients
→ Be aware of assessment strategies to guide the collection of data for assessing patients and clients and use assessment tools under guidance.
→ Discuss the prioritisation of care needs.
→ Be aware of the need to reassess patients and clients as to their needs for nursing care.

Contribute to the planning of nursing care, involving patients and clients and, where possible, their carers, demonstrating an understanding of helping patients and clients to make informed decisions
→ Identify care needs based on the assessment of patient or client.
→ Participate in the negotiation and agreement of the care plan with the patient or client and with their carer, family or friends, as appropriate, under the supervision of a registered nurse.
→ Inform patients and clients about intended nursing actions, respecting their right to participate in decisions about their care.

Contribute to the implementation of a programme of nursing care, designed and supervised by a registered practitioner
→ Undertake activities which are consistent with the care plan and within the limits of one's own abilities.

Demonstrate evidence of a developing knowledge base which underpins safe nursing practice
→ Access and discuss research and other evidence in nursing and related disciplines.
→ Identify examples of the use of evidence in planned nursing interventions.

Demonstrate a range of essential nursing skills, under the supervision of a registered nurse, to meet individuals' needs, which include:
→ Maintaining dignity, privacy and confidentiality, effective communication and observational skills, including listening and taking physiological measurements, safety and health, including moving and handling and infection control, essential first aid and emergency procedures, administration of medicines, emotional, physical and personal care, including meeting the need for comfort, nutrition and personal hygiene.

Contribute to the evaluation of the appropriateness of nursing care delivered
→ Demonstrate an awareness of the need to assess regularly a patient's or client's response to nursing interventions.
→ Provide for a supervising registered practitioner, evaluative commentary and information on nursing care based on personal observations and actions.
→ Contribute to the documentation of the outcomes of nursing interventions.

Recognise situations in which agreed plans of nursing care no longer appear appropriate and refer these to an appropriate accountable practitioner
→ Demonstrate the ability to discuss and accept care decisions.
→ Accurately record observations made and communicate these to the relevant members of the health and social care team.

Domain 3
Care management

Contribute to the identification of actual and potential risk to patients, clients and their carers, to oneself and to others and participate in measures to promote and ensure health and safety
→ Understand and implement health and safety principles and policies.
→ Recognise and report situations which are potentially unsafe for patients, clients, oneself and others.

Demonstrate an understanding of the role of others by participating in inter-professional working practice
→ Identify the roles of the members of the health and social care team.
→ Work within the health and social care team to maintain and enhance integrated care.

Demonstrate literacy, numeracy and computer skills needed to record, enter, store, retrieve and organise data essential for care delivery

Domain 4
Personal and professional development

Demonstrate responsibility for one's own learning through the development of a portfolio of practice and recognise when further learning is required
→ Identify specific learning needs and objectives.
→ Begin to engage with and interpret the evidence base which underpins nursing practice.

Acknowledge the important of seeking supervision to develop safe nursing practice

Reproduced by kind permission of the Nursing and Midwifery Council (2002).

References

Connolly, C. and Seneque, M. (1999) 'Evaluating problem-based learning in a multilingual student population', *Medical Education* **33**(10), 738–44.

Duch, B. J., Groch, S. E. and Allen, D. E. (2001) *The Power of Problem Based Learning: A practical 'how -to' for teaching undergraduate courses in any discipline*, Stirling, Va., Stylus.

Gibbs, G. (1988) *Learning by Doing: A guide to teaching and learning methods*, Oxford: Further Education Unit, Oxford Polytechnic (New Oxford Brookes University).

Glasper, E. A. (2001) 'Child health nurses' perceptions of enquiry-based learning', *British Journal of Nursing* **10**(2), 1343–9.

Humphris, D. and Masterson, A. (eds) (2000) *Developing New Clinical Roles: A guide for health professionals*, Edinburgh, Churchill Livingstone.

Long, G. and Grandis, S. (2000) 'Introducing enquiry-based learning into pre-registration nursing programmes', in Glen, S. and Wilkie, K. (eds), *Problem-Based Learning in Nursing Programmes: A new model for a new context*, Basingstoke, Macmillan.

Long, G., Grandis, S. and Glasper, E. A. (1999) 'Investing in practice: enquiry- and problem-based learning', *British Journal of Nursing* **8**(17), 1171–4.

McGill, I. and Brockbank, A. (2004) *The Action Learning Handbook*, London, RoutledgeFalmer.

McMaster University (1996) *Tutor Handbook*, Hamilton, Ontario, McMaster University.

Morales-Mann, E. T. and Kaitell, C. A. (2001) 'Problem-based learning in a new Canadian curriculum', *Journal of Advanced Nursing* **33**(1), 13–19.

Newman, M. (2000) Project on the effectiveness of problem based learning (PEPBL) [online] www.hebes.mdx.ac.uk/teaching/research/PEPBL/index.htm (accessed 23 December 2008).

Nursing and Midwifery Council (NMC) (2002) 'Nursing competencies', Section 3, pp. 9–21 in *Requirements for Pre-Registration Nursing Programmes*, London, NMC.

O'Neil, P. A., Morris, J. and Baxter, C. M. (2000) 'Evaluation of an integrated curriculum using problem-based learning in a clinical environment: the Manchester experience', *Medical Education* **34**(3), 222–30.

Penfield virtual hospital (2007) [online] http://www.hud.ac.uk/hhs/departments/nursing/penfield_site/default.htm (accessed 23 December 2008).

Rhem, J. (1998) 'Problem-based learning: an introduction', *National Teaching and Learning Forum* **8**(1) (December) [online] http://www.ntlf.com/html/pi/9812/pbl_1.htm (accessed 23 December 2008).

Schon, D. A. (1983) *The Reflective Practitioner: How professionals think in actions*, New York, Basic Books.

Steele, D. K., Medder, K. D. and Turner, P. (2000) 'A comparison of learning outcomes and attitudes in student versus faculty-led problem-based learning: an experimental study' *Medical Education* **34**(1), 23–9.

United Kingdom Central Council (UKCC) (1999) *Fitness for Practice*, London, UKCC.

Woods, D. R. (1994) *Problem-Based Learning: How to gain the most from PBL*, Hamilton, Ontario, McMaster University.

Insights into the context of caring

Chapter

1

Study skills

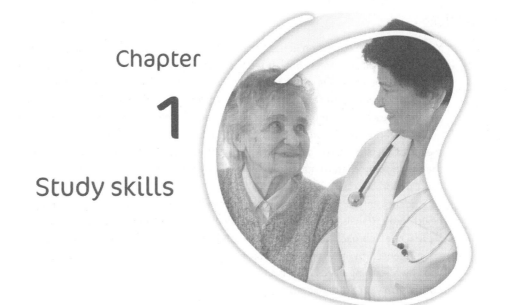

Colin Rees and Alan Glasper

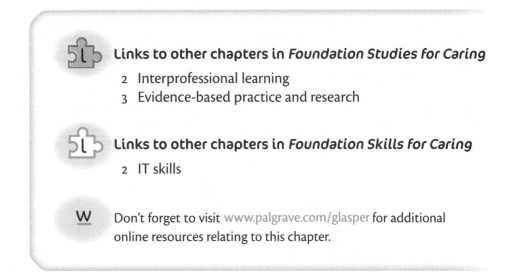

Links to other chapters in _Foundation Studies for Caring_

  2 Interprofessional learning
  3 Evidence-based practice and research

Links to other chapters in _Foundation Skills for Caring_

  2 IT skills

W Don't forget to visit www.palgrave.com/glasper for additional
online resources relating to this chapter.

Introduction

Your professional education in healthcare is an active method of preparing you for your future role as a healthcare professional. It requires the ability to think logically, and use a number of key skills to pull together a vast range of knowledge, and apply it to complex situations. Study skills are a major part of that activity. They consist of a range of techniques and methods for advanced reading, writing and critical evaluation, as well as methods of organising your time.

You will find your student life is easier if you acquire good study skills, as they provide a means of keeping on top of academic work. They help by providing a system and method for the processes needed to make sense of the knowledge and skills that have to be absorbed in a short period of time.

Student-centred learning is rapidly becoming a popular way of structuring learning for health professionals, as it develops the skill of identifying personal learning needs, and taking a proactive approach to learning. Both student-centred learning and professional education are influenced by how organised you are, and the extent to which you identify and satisfy your own learning needs. This chapter is an essential first step in helping you to a successful outcome in your academic work.

The aim of this chapter is to provide an insight into studying for a professional qualification. It covers essential features of study skills – in other words, how you learn to learn, and particularly how you can make tackling assignments easier. These skills will prepare you for some of the activities you will face early in your course.

Learning outcomes

The chapter will enable you to:

- outline the features of professional education
- describe the key features of student-centred learning
- outline a planed approach to learning
- describe key features of time management for assignments and projects
- identify the range of learning situations encountered in professional education
- describe the main features of reading for assignments
- demonstrate how to search for material on the web
- carry out a review of the literature
- demonstrate how to critique research articles
- outline the basic features of academic writing
- construct a references list using the Harvard system
- describe how to prepare seminar feedback
- summarise how to construct a poster presentation
- outline how to make appropriate use of supervisors.

Concepts

- Professional education
- Student-centred learning
- Sourcing literature and evidence
- Primary and secondary sources
- Reviewing the literature
- Critiquing research articles
- Academic writing
- Assignment work
- Plagiarism
- Referrals
- Reading styles
- Harvard system of referencing
- Seminar participation
- Poser presentations
- Supervisor support

[S] Scenario: Introducing Sue

Sue is 32 years old and starting her nurse education programme, after having worked part-time as a care assistant in a local home for the elderly for the last four years. She has two children aged 9 and 7. Adult nursing has always been her ambition, but when the children came along she had to put thoughts of becoming a nurse on hold until they were fully settled in school. She has some NVQ qualifications but not a great deal more.

Sue is excited about finally starting her nurse education, but is apprehensive about the academic side of it. She feels intimidated by younger students, and imagines they will be computer literate, and very bright. She sees herself as a slow learner. It is a long time since she has done any studying at this level and she does not have a great deal of self-confidence in her academic abilities.

There is a computer at home, which she bought with the children's education in mind. She does use the web for weekly shopping, and buying household bargains. She has a new pencil case, an A4 note pad, and a neat backpack, so feels ready for the challenge. On commencement of the course Sue is allocated to a student learning group.

a) Learning activity

What do you feel are some of the common feelings and concerns of people starting an academic health professional course like yours? You may wish to undertake this activity as part of your initial learning group activities.

The start of any course can be overwhelming. Once you are provided with the details of course and module content, there seems so much to learn, and assignments and exams seem to require so much understanding and work. Even understanding the question of some assignments can feel like a huge challenge.

The world of education has also to fit in with life outside the university, where there can be other demands such as family and social commitments. Managing your learning can mean a lot of juggling commitments and opportunities, and deciding on priorities so everything exists comfortably together.

At the start of any course it is important to decide on some principles to follow in your academic work. The temptation is to become immersed in student social life and let the structure of attending lectures, seminars and tutorials just happen. On the other hand, you may find yourself squeezing your academic life into the time left over from looking after a family. Situations like this will result in tensions and difficulties in your life and need to be avoided.

Time management

Organising your time is one of the most important skills to develop early in a course. This means using diaries, calendars and 'to do' lists to ensure that you pace everything and successfully attend modules, meet deadlines and are at the right place at the right time. There are many tools to help you achieve this, such as:

- electronic palm-held organisers/mobile phone organisers
- notepads
- diaries
- wall calendars
- combinations of all these.

Choose a method that suits you, but be self-disciplined and consistent in its use. Have a clear system to record key events, times and places such as lectures, seminars and clinical placement details. You will find that you have to consult noticeboards for details of venues, or check the university website or virtual learning platforms such as 'Blackboard' for modules for changes or information on where you should be, and what you will need to bring with you, or wear.

One of the keys to being a successful student is taking responsibility for yourself, and ensuring that you are well prepared for daily life and for assignment and other academic work.

Becoming a good learner

Professional education means *engaging* with knowledge and skills that will provide the basis of your professional role. You will always be learning new things. Knowledge is not something that you empty out of a box and capture as a 'one-off' event. The secret of success is learning how to learn. That means developing skills that allow you to develop new understandings and put together, by synthesising, knowledge that can be applied to daily work. It also means being proactive in applying learning skills in all the situations in which you find yourself.

To engage with knowledge is more than learning something by heart, or rote learning. This is because learning something by heart does not mean you understand it, or can adapt it to different situations. You are limited to using such information in the way that you learned it; in other words, the knowledge or skill is not transferable. This chapter covers the ways in which the main forms of engagement take place. They include:

- thinking
- reading
- thinking
- writing
- thinking.

The repetition of 'thinking' is deliberate. The key to engaging with knowledge is through thinking and reflecting on meaning, so that you can join areas of knowledge together and create your personal understanding. In your course, you will demonstrate that you have achieved understanding by writing about it, talking about it, and perhaps answering exam questions, as well as carrying out practical activities to demonstrate your grasp of information and skills.

Types of learning setting

> **S** Scenario continued
>
> Sue's previous education consisted of her school years, and the NVQ course she undertook. Her thoughts about the possible differences between nurse education and her past experiences were a little hazy. When she started the course she was surprised at the size of the student group in lectures. She was also unprepared for the variety of forms in which learning takes place.

There are a number of different ways in which your learning will be structured. These include:

- lectures
- seminars
- tutorials
- workbooks
- student-centred learning
- group work and activities
- reflective accounts
- e-learning
- poster presentations.

Each of these depends on similar processes, although the way the student demonstrates that learning has been achieved may differ. The basic process is to:

1 Identify the learning outcome (aim).
2 Collect information and process it (or in the case of a skill, practise it).
3 Structure an answer to satisfy the aim or carry out a skill that has been demonstrated or described.
4 Reflect on what has been learned.

Throughout this chapter we show you how this is achieved in different situations. We concentrate mainly on thinking skills rather than clinical skills. Whatever the setting, it is important not to lose sight of the bigger picture of your course and how each part makes a contribution to your professional education. In other words, do not treat each part of your course as a 'stand alone': they are all meant to fit together, although at the time they might not seem to.

E-learning

S   Scenario continued

Sue has a home computer but leaves its use mainly to her husband, Simon. The children love it, and find little difficulty in using it for games and entertainment. Sue occasionally 'borrows' it for supermarket shopping to save time. She has some keyboard skills but feels she is a little slow. Now she is on the course she is surprised to find how much students are expected to use the computer. They need to use it not only to write and submit assignments, but to communicate with lecturers through email and access learning programmes. This is yet another area of the course she finds a little stressful.

E-learning is any form of learning that takes place through electronic means. This includes everything from computers to learning programs on compact discs (CDs). However, more usually it focuses on computers and web-based methods of learning.

People vary in their skill and familiarity with computers, but whatever your level of skill, the best plan is to make it work for you. You will find computers make almost every aspect of being a student easier:

- writing in all its forms, including preparing assignments, emailing other students and university staff
- finding out what information is available on a topic
- getting hold of published and web material
- sending drafts of work to lecturers for comments
- using software such as referencing programs to make putting work together easier
- increasing understanding of topics through material available on websites and CD packages
- taking part in noticeboards or discussion pages on the web, often part of the university website
- working through learning packages on the web.

Practice placements

S   Scenario continued

Sue is allocated to her first placement, where she meets her mentor for the first time. She is apprehensive about what she is supposed to do.

Getting the most from your mentor

All healthcare students are allocated a mentor when attending practice placements. The role of the mentor is to support students in meeting their practice learning outcomes. Practice learning outcomes are an integral part of the curriculum, and in some courses such as nursing, the practice component makes up to 50 per cent of the programme. All healthcare students should expect full support from their mentor, who will have undertaken a programme of study to equip them for this role. In some programmes such as nursing the mentor has to directly provide supervision to a student for at least 40 per cent of their allocated duties. It is the mentor's responsibility to plan and coordinate the student's learning experience and help them achieve their stated competencies. These competencies are prescribed by healthcare regulators such as the Nursing and Midwifery Council.

You are advised to make contact with your allocated mentor before starting the placement. This will enable you to coordinate your shifts to mirror those of your mentor.

t☆
Practice tip

One of the valuable student skills is being able to use a computer effectively.

During your placement your mentor will help you experience and demonstrate competence in a range of clinical skills. Always endeavour to ask your mentor for help when you feel overwhelmed in a particular clinical situation. You are a student and they are experienced practitioners who want to help you achieve your professional goals.

Improving your skills

Computer skills

You will need (as a minimum) to be familiar with word processing programmes, accessing the web and downloading material. It also helps if you have good keyboard skills and can type using all fingers rather than a 'two-finger stab'. There are a number of programmes to develop your typing skills, and these are well worth buying and persevering with, as the time you spend in learning will be more than repaid in the time saved later. Many universities insist that students undertake the European Computer Driving Licence (ECDL). This is an extremely valuable course: you will find it easy to grasp and very worthwhile. The more you use the computer, the more valuable you will find it in every aspect of student life. Start with a positive view of using the computer, and develop your skills as much as you can throughout the early stages of the course.

Writing skills

During your course you will write for a variety of reasons and in a number of different ways. For example, you will:

- make notes in lectures
- make rough notes for assignments or tutorials
- take notes from articles or websites
- do assignment work
- note down reflections on your work for an assignment or private reflections
- prepare notes for a student-centred learning group meeting.

It is worth spending time to learn how to do all these different forms of writing effectively.

Making lecture notes and planning assignments

> **S** Scenario continued
>
> In lectures, Sue is unsure whether to sit and listen and makes notes later, or write down what the lecturer is saying at the time. Often lecture notes are available in hard copy for students after lectures, or can be downloaded from the university website. Other students seem to do a variety of things, including scrawling all over their notepads and producing something that looks like a spider's web. Sue wonders whether there is a right or wrong way to make notes.

It is common to take notes in lectures, but Race (2005) makes the distinction between 'note taking' and 'note making'. Note taking is like 'dictation' where we can be on automatic pilot, just going through the motions of taking notes. The results will not be very meaningful to us. In contrast, where we understand what is going on and want to ensure that we don't forget that understanding, *making* notes will allow us to recall that understanding.

There are a number of ways you can simplify note taking. Usually writing down the main words or key phrases will be enough to act as a trigger to remembering the most important aspects of a session. If you find it difficult to concentrate in lectures, taking some notes of the key points can help you keep tuned in to the main point of the lecture. Do not write down the content of PowerPoint presentations, as they will usually be made available to you, either as PowerPoint notes, or for download from the university website.

One interesting way of making notes, not only from lectures but also for planning assignments, is using 'mind maps'. These are the 'spider diagrams' Sue saw someone making. Key words, perhaps enclosed in bubbles, are linked with lines and arrows, producing something rather like an underground map. Mind maps were originally developed by Tony Buzan, and he discusses how to use them in a number of books: for example, Buzan (2006).

Lectures are meant to be incomplete, in that it is not possible to cover everything you need to know in a lecture, and they are not always a good way to learn. The content of a lecture should provide the basics; you need to add to the information by reading source material and giving plenty of thought to what it all means. Use the lecture as a means to trigger questions and connections in your mind. It is just as important to write down your own ideas and questions during the lecture, to follow up later. Fill out your lecture notes with material taken from books and articles, and also add your own reflections and comments. In written assignments, do not simply repeat back to a lecturer their own words. This is not what they want to read: they want to know what you can add to the basic information they gave you. The key activity in university learning is reading: reading around the topic to show that you are an independent learner. Concentrate on this aspect of developing your own knowledge to gain good marks.

During your course you will effectively learn a new 'language': the vocabulary of your chosen profession. Many of the words will be new to you, and other familiar words will be used in a more specific way. In lectures, or as you read, each time you encounter a new word or phrase, record it in a specific 'vocabulary' notebook for future reference. Concentrate on producing a definition for these words. Make sure you can spell them correctly, and use them appropriately as part of a sentence. Read through your 'vocabulary' notebook regularly so that the words become familiar.

> **t** ☆
> ## Practice tip
> It is a good idea to keep a vocabulary notebook.

Academic writing

Using ideas and words from published sources such as books and articles is a big part of 'academic' writing: that is, formal writing such as in written assignments. This is because it shows that you have taken other viewpoints into account, and that where possible, you have read and considered what experts on a particular topic have learned or said about something.

Academic writing follows some important rules and principles. If you learn these, and follow them closely, it will make everything a lot easier for you, and help you develop a good writing style.

Plagiarism

> **C** ## Professional conversation
>
> Sue comments: 'I was asked by another student from a different learning group in the second year whether I wanted to borrow her assignment from the first year. She said she would give me a copy the next time we met at the coffee point. As I was nervous about writing this assignment I was grateful for the offer. When I told my mentor about this the following day she became quite concerned, and told me that I might stray into potential plagiarism. I did not know what she meant, but when she explained, I was relieved that I had not actually taken the assignment from the other student. When I met the student again the following week she had forgotten all about the offer, and I never mentioned it again.'

One very important rule is that you must avoid plagiarism. This means using someone else's words and thoughts as if they were your own, without acknowledging where you got them from. Your student handbook will probably include some advice on this. Academically it is seen as a form of dishonesty, as it is intended to deceive people into thinking you are giving your own thoughts in your own words. Avoid this all costs, as the academic consequences if you are caught plagiarising someone else's work are quite severe, and at the worst you might be asked to leave the course.

It is easy to avoid plagiarism. Do not stop introducing other people's ideas into your work, but do make sure you acknowledge where they come from every time you do so. Keep track of where you get material from, and always make sure when you include someone's ideas that you give full details of the publication (if the source is a book, article or website), or of the person providing the idea if it was not from a published source.

Where you use other people's ideas and words you will gain good marks if you discuss and analyse them, rather than simply repeat them. Say what ideas you agree with, or have found that others agree with. If you or others disagree with the author or have a different viewpoint, explain why. That is, you need to provide evidence or illustrations to support your comments.

Assignment work

> **S** **Scenario continued**
>
> A major worry for Sue is writing assignments. She feels she has little to say and worries that she will end up just repeating what has been said in lectures or what other people have written. She has been told that to get good marks she must develop an 'academic writing' style. In particular, she has been told she should be analytical, not simply descriptive. If she knew what all this meant, she feels she might stand a chance! At the moment it all seems intimidating and she really does not know where to start with her first assignment.

Like all forms of writing, there are a few simple rules that will help you get a good mark for your assignments. These include:

- Understand what is required by carefully studying the question or title.
- Check the learning outcomes for the module to work out what you are being testing on through the assignment.
- Produce a timetable that will give you time to work on the assignment.
- Gather material that will be useful.
- Work to an assignment structure.
- Be prepared to spend time on editing the work several times.
- Ensure that the question or title has been fully answered.
- Reflect on what has been learned through the assignment.
- Always carry out a final check for simple errors, especially referencing errors, before submitting the work.

> t★
> **Practice tip**
> Always follow the stated learning outcomes for the assignment. Each learning outcome must be addressed.

One of the unspoken rules for students regarding assignments is, 'First find out what they want, then give it to them!' It will help if you take some time at the beginning of an assignment to ensure that you understand what is being asked, and plan how you are going to answer it. You will save time overall by doing this. Once you feel confident that you know the 'angle' the assignment should take, you can calculate how much time will be required to complete the rest of the steps:

1 Write an assignment plan starting with 'Beginning/Middle/End' as a rough structure. You should not use these headings in the final version but they will help in the early stages of the work.
2 Gather material to slot into the various sections.
3 Write a first draft.
4 See your supervisor and get some feedback.
5 On the basis of the feedback you receive, edit the draft into the final version.
6 Check that you have followed the assignment brief and answered the question within the word limit set.
7 Make a final check for simple errors, including ensuring that references are complete and accurately presented.
8 Submit your work in the university agreed font style, size and spacing. Avoid exotic font designs and fancy layouts: remember you are writing an academic assignment.

Seeking an extension/mitigating circumstances

Through no fault of your own, circumstances may occur which prevent you from meeting your assignment deadline. Most universities will grant a one or two-week extension provided you contact the assignment leader at least a week before the deadline. If they agree to give you an extension, the assignment leader will complete a student assignment extension form, a copy of which will be sent to you. This copy must be appended to your work at the point of submission.

Clearly it is not always possible to let your assignment leader know that you will be late completing more than a few days in advance of the assignment deadline. For instance, personal or family illness might occur suddenly. However, it is always better to give a reason for your inability to meet a deadline, rather than simply to submit late without explanation. This is known as 'mitigating circumstances'. A sudden serious illness provides strong mitigating circumstances, but 'the dog ate my hard drive' is a weak mitigating circumstance, and you will not be given much sympathy, even if you are able to provide authenticated photographic evidence! To avoid the dog scenario, buy a data stick and back up your work. Most universities sell low-cost data sticks to students.

It is much better, of course, to ensure the work is finished on time. It is a good plan to work backwards from the submission date and schedule the tasks you need to carry out, allowing plenty of time to achieve each stage, and to cope with any mishaps along the way.

One way to save time is to write your assignment plan and your draft material straight onto a computer, in a file marked clearly with the assignment name. If you make notes by hand then transfer them onto the computer, you will waste a lot of time. Once the material is on the computer it can be moved around, extended, or reduced, and you will already be quite a few words closer to your final draft.

Structuring your work

Your work will need a structure: that is, a way of logically dividing up the work. Unless you are writing a very short assignment, it is a good idea to use subheadings. This helps you to plan it all out, and it also helps the reader to find their way through the work. You can build on the simple structure of beginning, middle and end suggested above, to produce a more detailed outline:

- In the beginning section, you look at the title and what it means. Is there a question you are asked to answer? If the title is not in the form of a question, it can help to define it as a problem that you need to solve. In this section you will clearly state the aim of the assignment. This is also the place to outline the structure of the topics you will consider in the middle section.
- The middle is the body of your work. This is where you consider the main themes under subheadings. You will collect information to present under each of the headings, then discuss and analyse it.
- The end is where you bring it all together. You need to give a clear answer to the question, or summarise what you have done in the assignment. Think of the end of assignment as the prize you are giving the reader: the statement, or conclusion they will value that has made it worthwhile.

As mentioned above, 'beginning', 'middle' and 'end' are not appropriate headings to use in your final draft: these three headings are for planning only. Your final draft will need appropriate headings, which might be 'Introduction', a heading and subheadings relevant to your main themes, often the prescribed learning outcomes and 'Conclusion'.

Table 1.1 Writing tips

→ Write the assignment question or aim on a piece of paper and place it somewhere you can see it when you are writing. This will keep you focused and avoid drifting aimlessly through the work.	→ Write a fast first draft so that you have something to work from. Use simple words. Where you know there should be a reference, indicate to yourself that something needs to be added.
→ Don't go for easy answers, just repeating what you have already heard in lectures. Try to be creative, or at least thoughtful.	→ Always expect to change your draft later, rather than trying to write the perfect sentence and paragraph first time.
→ Think about the question and what the topic means to you.	→ Look at the way other writers craft their work: how they introduce the names of other authors, how they start sections and paragraphs and so on.
→ Gather examples to support your statements and add definitions where specialist words are used.	→ Check drafts for notes to yourself you have not removed, repetition of words, and jumbled material.
→ Make your references as up-to-date as possible.	→ Avoid over-using the same words like 'important' or 'key', and avoid starting sentences that are close together with the same words or phrases (such as 'It is').
→ Use a variety of books or articles to show you have read around the subject.	
→ Don't over-use 'cited in': that is, giving second-hand references from someone else's work.	→ Look out for superfluous phrases such as 'as was said earlier', and delete them, as they do not add anything to the work.
→ Each time you mention an author, add the reference to the 'References' section at the end of your draft. Then when you have finished your draft, you will also have finished your references section. This will also save you from omitting references.	→ Put your nearly completed draft out of mind and don't look at it for a day or two. Then you can take a final look at it with fresh eyes.
→ Take care over spelling, grammar, punctuation and referencing. Mistakes in these can all lose you marks. Make sure your automatic spell check and grammar check are switched to English UK and not English US.	→ Write from a reader's point of view; would you be interested in reading it?

Housekeeping

Whenever you work on your computer, it is essential to back up your work as you go along. Save a copy onto a data stick, a CD or a different computer. There is nothing more upsetting than completing a lot of hard work on a draft and then losing it because the computer has crashed or a similar tragedy has struck. Even if your program autosaves, also save the work manually from time to time, and close the file, so that you are certain the material has been saved.

Label your files clearly with a file name that you will recognise in relation to the assignment. If you include a date in the file name (for instance, 'Assignment B 24 June') it will allow you to quickly identify different drafts on the same topic.

Receiving a referral for an assignment

Not everyone passes an assignment first time: sometimes you might be given a referral, which means that you are asked to do some extra work on the assignment to bring it up to the required standard.

It is useful to consider what you should do if you get a referral rather than a pass. The important thing is to get the work back, along with the comments. Read them carefully (and read through your work again) so that you understand what problems or failings the assessor(s) identified. Then make an appointment to see your supervisor, to discuss what you should do. You should already have learned something from the feedback, and have some ideas on how you can improve the work, but your supervisor should be able to advise you further.

There are a number of areas you may need to focus on, depending on the feedback you have received. The most obvious is, did you answer the assignment question by addressing each of the learning outcomes? You need to have an explicit answer to the question or issue in the assignment title or brief. You also need to consider how much evidence you included in the assignment. Did you give your own opinions without backing them up adequately, or did you include sufficient examples and references from the literature to support your ideas?

A common problem highlighted in feedback comments is that students tend to describe things rather than include critical comment. In other words, you should not just repeat what other people have said. You need to say what *you* think about what they have said, and how convincing you feel their arguments are. In this context, being 'critical' does not mean being negative: it means looking thoughtfully at something. An important part of criticism is to explain why something has been successful, or why you agree with an author's viewpoint. Of course, if you disagree, you can say so too, but you should avoid making offensive comments about the authors whose work you discuss, and you need to provide reasons to back up your opinion. So it is not sufficient to say, 'I don't agree with this', and unwise to say, 'This author is wrong.' It is much better to say, for example, 'There is a lack of evidence provided by the author to support this view.'

Referral comments might also mention poor grammar, punctuation, style and referencing. Referencing is seen as very important in academic work: it is discussed on pages 13–16. Getting your referencing right is a mechanical job – you just need to be more thorough and systematic – but it is not so easy to improve your grammar and punctuation, if they are not up to the required standard. The best approach is to identify your blind spots and get hold of some easy to understand books that will help you overcome them.

Do not resubmit the work until you are confident that you have dealt fully with the comments you received. This time around the work should look and read differently. Use the feedback sheet to identify and number the points the assessor(s) suggested should be improved, and before the resubmission, go through the sheet again and tick them off once you have addressed them.

You will find further useful ideas on this in Price (2004).

Getting the best from your academic personal/link tutor

Most universities have a system of link and personal tutors (often the learning group leader). The university should provide you with a student handbook which gives details of how to contact your personal tutor. These individuals are there for your benefit. The link tutor will act as the intermediary between your mentor and the university, and the personal tutor will help you primarily with your academic assignments. Their responsibility is to help support the link between practice and the university department or school. Both are mandated to help you achieve your goal of becoming a healthcare professional. Remember most personal tutors are very happy to meet and help students.

Seeking academic support if you have a learning difference

If you believe, or your tutor believes, that you might have a learning difference such as dyslexia, you can be referred for a learning assessment to your university Learning Differences Centre. It is important for you to understand that all students have different learning styles. Being referred to a centre is not a reflection of your intellect: it simply means that steps are being taken to ensure you are able to benefit to the full from your education. If you are subsequently diagnosed as dyslexic you will be in good company: among the famous dyslexics are Zoe Wanamaker, Steve Redgrave and Brian Conley. If your assessment suggests that steps need to be taken to deal with a learning difference, you and your tutor will be kept informed by the centre.

Referencing skills

When collecting material from any source, remember that if you subsequently use it in your work you will have to provide a full reference for it. Always ensure you have recorded all the information you will need to complete the reference. This is equally true whether the material is a hard copy or electronic (such as information from a website).

There are a number of different referencing systems, but all of them provide essentially the same information. The differences are in the way the information is given in the references section, and how the reference is given in the body of the work.

The most popular system in UK academic schools is the Harvard system, and this is the system outlined below. In this system, references are listed in alphabetical order of author's surname in the references list, and the author's surname and date of publication are used as a reference in the body of the work. The main alternative is the Vancouver system. This uses numbered note markers in the body of the work, and a references section with corresponding numbered entries.

There are a number of variations in the Harvard system. It is important that you use the system recommended by your academic institution, so the discussion here is intended to show you the broad principles. Refer to university sources to ensure that you are aware of any differences between your university's standards and the one used here, or to more detailed books if you need to know how to phrase more complex references, since this provides only a general outline.

A simple guide to the Harvard referencing system

In order to provide a reference to a book you will need details of:
- the surname(s) and initial(s) of the author(s)
- surname(s) and initial(s) of the editor(s) if any
- year of publication (see below)
- title (in italics)
- number of the edition if second or greater (first editions are not indicated)
- place of publication (where several places are given, use the first in the list)
- the publisher (not the book printer).

This information should all be available in the book itself. The cover and spine will give you details of the author(s), title and publisher, and the remaining information is usually on a left-hand page near the start of the book. Where there have been several editions of a book, this 'imprint' page will list all of them: it is the most recent that is required. (A reprint is not the same as a new edition, and details of reprints are not needed: what you should give is the year in which the edition to which you are referring was first published.)

For example, in the references section the entry might be:

> Michaels, J. and Owen, D. (eds) (2008) *Professional Education in Healthcare* (2nd edn). Oxford: Blackwell.

In the body of the text, you will give a reference such as (Michaels and Owens, 2008: 25), where 25 is the page reference for a passage you have quoted. (If you are not quoting the text but just discussing it or giving it as a source of information, it is not always necessary to reference a specific page or page span, but it is good practice to do so whenever it is appropriate.)

If you are referring to a specific chapter in a book (for instance, an edited collection of chapters contributed by different authors), you will also give the title of the chapter and (according to some standards) the page span within the book. For example:

> Johns, M. (2008) 'Assessing pain in the young', pp. 24–47 in Davies, O. (ed.), *Pain and its Treatment*. London: Routledge.

The text reference is the same as for a book, for example (Johns, 2008: 31).

Note that each reference is given on a new line, running right across the page. The references are normally presented as continuous text, not in table format, and are not fully capitalised.

For referencing a journal article, you will need the:
- surname(s) and initial(s) of the author(s)

- year of publication
- article title
- name of journal in full (in italics; do not use abbreviations)
- volume number
- number within the volume
- page numbers over which the article is spread.

For example:

> Hauxwell, B. (2008) 'Study tips for students', *Nurse Education Today* **36**(4), 26–30.

The volume number here is 36, the number in the volume is 4, and the page span is 26 to 30. Note that there is no need to use 'vol', 'no' or 'pp.' unless this is the style specified by your educational institution. The text reference to this will be, for example (Hauxwell, 2008: 27).

For website material you should give the:

- author's name, or name of organisation if no individual author is credited
- year if indicated ('not dated'/'nd' if not)
- title of page or article
- name of organisation or website
- web address (listed at top of screen or bottom of printout page): your computer will probably automatically underline this, and that is fine
- date accessed (usually automatically printed at the bottom of a printout of an article, unless it is a pdf).

For example:

> Royal College of Midwives (RCM) (2004) *Position Statement Number 4: Normal Childbirth*, RCM [online] http://www.rcm.org.uk/info/docs/PS4-Normal-Childbirth.doc (accessed 21/5/09).

For this the text reference would be (RCM, 2004). Although we have covered books, articles and websites separately, in the Harvard system it is usual to combine the entries in one alphabetical sequence and not separate them by category.

The difference between a references section and bibliography is that references are all the works you refer to in your assignment. A bibliography also lists material you have read or referred to in the course of your research, but not made specific reference to in your work. Although some courses ask students to provide bibliographies with their assignments, their ability to show learning is questionable. They could be the first 20 titles you spot walking into a library, since the body of the text will not provide any evidence that you have read them.

There are some variations in the referencing in the main part of the assignment depending on the use you have made of the material. If you are directly discussing a work, you would phrase it as, for example:

> Francis (2008: 94) feels that the problem is easily overcome.

If you are giving a source for some information you provide but not discussing it directly, you would phrase it as:

> Although it is felt that the problem can easily be overcome (Francis, 2008: 94) …

'Cited in' and 'et al.'

This part of the chapter covers only some of the main principles, but two points that frequently cause confusion need attention.

You might read an article by, say, Lee (2009), who mentions some interesting points made by another author, Peters (2008). The point you want to include in your assignment is one made by Peters, and not an original observation by Lee, so you need to make this clear in your reference. In the body of your work you would say:

> Peters (2008, cited in Lee, 2009) suggests that the key points include …

The idea of referencing is to direct the reader to your own source material, so in the references section there will be no mention of Peters, as you did not read Peters' original work. You would reference Lee in the usual way, as that is where you got your information.

'Et al.' is short for the Latin *et alia*, which means 'and others'. It is used when there are three or more authors for a piece of work. To save cluttering the body of the assignment (and using up the word allowance) by listing all the authors' surnames, you give the name of the first author, followed by 'et al.' and the year of publication. (There is a full stop after 'al.', because it is an abbreviation which does not end with the final letter of the original word: sometimes in the modern style this is missed out, as are the full stops after authors' initials.) However, the references section should give all the names. So for an article by Emerson, Lake and Palmer (2009), the text reference could be:

Work by Emerson et al. (2009) illustrates the use of this technique.

The use of Latin abbreviations like this is sometimes discouraged today, and it is usually acceptable to use 'and colleagues' or 'and others' if you prefer, but et al is the academic norm.

You can lose up to 10 per cent of the available marks for the incorrect use of references in an assignment, so it is worthwhile to have a checklist of all the elements in the Harvard system with you on a card, or electronically, while you are doing your research, and ensure you record the reference information at the same time as the material you want to use. Otherwise, when you come to add the material to your assignment, you might find you do not have an essential detail, and you will have to go back to the reference, or do a web search, to find it.

Common problems include a missing year of publication, place of publication, publisher or website address. If you use a photocopier, essential information such as page numbers can be missed off the copy. When you photocopy sections from a book, it is a good idea to photocopy the imprint page too.

Practice tip

Get into the habit of systematically checking that all this information is present as soon as you source the material, whether it is from a library or from the web.

Learning activity

To avoid grade penalties for the incorrect use of references in assignments, in your learning group take a selection of books and papers and practise developing a reference list.

Gathering information

Assignments depend on your gathering information that will help you in putting an answer together. An important consideration is the source of that information, as that can influence the weight you put on the information or views it contains. Some sources of information are more trustworthy than others.

Learning activity

If you were looking at a public health topic such as the problems associated with smoking or drinking, think what kind of information might you gather? What sources would you feel were more trustworthy or reliable than others?

Sources of information include:
- published articles
- books
- websites
- leaflets
- expert opinions
- personal written accounts.

When it comes to organising your thoughts about a topic, whether it is to take notes ready for an assignment or exam question, there is a structure that will help in most situations. This takes the form of answering these questions:

- What?
- Why?
- How?
- Who?
- When?
- Problems?
- Solutions?
- Implications (for practice/the assignment/the future)?

Part

I

> **(a) Learning activity**
>
> Look back on your thoughts on the public health topic such as the problems associated with smoking or drinking, and the kind of information might you gather. Try to organise your thoughts on how you might look at information on the topic to answer some of the questions in the list above (what? why? how? and so on).

All the knowledge you gain needs to be thought of in terms of what it says and how it fits together, and how much weight you are prepared to put on each part.

Published articles

A major consideration here is the journal in which they are published. Journals are taken more seriously if they take steps to control the quality of the information they publish. Good-quality health journals are 'peer reviewed'. That is, when articles are submitted for publications, they are first sent to an expert on that topic to ensure that the content is sound. Although this is a useful form of 'quality control', you should be aware that it does not guarantee accuracy. However, knowledge gathered from peer-reviewed journals stands a better chance of being accurate and dependable.

Much the same considerations apply to websites. Information from 'official' sites, such as the Department of Health, an academic department or professional body, is considered to be more reliable than information from a commercial site, or one where it is not known whether the material has been subject to review.

With journal articles the age of the material is a further consideration. Information does have a 'sell-by' date, in that our knowledge advances so quickly that what was believed to be true some years ago might now be known not to be true. It is usual to try to ensure that articles cited are less than five years old. The closer they get to ten years, the less likely the information is to hold true, where it is based on opinion or research knowledge.

> **(a) Learning activity**
>
> Visit your academic library and look at a small number of professional journals. Examine articles to see whether they say, 'This article has been subject to double-blind review.' This means that the person who was sent an article for comment did not know who the author was, and so was not influenced by their reputation, or lack of one. This form of review is called 'double-blind' as the author also does not know the identity of the reviewer. Double-blind is a common form of peer review (which means, review by someone of similar status to the author). Are most of the journals you consult peer reviewed?

There are some clear exceptions to this, and some research studies of much earlier date are still accepted as reflecting the current level of understanding. These are known as 'seminal' studies or papers, and have proved to be reliable. In general, however, age is an indicator of the weight you should put on the information.

The country in which a study or opinion is carried out should also influence its value to your assignments. Healthcare systems vary throughout the world, and cultures vary in their attitude towards health and healthcare. Different populations also vary in lifestyle patterns, and this might influence the effect of conditions and treatments. This means that some information that is sound in one country might not be transferable to another. It is useful to show that you are aware of these problems, but if you refer to material of which this is true, it is unwise to say that the information cannot be used because it is biased/out of date/

unreliable. It is better to say, 'There may be limitations to its use', and to then spell out what you consider them to be.

Reading

S   Scenario continued

Each module Sue undertakes seems to have a vast reading list. In many of the lectures, further references are given, and handouts similarly seem to give long lists of things that have been referenced. The question going through

Sue's mind is, when is she supposed to find time for all this reading? Do they want her to read every single reference? If so, what is she supposed to do with it if she reads it?

Traditionally, university students have talked about 'reading' for a first or higher degree. This is because education at this level has mainly been based on knowledge gained from books, rather than simply attending lectures. Students quite literally 'read' for their qualification. However, it is not possible to read every single reference that is given to you, although you will be expected to read key authors and sources of information. Where you are given 'indicative reading' lists you will be expected to choose from among the sources given, so that you follow up the information given by lectures.

The purpose of all these references is to provide you with the primary sources of the ideas or research that underpin the course. 'Primary sources' are those in which a point was first made or research evidence presented. 'Secondary sources' are pieces by other writers that report on or discuss the material in the primary sources.

It is always best to try to read and use primary sources in your work, as those producing the secondary information might have been selective, or had a personal interest or agenda which helped determine which information they included in their work. In others words, there are issues of accuracy and bias in the use of secondary referencing. Sometimes where a book or article is out of print or too difficult to get hold of, discovering what it said from a secondary source may be the only option open to you, but as a general rule you should avoid secondary sources.

Reviewing the literature

S   Scenario continued

Sue develops a method of 'reviewing the literature', as she has been advised to do. This consists of her getting hold of as many books and articles on a subject as possible, copying out relevant passages, then sitting down and joining it all together, keeping the words copied from the articles and books intact as far as possible, but not

making it clear that they are someone else's words, rather than her own. She then sums up with a conclusion she writes herself. Her tutor says this is totally wrong. Sue is now confused and does not understand what she has to do. Her tutor explains that she needs to paraphrase.

A common task that is given in assignments or module activities is to review the literature on a particular topic. This is a skill that you will need to develop. It will be easier if you understand what is meant by a literature review, and the principles to follow in conducting one.

A literature review does not mean copying down as much information as possible on a topic, then putting it together in an assignment (using direct quotes) to form a new version, a bit like a collage or mosaic. A review should be written to answer a specific question. It should contain a description of what you have learned about a topic, and in parallel, include your comments, thoughts and views on that material. This should address both what it says and how convincingly, or persuasively, it says it. You can make some direct quotes from your source material, but it is not wise to do this in excess (they should make up a minority of your piece, not the bulk of it), and you must always make it clear that they are not your own words, or you will be guilty of plagiarism.

Collecting information for a literature review

Like so many other activities described in this chapter, reviews are also better if they are carried out systematically following a logical process. Here are some tips on organising the literature review.

You must be clear on themes to be covered, so start with a clear statement or aim of the review. This will provide the search terms you will need to search for information from databases. Using the key word of your topic, consider the list of key words for organising a review mentioned earlier (the 'what, why, how, problems, solutions and so on) and decide which might help you decide on areas to be covered in your review. This will help you decide on the theme subheadings that will divide up your review and help you see the relationship between the sections. These words will also give purpose to your reading once you have the articles, as it means you can speed read through much of an article and slow down once it starts to cover an aspect that can be placed under one of the key words.

When you write up your review, you may be required to include information on how you went about gathering information. This usually includes:

- key words you used to search databases
- the names of the databases or search engines you used
- time frame, that is the years between which most of the information was published
- inclusion and exclusion selection criteria, if you specifically searched for information from certain countries or aspects of information (for instance, including information about relatives or carers as well as patients/clients).

Search the databases following your plan, and note any changes you find you need to make or difficulties you encounter, such as different spellings of words for American sources, or unanticipated phrasing in the literature. For example, an initial search for information on teenage pregnancies using the word 'teenage' might show you that information is easier to locate if you use the word 'adolescent'.

Using your key words, you should first search for articles that have relevant titles. If there is a summary, check it for relevance (discard the item if it is clearly not relevant to your topic). If you search online databases you may be able to directly download some of the articles you find listed. You will probably find it best to search for information on two or three occasions, and reconsider the relevance of some of the articles you have already found.

When you read articles, give them a 'star' rating out of 5. Note this down on the cover or first page, at the top right or left, whichever you prefer. A 5 rating will mean 'brilliant – lots of good material' and a 1 rating, 'very little relevance'. Keep articles with similar star ratings together, and concentrate initially on the high-star articles when you start putting the material together. You might find you get enough information from these, and do not need to go through the low-star pieces.

Look carefully at the reference sections in the articles you have gathered. These often provide details of articles you could add to your search.

If you think you will use an article, list the details in a 'references' file or on index cards, using the Harvard system. This can also be used to check whether you have already reviewed an article, if the title comes up in a future search.

Once you have your material, you need to extract relevant 'quotes' and comment on them. These will form the basis of your ideas and material for your work. It is a big advantage if you

Practice tip

What is paraphrasing? It is simply a restatement of concepts and ideas from published work which is put into your own words (with acknowledgement of your sources).

Practice tip

When you have got hold of some articles, do not stockpile them but scan them quickly to look for information relevant to the theme headings under which you will structure the review. You might want to use a highlighter pen for this.

can put this material together under theme headings so that you can see it and identify any possible agreements between the writers (a consensus of opinion) or any differences.

Your aim is to compare, contrast and comment on the literature as a whole under these theme or sub-theme headings. In writing the review, it is important that the reader hears your voice talking them through this literature, and not a large number of other voices as a result of your simply summarising all the studies or providing a series of 'sound-bites'.

In writing up the review, you need to tell the reader the results of your examination of the literature. This will include what the literature says, how well it says it, and the strengths and limitations of the available literature.

Critiquing research articles

Professional knowledge is based on the strongest evidence possible, and often that takes the form of information derived from research. Research is a vast topic, and you will probably have sessions on this subject. We recommend you to use that knowledge in conjunction with the research textbooks recommended to you. Here, we concentrate on research articles you may have to read and make sense of as part of your course. This is called *critiquing* research.

Critiquing has been defined by Rees (2003) as 'the careful consideration of both the strengths and limitations of a published piece of research'. It is not simply 'criticising' or being very negative about a study.

In order to successfully critique an article you will need a systematic framework for critiquing, and some essential research knowledge. There are a number of critique frameworks, which all provide a systematic checklist of important areas to consider in a research report.

Table 1.2 Critique structure

1 Focus What key words sum up what this is about? Look for key words in the title. **2 Background** Why did the researchers choose this topic? What literature do they use to support the issue? **3 Aim** What is the statement or question the researchers want to answer through the data collected? (It usually begins with the word 'to': to examine/compare/determine, for example.) **4 Methodological approach** Is it quantitative/qualitative? Is it descriptive, or does it look for relationships between variables? **5 Tool of data collection** What was used to collect the information? Questionnaires, interviews, observation, assessment scales, physiological measures? If it is quantitative research, did the researchers pilot the method?	Do they consider the reliability and validity of the tool? What has actually been measured by the tool? (Qualitative research works a little differently: refer to research textbooks for more on this.) **6 Ethics** Was the research considered by an ethics committee (REC in the United Kingdom, or in the United States an IRB)? Did the researchers get informed consent? Were possible risks to the individual(s) considered? **7 Sample** On how many subjects are the results based? How did the researchers choose them? Were there specific inclusion and exclusion criteria? Did anyone drop out of the study, or what percentage response rate did the researchers achieve? Do you feel those remaining were typical/representative of the group? **8 Data presentation** How did the researchers process the information collected? How do they present it? Is it understandable like this? Is it explained?	**9 Main findings** What data answers the aim (the results)? **10 Conclusion** In the author's own words, what sums up the answer to the aim? **11 Recommendations** What do the researchers suggest should happen now? Who should do what? **12 Readability** Did the researchers make it easy to read by explaining technical aspects? Was it interesting? **13 Strengths/limitations** Summing up, what were the good aspects of the method? What were its weaker areas? **14 Implications for practice** What do you feel are the messages for practice? What is the 'so what?' aspect for you?

The system introduced in Table 1.2 outlines the main headings used by Rees (2003). The framework comes in two versions, depending on the type of research being examined, but Table 1.2 provides just the basic quantitative framework. (Do look at the qualitative framework in Rees (2003) if that is the kind of study you are examining.) It is not essential to use this specific framework, provided you use one that covers the relevant issues, and that you find easy to apply. Without a system, it is easy not to notice that important elements are missing from a study.

As part of your course you will learn some of the fundamental principles of research. This is important if you are to assess whether the research has been carried out soundly, and can be compared to the best of its type. In other words, you need to be confident that the researcher(s) have rigorously followed good research practice. If they have, the result will be 'robust' in the sense that it gives strong and reliable findings. It should then be possible to apply the results safely in a variety of appropriate settings.

The advice here should be supplemented from a research textbook from your course booklist.

Essential pointers to remember when critiquing

One research study rarely provides the definitive answer to what should be done in a clinical setting. That is why replication studies – ones repeating an original study under the same or slightly different conditions – are important to ensure that initial results are reliable. Research is seldom undertaken under perfect circumstances, so it will never be flawless. However, when you comment on any limitations, remember not to be over-critical. Try to suggest an alternative that could have been used if you feel there were weaknesses in the work.

Although you must remember that there are possible limits to knowledge produced by research, and no published research is beyond criticism, relying on research results is always better than unquestioned faith in interventions that have not been subject to enquiry or testing.

Among the common classifications of research is a broad division into quantitative and qualitative approaches. Although some academics do not like this distinction, if you are new to critiquing it certainly helps to understand some important differences in study designs. Quantitative research focuses on measurement and the relationship between things of interest (variables). It is relatively easy to spot this approach as the results are numerical: provided for instance in tables, bar charts or pie charts.

Qualitative research is not about 'quality', nor should it offer subjective views. It is about experiences, understandings and interpretations. It explores human situations and events through the eyes of those concerned, using their language and descriptions of things. The findings sections will be in the form of words rather than numbers.

The most important aspect to identify when critiquing is the aim of a study. This usually begins with the word 'to' and will be phrased as, for example, 'the aim of this study was to determine/examine/identify/describe …'. There may be more than one aim, and if that is the case, it is worthwhile naming them as part 1, part 2 and so on. As you read through the study, you should ensure that each part is followed up in the results section and the conclusions. It is easy for the researcher to start off with an impressive list of aims and not address them all.

The importance of the aim is that it influences the form and nature of many other aspects of a study, such as the broad research design, the tool of data collection, and method of analysis and sample. At the end of the study, part of your judgement will be how well the author has achieved the aim.

It is crucial to look for ethical considerations in a study. An ethics committee should have approved studies involving patients/clients, or health staff, unless the study is an audit. In the United Kingdom this committee is a Research Ethics Committee (REC). In the United States it is an IRB (Institutional Review Board). You will also want to see it confirmed that informed consent was given by those involved, and that they were treated with dignity throughout.

The use of numbers and statistical processes in research articles intimidates many readers. Although you should not take it for granted that figures are right, in a peer-reviewed journal someone should have considered whether appropriate statistical techniques were used, and might have checked the accuracy of calculations. It is not good practice to avoid having anything to do with numbers or charts. You need to look at the figures and try to work out what they show. Usually the writer will explain in the article what the numbers represent and their interpretation of them. It is very important to give attention to the researcher's interpretation as well as to the data provided. Try to make your own interpretation of the results, then compare it with the researcher's interpretation.

Similarly, do not be put off by the specialist language of research; each health professional group has its own jargon. When in doubt of the meaning of words, you should use the glossary section of research textbooks.

There are a number of different research tools that can be used to collect data. Each one has advantages and disadvantages, and is better fitted to some settings than others. You need consider whether the researchers' choice was reasonable given the aim of the study and the target sample group. Do they justify their choice? Have they made allowances for the limitations of the chosen tool(s)? Do you think an alternative tool might have been more appropriate?

A tool used for a quantitative study should have been either used in previous research, so it is known to be accurate, or piloted to test how consistently and accurately it worked. Check on whether the researchers have demonstrated one of these alternatives. A related issue is validity, which relates to what the tool measures, and how appropriate this is to the aims of the study. Often in the discussion section, the results of similar studies using the same tool are compared to suggest that validity has been demonstrated.

Qualitative research does not use such standardised tools. One feature of qualitative tools and approaches to data collection is that they are very fluid and flexible. This makes piloting difficult, as qualitative studies do not seek standardisation. Although many readers are uncomfortable with this flexibility, qualitative research can and should be carried out in a rigorous way, especially during data analysis.

Look closely at the size of the sample, and how this compares with other studies mentioned, or known to you. Sometimes it is very small, even under a dozen. The research can still be valid and relevant because of the depth of data produced. In quantitative studies, the general rule is that the bigger the sample the better, as this makes generalisations more acceptable. However, this does not apply in qualitative studies; the core question is whether the sample provides sufficient information on the topic.

The way the sample is selected for inclusion in a study can vary enormously. Each sampling method too has advantages and disadvantages. The main consideration in quantitative research is whether the sample is an accurate representation of the 'population' it is derived from (which can itself be defined in various ways). Consult your research texts for more information on this.

The crux of a study is its findings: the answer to the question the researchers set out to explore. Do not just read what the authors say they found: look at the results (the tables, charts or quotes they present).

The discussion section will raise issues arising from the results. It may start out by discussing the limitations of the study. You should take this as a positive feature: it means the researchers are trying to help you determine how much emphasis you should put on the results.

The final section of a research paper includes the conclusion and recommendations. These round off the study, and should answer the aim. In some cases, the conclusion consists of the recommendations, and you have to look to the discussion to find the answer to the aim. The recommendations should make proposals for who should do what now, and how, based on the researchers' interpretation of the results.

The most important part of the critique is deciding whether the study is fit for purpose.

You need to consider whether you feel the results can reasonably be applied to practice. In some cases articles specifically refer to this, perhaps in a box at the end.

To sum up this section, critiquing is a core professional skill that will inform your clinical practice. It is not just an academic exercise that you will carry out during your time at university. All healthcare professionals need to be careful about accepting the results of research without question. Do not accept research simply because it has been published. Part of the responsibility of researchers is to share their findings so that they can be debated and weak areas identified and strengthened. In other words, you have a right (and a duty) to consider how a study was undertaken as well as what it found. The most important point is to consider how the research can make a contribution to practice.

When you have critiqued a study you should be able to explain verbally or in writing the following main areas. These can form the summary of your critique:

- The aim of this study was to (aim) …
- It did this by means of (this kind of study), and (this kind of data collection method), on (this number of) people (design and method) …
- They found (main results) …
- The conclusion was …
- The strengths of the study included …
- The limitations were …
- The implications this study has for practice include/are …

If you are able to structure your thoughts in this way, you have achieved a balanced critique of the study. Critiquing is a skill, and the more you practise it, and talk to others about your thoughts, the more proficient you will become.

Seminar/learning group presentations and poster presentations

Learning takes place through many different activities on a course. Different people will have different favourite methods, but the course will ensure that you develop a range of skills. Throughout your course you will use a range of presentations in your student-centred learning groups, including seminar and poster presentations. Each has a variety of forms, so here we consider some general principles.

Seminar/learning group presentations

The idea here is that instead of learning coming from a lecturer, the students take on the responsibility for preparing and presenting material, with the lecturer adding to the discussion as appropriate. As with other forms of learning, what you get out of these sessions is influenced by what you are prepared to put into them.

Although some people are reluctant to speak out in a group, once you have qualified you will be expected to present information to others, and to do so to a high standard. Seminars are topic or question based, and you will be given guidelines on what to read as background to the discussion, or what you are expected to present at the session. As for assignments, you will be expected to add your views and not simply present the material you look at.

Among the skills you need to develop are the abilities to grasp the essential points in the material you read, reflect on it and develop some views, and get the main points over in a structured, systematic way. If you are asked to stand in front of the group, you must project a confident image, and be able to talk clearly, succinctly, and at a speed that allows people to follow what you are saying. Where you are arguing a case, you also need to be able to make it interesting and engage people's attention.

t ☆

Practice tip

If you are asked to present material at a seminar or learning group you need to prepare what you are going to say, and rehearse how you are going to present it.

Preparing for a seminar or a learning group is similar to preparing for any other kind of work, in the sense that you need to be clear on the aim, and work out how you will achieve it. You should make be easy to identify points, backed up with evidence or argument. Your 'script' should be put on cards, or a PowerPoint presentation. Do not write out what you will say in full, then read it word for word: be prepared to talk around key phrases or bullet points.

Rehearse what you are going to say out loud, either to yourself, or even better to a few friends or family to give you the feeling of a 'live audience'. They will probably interrupt less than the seminar members, so this rehearsal is likely to be shorter than the live presentation.

When you present in the seminar, do not keep your head down, reading off cards, piece of paper or a computer screen all the time. Project your voice so that everyone can hear you, and swing your gaze round the room so that everyone feels included in the conversation. This is called the 'lighthouse effect'. Make sure your contribution has a clear beginning, middle and end, and make good use of pauses to emphasise important parts. Do not try to say it all in one breath.

Before you start to speak, take a big breath and let it out slowly, getting rid of any tension or stiffness in your body, and start with a smile. If you get any questions, thank the questioner and do not be defensive. Answer honestly. If you don't know the answer to a question say so, and ask whether anyone else can contribute information or an opinion. Afterwards, consider what aspects you did well, and what you might have changed in retrospect. Above all do not be over-critical of yourself. If you did your best, you can be proud.

Poster presentations

Poster presentations are a popular method of communicating research and practice developments at many health professional conferences and in learning groups. During the first decade of the 2000s they have also become a frequently used learning method in university schools of health, and they form part of formative assignments on some courses. Part of their popularity is due to their flexibility and creative element: they can provide a more stimulating way of engaging students with topics. They are ideal as a feedback method to demonstrate knowledge and skills, as they require you to be very clear on the messages you are trying to convey, and allow you to use pictures, images and other visual means to complement simple text.

Poster presentation sessions are very interactive, and stimulate plenty of questions and feedback between the presenter and the audience. Some of this is a result of the increased physical proximity between the two. Posters can be designed on an individual or group basis. This makes them far more enjoyable than more formal methods of verbal or PowerPoint presentations.

Designing your poster

Designing a poster involves deciding what goes into it (content), and how it will look (presentation). The content must fit the instructions or 'brief' you will be given for the poster. The selection of the material will be influenced by the space you have available. The key is to think about the main statements or issues you need to cover, to lead up to your main point.

Think about the content as a series of 'pages' or areas of information that will need to be laid out on the poster in a logical way. Posters can be displayed as wider than they are tall (known as landscape orientation) or taller than they are wide (portrait orientation). This has a bearing on how the information is set out. The poster should have a strong visual appeal and high impact. This can be achieved through well-selected graphics, strong colours, and a good choice of attention-grabbing wording. All these should contribute to the message of the poster.

It is best to avoid lots of writing or text, as this is too difficult to read and looks unattractive. Ensure you look at the poster from the viewer's perspective, and make it an interesting and challenging presentation.

Content can be handwritten or printed from a computer. The latter will give you a range of fonts, colours, clip art and pictures. Illustrations can be drawn directly onto a poster by hand, or photos or other images stuck on, as well as generated by computer.

Where posters are a group effort, make sure that each group member has the opportunity to use their talents and imagination to contribute to the finished project. Make sure everyone agrees on the basic message and approach.

Some of the problems relating to posters are outlined in Table 1.3.

Table 1.3 Poster presentation problems and solutions

Problem	Solutions
No clear aim or message	Make sure both are explicitly stated, and use a title that explains the purpose.
Too much information presented in a confusing or boring way	At the design stage split material into 'pages'. Keep the content succinct and use space and graphics as much as possible.
Unimaginative appearance	Go for impact, colour, bold titles and graphics, supporting clear ideas.
Unreadable	Writing should be seen clearly from 2 metres away. Try 18-24 font sizes.
A jumble of items	Ensure logical progression of ideas. Indicate the order in which the items should be read with arrows, lines or numbers.
Takes a long time to read	Avoid using only capital letters as text, as the eye tends to stop at each letter and slow down reading. Write in both upper and lower case throughout.

S   Scenario continued

Sue has to present a poster as part of her public health module. It came as a surprise to her that her initial feelings of bewilderment of how to approach this disappeared once she realised that the format was very similar to all the other activities she had engaged in on the course. At this point she realised that perhaps of all the things she had learned, the study skills were the most important, as they provided her with the tools to do the job.

She now finds her modules challenging, but is clear on what is expected of her, and how she will tackle all demands on her to demonstrate her understanding of the course content. She feels these skills will continue to be important to her, once she has qualified and is required to continuing learning as part of her professional development.

a   Learning activity

In your learning group design a poster presentation format which you can adapt and use for future learning group presentations.

Conclusion

Being on a course calls for more than just remembering everything that is said or done; it involves developing an understanding of how it all fits together and shaping your own knowledge. To achieve this you need some process skills and tools. This chapter has presented some of the key elements you will need to make the learning process enjoyable and get the most out of it.

References

Buzan, T. (2006) *The Buzan Study Skills Handbook: The shortcut to success in your studies with mind mapping, speed reading and winning memory techniques (mind set)*. Harlow, BBC Active.

Price, B. (2004) 'Effective learning number 20: retrieving an assignment' (Supplement), *Nursing Standard* **18** (31).

Race, P. (2005) *Making Learning Happen*, London, Sage.

Rees, C. (2003) *An Introduction to Research for Midwives*, Edinburgh, Books for Midwives.

Chapter 2

Interprofessional learning

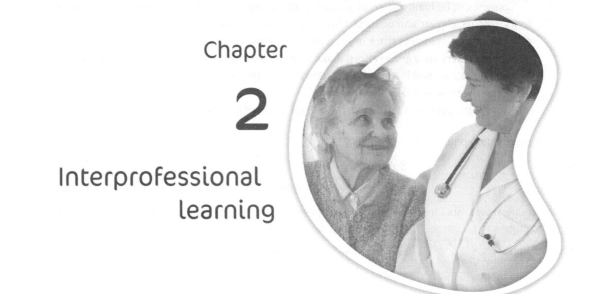

Jane Morgan

 Links to other chapters in *Foundation Studies for Caring*

1 Study skills
3 Evidence-based practice and research
4 Ethical, legal and professional issues
28 Rehabilitation

 Links to other chapters in *Foundation Skills for Caring*

1 Fundamental concepts for skills
2 IT skills

W Don't forget to visit www.palgrave.com/glasper for additional online resources relating to this chapter.

Introduction

A broad range of changes are occurring in society which influence healthcare practice today and will influence practice in the future. A significant change to healthcare practice is the development of interprofessional practice, brought about by calls for closer communication and collaboration between healthcare practitioners who are members of different professions. This has escalated over the last decade. Both interprofessional practice and multiprofessional practice are terms used to describe the process when healthcare practitioners from different professions practise as members of a single team.

Interprofessional learning is the term used to describe the process of learning that aims to prepare future healthcare practitioners to develop specific knowledge, skills and attitudes to communicate and interact with members of the health and social care professions. This process is often referred to as 'learning with and about healthcare professions' in order to practise successfully as a team member.

This chapter is divided into four parts, The first part introduces the concept of multiprofessional practice, and traces its historical development, emphasising what it means for today's practitioners. The differences between the concepts of 'multiprofessional practice' and 'interprofessional learning' are explored.

The second part considers why interprofessional learning is so important for all future practitioners. It focuses on recommendations from national enquiries into preventable deaths, which explain what multiprofessional practice should achieve for patient care. The aims and intentions of interprofessional learning are drawn from such recommendations.

The third part concentrates on what interprofessional learning is about, and the final section of the chapter suggests ways to be successful in interprofessional learning.

Learning outcomes

This chapter will enable you to:

- discuss the historical development of multiprofessional practice over the three decades prior to 2009
- explain the meaning of successful multiprofessional practice
- explain how successful multiprofessional practice can influence patient/client care and healthcare delivery systems
- explain the meaning of interprofessional learning, including its underlying aims and principles
- explain how successful multiprofessional practice is achieved
- discuss barriers to achieving successful multiprofessional practice
- explain how you can increase your success in interprofessional learning.

Concepts

- Interprofessional practice
- Multiprofessional practice
- Uniprofessional practice
- Interprofessional collaboration
- Teamwork
- Client-centred care
- Professional systems
- Active learning
- Healthcare professional systems
- Healthcare professional identity
- Healthcare professional regulatory bodies
- Healthcare professional stereotypes

Defining key terms

It is important to become familiar with the terms used in this chapter before you start reading. This section sets out a number of terms that have significant meaning when used in relation to interprofessional learning. It will help you to gain a clear understanding of the meanings of these terms. By completing the activities you will create your own set of notes of key terms, a glossary and a bibliography. Once created, you will need to refer to them to remind yourself of the meanings of different terms as you progress through the rest of this chapter. This section helps you to complete the first learning outcome.

> ### [S] Scenario: Sue's interprofessional learning
>
> Sue (whom we first met in Chapter 1) has just arrived for her first interprofessional leaning group activity. She is bewildered by the terminology.

Definitions

'Multiprofessional' and 'multidisciplinary'

These are terms to describe a group of colleagues from two or more disciplines who coordinate their expertise in providing care to patients/clients (Farrell, Schmitt and Heinemann, 2001). They are used interchangeably: that is, they mean the same thing. Multidisciplinary colleagues join together to enhance healthcare expertise to plan, implement and evaluate the delivery of care. Another term used to indicate a team that contains members of more than one profession is 'interdisciplinary'. This distinguishes them from 'uniprofessional' teams, in which groups of qualified professionals from the same profession work together.

'Interprofessional'

'Inter' refers to interchange, between and among people. Interprofessional is a term for a learning process. In interprofessional learning, learners who are studying to join different healthcare professions join together in a unique process of learning. They study specific subjects that are designed to prepare them to practise as members of a multiprofessional team. This unique learning process is described as 'learning with, about and from each other'.

Team

'Team' is a frequently used concept that has meanings about special ways of working and specific behaviours. It indicates that a number of critical factors are present which influence what can be achieved. Multiprofessional healthcare team work has the potential to achieve healthcare outcomes that could not be achieved by individual professionals working on their own.

When a team is made up of different healthcare practitioners it is termed a 'multiprofessional team', as opposed to a 'uniprofessional team' which is made up of practitioners of the same profession. The concept of a multiprofessional team is unique, and there are some essential factors if it is to be effective. These factors are like the essential ingredients of a cake: if any of them are missed out, the cake will fail to bake properly and be inedible. Understanding how multiprofessional teams work effectively in practice is the very foundation of interprofessional learning. The subject of teams is discussed in more detail later in this chapter.

Organisations generally are reliant on effective team work, and this is especially the case for the National Health Service (NHS) (Robinson and Kish, 2001). The benefits to both patients/clients and the professionals involved have been described in the literature as complex in their outcomes. These too are discussed later in the chapter.

The team-working processes in multiprofessional practice are unique and have been studied. Different authors present findings in the literature that explain this process in detail, and again, these are discussed in more depth later in this chapter.

Other terms related to this subject include 'healthcare practitioner', 'healthcare practice' and 'healthcare team'. If you are not familiar with the meaning of these terms, now is a good time to read about what they mean.

(a) Learning activities

It is now a good time to consider your individual learning by completing the first set of learning activities in this chapter. You might like to also look at the material on the companion website.

List as many definitions as you can find in the literature of the term 'multiprofessional practice'. Add the name of the author for each explanation. This list forms the start of your 'glossary of terms'. Keep this record safe so that you can add to it as you work through this chapter. We suggest you create a new electronic file to hold this list with a title such as 'IPL Glossary'.

Now review the literature again and list definitions of 'interprofessional learning'. Add the names of authors for each explanation and add it to your electronic glossary. You will find helpful guidance on

www.commonlearning.net   W

Finally, write a brief explanation of the difference between interprofessional learning and multiprofessional practice. Include a definition for both terms.

Why interprofessional learning is important

This section considers the reasons for the development of multiprofessional practice. It sets out why multiprofessional practice is so important and why interprofessional learning has been included in your programme. It will help you to complete the first two chapter learning outcomes.

It is important that you know that interprofessional learning is about learning with and about other healthcare professions, and how this learning takes place, but you first need to know *why* this is so important today. This means understanding what has happened over the last decades and how it has impacted on professional practice. You need to know the contextual background that explains when and why multiprofessional practice has succeeded or failed in the past. This helps you to understand why interprofessional learning has been designed in the way it has. You will then appreciate why you study what you do.

(c) Professional conversation

While on placement Sue overhears a doctor discussing with a physiotherapist the best way to mobilise a patient who has had a stroke. She comments, 'I was on duty when I overheard a discussion between one of the doctors and a physiotherapist and heard the physiotherapist explain how she wanted the patient to be mobilised. I questioned my mentor about this later that day. She was very helpful and reminded me that one of the main aims of the interprofessional healthcare programme operating in my university was "to foster an appreciation of the differing roles of healthcare professionals and an understanding of how each profession should call on the expertise held by other professionals when planning their care to ensure the patient benefits from the collective expertise available".'

A recurring message over the last five decades, particularly when health and social care goes wrong, is that there has been a lack of communication and collaborative teamwork between professionals and/or agencies. Lack of communication or ineffective communication has been identified as both a symptom and a cause of poor healthcare practice (Ovretveit, Mathias and Thompson, 1997). It is an imperative today to find ways to continually improve healthcare services, and multiprofessional practice is considered one of the best ways to improve health and social care. Calls for collaboration (close communication, interaction) across health and social care professions and agencies are not new, they started as early as the Beveridge Report in 1942. Calls for collaboration have resulted from a number of important changes that are influencing societies worldwide today.

These changes have resulted in calls for active collaboration of all professions nationally and internationally. This in turn calls for all future healthcare practitioners who are preparing to join their profession to be prepared to practise in a changing climate, adapt to ongoing changes and work more closely together.

Changes from 1990 to 2008

Before considering what interprofessional learning involves, it is important to consider what has led to calls for introducing interprofessional learning to your programme. The causes lie in a number of significant changes that have occurred. These changes fall into three broad categories:

- professional changes
- failures in healthcare delivery
- social and scientific changes.

Professional changes

UK healthcare practitioners have experienced major changes since the Second World War, after which the the National Health Service was first introduced into the United Kingdom. Recent changes have influenced their roles significantly more. More recent changes include:

- a better informed public, which changes relationships between patients/clients and professionals
- shortages of professional expertise
- increasing complexity of healthcare practice
- catastrophic failures in healthcare delivery which have led to calls for closer collaboration and teamwork between professions.

All healthcare practitioners are challenged and questioned by a better-informed and more assertive public. There has been a shift away from the relatively passive acceptance of authority by society. The general public can access health information that was once not available to them. Added to this, the public are more likely to challenge received opinion. There is growing public pressure for the relationship between health professional and patients to be open and on an equal status and power basis. Learning to work in partnership-style relations with patients and clients, and placing patients/clients at the centre of care, are important aspects of interprofessional learning.

Shortages of professional expertise

One of the most pertinent reasons for today's problems with professional practice is a crisis in human resources for healthcare (Barr, 2002). This crisis is created by a shortage of well-trained health practitioners in some parts of the world, as a result of regional underproduction accompanied with overproduction in other places, migration from poor to rich countries, and stress and insecurity among healthcare practitioners. More details can be found in the report by Dr Lee Jong-Wook, Secretary General of the World Health Organization (WHO), *The World Health Report 2006: Working together for health* (WHO, 2006).

> **a Learning activity**   **W**
>
> In your interprofessional learning group take some time to read this report in more depth. You can access the WHO report by visiting the companion website.

Complexity of practice

Good interactions, relationships and communications based on mutual respect between health professionals and patients become more important as practice becomes more complex. There are a number of reasons that practice is increasingly more complex. They include the requirement for advanced technical ability. As an emphasis on technical competence has grown, there has been a shared concern among patients and health professionals that the central human dimension of relationships has been weakened. Calls are made for a new and more understanding relationship between professionals to compensate for and correct the negative effects of technology on human relationships. Changes in law have moved some role responsibilities from one healthcare practitioner to another. This means that some practitioners are required to learn new and extended skills, and these changes influence their relationships with each other.

Healthcare failures

A greater degree of media scrutiny is subjecting all healthcare professions to closer examination of the way they practise. Both nationally and internationally, the period around the end of the twentieth century has seen a series of high-profile and controversial cases which have sent shockwaves through healthcare practitioners, their regulating bodies and public thinking. These cases called for urgent and major changes to practice. Names like Beverley Allitt and Harold Shipman are now fixed in the public memory. The inquiries into these cases, along with the Bristol Royal Infirmary Inquiry, have led to growing doubt in the public's mind about the adequacy of arrangements for professional regulation.

Recommendations for changes to professional practice are based on an understanding that patient care is a shared responsibility for healthcare teams. Recommendations from national enquiries into preventable deaths provide the most influential and convincing rationale for multiprofessional practice. Enquiry outcomes in a number of specific cases clearly state that deaths could have been avoided if health and social care professions had worked collaboratively, shared the information they held on cases and understood each other's roles better. Recommendations were made that interprofessional practice should be improved dramatically as a matter of urgency. Messages of such urgency have been interpreted as signalling crises in health and social care services. The most serious evidence came in:

- the Bristol Inquiry (DH, 2001b)
- the Victoria Climbié Inquiry (DH, 2003)
- the Shipman Inquiry (DH, 2005).

The Bristol Inquiry, chaired by Ian Kennedy, was one of the most far-reaching and detailed investigations into the National Health Service (NHS) ever undertaken. It addressed fundamental issues of clinical safety and accountability, professional culture and patient rights, and made specific recommendations for multiprofessional practice which have been used to develop interprofessional learning.

The Victoria Climbié Inquiry examined the death of an 8-year-old girl in London as a result of abuse by her carers. This was the most extensive investigation into the child protection system in British history. The government ordered a statutory inquiry into Victoria's death headed by the former chief inspector of social services, Lord Herbert Laming. The investigation was public, and was the first tripartate inquiry into child protection, investigating the role of Social Services, the NHS and the police, under the Children's Act, NHS Act and Police Act. Lord Laming pledged that Victoria's suffering would mark an 'enduring turning point in ensuring proper protection of children in this country'.

The inquiry revealed that child protection staff missed at least 12 chances to save Victoria. It also exposed a complete breakdown in the multi-agency child protection system. Health, police, housing charities and social services failed to work together effectively to protect the girl. The report made 108 recommendations in total. One major recommendation included setting up a national database recording every contact made by a child under 16 with the police, health and local authority services, to prevent children from getting lost in the system.

The Shipman Inquiry followed the conviction of a general practitioner, Harold Shipman, at Preston Crown Court on 31 January 2000 for the murder of 15 of his patients. He was originally charged with one count of forging a will, and was sentenced to life imprisonment.

> **ⓐ Learning activity** W
>
> In order to become familiar with the issues surrounding these cases it is important to read each report. They can be read online, or downloaded. The companion website for this chapter gives the web addresses.

In September 2000, the Secretary of State for Health announced that an inquiry would be held in public to establish what changes to current systems should be made in order to safeguard patients in the future. The Inquiry's reports (19 July 2002 and 27 January 2005: see DH, 2005) recommended changes to the way professions work together, including monitoring of professional competence, and calling on clinical governance as a way of ensuring that healthcare practitioners support and report on the professional competence of their team members.

Social and scientific changes

Changes in social and economic structures have had considerable impact on the health and well-being of populations. Some examples are expanded population numbers; increasing pollution of air, water and soil; and growing nationalist, political and religious extremism, possibly leading to social destabilisation. All these impact on the way professions share information and work together.

The emergence of new diseases and an increase in antimicrobial resistance present challenges for both the NHS system and its professionals, which call for more input of both money and expertise.

The healthcare needs of populations are constantly increasing and set to grow significantly more since there are ever greater numbers of elderly people.

Continuing advances in technology tend to increase the public's expectations of healthcare practitioners. They offer potential new ways for professionals to communicate with each other and share information. Conflict between what is possible and what is achievable in terms of skills and time presents professionals with professional challenges and ethical dilemmas.

Multiprofessional practice as a way of improving patient care

This section explores how multiprofessional practice links to and improves patient care. It should help you to gain a deeper understanding of why multiprofessional practice is so important, and assist you to complete the second learning outcome.

Many propositions and initiatives rest on the premise (that is, the assumption) that multiprofessional practice improves patient care outcomes.

Evidence has indeed been put forward that the outcomes of care are improved when care is delivered by a multiprofessional team who achieve effective multiprofessional practice. The NHS Plan (DH, 2000a) uses this evidence to promote the development of multiprofessional practice. Interprofessional learning includes learning how to develop close partnerships and how to collaborate with other professions at all levels. The overall aim is to ensure a seamless service for patient-centred care.

Two slightly different points are made here: first, that multiprofessional practice is a way of improving professional practice, and second, that multiprofessional practice is a way of improving patient care outcomes. The question that will now be explored is, 'In what ways can successful multiprofessional practice influence (and improve) the quality of professional practice and the quality of health and social care outcomes for patients/clients?'

Improved professional practice

The WHO argued the case for multiprofessional practice in the late 1980s, on the basis that it improves working relationships and improves the quality of healthcare outcomes, issues that remain relevant today. Some common messages have emerged suggesting that multiprofessional teams who share discussions on the needs of patients/clients improve the quality of the healthcare (Wilcock and Headrick, 2000). Among the perceived improvements are:

- taking a more comprehensive approach to patient/client care
- discovering new ideas for improving care
- creating realistic improvement projects to test in practice.

This kind of evidence is still emerging, and as yet there is no agreement between all of the lead authors in the field. As yet interprofessional learning is not common to all health professional education programmes, although it may well be in the near future, and multiprofessional practice is not the norm across all NHS regions.

To achieve close partnerships and a seamless service, the *NHS Workforce Strategy* (DH, 2000b) recommends joint training programmes across the professions to promote team work, partnership and collaboration between professions and agencies. This is the basis of interprofessional learning. A paper entitled 'Towards a European approach to an enhanced education of the health professions in the 21st Century' (CAIPE, 2000) details the ideas and recommendations that have been made for interprofessional learning. You might like to read this paper and follow it with the adjacent activity.

What interprofessional learning is about

This section introduces you to the concept of interprofessional learning and helps you to gain an understanding of what interprofessional learning is about, what subjects are studied and what is required of you as a learner. This section assists you to complete the third learning outcome for this chapter. It is essential to study this section before moving on to read about how you can increase your success with interprofessional learning.

The concept of interprofessional learning

The process of interprofessional learning/education is defined by Barr (1997) as:

> Occasions when two or more professions learn from and about each other to improve collaboration and the quality of care.

A wide range of professions may be involved, including audiologists, social workers, podiatrists, physiotherapists, occupational therapists, nurses, midwives, radiographers, doctors, pharmacists, speech and language therapists, complementary therapists, psychologists and art therapists. You are likely to meet members of some or all of them during your learning experiences and future practice. This section will help you to gain a clear understanding of the roles of different health and social care professions, and of their professional regulatory bodies. It assists you to complete the third and fourth learning outcomes.

Universities in the United Kingdom and Canada are the first in the world to develop interprofessional learning, and the subject as a whole is still developing theoretically. The UK government takes responsibility for ensuring that university programmes prepare future professionals for multiprofessional practice, with the expectation that they will then contribute to increasing the quality of healthcare delivery, adapt to change individually and contribute to the ongoing future changes to their chosen profession.

Interprofessional learning in pre-qualifying comprises themes, modules and/or placements. In some cases, interprofessional learning is referred to in programmes and filtered into the content and culture of the programme but there is no specific module or unit. In other cases, interprofessional learning takes a more prominent focus and is a formal part of a programme. It is assessed and contributes to students' academic and professional awards. Interprofessional

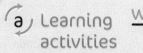

Learning activities

Read the recommendations of the CAIPE report by going to www.caipe.org.uk. Make notes on the key points, with accompanying references.

In your learning group, consider and list the ways that multiprofessional practice might improve the care given to patients/clients. Include, as evidence, references from the literature you have read, naming the authors of the ideas. Present your findings and initiate a group discussion.

learning in such cases uses 'active methods of learning and facilitation to guide and support learning', requiring students to engage in learning with students from other professional courses as well as their own. For example, the universities of Southampton and Portsmouth join together to offer interprofessional learning that brings together students from every one of the above professional groups. Different universities offer different courses, some may offer opportunities for all of these professions to learn together, and others may include a smaller representation from professional groups.

W   The chapter website lists all UK education institutions currently offering interprofessional learning. This information is also available at www.commonlearning.net.

Learning about interprofessional and multiprofessional practice

This section involves you in a process of deconstruction. That means that the terms 'interprofessional' and 'multiprofessional' are broken down in order to examine their parts in greater depth. For example, 'collaboration', 'team work' and 'personal communication and interaction' among other terms are examined more closely.

The activities earlier in the chapter explored the impact of changes on future healthcare practitioners and what is needed in order to practise effectively in the future. The reports cited recommended closer working relations between professions, and used such phrases as 'collaboration between professionals', 'working together' and 'sharing important information', suggesting that there is a need to improve existing practices and find new types of practice in the future.

When reading about what creates successful multiprofessional practice you will also find discussion on how existing practice goes wrong, how it can be improved in future and how practice contexts (organisations and management structures) need to change in order for interprofessional and multiprofessional practice to develop successfully in the future. You will find scepticism and criticism which it is useful to read and draw on in order to create a balanced argument when writing about this subject. Bear in mind that what is known today will be continuously added to as more research is completed and new ideas emerge which influence what is considered to be the best way to practise in a multiprofessional and interprofessional team.

Successful interprofessional and multiprofessional practice is based on a body of knowledge, skills and attitudes that are considered to be essential:

1 Collaboration. Examples of successful collaboration include being able to:
   - negotiate
   - create a climate of openness
   - create equality between professionals
   - put team resources (space and time for positive conflict management) in place
   - put administrative support in place
   - create effective communication and coordination systems (physical proximity and electronic communication technology).

2 Team work. Examples of successful team work include being able to:
   - trust other practitioners
   - build effective interpersonal relationships
   - lead others
   - know how professionals work together successfully in groups.

3 Professional systems. Examples include knowing about:
   - client-centred practice
   - reflective practice
   - your own and other professions' roles
   - your own and other professions' organisational systems.

4 Self-awareness. Examples of the personal characteristics to develop are:
   - effective communication and listening skills
   - clear understanding of your own beliefs, attitudes and stereotypes
   - reflection on your experiences
   - willingness to collaborate
   - understanding of how your behaviour impacts on other members of a group and vice versa.

5 Active and self-directed learning. Examples of successful active and self-directed learning include being able to:
   - be proactive
   - understand the information, communication and technology systems and processes used in interprofessional practice
   - plan your study
   - ask for help with your learning and help others with their learning.

Interprofessional learning courses have been designed to include the five categories of skills, attitudes and knowledge shown above. They are discussed in more depth in the next section.

The process of learning different subject areas is summarised as 'learning with, from and about your own and others' behaviours and your own and others' professions'. The prerequisite knowledge, skills and attitudes, listed above, form the basis of interprofessional learning. The subjects studied that are common to all programmes are drawn from these five areas:

- collaborative practice: how effective collaborative practice is developed and potential restrictions
- team work: how effective teams work in health and social care practice, and potential barriers
- professional systems: the influence of professional and organisational structures, systems and roles on team work and collaboration
- self-awareness: your own beliefs, attitudes and values, and their influence on team work and collaborative practice
- active learning: how to be proactive and self-directed in your own learning to achieve successful lifelong learning and become an effective multiprofessional team member.

Table 2.1 sets out a number of essential components for success for each of the subjects studied in interprofessional learning.

Table 2.1 Subjects and their components for successful interprofessional learning

Subjects studied in interprofessional learning	Subject components
How to develop effective collaborative practice and recognise real and potential barriers	**Collaboration** includes: → equality between professionals → negotiation → climate of openness → team resources (space and time for positive conflict management) → administrative support → effective communication and coordination systems (physical proximity and electronic communication technology).
How to develop effective team work and recognise real and potential barriers	**Team work** includes: → trust → effective interpersonal relationships between team members → leadership → knowledgeable about how professionals work together successfully in groups.
Knowledge of your own and others' professional and organisational systems, roles and structures and their possible negative impact on successful multiprofessional practice	**Professional systems** include: → client-centred practice → reflective practice → knowledge of own and other's professional role.
Knowing yourself, reflecting on your own beliefs and attitudes, recognising those that inhibit and promote successful multiprofessional practice	**Self-awareness** includes: → effective communication and listening skills → self-awareness → reflection → willingness to collaborate.

Subjects studied in interprofessional learning	Subject components
How to be proactive and self-directed in your own learning to achieve successful multiprofessional practice, recognising how without self-direction multiprofessional practice is impaired	**Independent and self-directed learning skills** include: → proactive → ICT literate → effective study planning skills → team player.

The subject areas here form the basis of interprofessional learning, and as you can see if you look back at the list of prerequisite criteria, your programme of learning aims to assist you to start your profession with appropriate skills, knowledge and attitudes gained from studying these areas, which are known to create successful multiprofessional practice.

Once you have read about your own course, talk to other students who have studied it before you. Ask what they most enjoyed and what they would do differently if they were starting again.

You can see from the subjects studied that multiprofessional practice is more than knowing a bit about what other professions do, or knowing who else to talk to about patient/client care. It is potentially more far-reaching than any previous change in professional practice. It involves different ways of practising in different contexts. Of course, experience plays a large part in helping you to become successful, and the skills and attitudes involved in multiprofessional practice need to be used and experienced in order to be developed fully, during which time your knowledge and understanding increases. After qualifying you will build experience which, when added to your knowledge, skills and attitudes, will enable you to guide others, both senior and junior colleagues, in the move towards building successful multiprofessional practice.

As interprofessional learning is a new and still developing subject, new views on what kind of interprofessional learning is best for interprofessional practice are continually being presented in the literature. Interprofessional learning courses and programmes are still developing, so recommendations on how interprofessional learning should be designed are being published today to inform new programmes that will be offered in the future.

> **⟳ⓐ Learning activity** W̲
>
> You may like to look at the course designed by the Common Learning team at the University of Southampton to see an example of an effective interprofessional learning course. www.commonlearning.net tells you what is learned and how learning is designed.

However, calls for interprofessional practice started in the 1940s, so there is sufficient history to inform the way education programmes are designed. These subjects associated with interprofessional learning are not new, they have been studied in all professional courses. The unique difference in interprofessional learning is an organisational one: it brings students from different professional courses together to study as one learning group. Learning as a member of an interprofessional learning group mirrors some of the important processes for practising as a member of a multiprofessional team.

Collaborative practice and team work

'Collaborative practice' is a term used to describe the nature of the interpersonal communication and interaction process between members of a team or group of professionals. It is central to successful multiprofessional practice. Collaborative practice involves team work and more. This section explores the meaning of collaborative practice, and explores in more depth the essential aspects for success. It shows similarities and differences between collaboration and team work.

For successful collaboration, all members of a team need a number of key interprofessional skills. The interpersonal skills required for successful collaboration are for all members of a team to be:

- respectful to each other
- trusting towards each other
- clear and open communicators between each other (including negotiation)
- assertive
- effective in coordinating self and others
- effective at making decisions based on best evidence
- willing to collaborate
- autonomous
- accountable and able to take responsibility for their own decisions and actions.

More can be read about essential interpersonal processes (also referred to as collaborative competency outcomes) in San Martin-Rodriguez et al (2005) and Way, Jones and Baskerville (2001).

Collaboration is sometimes confused with contact with others. However, contact with others in itself is not enough. Hewstone and Brown (1996), point this out in their findings on this subject. It is important to create a number of necessary conditions for contact to be effective.

Learning how to collaborate effectively is important for achieving multiprofessional care, but it is also an important aspect of learning your own professional practice. It involves increasing your knowledge and understanding of yourself and how you interrelate with others. It involves recognising your existing values, beliefs and attitudes and how they impact on others, along with how others' beliefs and attitudes impact on you. Interprofessional learning is organised in a specific way in order to give you opportunities to do this. Students from different professions join together in groups or teams to work collaboratively to achieve shared tasks and outcomes. These activities give you opportunities to learn from experience about your and others' attitudes, beliefs and ways of viewing the world. By attempting a shared activity you learn how well your group as a group of individuals in partnership can achieve a shared goal.

Successful collaboration is dependent on each individual's willingness to take part. Two important influences on willingness to collaborate are pointed out by Borril et al (2002). These are understanding the benefits of collaborating learned through education, and shared objectives within the team/group. The first depends on spending time reading and learning: for example, using this chapter with all its additional reading and activities. The second depends on negotiating with other members of the team/group to reach agreement on shared goals and objectives. So you need to think through what will increase your motivation to collaborate with others, and what will sustain your motivation.

ⓐ Learning activity

In your interprofessional learning group, independently write a list giving four reasons that you might not be willing to collaborate in a group/team of students from other professions. Discuss your reasons with your fellow group members. Now write a list of four reasons that you would want to collaborate in a group/team. Discuss this too with your colleagues.

The next time you are on placement, ask your mentor to examine your lists. Talk about your list and ask your mentor the following questions:

- In your experience, why would a practitioner not want to collaborate in a group or team with other professions?
- Why would a practitioner want to collaborate?

The terms 'collaborative practice' and 'team work' are often used interchangeably. However, there are differences that you need to be aware of. Effective team work contributes to collaborative practice and so is an essential part of collaboration. Successful collaborative practice, however, requires more than effective team work.

The team-working processes involved in multiprofessional practice have been studied, and different authors have explain their findings on them in detail (for example, Miller, Ross and Freeman, 1999; Baker et al, 1995; Irvine, 1998; Borrill et al, 2002). Effective team work is more complex when it contributes to successful multiprofessional practice.

Skills of negotiation for interprofessional communication

Successful team work requires each member of the team to be skilled at negotiating. How to negotiate is an area of communicating that is particularly important for interprofessional learning. Pointers to improving your general communication skills are not discussed in this chapter as they are addressed specifically in Chapter 5.

Professional systems

This aspect of interprofessional learning is about developing an understanding of your own professional roles and responsibilities as well as those of other professions. These are set out by the professional regulatory bodies. This is an aspect of interprofessional learning that can often be the most challenging. It is essential to understand your own and others' roles in order to be able to understand why possible differences and misunderstandings arise when working together towards shared goals for patient care. To be successful in this area of learning enables you to respect other members of both your own and different professions.

The question arises, when is the best time to start interprofessional learning? If you start in the early part of your programme it is more likely that you will avoid developing negative stereotypes of other professions (Leaviss, 2000). Some students start their programme after they have developed stereotypes of healthcare practitioners, and most have fixed ideas about what the professions are like (that is, stereotypes), gained usually from the media or past experiences. Such fixed ideas may make it more difficult for you to achieve the interpersonal skills necessary for successful collaborative practice.

The term 'systems' is important here. Being systematic means following a system, pattern or step by step process, accepted as the best way of doing something. Some of the systems that you learn about are specific to your profession. For example, a future nurse will learn about the Nursing Process, which is a stepped process that ensures you deliver care in a systematic way. You deliver care in the same way regardless of the day or year in which you practise, the patient receiving the care or the place you give care. This particular system aims to ensure that all patients receive the same quality of care regardless of who they are, who cares for them, where and when. Systems are learned in the same way as roles, and as pointed out earlier, you need to understand the systems that are specific to your own profession, and to be aware of the different systems across different professions. So which comes first, understanding your own or others'? The two are likely to develop alongside each other, increasing in depth as you progress in your programme or course.

It is essential to have contact with students from different professions, to talk and exchange understandings with them. It is important that you read and learn about your own and others' professional systems, then talk again with members of your interprofessional group as part of an ongoing cycle. Interprofessional learning programmes are organised to provide you with opportunities to undergo this cycle of events and activities.

Professional regulatory bodies

Each profession has a regulatory body which influences its culture, values and structure. This section introduces you to the regulatory bodies, their roles and functions. It is important to know about all of the health practitioner regulatory bodies, not just your own, because their influence is far-reaching. Each body has a set of statutory roles: that is, its members are given powers by the government to carry out particular functions. Each one regulates a particular profession and influences it in ways that are positive for that profession. However, their influence might also act as a barrier to interprofessional working. This section explores the functions of the regulatory bodies in light of recent government directions following the Shipman case, and considers implications for interprofessional learning.

Professional regulatory bodies include:

- Health Professions Council
- Nursing and Midwifery Council
- General Medical Council
- General Dental Council
- Royal Pharmaceutical Society of Great Britain
- General Osteopathic Council
- General Optical Council
- General Chiropractic Council
- Pharmaceutical Society of Northern Ireland.

Professional regulatory bodies have common core functions. These are based on establishing and continually improving standards of care. The functions common to the different professional bodies are:

- setting and promoting standards for admission to the register and for remaining on the register (these include guidelines for conduct, performance and ethical standards)
- keeping a register of those who meet the standards, and checking that registrants continue to meet them through a recognised process of continual professional development (CPD)
- administering procedures for dealing with cases where a registrant's right to remain on the register has been called into question (considering allegations of misconduct)
- checking and ensuring high standards of education for the health professionals that they regulate
- providing free and confidential professional advice.

The primary purpose of professional regulation is to ensure patient safety. As such, it is a vital component of the overall framework in the United Kingdom for ensuring the highest quality healthcare for the public, but it is only one component of a much wider system to sustain and improve the standard of care that patients take for granted. The government has a programme for ensuring the quality of healthcare in England, and there are similar strategies in Scotland, Wales and Northern Ireland.

The recommendations of the Shipman Inquiry include important messages for professional regulatory bodies. For example, the effectiveness of professional regulators in providing objective scrutiny of practitioners was called into question. Reviews of professional regulation are ongoing and a number of white papers have since been published. This is likely to continue as efforts are made to improve standards of professional practice.

The proposed reforms were intended to ensure that there were systems in place to deal fairly, quickly and effectively with potential threats to patient safety.

a Learning activity

It is valuable to read two DH papers at this stage in order to learn more about the roles, functions and influence of professional regulatory bodies: *Good Doctors and Safer Patients: The regulation of the non-medical healthcare professions* (DH, 2006) and *Trust, Assurance and Safety: The regulation of health professionals in the 21st century* (DH, 2007). The references section of this chapter gives the website addresses.

One key recommendation was to ensure that multiprofessional practice is put into place:

> Effective healthcare in the 21st century is usually dependent on multiprofessional teams and the contributions of many health professions. Good quality healthcare depends on a large and diverse team of professionals. In order to assure a safe and high-quality experience for patients across the spectrum of their encounters with health professionals, we need to ensure proportionate arrangements for all the professions involved. There can be no weak links in the chain of care. In a multi-disciplinary environment where health professionals frequently work together, their ability to work co-operatively in the best interests of their patients is as much a measure of clinical quality and good patient care as the individual strengths and weaknesses of the professionals within the team.
>
> (DH, 2007)

The reforms have already been far-reaching, particularly in relation to new regulatory arrangements and the introduction of new requirements for continuing professional development. It falls to professional bodies to ensure that a range of professional standards are met at all times.

Professional regulatory bodies and their influence on professional identities

This section describes a range of different views published in the literature on the influence of regulatory bodies on professional identities. The impact on interprofessional learning is considered. This section helps you to gain a clear understanding of professional identities, and introduces you to the concept of stereotypes, which is important to understand for interprofessional learning.

Each healthcare profession has its own characteristics based on a different culture. Each of the professions' cultures includes a set of values, beliefs, attitudes, customs and behaviours. Professional cultures evolved over time as the different professions developed, showing historically based, social class and gender differences. Educational experiences and the socialisation process that occur during the training of each healthcare professional tend to reinforce the values, attitudes, beliefs, customs and behaviours of the chosen profession. For example, the problem-solving approaches and language/jargon used by each profession are learned during professional education. Increasing specialisation has lead to even further immersion of students in the knowledge and culture of their own professional group.

a Learning activity

W

To explore the rather complex subject of professional identity, find an experienced practitioner (perhaps one of your mentors) and ask questions that will help you understand common feelings among your profession, such as:

- What are the professional values, beliefs and customs promoted in our profession?

- In what ways have you changed as a person as a result of becoming a qualified practitioner in our profession?
- How do our professional values, beliefs and customs differ from those of other professions?

You may like to find some answers to these questions by reading appropriate texts and articles. See the 'resources' section on www.commonlearning.net

Professional cultures may create opportunities for effective interprofessional practice, or they may create barriers, in that professional systems can promote values of domination and autonomy which run counter to the spirit of collaborative practice (Hanson et al, 2000). Instead, professionals need to be interdependent (each one dependent on the other in order to achieve high standards of care) and accept that their contributions to care may overlap (Henneman, Lee and Cohen, 1995).

Some organisations may harbour deep cultural values that run counter to the spirit of collaboration. For example, a strong belief in the right to be autonomous will tend to foster individualism and specialisation rather than collaborative practice – as pointed out by Glen (1999). The signals and messages about what is approved of that are sent to a workforce by senior managers or senior professionals will tend to be adopted as the norm. The extent to which collaboration is adopted as the best way to practise will be influenced by existing professional and organisational values. A study by Arslanian-Engoren (1995) found that where nurses are considered equal partners with physicians, collaborative relations are more likely to be established.

It is vital then that because of the nature of the characteristics of collaborative practice, you consider your existing beliefs, values, views, stereotypes and attitudes, and ask yourself whether they will assist you or hinder you in achieving successful interprofessional collaborative practice.

Stereotypes

When students from different professions are brought together to learn about each other, stereotypes are challenged, both openly as part of group discussions and in a closed way when individuals reflect on the beliefs they hold. Understanding how stereotypes are formed and/or changed is part of the subjects of sociology and psychology. You are not expected to understand these complex processes in depth, but you do need to know the meaning of the term 'stereotypes', as well as common stereotypes held by your profession and other professions. You also need to recognise the stereotypes you hold and the way in which they are likely to influence your ability to work as a member of a team/group and collaborate successfully in your future practice.

It is important to understand the term 'professional stereotypes' because as we establish the attitudes as well as knowledge and understanding of our profession, we develop greater understanding of the differences between our own professional attitudes and those of other health and social care professions. It is essential to recognise changes in your own attitudes as well as those of others. The concept of an 'archetype', used to refer to the inherited patterns of emotion, thought or behaviour that operate in the subconscious minds of individuals, is important to understand and recognise. Individuals subconsciously function by seeing and interpreting events within the environment in certain ways. For example, men are predisposed to certain ways of knowing and understanding women, and vice versa. Through the study of groups, it has become clear that a sense of kinship and a shared sense of both self and others is an important characteristic for group cohesion (Nytanga, 1998). In a study of perceptions amongst healthcare students working in groups, Pietroni (1996) found evidence of 'in-group' and 'out-group' behaviour, demonstrating views of 'us' and 'them'. Accompanying the 'us and them' views were a range of negative and positive stereotypes of both their own and other groups. Similarly, sentiments about professional boundaries and role differences reflect archetype and stereotype views.

Increasing your success in interprofessional learning

The final part of this chapter considers how to increase your success in interprofessional learning. It builds on earlier parts of the chapter and complements other chapters in this book. It looks at areas of learning that are required for success which relate to you as an individual. These include self-awareness and independent self-directed learning. Skills of reflection are vital for your success. To develop awareness of your attitudes you need to reflect on your own thoughts, ideas and understandings, including your assumptions and existing stereotypes. Self-directed learner skills are also essential if you are to be successful in interprofessional learning.

Skills of reflection for interprofessional learning

You need to be skilled in reflection in order to learn from your experiences of collaborating in a team/group. Reflection forms a central part of learning for all professions involved in interprofessional learning.

The overriding skill for interprofessional learning is self-awareness. This means being skilled at looking at who you are, what your beliefs, views and attitudes are, and even more important, how your beliefs and attitudes influence how you interact with others and how they interact with you. You can achieve this understanding by using the process of reflection.

Your personal characteristics as a practitioner will develop over a period of time during your course, regardless of the stage at which you start. You may think you know yourself well, but by exploring previous experiences systematically, you will find much more about who you are now and who you are becoming as you change throughout your course. Remember, it may not feel like it, but you change as a result of each and every course experience, and you emerge from the course as a practitioner demonstrating specific professional characteristics.

(a) Learning activities

To learn more about how you as an individual are changing, reflect on times in the past when you demonstrated some of your personal characteristics to others, and how your behaviour impacted on others at the time. Think about how others have behaved towards you in previous situations. In what ways has your behaviour changed over recent years? Make a list of the characteristics you have demonstrated, and consider how these have changed over time. You will find it useful to recall what happened when you were with a group of friends, members of your family, organisation groups or groups at work several years ago. Then compare your personal characteristics then with those of today.

Before you meet others in an interprofessional learning group consider who you are. Ask yourself the questions below. If you have not thought of these questions before, or struggle to think of an answer, you need to consider how you can best increase your understanding of yourself. Try to answer the questions as truthfully as possible:

- How confident am I interacting with others in the group?
- How are my past experiences influencing the way I interact with others in my group today?
- What stereoptypes do I hold? How are they influencing how I interact with others in my group?
- How do I feel about my own professional identity at this point in my course?
- How do I feel about the professional identity of others in my group at this point in my course?
- Have my feelings about professional identities changed, and if so what influenced the change?
- How do I feel about hierarchies in groups?
- Where do I fit into any hierarchies? What impact does that have on me?
- How do I feel about tension or conflict?
- How do I feel about negotiating with others?

In order to learn successfully, you need to focus on who you are and what others can learn from you, as well as who others are and what you can learn from others in the group. For you to learn with and from other members of the group, a particular climate must be created. Each member of the group should contribute equally towards creating a climate of openness, approval of others, mutual trust, respect, active listening and clear communication, balanced with positive conflict management. When each member of the group focuses on building such an environment, it is considered to equate to a willingness to collaborate.

It stands to reason that if interprofessional learning is aimed at learning with, about and from others, the teaching strategies designed to assist you to learn are predominantly active and interactive. Examples of interactive teaching methods are case-based and scenario-based learning, problem-based learning and observation-based learning, all using small group formats. Teaching strategies include presenting a group with a patient or group of patients/clients or a consumer group scenario, and a question or set of questions for the group to explore, review and discuss in order to share understandings of each other's professional roles.

Groups may be asked to carry out case interviews with patients/clients in order to explore the patients' priorities and concerns. As well as case studies, in some courses, simulation, role play and video are used to assist group members to learn with and from each other about professional roles. Care is taken to include problems that lead the group to explore different professional roles. Other learning opportunities you may be involved in include group presentations, self-assessment and peer assessment. It is essential to take a proactive attitude to learning and to take responsibility for building your individual effective study skills.

Your interprofessional learning is designed to provide you with opportunities to write and keep a record of your reflections. Each interprofessional learning group of students has their own facilitator who is skilled in guiding the group to work through the knowledge-gaining process in their own way as active learners. Each individual student is asked to carry out frequent reflections (following guidance on how to reflect) and to use them to analyse how their attitudes, values, opinions and ideas about others change as a result of completing the course of interprofessional learning.

W

To review the range of learning activities you can expect to undertake in interprofessional learning please go to www.commonlearning.net

Conclusion

As I hope you can appreciate, after reading this chapter and additional texts, working through the activities and reviewing the supporting website material, multiprofessional practice is more than knowing a bit about what other professions do or knowing who else to talk to about patient/client care. It is potentially more far-reaching than any other change in professional practice to date.

It involves a different form of professional practice in a different professional context. Interprofessional learning aims to promote sharing and integration of the knowledge of different professions, in order that all those involved can be familiar with, understand and value the roles played by all of the professions in order to achieve high-quality health and social care practice. This sounds straightforward but it is not just about learning what other professionals do. It is about interacting with others with attitudes, understanding and knowledge that will contribute to achieving set outcomes.

This chapter is an introduction to interprofessional learning. It emphasises the basis of interprofessional learning as a process of collective learning. Learning with, about and from others is a simple description of interprofessional learning but one that implies great demands from you as a learner.

The first part of the chapter introduced you to the term 'multiprofessional practice' and described how it developed at the end of the twentieth and start of the twenty-first century. Particular emphasis was placed on a number of professional, social, economic and scientific changes. The meaning of successful multiprofessional practice and its potential impact on patient care were explained.

The next part of the chapter introduced the concept of interprofessional learning and what it means for you as a learner. Although there are slight differences between courses across the United Kingdom, the main subject areas studied in interprofessional learning and their importance for multiprofessional practice are the same throughout. These were listed and explained in order to make clear what is meant by successful multiprofessional practice.

The rest of the chapter concentrated on how to increase your success in interprofessional learning. It explained the key areas of knowledge, skills and attitudes you need to learn. Of course, experience plays a large part in helping you to become successful, and the new knowledge, skills and attitudes you acquire from interprofessional learning should be used and revised regularly in order to achieve a high standard of both multiprofessional and uniprofessional practice.

On a final note, multiprofessional practice is today in its infancy, and experienced, proficient practitioners acting as experts in their field of practice may not be as familiar with its meanings and ways as you. Remember you may well be involved in guiding others, both senior and junior colleagues, while still learning yourself. Once qualified, you will have a particular responsibility to ensure the intended aims of interprofessional learning are achieved and practised on a day-to-day basis. It is up to you to achieve the highest standards of multiprofessional practice in order that patients/clients and healthcare systems benefit to the greatest extent possible. I hope this chapter contributes to your learning and helps you on your way to achieving the highest standards.

References

Arlsanian-Engoren C.M. (1995) 'Lived experiences of CNSs who collaborate with physicians: a phenomenological study', *Clinical Nurse Specialist*, 9, 68–74.

Baker, R., Sorrie, R., Reddish, S., Hearnshaw, H. and Robertson, N. (1995) 'The facilitation of multiprofessional clinical audit in primary healthcare teams – from audit to quality assurance', *Journal of Interprofessional Care* **9**(3), 237–44.

Barr, H. (1997) 'Interprofessional education – a definition', *CAIPE Bulletin* 13 [online] www.caipe.org.uk (accessed 26 February 2009).

Barr, H. (2002) *Interprofessional Education. Today, Yesterday and Tomorrow: A review commissioned by the Learning and Teaching Support Network for Health & Practice and the UK Centre for the Advancement of Interprofessional Education* [online] www.caipe.org. uk (accessed 26 February 2009).

Beveridge, W. (1942) *Social Insurance and Allied Services*, CM 6404, London, HMSO.

Borrill, C., West, M. A., Dawson, J., Shapiro, D., Rees, D. and Richards, A. (2002) 'Teamworking and effectiveness in healthcare. Findings from the healthcare team', Effectiveness project. Aston Centre for Health Service Organisation Research [online] http://homepages.inf.ed.ac. uk/jeanc/DOH-glossy-brochure.pdf (accessed 26 February 2009).

Bristol Inquiry (2001) Final Report of the Bristol Royal Infirmary Inquiry [online] www.bristol-inquiry.org.uk/final_report/index.htm (accessed 26 February 2009).

Centre for the Advancement of Interprofessional Education (CAIPE) (2000) 'Towards a European approach to an enhanced education of the health professions in the 21st Century' [online] www.caipe.org. uk (accessed 5 February 2009)

DH (2000a) *The NHS Plan*, London, The Stationery Office [online] http://www.dh.gov.uk/en/index.htm (accessed October 2007).

DH (2000b) *NHS Workforce Strategy*, London, The Stationery Office [online] http://www.dh.gov.uk/en/index.htm (accessed 5 February 2009).

DH (2001a) *Working Together, Learning Together: A framework for lifelong learning in the NHS*, London, The Stationery Office [online] http://www.dh.gov.uk/en/index.htm (accessed 5 February 2009).

DH (2001b) *The Bristol Inquiry*, London: The Stationery Office [online] http://www.dh.gov.uk/en/index.htm (accessed 5 February 2009).

DH (2003) *The Victoria Climbié Inquiry: A report of an inquiry by Lord Laming*, London, The Stationery Office [online] http://www.dh.gov. uk/en/index.htm (accessed 5 February 2009).

DH (2005) *The Shipman Inquiry, Fifth Report Safeguarding Patients: Lessons from the past – proposals for the future*, London: The Stationery Office [online] http://www.dh.gov.uk/en/index. htm (accessed 5 February 2009).

DH (2006) *Good Doctors, Safer Patients: The regulation of the non-medical healthcare professions*, London, The Stationery Office [online] http://www.dh.gov.uk/en/index.htm (accessed 5 February 2009).

DH (2007) *Trust, Assurance and Safety: The regulation of health professionals in the 21st century*, London, DH [online] http://www. dh.gov.uk/en/index.htm (accessed 5 February 2009).

Farrell, M., Schmitt, M. and Heinemann, G. (2001) 'Informal roles and the stages of interdisciplinary team development', *Journal of Interprofessional Care* **15**(3).

Glen, S. (1999) 'Educating for interprofessional collaboration: teaching about values', *Nursing Ethics* 6, 202–13.

Hanson, C. M., Spross, J. A. and Carr, D. B. (2000) 'Collaboration', pp. 315–47 in Hamric, A. B., Spross, J.A. and Hanson, C. M. (eds), *Advanced Nursing Practice: An integrative approach*, 2nd edn, Philadelphia:, W. B. Saunders.

Henneman, E. A., Lee, J. L. and Cohen, J. L. (1995) 'Collaboration: a poststructuralist view', *Journal of Advanced Nursing* 21, 103–9.

Hewstone, M. and Brown, R. J. (1986) 'Contact is not enough; an intergroup perspective on the "contact hypothesis"', in Hewstone, M. and Brown, R. J. (eds), *Contact and Conflict in Intergroup Encounter*, Oxford, Blackwell.

Irvine, D. (1998) 'Team working and quality assurance', *Kings Fund News* 21(4), 1–2.

Leaviss, J. (2000) 'Exploring the perceived effect of an undergraduate multiprofessional educational intervention', *Medical Education* 34, 483–6.

Miller, C., Ross, N. and Freeman, M. (1999) 'Researching professional education: shared learning and clinical teamwork: new directions in education for multiprofessional practice', Research Report 14, London, English National Board for Nursing Midwifery and Health Visiting.

Nytanga, L. (1998) 'Professional ethnocentrism and shared learning', *Nurse Education Today* **18**(3), 175–7.

Ovretveit, J., Mathias, P. and Thompson, T. (1997) *Interprofessional Working for Health and Social Care*, Basingstoke, Macmillan.

Pietroni, P. C. (1996) 'Stereotypes or archetypes? A study of perceptions among healthcare students', in Pietroni, P. and Pietroni, C. (eds), *Innovations in Community Care and Primary Health*, Edinburgh, Churchill Livingstone.

Robison, D. and Kish, C. P. (2001) *Core Concepts in Advanced Practice Nursing*. St Louis: Mosby

San Martin-Rodriguez, L., Dominique-Beaulieu, M., D'Amour, D. and Feerrada-Videla, M. (2005) 'The determinants of successful collaboration: a review of theoretical and empirical studies', *Interprofessional Education for Collaboration Patient-Centred Care: Canada as a Case Study* **19**(Supplement 1) (May), 132–47.

World Health Organization (WHO) (2006) *The World Health Report 2006: Working together for health*, Geneva, WHO [online] http://www.who.int/whr/previous/en/index.html (accessed 26 February 2009).

Way, D., Jones, L. and Baskerville, N. B. (2001) 'Improving the effectiveness of primary healthcare through nurse practitioner/ family physician structured collaborative practice', University of Ottawa.

Wilcock, P. and Headrick, L. (2000) 'Interprofessional learning for improvement of healthcare: why bother?' *Journal of Interprofessional Care* **14**(2).

Useful websites

Visit the resources section at www.commonlearning.net
www.caipe.org.uk

Chapter

3

Evidence-based practice and research

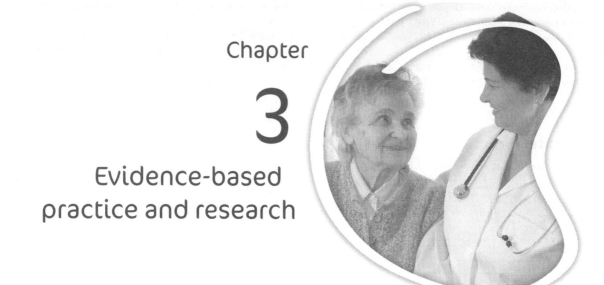

Theresa Pengelly

 Links to other chapters in *Foundation Studies for Caring*

1 Study skills
2 Interprofessional learning
4 Ethical, legal and professional issues
8 Healthcare governance

 Links to other chapters in *Foundation Skills for Caring*

1 Fundamental concepts for skills
2 IT skills

W Don't forget to visit www.palgrave.com/glasper for additional online resources relating to this chapter.

Introduction

Evidence-based practice (EBP) is a term that applies to all aspects of healthcare provision. The use of appropriate evidence to support decision making is now recognised as being the responsibility of all healthcare practitioners. *The New NHS: Modern, dependable* (DH, 1997) set out the modernisation agenda for the United Kingdom, with EBP being an integral part of its implementation. The development of Clinical Governance, National Institute of Clinical Excellence (NICE) and National Service Frameworks are all reliant on healthcare practitioners being able to understand and apply the most appropriate evidence to their practice setting.

The concept of using the best-quality evidence to support care is one that initially appears quite straightforward. However deciding which is the best and most appropriate type of evidence can be daunting if you do not understand the basic aspects of EBP. This chapter gives simple explanations of what constitutes evidence and how to appraise which is best for any specific circumstances. The use of research studies plays a major part in EBP. The research process is broken down into easy to understand terms and the most common research designs are explained. Audits, benchmarking and the use of integrated care pathways are also explained in relation to everyday practice. The scenario follows a person's journey through the healthcare system, demonstrating the different ways in which EBP can be undertaken.

EBP can sometimes be perceived by healthcare practitioners as not always closely related to what actually happens in practice. The terminology used, especially when discussing research, can be difficult to understand at first, but the use of evidence is central to everyone's practice whatever role they have. The use of EBP can very satisfying: it is a key factor in providing high-quality healthcare tailored to the individual's needs. The aim of this chapter is to explain EBP in a way that you will find interesting, and help you to develop skills in selecting and using the most appropriate evidence for your practice.

Learning outcomes

This chapter will enable you to:

- discuss the different sources of nursing knowledge
- define evidence-based practice (EBP)
- explain the different types of evidence available and how they can be appraised
- discuss what is meant by research and explain the research process
- state the most common research designs used in both qualitative and quantitative research
- describe the concepts of audits, benchmarking and integrated pathways.

Concepts

- Types of evidence
- Clinical effectiveness
- Audit
- Hierarchy of evidence

- Qualitative research
- Quantitative research
- Systematic reviews
- Appraisal tools

- Integrated care pathways
- Benchmarking

Good-quality healthcare needs to meet the specific needs of each individual. *The NHS Improvement Plan* (DH, 2004) stresses the importance at looking at the whole of the patient's journey, with the ultimate aim of seamless and consistent care provision. The use of appropriate evidence is central to this goal as it provides the rationale for care interventions, helping to ensure that each person receives the best possible care.

S Scenario: introducing Lisa

Lisa is a 20-year-old secretary who lives with her partner Tom, a mechanic. Lisa's parents live nearby. Lisa has now lived with Tom for a year, having previously lived with her parents and two younger sisters.

Lisa has had asthma since she was a child. It is well controlled, and she attends the respiratory clinic at her health centre on a regular basis. When she last attended she was surprised that her peak flow was not as high as normal. She chatted this through with the practice nurse to see whether there were any changes in her life that could have precipitated it.

Lisa discussed how moving in with our partner had been a much bigger change than she had anticipated. She now realised how reliant she had been on her mother to provide her with a healthy diet. Her partner works very long hours and has not shown much interest in helping with either shopping or cooking. Lisa has really struggled with this, and has found that many days of the week they ended up having take-away meals.

The practice nurse explained that it was quite possible that her weight gain could be one factor affecting her peak flow rates. She suggested to Lisa that she saw her GP to discuss the management of her asthma, and Lisa did so.

Lisa thought about her weight gain over the next few weeks. She decided that she would really like to lose weight, and to try out the weight management clinic at the health centre. This worked out well. She persuaded a friend to go with her and was really pleased with her steady weight loss over the next few weeks.

Lisa developed mild abdominal pain just as she arrived for work one morning. Initially she thought that it was because of her change of diet, but within a few hours the pain began to be quite severe, and moved to her right side. Her manager thought she was looking very unwell, so she took her to the local Accident and Emergency Department. Appendicitis was diagnosed. Lisa had an appendectomy late that evening. She made a good recovery and was discharged home two days later.

a Learning activity

At every stage of her journey Lisa will have seen healthcare practitioners wash their hands. This is an activity which in practice you will have undertaken out several times a day, not just as a healthcare practitioner but as part of everyday living.

Think back to the last time that you washed your hands while on a clinical placement. Write down how you washed your hands and why you did it that way. Then list the reasons you chose that method. You may be surprised

at the length of the list for what appears on the surface to be a very simple task.

The *why* part of the activity is what EBP is in a nutshell. This is EBP at a very simple level. It provides a list of different types of evidence, but at this stage there is no attempt to break down the different types and decide which is the most suitable. This will be undertaken in further activities.

Background to EBP

EBP is not a new concept. In 1972 the epidemiologist Archie Cochrane wrote what is now considered to be a groundbreaking book *Effectiveness and Efficiency: Random reflections on health services*, which called for scientific proof to underpin medical interventions. He also set up a central register for clinical trials, which saw the beginning of a more collaborative approach to the sharing of research outcomes (Greenhalgh, 2006). In the same year the Briggs Committee on Nursing (DHSS, 1972) stated the need for nursing to become a research-based profession (Upton, 1999). The need for a massive development in the use of research to underpin all healthcare was also highlighted in a report that set out a research strategy for the National Health Service (NHS) (DH, 1991).

This approach has continued to be developed. The white paper, *The New NHS: Modern, dependable* (DH, 1997) set out a ten-year modernisation plan which was heavily reliant on the use of EBP to implement the underpinning strategy of clinical effectiveness. There are also financial reasons for the implementation of EBP. It is anticipated that the integration of EBP throughout all healthcare provision will mean a far higher degree of clinical effectiveness, and massive savings in costs in an overburdened healthcare system (Parahoo, 2006).

The meaning of EBP

There is no one set definition of EBP, which is sometimes called evidence-based medicine or evidence-based nursing. These are three variations:

> The conscientious, explicit, judicious use of current best available evidence and about the care of individual patients. The practice of evidence-based medicine means integrating individual clinical experience with the best available evidence from systematic research.
>
> (Sackett, 1996: 71)

> Evidence-based medicine is the use of mathematical estimates of the risk of benefit and harm, derived from high quality research on population samples, to inform clinical decision making in the diagnosis, investigation or management of individual patients.
>
> (Greenhalgh, 2006: 1)

> Evidence-based nursing is the term that is used to describe the process that nurses use to make clinical decisions and to answer clinical questions and uses four approaches:
> Reviewing the best available evidence, most often the results of research.
> Using the nurse's clinical expertise.
> Determining the values and cultural needs of the individual.
> Determining the preferences of the individual, family and community.
>
> (Macnee and McCabe, 2006: 4)

(a) Learning activity

The three quotes show that the common ground in EBP is that the use of evidence is important. However what evidence is and how it used does seem to differ.

Read through the quotes a few times, and jot down the similarities and differences. Think about which definition is most relevant to your own clinical practice and why.

Clinical effectiveness

Clinical effectiveness is a term often used in conjunction with EBP. It is defined as 'The extent to which specific clinical interventions, when deployed in the field do what they are intended to do i.e., maintain and improve health and secure the greatest possible gain from the available resources' (NHS Executive, 1996). Cranston (2002) describes clinical effectiveness having three distinct parts:

- obtaining evidence
- implementing the evidence
- evaluating the evidence.

(a) Learning activity

Clinical effectiveness covers all types of clinical interventions, not just specific treatments. Look back on your notes on hand washing from the first learning activity. In your next clinical placement find out about the trust's policy on hand washing, what resources are used to implement this and how it is evaluated.

What is evidence?

A very important aspect of EBP is what evidence actually is, what can be used and whether some evidence is better than others. This is important because you need to be certain that you have selected the right evidence to back up an individual's treatment, not just in terms of clinical effectiveness but to meet all the needs of the individual.

Evidence for healthcare interventions is likely to come from a wide range of sources. Research is considered to be the most reliable because of the systematic way that it is undertaken, but it is unrealistic to expect every single aspect of healthcare to have up to date and relevant research to support it. It used to be assumed that evidence in a healthcare context meant scientifically based research, but this is no longer true. In order to provide care that is person-centred it is important to look at all the different types and levels of evidence, then make the decision on what is appropriate in a particular situation (Rycroft-Malone and colleagues, 2004).

Experienced healthcare practitioners often have vast amounts of knowledge of dealing with particular situations. Although obviously the most up to date literature is very important, their knowledge and skills should not be overlooked when considering evidence. In the quest to find the most relevant evidence it is also easy to forget the person requiring the healthcare intervention, the service user, but their personal experience can be a valuable source of evidence too. It is therefore important to develop skills in assessing all available evidence. One way of doing this is to use a framework that helps you to take into consideration different types of evidence.

Rycroft-Malone and colleagues (2004: 83) define evidence as coming from four main sources:

- research
- clinical experience
- patients, clients and carers
- the local context and environment (including audit and evaluation data, local professional networks, and feedback from quality assurance programmes).

This framework is a useful starting point for explaining what constitutes evidence. This is important because in each situation you should be looking at what evidence is best. It is likely that you will draw on more than one source. Below is an overview of the sources.

Research

Out of all the available evidence, research will be the most reliable. Research can appear very complicated but the principles are simple. It is systematic inquiry that uses specific methods to answer a particular question (Polit and Beck, 2007). Because research is carried out in a set way, the information obtained is likely to be higher quality than that acquired by nonresearch methods. It is however important not to assume that all published research provides suitable evidence to support your practice. In addition to understanding the main concepts of research, you also need to be able to appraise a study to gauge its usefulness. This vital skill is covered later in the chapter (and also see Chapter 1).

Clinical experience

The skills and knowledge of healthcare practitioners are an important aspect of EBP. Healthcare knowledge will be individual to each practitioner. The skilled practitioner will be able to draw on their knowledge base and use the appropriate combination for each individual situation.

There are various kinds of knowledge that derive from clinical experience. *Empirical knowledge* is based on hard facts. As well as research this involves theoretical knowledge: for example, in order to care for patients it is important to understand anatomy and physiology. *Aesthetic knowledge* is about trying to gain insight into the human experience. This can be used to try to provide care that meets the individual's wider needs. Sometimes this is called 'adding the small touches'. *Personal knowledge* is linked to self-awareness. This is about using your life skills and experience to aid clinical decision making. Personal knowledge can also encompass two other terms, experiential knowledge and intuition. *Experiential knowledge* is knowledge based on previous experience, which you can draw on to deal with a situation. It can derive from your broader life experience, such as a family member being ill in hospital, or directly from your clinical experience (Edwards, 2002). *Intuition* is described as knowledge that comes from the subconscious: we do not know how we acquire this kind of knowledge. For example a skilled healthcare practitioner may be able to predict that a patient is about to experience a crisis before there are any physical signs or symptoms to base the prediction on. In reality, they are probably drawing together all their vast range of knowledge and experience to come to this judgement.

Information derived from the experiences of practitioners can obviously be found in journals, books and websites. It is however also really important to remember to ask about the experience of clinical colleagues in your placements. For example, working with your mentor will provide you with a rich source of evidence.

Patients, clients and carers

The importance of consulting service users and their families when planning and undertaking care is central to EBP. There are now an increasing number of research studies which involve service users, but all decision making should include the views and often vast experience of the individual undergoing the care and treatment. The importance of valuing and respecting the knowledge base of service users is being increasingly recognised by the Department of Health. The Patient Advice and Liaison Service (PALS) helps service users to ensure that their voice is heard in the decision-making process. The specific needs of people with long-term illness have also been recognised. The Expert Patient programme (DH, 2001b) seeks to ensure that people with chronic illness are encouraged to take more control of their care and treatment. One aspect of this is that the healthcare practitioner needs to remember that the individual will often have a huge insight into their condition. Their input should always be taken into account when planning, implementing and evaluating care.

The local context and environment

There are local guidelines and policies for many areas of practice. These are drawn up locally but will often incorporate national guidelines such as those produced by NICE. Audits are often used locally. They are an excellent way of gaining information about service provision that may not always be captured in research studies, which are unlikely to be local to that clinical area.

The major difference between research and an audit is that research seeks to explore a problem whereas an audit measures what has already occurred against a predetermined standard (Lindsay, 2007). Because of this audits are limited: they cannot be used for testing new interventions. They are however very flexible and can be used in number of ways by both healthcare practitioners and service users.

It is likely that the majority of locally sourced evidence will be unpublished. This can be limiting because it means that it is unlikely to have been subjected to external scrutiny. However it still very useful evidence and may well cover local factors that are not represented in published evidence.

The collective term for unpublished written evidence is *grey literature*. The use of this type of evidence is increasing, partly because the rapid development of the internet means that it often easily accessible. Coad, Devitt and Hardicre (2006) explain that this can be a very rich source of evidence which should not be overlooked.

⟨C⟩ Professional conversation

Aisha, a staff nurse, says, 'I admitted Lisa to the ward when she came in for her appendectomy. She looked very apprehensive and worried so I took a bit of time to chat and put her at her ease. She then told me that a major worry for her was her asthma. Because she had never had an anaesthetic she was worried that this could trigger a severe asthma attack. I was able to reassure her that this information would be recorded and that all healthcare professionals would be aware that she had asthma.'

Asthma is a common condition and one that can vary in severity. It is very likely that wherever you have worked you have come in contact with people who have asthma. You may have asthma yourself or have close friends or family who do. Using Rycroft-Malone and colleagues' framework (2004) as a guide, keep a diary over the next few weeks about all the different types of evidence that you can find about asthma. As you collect each piece of evidence, make notes about what you think are its strengths and weaknesses.

Where to look for evidence

Looking for specific evidence can be a daunting task. There is an ever-increasing amount of different sources which at first can be bewildering. It can also be quite time-consuming. However, taking time to search for the most appropriate information is important. You will also need different types of information for different situations. The following sources all have their place but it is important to be able to understand the main strengths and weaknesses of each one. What might be the quickest way of obtaining information does not always provide the most accurate information; remember that an unreliable source could have implications for safe practice.

Journals

There are masses of journals ranging from weekly general magazines to more specialist academic journals. They are an excellent way of keeping up to date with healthcare in general. It is a good idea to find a journal that is linked to your area of practice and to look through each issue. Keeping up to date in this way should not be underestimated. Greenhalgh (2006) explains that browsing through literature accounts for quite a large proportion of knowledge gained, and also means that you can gain information that you would miss solely by undertaking focused literature searches. The types of article in journals vary from personal opinion to research studies. You are best advised to stick to peer-reviewed journals; this means that the article has been reviewed by an expert in that field prior to publication. Journals are not always the most up to date source of information: publication in a specialised journal can take about a year.

The internet

This is generally a means of accessing information rather than an actual source (Beechcroft, Rees and Booth, 2006). It can be an excellent means of gaining up to date information. However it needs to be used with caution. Because the internet is so accessible, anyone can set up a website, so you need to check carefully that the information is from a reliable source.

You will also often find when using search engines that vast amounts of information come with one mouse click. However trying to decide what is suitable evidence can be daunting and time-consuming. There are many reliable websites which are well managed and are updated on a regular basis. If you are not familiar with accessing websites a good starting point is the Department of Health website (www.doh.gov.uk).

An alternative to using a search engine to find relevant websites is to use a gateway: a resource that provides access to specific websites. A very good example is that of the National Library of Health (NELH) (www.library.nhs.uk) which provides access to a vast range of health-related information.

Books

Books are a useful resource. They can be really good for providing an overview of vast topics. Many books now give pointers on where to find more detailed information, and provide activities to motivate you to find out more about a subject. More specialist books often give very helpful insights into specific topics. Books do have limitations, however. They often take a long time to be published and are not always the most up to date source of information. For this reason they should generally be used in conjunction with other types of evidence.

(a) Learning activity

This builds on the information gained in the previous learning activity. Go though the written evidence that you have obtained and allocate it to three categories:

- journals
- the internet
- books.

If you do not have examples from each you will need to collect some more evidence. Read through a selection of the evidence. For each item, consider how you can decide whether it is reliable and up to date. If there are differences, for example in recommended treatments, which one would be the best to follow and why?

Using a question to find evidence

You will have found that choosing evidence can be difficult as it often means sifting through vast amounts of information. This can be very frustrating and time-consuming. You may have found in the last activity that so much information was generated it was quite tricky to decide which to select.

One way of making your searching more effective is to formulate a search question. Doing this will mean that you are more focused. The PICO framework is the most widely used (Sackett et al, 1997):

- Patient or Population
- Intervention
- Comparison
- Outcome.

It can be used as question for one person or a group of people. There are drawbacks, however. It works best when there is cause and effect in the question. It can be very useful, and help guide your thinking to cover the required aspects.

For example, Lisa will need to fast before her surgery. The clinical area should have guidelines on how this should be done, which should be based on the best available evidence. If you want to find out for yourself what the evidence tells us, PICO could be used in the following way:

> What is the correct fasting procedure for adults undergoing surgery?
>
> Patient/population = Adults fasted for surgery
>
> Intervention = fasting
>
> Comparison = different fasting times
>
> Outcome = safely prepared for anaesthetic.

We have now outlined the concept of EBP and the different types of evidence that can be used. It is important to consider all available evidence, but the use of research studies is particularly important. The advantage of research above other evidence derives from the way that research is carried out. The next section explains why, then gives an overview of the most common types of research.

(a) Learning activity

Read through the scenario about Lisa again and select an aspect of her care that would be suitable to use with the PICO framework. Design a question to be answered and break it down into the different parts of the framework.

Research studies

Research can appear complicated and offputting but the principles are really quite straightforward. All of us gather evidence in a variety of ways, and make decisions based on it in our professional lives. Of all the available evidence, that derived from research will be the most reliable. This is because research is a systematic inquiry that uses specific methods to answer a question (Polit and Beck, 2007). There are certain steps that need to be followed in order to carry out research. This is called the *research process* (see Figure 3.1).

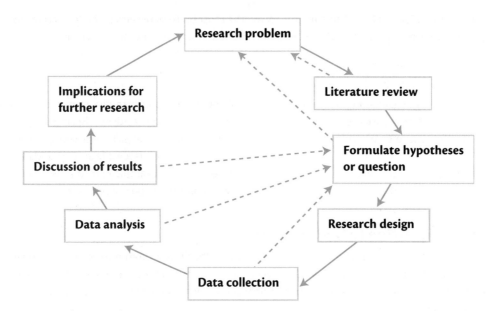

Figure 3.1 The research process

There may be slight deviations according to the type of research but all research studies follow this broad process. The stages are briefly explained here, and discussed in more detail towards the end of the chapter.

- Research problem: there must obviously be a topic that is to be explored.
- Literature review: the researcher carries out a comprehensive search of all literature pertaining to the topic to find out what is already known about it.
- Formulate question or hypothesis: the researcher needs to draw up a specific question to be answered by undertaking the research, or frame a hypothesis: a statement about the possible outcome of the study, which the research will either prove or disprove.
- Research design: this means drawing up the framework that is used to structure the study.
- Data collection: this covers deciding how the information from the research study is to be obtained, then actually obtaining it.
- Data analysis: the researcher then decides how the information gained from the research study is to be broken down and presented, and does so.
- Discussion of results: this is the stage for discussing what the findings are and how they fit into what is already known.
- Implications for further research: finally, the researcher should consider what aspects of this topic need further research.

There are two main approaches to research, the qualitative and quantitative. They are very different but are both important in getting a better understanding of healthcare, as they offer quite different perspectives.

Qualitative research

The goal of qualitative research is to increase understanding of people's experiences by collecting information directly from people who have undergone a specific experience (Macnee and McCabe, 2006). This type of research is based on the belief that the complexities of human experience cannot be represented just by the use of figures. Qualitative research can be carried out in a number of ways but the most common method is interviewing people. This research approach is now considered very important in healthcare because it contributes to gaining more insight into what individuals think and feel about their specific experiences.

There are limitations to qualitative research. In general because the information gathered tends to be very detailed it is often obtained from a small number of people. This means that although it is very valuable it cannot be generalised (that is, assumed also to apply to a much wider population).

Quantitative research

The aim of quantitative research is to gain more knowledge by investigating phenomena that can be precisely measured and quantified. Quantitative research uses empirical data: that is, evidence that is based on an observation, which is gathered using a structured measuring instrument (Polit and Beck, 2007). This traditional scientific method produces numerical information which is then analysed. This can vary from quite simple statistics to very complex comparisons of the different data. Much quantitative research seeks to generalise: this means that the result of the study are intended to relate to a wider population.

There are limitations to quantitative research too. Often the research looks at quite a narrow aspect of a complex situation. This is sometimes described as sedimented, meaning that it does not capture the complete human experience (Polit and Beck, 2007).

The use of quantitative and qualitative research in healthcare

Many healthcare research questions cannot be fully answered without using both approaches. This is because many health situations are complex and involve human experiences which cannot be fully represented using statistical information. On the other hand, there is a clear role for statistical information (most obviously, for example, on drug dosages), which provides a basis for safe and effective care.

(c) Professional conversation

Emma a first-year student nurse, says, 'I was allocated to care for Lisa the day after her surgery. I was apprehensive at first. Lisa seemed very keen to chat and it became clear that she was very self-conscious about being overweight. I was very careful to make sure that I did not draw attention to this when caring for her. She chatted about it quite a bit, explaining how glad she was that she had found out about the weight management clinic at the local health centre.

My mentor gave me very positive feedback at the end of the shift. She had observed how I gained a good rapport with Lisa. She also explained that she was unaware of weight management clinics but would be finding out more about them as part of her professional development.'

(a) Learning activity

Lisa has sought help regarding her weight gain. Obesity is a major problem today, with an increasing number of people becoming overweight. This is an area that is now being widely researched. Undertake a literature search and select some qualitative and quantitative research studies. Read through the abstracts and the findings. Make notes of what information the different studies contain and how they could enhance your practice.

When you search for articles you may come across research studies that have used both quantitative and qualitative approaches. Keep these back for the next activity.

Mixed method studies

Mixed method studies combine quantitative and qualitative research. This can work well and produce research studies that address the weaknesses associated with using just one approach. The number of mixed method studies is increasing. It is now recognised how valuable it is for researchers of different backgrounds to work together and produce cohesive research that meets the entire research question (Parahoo, 2006).

Trying to understand research is often easier if you use a step by step approach. It is quite common for students to become very frustrated by the terms used in research studies. They can be confusing and put people off from further developing their skills. So far you will have read through articles and looked at the abstracts and findings but not looked at the methods used. The next section looks at the most common types of research designs and methods.

Research designs

In all research there needs to be a overall plan of the type of sample, and the data collection and analysis methods. This plan will assist the researcher to overcome issues that may arise in the research process. It is called the *research design*. It needs to be the most suitable to answer the research question, and forms the structure of the study. In quantitative research the designs tend to be rigid. In qualitative studies there is sometimes a more flexible approach to interpretation (Polit and Beck, 2007).

Design and methods for qualitative research

The most common qualitative research methods are based on:

- ethnography: a holistic viewpoint of a specific culture, examining all the different aspects in depth
- grounded theory: the way in which people make sense of social interactions
- phenomenology: the interpretation and meaning of an individual's experience
- discourse analysis: to uncover the values, meanings and intentions in interactions between people.

We outlined the research process in general terms earlier in the chapter. It is now explained in more detail in relation to qualitative research.

Research problem

This is the topic that is to be explored.

Literature review

The depth of the literature review may vary. Sometimes only a modified literature search is carried out. This happens when it is thought that finding out too much in advance of the data analysis could cause the researcher to have preconceived ideas and possibly lead to bias.

Formulate a question or hypothesis

It is rare for a hypothesis to be used in qualitative healthcare research. Usually there is either a research question or a stated aim.

Research design

There is not always a definite research design. Some but not all elements of a research design may be used. There can also be different interpretations of the research design.

Data collection

Sample sizes are often small. This is because the data is often very rich and detailed. The most common form of sampling is purposive: in other words, the participants are specifically selected (rather than being, for example, chosen at random out of the population of interest). Data are usually collected by holding interviews or focus groups. Other methods are observation, questionnaires and the use of drawings.

Data analysis

The analysis can be undertaken manually. There are some software packages but they are still limited when it comes to using qualitative data. The most common form of analysis is to sort the data into themes. This is known as *thematic analysis*.

Discussion of results

The results should be presented in a clear format. It should be easy to see how the research aim or question has been answered. Excerpts from the data should be included. These should be direct copies of the original data (for instance, transcripts of what the interviewees said). It may not always be possible to give recommendations for practice. If they are relevant and practicable, the implications should be highlighted.

Implications for further research

The researcher should consider and comment on aspects of the topic that will need further research.

Design and methods for quantitative research

The most common research methods in quantitative research are:
- Randomised controlled trial: an experimental study which uses a randomised proportion of the population to try out an intervention on. There is always a control: that is, some or all of the remaining section of the population must be considered, so it is apparent what difference the intervention has made.
- Quasi experimental: this is not a true experimental study. There is always an intervention, or there would be nothing to study, but there is not always a control. Participants are not always randomised but might be selected in some other way.
- Survey: this is a nonexperimental study which obtains descriptive information about populations.

Research problem

Again, this specifies the topic that is to be explored.

Literature review

There is always a literature review. The aim is to find out as much as possible in advance of undertaking the study.

Formulate a question or hypothesis

A research question can be used to structure the study, but in experimental studies a hypothesis is always used.

Research design

There is always a definite and fully specified research design for quantitative research, and it should always be followed closely.

Data collection

The sample size is very important, and should not be too small. This is because often the researchers want to be able to generalise their findings, and they must use a sufficiently large sample to be able to do so reliably. Samples often need to be representative of populations. For that to occur they need to be randomised, and not selected in a way which might make them unrepresentative.

Data analysis

The analysis always involves numerical data, and to make it simpler and faster a software package is always used.

Discussion of results

The results should be presented in a clear format. All the analysed data should be apparent in the findings. If there is a hypothesis the discussion should indicate whether this has been proved. There should be recommendations for practice.

Implications for further research

Again, the researcher will need to consider what aspects of the topic need further research.

Systematic reviews

In general most individual research studies are too small to completely answer everything about a particular topic. A systematic review is a higher-level study, a kind of synthesis of other studies. It is undertaken by reviewers who look in depth at the existing research evidence on a specific topic. The research is appraised using specific tools, and the reviewers provide summaries of their findings for readers (Webb and Roe, 2007). A systematic review has some similarity to a literature review, but there are important differences. The evidence accessed is analysed and appraised, and not just used to discover what has been done before, and the way the review is undertaken means that there are far stricter criteria for inclusion (Lindsay, 2007).

Systematic reviews can cover both quantitative and qualitative research, and can be an excellent way of gaining an overview of research in a specific area. They are very good as a first point of reference. There are not systematic reviews available for every aspect of healthcare, but their numbers are increasing. The most comprehensive collection of systematic reviews in healthcare is the Cochrane Library (www.cochrane.org). This is a huge collection, and it can be rather daunting to use at first. Many libraries offer specialist training on how to get the best out of it.

W

a) Learning activity

Lisa will require management of her pain, and also wound care following her surgery. Search for a systematic review on both of these topics. Select one systematic review, and answer these questions:
- How easy were the reviews to find?

- Was one topic easier to find reviews on than the other?
- What evidence was included in your selected review?
- What was excluded?
- How helpful are the summaries to the development of your practice?

Ethical issues

All research studies within the healthcare field are required to address ethical issues. The principles are set out in the Research Governance Framework for Health and Social Care (DH, 2005). Readers can tell that the framework has been applied because the research report will state that ethical approval has been obtained. The guidance for what studies require ethical approval has recently changed so this statement may not be included in older studies.

Researchers must take responsibility for the welfare of participants and ensure that everything is done to ensure that their welfare is considered throughout the study. It is highly likely that you have already been in contact with service users who are participants in a research study.

It is important that all healthcare practitioners have an understanding of the main principles of research ethics. Williamson (2007) explains this from a rights perspective. This is a very good starting point as it breaks down the different factors that need to be considered. The list seems lengthy, which indicates how complex it can be to ensure that people's rights are not infringed during the research process.

Right to be informed

All participants need to appreciate exactly what the study involves. For some groups of people

– for example children and the mentally ill – specific measures need to be taken to ensure that this happens. All studies are required to provide a written information sheet that can be understood by all those taking part.

Right to withdraw

Participants have the right to change their minds and to withdraw at any stage of the study. This needs to happen in such a way that their standard of care and their relationship with healthcare practitioners who may also be involved in the research are not adversely affected.

Right not to be harmed

There is always some potential for harm when treatment is given (and often when it is not, too), but this needs to be managed very carefully. For example asking people about difficult situations may cause considerable distress. The researcher needs to try to find the research design that provides the most sensitive approach in order to minimise this. Researchers also need to know when to withdraw participants for their own safety or even to stop the study, if for example it is very clear that an intervention is not working as was hoped.

Right to be researched

It is important that steps are taken to ensure that particular groups within the general population are not excluded from research studies. This can sometimes happen because of a lack of resources: for example if there are no translation facilities, this could lead to an under-representation of minority ethnic groups whose first language is not English. Allocation of funding can also mean that some groups of people (for example those with heart disease) are more likely to be involved in research than those with other conditions.

There is also a fine balance between protecting vulnerable people and allowing them to be involved in research studies with the appropriate support.

Right not to be over-researched

The government designates priority target areas for research, for example cancer services, and this can result in some people being frequently involved in studies. Consideration needs to be given to the fact that often the participants may be very frail. In these situations careful thought needs to be given to the research design so that they are not overtaxed.

Right to payment

Participants need to be made aware that they do not generally have a right to payment, although often travelling expenses are paid, and if the study involves long periods of input, sometimes participants are paid a small amount to compensate for the time that is taken.

Rights of ownership

The data from a study belongs to the researcher. However they have a responsibility only to use it as was agreed and not for example to keep it for other uses.

Right to confidentiality and anonymity

Participant details need to kept securely by the researcher. It is important that individual participants cannot be identified in published findings. Organisations that participate in research often choose not to have their exact details given for similar reasons. It is sufficient to provide an indication of their size and geographical location.

> ### a Learning activity
>
> Lisa is known to have asthma. Imagine that she has been asked to take part in a randomised controlled trial that is comparing different types of inhalers. Make a list of the concerns that Lisa might have with regard to taking part in the study.
>
> What steps do the researchers need to take to address these possible concerns?
>
> There are many factors that can make people vulnerable with regard to taking part in a research study. Groups such as the mentally ill, children, the elderly and people with learning disabilities are particularly vulnerable. How could their special needs and vulnerabilities be taken into account by the researchers?

Appraisal of research studies

The hierarchy of evidence is a useful tool in understanding the different levels and types of evidence, but it should not be used in isolation. Before you decide whether to apply the results of a research study to your practice, you need to look carefully at the information that is available on the study, and be able to make a decision about the quality and whether it is applicable to the particular practice situation. This is called *critical appraisal*. It is an area that most people find difficult and time-consuming at first. However it is a really important skill to master, as without this you cannot make an informed judgement about a research study. A step by step approach will help you gradually master the skill so that it is less daunting.

(C) Professional conversation

Anne, a ward manager, says, 'About a year ago I set up an interprofessional working group to look at developing a fasting policy. This has proved very challenging as not everyone was enthusiastic about changing their practice. The policy has now been agreed by all group members. I feel a real sense of achievement that patients will no longer be starved for unnecessarily long periods of time.'

(a) Learning activity

Lisa will have been fasted prior to her appendectomy. Using the guidance provided in this chapter, undertake a literature search. Select a small set of research studies on this subject. Read through the abstract, introduction, findings and conclusion of each study and make notes. Decide which you think is the most useful study for your practice and why.

The steps outlined in the learning activity are a good starting point for critical analysis. Reading through the abstract, introduction, findings and conclusion can give a guide to the suitability of a research study. This can save time in that you may well discount some articles at this stage, and will not need to read the body of the text. However this partial review cannot be used to make a complete decision on the value of the study. You now need to systematically go through the information provided on the research methods used. Unless you do this you might miss out on vital aspects of the study.

Critical appraisal basically involves answering a set of questions about the research study. It is not about undermining the researchers and trying to find fault, it is about being certain about the value and relevance of the study before using it to support your practice. Many different tools have been designed to help you do this. They are useful because they provide structure and help make sure that you cover everything in your appraisal. The main parts of a critical appraisal framework designed by Hek, Judd and Moule (2002: 131–3) are:

- the purpose of the research study
- research problem
- literature search
- sample selection
- data collection
- results and analysis of findings
- conclusions, recommendations and limitations
- dissemination
- general points.

There are several frameworks to choose from, so it is not necessary that you use this specific

one. They differ so it is a good idea to look up a few and select the one that you find the
easiest to use. An increasing number of them are available online, including:

W
● Public Health Resources Unit (PHRU) CASP appraisal
tools: www.phru.nhs.uk/Pages/PHD/CASP.htm (accessed
31 October 2008)

W
● Healthcare Practice Research and Development Unit,
University of Salford (2003_ Assessment tools: www.fhsc.
salford.ac.uk/hcprdu/critical-appraisal.htm (accessed
31 October 2008).

If you find the idea of critical appraisal daunting, doing the
activity in pairs or small groups often helps. You might also find
that there are journal clubs in your practice area or university.
A journal club meets at regular times, and members take turns
to present papers, leading a discussion on the information
that the journal provides. They are a really good way of gaining
knowledge with like-minded colleagues, and often welcome
students to observe at meetings.

> **ⓐ Learning activity**
>
> Read through the different appraisal
> tools and select the one that you
> feel the most comfortable with.
> Appraise a study that you looked
> at in the previous learning activity.
> Compare what you have found from
> undertaking the appraisal with what
> you found from just reading through
> it. In view of what you have now found
> out about the research methods, make
> a list of the additional points you have
> discovered about the study.

Audits

Audits are now commonly used in healthcare. Using them can be quite confusing, but it is a
necessary skill for you to acquire. Audits always measure current practice; they do not seek to
explore options in the way of a research study.

There are some fundamental differences between research and audit. Table 3.1 outlines the
main ones.

Table 3.1 Differences between research and audit

Research	Audit
Explores what is the right action	Explores whether the action meets the right standard
Often looks at new ideas and concepts	The ideas and concepts are already in place
A systematic investigation of a topic	A systematic review of current practice
May involve new interventions that have been untested	Never uses interventions that have been untested
May include health service users	May include health service users

Audit is a very important aspect of EBP. It is one of the key ways in which trusts monitor
the quality of healthcare interventions at a local level. Audits have been used for this purpose
for a long time but there are now Department of Health recommendations that stipulate that
clinical audit must be fully supported by all trusts, which must have a central audit office to
coordinate all activities. All healthcare professionals are required to partake in clinical audit
activities as part of their contract of employment (Watson, 2006).

> **ⓐ Learning activity**
>
> Find out how clinical audit is managed in your current
> placement. There will be information on the trust intranet
> system, or alternatively you could contact the clinical
> audit office to find out more. The results of local audits
> are often made widely available.
>
> Read through the scenario and jot down all the aspects
> of Lisa's healthcare experience which could be audited
> (there are several). Select one and imagine that you are
> involved in undertaking this audit. Think through how
> this could be done, and how you could ensure that all the
> relevant professionals are involved, and how healthcare
> service users like Lisa could contribute to the audit.

Part

I

Hierarchy of evidence

There is a wide range of evidence that can be used for practice, and deciding which is the best evidence can be difficult. A hierarchy of evidence is one tool that can be helpful. It is a framework that ranks evidence according to its strength. One ranking that is often used (Muir Gray, 1997) is:

1 Strong evidence from at least one systematic review of multiple, well-designed, randomised controlled trials.

2 Strong evidence from at least one properly designed randomised controlled trial of appropriate size.

3 Strong evidence from well-designed trials without randomisation, single group, cohort, time series or matched case-control studies.

4 Evidence from well-designed nonexperimental studies from more than one centre or research group.

5 Opinions of respected authorities based on clinical evidence, descriptive studies or reports of expert committees.

There are many different hierarchies, but they work on the same principle. They put evidence in an order with the most reliable evidence at the top. They do not differ in the order, so much as in the number of categories: the more rigorous types of evidence (for example, systematic reviews and randomised controlled trials) are always at the top of the hierarchy. The hierarchy of evidence is a really important framework, but it should not be used in isolation to decide which evidence is best to use. This is because healthcare is a very complex area. If you wish to provide care that is holistic and meets the needs of each individual, you need to give consideration to evidence on each tier of the framework. Reliance just on 'gold standard' evidence, for example systematic reviews, can mean that a great deal of high-quality evidence is missed. In practical terms you might also find that research has not been undertaken for some aspects of care, so it is necessary to use lower standards of evidence to back up your practice.

> **Learning activity**
>
> By undertaking all the different activities you will have amassed a great deal of different types and levels of evidence. Match them against the hierarchy of evidence (Muir Gray, 1997). This demonstrates the wide range of evidence that is required in order to make sure that all aspects are covered.

Integrated care pathways (ICP)

Integrated care pathways are multidisciplinary outlines of care which provide guidance on what care and treatment people should receive during their journey of care. They help prevent inconsistencies in care, and are often used as a tool to incorporate both local and national guidelines (Middleton, Barnett and Reeves, 2001). There is national guidance on ICPs. The most comprehensive is the ICP database at the National Electronic Database for Health (NELHS).

In order to be effective, ICPs need to be specifically designed for local needs. In line with all local policies they must be supported by appropriate evidence that justifies the specified interventions. The use of the most up to date and reliable evidence is central to an effective ICP. They also need to be written in a way that is clear to all involved professionals. In view of how quickly healthcare practice changes, as with guidelines and policies they need to be updated regularly.

> **Learning activity**
>
> Go to www.library.nhs.uk and locate the ICP database. Select an ICP that covers one or more elements from the scenario (for example asthma, or care of the patient undergoing surgery). Examine the supporting references. Are they up to date? Do the references represent all the tiers of the hierarchy of evidence? How easy is the ICP to follow? Could it be understood easily by a service user?

Benchmarking

Benchmarking is a process in which best practice is identified and a continuum designed so that the standard of practice can be measured. Benchmarking can be at either a local or national level. This is based on the principles of audit. The most widely known benchmarks are those termed *Essence of Care* (DH, 2001a). These national benchmarks were designed to cover basic needs. They have since been further developed to cover other areas such as health promotion, but were originally designed because there was concern that basic needs were not always met to a high standard. They are commonly adapted for local use.

> **ⓐ Learning activity**
>
> Locate the most recent Essence of Care document. There may be a copy in your clinical area or it can be accessed from the Department of Health website.
> - What are the key aims of Essence of Care?
> - How do the benchmarks relate to Lisa's care?
> - Find out how essence of care is being implemented in your current placement.

Conclusion

This chapter has identified and explained the key aspects of evidence-based practice. It has used Lisa's healthcare experience to illustrate this. The aim of doing this was to ensure that EBP is seen as an integrated part of healthcare provision, and one that should be developed alongside clinical skills. If you do this you will become a skilled healthcare practitioner whose practice is of the highest quality, utilising the most relevant and up to date evidence in a way that meets the needs of the individual.

The majority of the activities in the chapter can be adapted to other clinical situations. This will help you to continue to enhance the knowledge and skills that you have gained from reading this chapter. The accompanying website contains further information to assist you.

References

Atkinson, T. and Claxton, G. (2000) *The Intuitive Practitioner*, Buckingham, Open University Press.

Beechcroft, C., Rees, A. and Booth, A. (2006) 'Finding the evidence', in Gerrish, K. and Lacey, A. (eds), *The Research Process in Nursing*, 5th edn, Oxford, Blackwell.

Burns, N. and Grove, S. (2003) *Understanding Nursing Research*, 3rd edn, Philadelphia, Pa., Saunders.

Coad, J., Devitt, P. and Hardicre, J. (2006) 'How to search for and use grey literature in research', *Nursing Times* **50**(102), 35–6.

Chambers, R., Boath, E. and Rogers, D. (2007) *Clinical Effectiveness and Clinical Governance Made Easy*, 4th edn, Oxford, Radcliffe.

Craig, J. V. and Smyth, R. L. (2007) *The Evidence-Based Practice Manual for Nurses*, 2nd edn, Edinburgh, Churchill Livingstone Elsevier.

Cranston, M. (2002) 'Clinical effectiveness and evidence based practice', *Nursing Standard* **16**(24), 39–42.

Department of Health (DH) (1991) *Research for Health: A research and development strategy for the NHS*, London, Research and Development Division, DH.

DH (1997) *The New NHS: Modern, dependable*, London, DH.

DH (2001a) *The Essence of Care: Patient focused benchmarks for healthcare practitioners*, London, DH.

DH (2001b) *The Expert Patient: A new approach to chronic disease management for the 21st century*, London, DH.

DH (2004) *The NHS Improvement Plan: Putting people at the heart of public service*, London, DH.

DH (2005) *Research Governance Framework for Health and Social Care*, London, DH.

DH (2006) *Essence of Care: Benchmarks for promoting health*, London, DH.

Department of Health and Social Security (DHSS) (1972) *Report on the Committee on Nursing* (Cmnd 5115, Briggs Report), London, HMSO.

Edwards, S. (2002) 'Nursing knowledge: defining new boundaries', *Nursing Standard* **17**(2), 40–4.

Gerrish, K. and Lacey, A. (2006) *The Research Process in Nursing*, 5th edn, Oxford, Blackwell.

Greenhalgh, T. (2006) 'How to read a paper', in *The Basics of Evidence Based Medicine*, Oxford, Blackwell.

Hamer, S. and Collinson, G. (2005) *Achieving Evidence Based Practice: A handbook for practitioners*, 2nd edn, Edinburgh, Bailliere Tindall.

Hek, G. (2002) *Making Sense of Research: An introduction for health and social care practitioners*, 2nd edn, London, Sage.

Hek, G., Judd, M. and Moule, P. (2002) *Making Sense of Research. An introduction for health and social care practitioners*, 2nd edn, London, Sage.

Jewell, D. (1995) 'Approaching the literature', pp. 6–18 in Jones, R. and Kinmouth, A. (eds), *Critical Reading for Primary Care*, Oxford, Oxford University Press.

Kania-Lachance, D., Best, P., McDonah, M. and Ghost, A. (2006)

'Evidence-based practice and the nurse practitioner', *Nurse Practitioner* **31**(10), 46–54.

Lindsay, B. (2007) *Understanding Research and Evidence Based Practice*, Exeter, Reflect Press.

Long, T. and Johnson, M. (2007) *Research Ethics in the Real World: Issues and solutions for health and social care*, Edinburgh, Churchill Livingstone Elsevier.

Macnee, C. and McCabe, S. (2006) *Understanding Nursing Research. Reading and Using Research in Evidence Based Practice*, 2nd edn, Philadelphia, Pa., Wolters Kluwer/Lippincott Williams & Wilkins.

Mallick, M., Hall, C. and Howard, D. (2004) *Nursing Knowledge and Practice: Foundations for decision making*, 2nd edn, Edinburgh, Bailliere Tindall.

Middleton, S., Barnett, J. and Reeves, D. (2001) *What is an Integrated Care Pathway?* New Market: Hayward Group Publications.

Muir Gray, J. (1997) *Evidence Based Healthcare: How to make health policy and management decisions*, Edinburgh, Churchill Livingstone.

Newell, R. and Burnard, P. (2006) *Research for Evidence-Based Practice*, Oxford, Blackwell.

NHS Executive (1996) *Promoting Clinical Effectiveness: A framework for action in and through the NHS*, Leeds, NHS.

Nursing and Midwifery Council (NMC) (2004) *The NMC code of Professional Conduct: Standards for conduct, performance and ethics*, London, NMC.

Parahoo, K. (2006) *Nursing Research: Principles, process and issues*, 2nd edn, Basingstoke, Palgrave Macmillan.

Pearson, A,. Field, J. and Jordan, Z. (2007) *Evidence-Based Clinical Practice in Nursing and Healthcare*, Oxford, Blackwell.

Polit, D. and Beck, C. (2007) *Nursing Research: Generating and assessing evidence for nursing practice*, 8th edn, Philadelphia, Pa., Wolters Kluwer/Lippincott Williams & Wilkins.

Royal College of Nursing (RCN) (2003) 'Promoting excellence in care through research and development: an RCN position statement', London, RCN.

RCN (2005) 'Perioperative fasting in adults and children: an RCN guidance for the multidisciplinary team', London, RCN.

RCN (2007) 'Research ethics: RCN guidance for nurses', London, RCN.

Rycroft-Malone, J., Seers, K., Titchen, A., Harvey, G., Kitson, A. and McCormack, B. (2004) 'What counts as evidence in evidence based practice?' *Journal of Advanced Nursing* **47**(1), 81–90.

Sackett, D., Rosenberg, W. and Gray, J. (1996) 'Evidence based medicine, what it is and what it isn't', *British Medical Journal* 312, 71–2.

Sackett, D., Richardson, W., Rosenburg, W. and Haynes, R. (1997) *Evidence Based Medicine*, Edinburgh, Churchill Livingstone.

Upton, D. (1999) 'Attitudes towards and knowledge of clinical effectiveness in nurses, midwives, practice nurses and health visitors', *Journal of Advanced Nursing* **29**(4), 885–93.

Watson, J. (2006) 'Ensuring quality and the role of clinical audit', in Glasper, A. and Richardson, J. A. (eds), *Textbook of Children's and Young People's Nursing*, Edinburgh, Churchill Livingstone Elsevier.

Webb, C. and Roe, B. (2007) *Reviewing Research Evidence for Nursing Practice: Systematic reviews*, Oxford, Blackwell.

Williamson, T. (2007) 'The theoretical and social context of research ethics', in Long, T. and Johnson, M. (eds), *Research Ethics in the Real World: Issues and solutions for health and social care*, Edinburgh, Churchill Livingstone Elsevier.

Chapter

4

Ethical, legal and professional issues

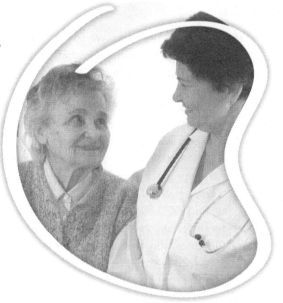

Lynda Rogers

Links to other chapters in *Foundation Studies for Caring*

2 Interprofessional learning
3 Evidence-based practice and research
6 Culture
8 Healthcare governance

Links to other chapters in *Foundation Skills for Caring*

1 Fundamental concepts for skills
2 IT skills
28 Routes of medication administration

W Don't forget to visit www.palgrave.com/glasper for additional
online resources relating to this chapter.

Introduction

Healthcare practitioners have to practise within a legal framework that is influenced and guided by the healthcare professions and their various codes of conduct and practice, such as the International Code of Medical Ethics (2003), and for nursing and midwifery *The Code: Standards of conduct, performance and ethics for nurses and midwives* (NMC, 2008). (The revised NMC *Code* became effective from 1 May 2008. Online copies can be obtained by accessing www.nmc-uk.org and following links to *The Code*.) These codes provide a framework that helps guide the practitioner in their decision-making processes with regard to the standards of care that are expected by each profession's governing body. The way in which we translate our practice and care will be influenced by our personal or moral code, which will have developed and been influenced by our cultural and social background.

W

Kitson (2007) highlights the importance of understanding that the interventions health carers undertake can be fraught with challenges to everyday practice. Dimond (2005) is careful to explain that although professional bodies such as the Nursing and Midwifery Council (NMC) consider that students are only 'responsible' for their actions (while after registration they become professionally accountable for them), the law regards all adults as having accountability for their actions and that ignorance of the law is no defence.

To help you understand some of the important areas of legal and professional practice, this chapter explores four important topics from a student or nonqualified healthcare practitioner's perspective:

- accountability of practice
- consent and capacity
- record keeping
- confidentiality.

The purpose is to help you gain knowledge and understanding of the issues related to these aspects of care.

Learning outcomes

The chapter will enable you to:

- understand the importance of legal and professional issues related to your practice
- understand the importance of working within a legal and professional framework, and the relationship between the ethics, the law and professional practice
- recognise how the law and the expectations of professional healthcare bodies influence healthcare practice
- appreciate the importance of patient/client/service-user-centred care
- reflect on your own developing healthcare practice with regard to legal and professional issues.

Concepts

- Professional practice
- Legal framework
- Professional accountability
- Consent
- Confidentiality
- Legal capacity
- Ethical principles and standpoints

Ethical principles and the relationship between the law and professional practice

> ## (a) Learning activity
>
> In your learning group examine the four core topics discussed in this chapter. Write down in your own words what each topic heading mean to you.
>
> Compare your ideas with each topic section in this chapter. You may be surprised and pleased to realise how much you already know and understand about these important aspects of care.

Dimond (2005) states that no one is above the law when they undertake healthcare practice. However we need to understand how the law and professional healthcare practice work, using an ethical framework to help and enhance our decision-making processes and developing knowledge of care.

Seedhouse (1998) in a seminal text argues that 'ethics is the heart of healthcare', and that practitioners need to understand ethical theories, principles and standpoints so as to practise with knowledge and understanding of the ethical issues that can arise in contemporary healthcare practice.

Hawley (2007) defines ethics as the study of people's moral behaviour. Their morals define a person's understanding and actions related to 'right' and 'wrong'.

It is suggested that a person's moral development arises from and is influenced by their social, economic and religious background (Hawley, 2007; Beauchamp and Childress, 2004). Ethics can be seen as the value and actions of a number of individuals working together to reflect a set of rules and regulations that encompass good, and reject, or not knowingly undertake, bad acts. This is referred to within ethics as *beneficence* (to do good where possible) and *nonmaleficence* (to not deliberately or knowingly do or intend harm) (Beauchamp and Childress, 2004).

Utilitarianism

Utilitarianism was first developed by two philosophers, Jeremy Bentham (1748–1832) and John Stuart Mill (1806–1873). This theory is sometimes referred to as 'consequentialist' in that an action is said to be right or wrong, good or bad according the outcome of the actions (the consequence of the action) (Tschudin, 2006). Bentham developed the 'principle of utility', which argues that all acts (actions) should be to promote 'the greatest happiness for the greatest number of people'. It may seem a good idea to try to provide as much (or the greatest) happiness for as many people as possible within healthcare, but in reality this might not be achievable. However utilitarianism can help healthcare practitioners to make choices between interventions by considering the 'best option' that would lead to the best outcome for as many people as possible.

For example, when helping a patient/client/service user (in this chapter, referred to as a client) decide where to go once they leave acute healthcare, the healthcare practitioner should consider the needs and wishes not only of the client, but also of the family or others who could be involved in the person's care. Are the family able to care for and support the person within their own home? Is there someone available when required, or would this move create 'happiness' for the patient but distress for the family because of family commitments and constraints?

Deontology

Deontology comes from two Greek words, *deon*, meaning duty, and *logos*, meaning dialogue or discourse. Immanuel Kant (1724–1804) first developed 'duty-bound' or deontological ethics. Kant believed that morality came from 'positive reason'; the highest moral reason was to 'do good'. He believed that the moral reason to 'do good' was so important that he called it the *categorical imperative*, or universal law (Seedhouse, 1998; Beauchamp and Childress, 2004; Tschudin, 2006).

Deontologists argue that the good of an outcome must be for all, and not only for some people. For example, if one person has a right to be cared for in their own home, them then it must be right and good for all people to have access to care in their own home. In contemporary healthcare there are number of reasons that this might not be possible. The healthcare trust might not have the money or resources to provide adequate or appropriate care for some people in their homes, but could support them in a specialised home or care unit. It could be questioned whether it is 'good' if some have certain access to home care and others don't. However if the intention is to 'do good' and provide good healthcare within the resources available, then the categorical imperative of doing good for all is maintained.

Virtue ethics

Virtue ethics is associated with Aristotle (384–322 BC), and became an important focus of moral reasoning during the eighteenth-century Enlightenment. It focuses on the character of the moral agent (Beauchamp and Childress, 2004). Crisp and Slote (1997) suggest that in order to act morally you must be a virtuous person and have, or strive for, a key set of characteristics such as temperance, courage, justice and prudence (Gillon, 2003). In order to follow this theory we need to make decisions according to conscience (or moral belief) and what we believe to be the right course of action. Therefore the outcome of whether a client stays in a specialist unit or is cared for at home could depend on the healthcare practitioner's, or group of healthcare practitioners', beliefs about what constitutes 'good' or 'best interest' for the client.

No one is above the law and ignorance is no defence. Healthcare practitioners must remain aware that although their practice is empowered through the law (Dimond, 2005; Jackson and Rogers, 2008), the law also has expectations that must be met. For example, no one should practise when their competency is not to an acceptable standard, and healthcare must be conducted within a framework that acknowledges legal, professional and ethical principles of good practice (Jackson and Rogers, 2006).

The NMC *The Code: Standards of conduct, performance and ethics for nurses and midwives* (2008) is an example of a set of rules that a group of professional health carers (in this case, nurses and midwives), are expected to adhere to within the course of their work. Hendrick (2004) argues that codes set standards which enable positive practice, whereas Dimond (2005) describes how the NMC code interprets the legal framework that the nursing profession is expected to work within.

Healthcare practitioners need to consider their practice and ensure that their actions are legal, professionally acceptable and ethically sound.

Accountability (responsibility) of practice

Accountability is defined as being responsible for something or someone, and being answerable for an action you take (*Collins Dictionary*, 2000). Thompson and colleagues (2006) argue that accountability and responsibility for your actions can only come from knowing and understanding your level of knowledge and skills competency to undertake and perform a task within an accepted framework of performance standards.

a Learning activity

a Learning activity

The first learning activity asked you *in your learning group* to write down your own meaning of accountability.

The definitions set out above may seem confusing and a little daunting to you, so you need to consider carefully in the context of care what accountability and responsibility mean to you, and the way you carry out your practice in healthcare environments.

Both Acts of Parliament such as the National Health Act 1948, and government policy and guidelines such as the white paper *The New NHS: Modern, dependable* (DH, 1997), require healthcare professionals to understand that they have a duty of care. This duty is based on a legal ruling by Lord Aitkin in the case of Donoghue v Stevenson 1932 (cited in Dimond, 2005), that a practitioner should take reasonable care to ensure that none of their actions result in foreseeable harm. This means that you should only undertake activities that you feel competent and confident in performing.

Confidence and competence come from having appropriate and knowledge, understanding and practice in the activity you are being asked to undertake. It would be unreasonable to ask a 3-year-old child to make a cup of tea if they have never been shown how to do it. It could also be very dangerous to ask such a young child to work with boiling water, as they could harm themselves and others. However once the child grows up and is able to understand the potential danger of boiling water, and has been taught how to use a kettle and transfer the boiling water safely to a teapot, it is reasonable to ask the child to perform the task and for them to agree. The competency of tea making will improve with experience and learning, and understanding the ways in which people prefer to take their tea, such as with milk and sugar or black with a slice of lemon.

This example might seem laboured, but put it into the context of performing a task for a healthcare client, and you can begin to understand the importance of knowledge, understanding and skills competency. When you are confident that you are competent to perform a task within an expected competency framework (see *The Essence of Care: Patient focused benchmarking for health practitioners*: DH, 2001a), you agree to undertake tasks and skills that are asked of you. Within a healthcare setting, you will do so knowing that you are responsible and legally accountable for your activities or actions. Examples are helping a client to have a bath, or assisting them to eat when they cannot hold a knife, fork or spoon themselves.

The NMC *The Code* (2008) states that a qualified nurse, midwife or specialist community public health practitioner is accountable for their actions, and that they have a duty of care to their clients who are entitled to receive safe and competent care.

Whether you are a student nurse, associate practitioner or a healthcare assistant, you should always consider whether you feel comfortable and confident to undertake the task that you are being asked to do. For example, have you been shown how to help a person to eat their food (nutrition needs)? Do you understand about hand hygiene, and know why you need to wash your hands before and after you have had contact with a client so as to reduce the risk of infection? Have you watched others perform a particular task you are being asked to carry out? Have people who are deemed competent watched you undertake the task and told you that what you are doing is safe, and that you have done it in a way that is acceptable both legally and professionally? You should ask yourself these types of question to ensure that you are practising in an insightful, competent and accountable manner.

a Learning activity

With regard to helping a person to eat, ask yourself:

- Do I know what to do if a person starts to choke?
- Do I know how to get help?
- Do I understand the person's religious and cultural dietary requirements?
- Do I feel comfortable assisting the client to eat so that they do not feel frightened or uncomfortable?

If you answer yes to these questions, you are demonstrating that you are responsible for your actions and are developing appropriate accountability of practice.

Learning activity

Think of a task you perform in your own area of practice. Using the example of the questions about eating, create your own checklist to assess your level of skills and competency.

Having reflected on your level of competency and skills acquisition, you need to consider a framework for learning, and checking your level of ability and development. Figure 4.1 is a learning cycle (adapted from Kolb's experiencing learning model) which could assist you to enhance your knowledge and skills with regard to various tasks. By being able to demonstrate your level of competency you are also showing a good level of responsibility and accountability of practice within a healthcare setting, as is expected of healthcare practitioners.

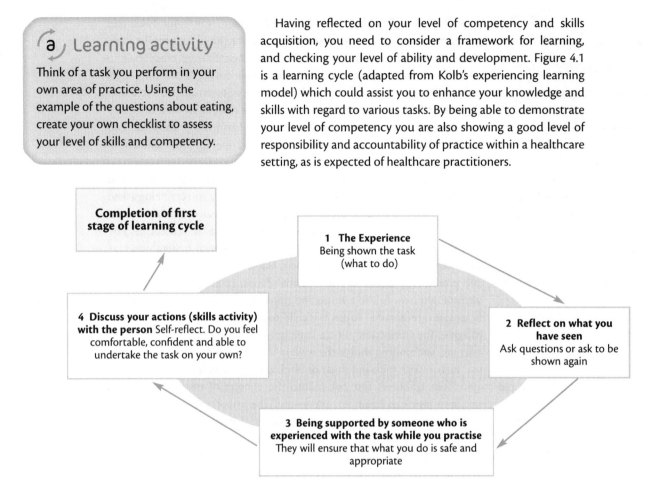

Completion of first stage of learning cycle

1   The Experience
Being shown the task (what to do)

4   Discuss your actions (skills activity) with the person Self-reflect. Do you feel comfortable, confident and able to undertake the task on your own?

2   Reflect on what you have seen
Ask questions or ask to be shown again

3   Being supported by someone who is experienced with the task while you practise
They will ensure that what you do is safe and appropriate

Figure 4.1 A learning cycle   Source: adapted from Kolb (1984).

Learning activity

In your learning group:

- Look again at what you wrote regarding the topic of accountability.
- Having read the part of this chapter related to accountability, do you feel that you have a better understanding of the meaning and actions related to responsibility and accountability of practice?
- Discuss the topic of accountability in your learning group.
- Find out how other people define accountability, and what they do to ensure that their actions are safe.

Some of the references at the end of this chapter will help you develop your ideas.

Consent

Whitney, McGuire and McCullough (2004) state that consent is a legal process used to promote patient autonomy. Dimond (2005) highlights the importance of gaining consent, and argues that if consent is not gained for a procedure, practitioners risk a claim of unlawful touching, which could result in a legal case being brought against them for trespass.

Consent is defined as the giving of permission (*Collins Dictionary*, 2000). *The Patients Charter* (DH, 1991) states that informed consent is the fundamental right of a client, and that they should be given clear information to help them understand the options or choices they have before they give their consent to a procedure or treatment.

As practitioners working in healthcare we need to understand the different types of consent, how consent can be given, what is meant by valid consent and when consent should be sought. We also need to possess an understanding of an individual's capacity to give consent.

The NMC argues that consent should always be informed. This means that the person giving the consent should understand what they are giving consent for and why they need to give that consent. Dimond (2005) argues that consent must be given voluntarily and without duress. The Department of Health, in its *Guidelines to Consent* (2001b), also stresses the importance of consent to healthcare practitioners.

There are three types of consent:

- **Verbal** (word of mouth). For example, a student tells a client that that they would like to take their temperature, and the client says, 'Yes, OK then.'
- **Written:** signing a set of statements, or a written agreement such as a consent form for surgical treatment. For example, a client has been offered therapeutic counselling. The practitioner clarifies what the sessions will entail, and that the client will attend the day centre at a given time for one hour each session, and is consenting to participate in the therapeutic sessions. The client is then asked to sign an appropriate form.
- **Implied:** this is a nonverbal form of consent. It can be argued that the actions of a person demonstrate a willingness to allow the activity to go ahead. For example, a healthcare assistant offers to help a client take a bath, and wash their hair. The person does not refuse, goes of their own free will to the bathroom, and allows the healthcare staff to assist.

a Learning activity

Think what information you would need to give in order to ensure that a client consents to let you help with their bath.

How would you know that the client had understood the information and explanation you provided? How would you explain the alternatives to having a bath (such as a shower, a bed bath, or simply staying dirty)?

Beauchamp and Childress (2004) argue that professionals should ensure that consent has been expressed by word or deed. They should also ensure that the consent is valid, and has been given without coercion or threat. They should ensure too that sufficient information is given about benefits and risks of the treatment, and that the client has had alternatives outlined and explained. It is important that the client can demonstrate an understanding of the treatment options and retain that information. Without clarity of knowledge and understanding, consent could be seen to be invalid.

Capacity to consent

The law and healthcare ruling bodies, such as the NMC and the Medical Council (MC), are clear that healthcare practitioners should always presume that a person has the capacity to consent. However, they also need to take appropriate steps to find out whether a person has any restrictions to their right to consent.

This is the case when the person falls under a section of the Mental Health Act 1983. (For further information regarding this Act, search for 'mental health act' at www.dh.gov.uk: a variety of leaflets are available.)

The Mental Capacity Act 2005 also deals with issues related to consent, and you should be aware of the relevant provisions.

Mental Capacity Act 2005

This Act outlines five key principles:

- A presumption of capacity: each person has the right to make their own decisions unless it is proven otherwise.
- An individual is supported to make their own decisions: this means giving practical help to ensure this is achieved.

- Unwise decisions do not mean that a person does not have the capacity to consent. You cannot overrule an individual simply because you disagree with their choice.
- Best interest: all actions must be taken with the best interests of the individual in mind at all times.
- Least restrictive option: things that are done for or on behalf of the person must be those that are least restrictive of their basic rights and freedoms.

There are three Parts to the Act:

- Part I defines how to ascertain mental capacity and incapacity, and best interest.
- Part II defines and clarifies the terms introduced: the Court of Protection, public guardianship, and Court of Protection visitors.
- Part III ensures that the Act conforms with the European Convention on Human Rights: in other words, that it is based on the principles of protection of private life, and protection of health and well-being.

The British Medical Association (BMA) *Guidance for Health Professionals* (2007) deals with the Act and clarifies some of its provisions. It states that it is a positive Act which enables healthcare practitioners to understand the boundaries of their right to act, what constitutes consent and where consent is not required for healthcare interventions. It also makes clear who can obtain consent, and where to go for support and help.

Capacity is defined in the Mental Capacity Act 2005 as 'the everyday ability to make decisions or take actions that influence their life'. This applies to both large and small decisions: anything from deciding what to eat for breakfast, to deciding whether to accept medical treatment or nursing intervention. It includes decisions that have an impact on others, such as financial or social decisions.

Incapacity is defined in the Act as 'a person being unable to make or communicate their decision because of an impairment or disturbance in the function of their mind or brain at the time a decision has to be made'. The question to be considered is whether the disturbance or impairment is sufficient that the person lacks capacity to make a particular decision. (The core test of this is whether the person can demonstrate knowledge and understanding related to an issue or question.)

So that healthcare staff can demonstrate that they have taken into account a person's capacity to consent, they need to use an assessment process that explains and justifies their decisions. The Act sets out a number of suggestions to help with this. For instance, in looking to decide whether the person lacks the mental capacity to make a decision, you would need to ask whether they fall into any or all of these categories:

- The person fails to demonstrate relevant understanding of the information given to them.
- The person cannot demonstrate retention of the information relevant to the decision.
- The person cannot demonstrate that they can 'weigh' (or question or consider) the pros and cons of information given to them.
- The person cannot communicate their decision by any means.

If this is the case, then it is seen as in the best interest of the person for a decision to be made for them. This is known as a *duty of care*.

A healthcare practitioner who makes a decision on behalf of a client in these circumstances is protected from what might otherwise be considered as criminal or civil liability by Clause Five of the Act. This clause refers to both lay and professional carers.

Children and consent

It is important to note that the Mental Capacity Act 2005 only relates to people over the age of 18 years. Subsequent legislation is being considered that would extend similar provisions to the care of children, but at the time of writing issues of a child's consent are governed by the requirements set out in the Children Act of 1989 and 2004. Other documents important to your practice are the *National Service Framework (NSF) for Children, Young People and Maternity Services* (DH, 2004), and guidelines set out in Gillick Competency, now known as Fraser Guidelines. Fraser Guidelines are the practice recommendations for identifying whether children (under 18 years old) have 'capacity to consent'. The recommendations are based on the common law case of Gillick which investigated the provision of contraception for under-16s. For a full explanation of Gillick Competency please read Dimond (2005, ch. 13); see also Chapter 1 of *Foundation Skills for Caring*.

Refusal or withholding of consent

It is important to note that unless a person is constrained by a section of the Mental Health Act, or it has been demonstrated that they lack the ability to consent for themselves within the framework of the Mental Capacity Act 2005, they have the right to withhold or refuse consent, and this includes withdrawing a consent that has previously been given. Unless a court of law gives power to healthcare professionals to carry out treatment, to attempt an intervention against a person's expressed wishes could be seen as unlawful assault and battery.

Considerations of good practice with regard to consent

Healthcare practitioners are consistently in the front line of contact with clients. Whitney and colleagues (2004) suggest that enhancing patient choice is a central theme of medical ethics and the law. Informed consent is a legal process that helps promote autonomy and respect for the person. To ensure good practice we must adapt strategies to ensure that client-centred care is promoted and demonstrated.

In this context, healthcare professionals should:

- ensure that they consider the person's capacity regardless of their age and apparent mental and or physical disability
- maximise opportunities for autonomous consent, such as giving adequate time for the client to think about an issue and express a view in their own way
- use different and innovative ways of communication (for example, sign language, or perhaps using electronic communication equipment) or forms of play to help both adults and children to present their views and choices in a safe, simple and familiar way.

Confidentiality

The contributors to Tschudin (2006) argue that confidentiality is one of the most important rules of healthcare ethics, and that healthcare practitioners need to understand that confidentiality of information demonstrates respect for the individual. Beauchamp and Childress (2001) concur with Tschudin's view, and agree that confidentiality is one of the four moral rules. An infringement of confidentiality is a breach of trust.

Clause five of the NMC *The Code* (2008) states that registered nurses, midwives and health visitors are personally accountable for their practice, and must protect all confidential information concerning clients. However the *Code* goes on to state that where required either by a court of law or in the wider public interest, disclosure is justified. The gulf between these two statements often proves difficult, not only in theory but in practice, when it leads to conflicts and dilemmas in care settings.

In the healthcare sector there is a clear expectation of maintaining confidentiality. In English common law there is no general right of privacy, but the Human Rights Act (1998), article 8, outlines the right to privacy and family life.

> **a Learning activity**
>
> In your learning group, consider how you would define a 'dilemma'.
>
> Think about your own beliefs regarding the issue of keeping confidences, and why and in what situations you may need to breach confidentiality.

Therefore, we need to clarify in a simple way how confidentiality can be maintained in practice, and recognise when and why it might need to be broken.

In general healthcare practitioners should ensure that all information provided by a client is recorded in a way that ensures it is not available to anyone who is not part of the person's healthcare team.

One relatively common circumstance in which it is necessary to disclose confidential information is when it is required by a court of law. For example, in a claim of negligence the court might require the disclosure of medical notes. In these cases, however, the information would be disclosed only to those who have a professional need for it, such as the claimant's and defendant's lawyers.

It is also sometimes necessary for public safety. For example, if you learn that someone has a notifiable disease (that is, a specific disease such as tuberculosis, for which healthcare professionals have a legal obligation to inform the authorities of occurrences), the duty to notify overrides the duty of confidentiality. This is because tuberculosis and the other notifiable diseases can be highly infectious, and all practicable steps need to be taken to prevent a wider outbreak.

In circumstances such as these where disclosure may be necessary, specific steps need to be followed. Among them is an obligation to inform the client at the earliest possible opportunity that the information must be shared, and with whom. This demonstrates good practice, accountability and consideration of best interest. It also shows how a duty of care is demonstrated in practice.

Thompson and colleagues (2006) point out that many clients are at first dismayed to realise how much sensitive and private information they need to give, and how many people in their healthcare team might have access to it. It may help to explain that this is necessary in order to ensure that the interventions chosen are appropriate to the person's needs. Thompson and colleagues (2006) also emphasise that the sharing of information is an issue of moral and ethical responsibility, and professional judgement.

Some specific legal requirement for disclose are noted below.

Road Traffic Act 1988

It is a requirement to inform the police in some circumstances when the Road Traffic Acts have been breached: for example, in cases of drink driving.

Prevention of Terrorism Act 1988

The police must be informed if a client is suspected of terrorism. As with other instances, there are specific procedures to be followed in these circumstances. A student nurse, for example, should not simply phone the police. The practitioner should share their information or suspicions with their senior manager, who in turn will discuss the situation with the trust or hospital manager, who makes the decision about disclosure.

Misuse of Drugs Act 1993

Informing senior managers of drug misuse is not a matter of personal judgement. Senior managers or other practitioners must always be informed, as confidentiality is overruled by a duty of care. If you do not tell other practitioners of a client's drug misuse, drugs might be prescribed that are affected by those taken previously.

Public Interest (Control of Disease Act 1988)

As mentioned above, it is the responsibility of a practitioner to ensure that information on incidences of notifiable diseases is passed to the local senior medical officer for health.

Abortion Act 1967

It is a legal requirement to ensure that all abortions, either illegal or illegal, are reported. When you report an illegal abortion, the correct authorities are notified and the woman who experiences the abortion can be cared for by those who are professionally qualified to do so. Abortions carry health risks, but if the woman receives medical attention, these can be minimised.

As healthcare practitioners we need to develop knowledge and understanding of the importance of maintaining appropriate confidentiality, but we also need to recognise that in some circumstances we must share the confidential information given to us. Your practice must not only be of a high quality, it must also be carried out within a legal framework. Understanding the issues and possible dilemmas related to confidentiality will enable you to demonstrate a high level of competent practice.

Record keeping

Melia (2000) argues that the patient-centred approach has emphasised the importance of record keeping within healthcare. Thompson, Melia and Boyd (2000) further state that accurate, meaningful record keeping can provide information that not only justifies an intervention, but also enables healthcare practices to be evaluated for the benefit of the client as well as the healthcare professional.

The NMC *Guidelines for Records and Record Keeping* (2004: 6) state that 'record keeping is an integral part of nursing, midwifery and specialist community public health practice .... It is a tool of professional practice and one which should help the care process.'

NHS governance frameworks such as *For the Record: Managing records in the NHS health trusts and health authorities* (1999) emphasise the need for accurate records. These guidelines suggest that greater involvement of client and their families and carers leads to a more client-centred approach.

Good record keeping can help promote best-quality practice, which underpins positive evidence-based practice. It also provides a safeguard for the professional, should things go wrong and an investigation need to be made. The information in properly kept records can demonstrate what was done, the rationale for interventions and their outcome. Poor record keeping can actually increase your and your colleagues' workload, since professionals who do not know what interventions have taken place previously or their outcomes will need to make lengthy further enquiries. Poor records could also leave a healthcare professional vulnerable to accusations of professional negligence or legal proceedings.

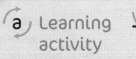

a **Learning**   W
activity

Read the NMC *Guidelines for Records and Record Keeping* (2004), online on www.nmc-uk.org.

c **Professional conversation**

Rishma, a first-year student nurse, is allocated to a medical ward. Chris is a band 5 senior staff nurse, and her mentor on this assignment.

Rishma says, 'When I came on duty this morning I noticed that the nursing record for my allocated patient had not been completed for the night before. I was not overly concerned, but when I was helping my patient get ready for his breakfast he told me about an incident that had happened in the night, when he had been given the wrong type of drug. Fortunately he said it was only another type of antibiotic. I was concerned about this, and after breakfast I approached Chris and discussed it with him.

'Chris explained to me the importance of documenting any incident, and told me he would discuss the issue with the night staff.

'After this event I read the copy of the NMC *Guidelines* that Chris gave me. I was pleased he had, as I now fully understand this important aspect of care practice.'

What constitutes client records?

Dimond (2005) is clear that anything that relates to a client within the context of their care can be seen as part of their healthcare records. This includes care plans (such as admission documents or care pathway documents), individual food or weight diaries, birth plans (related to maternity care), and temperature, pulse and blood pressure records (often referred to as TPR charts).

It is important that all documents are accurate and timely, written during or near the time of the interaction. These are sometimes referred to as contemporaneous records or notes. It is not always easy to keep track of record keeping, and it is harder if you leave it a while to remember exactly what was said and done on a specific occasion. However, forgetting to complete documents, or failing to put down a clear account of events, can have devastating consequences for the client and/or the professional.

[S] Scenario: Introducing Molly

Molly is an associate practitioner in an acute hospital assessment centre. One client who is admitted is assessed as needing help with her hygiene.

Molly is given this task, and asks the client if she would like her to help her take a wash, bath or shower.

The client says she doesn't need any help, she can manage if someone takes her to a bathroom, so this is what Molly does.

The next day Molly is told the client has complained that no one helped her with her hygiene needs: she was just left in a bathroom to cope on her own.

[a] Learning activity

Note two things Molly could have done to ensure it is known that she offered help and it was declined. Consider your answer before you read on.

[a] Learning activity

Think about the clients you have contact with. How do you cope with situations similar to those experienced by Molly?

What do you do differently, or what will you do differently in future?

In the scenario case, Molly should have recorded in the client care notes (which might be either electronic or paper documents) what help and support she has offered the client, what the client has accepted, and the outcome of the interaction.

As she is an associate nurse she might have needed someone to countersign her entry.

She should have also shared the fact that she had offered help and had it refused with the person who had given her the assignment. This more senior person could then have made a decision whether the refusal was appropriate, in the light of the client's assessment, or whether further action needed to be taken.

The scenario demonstrates how a simple situation can easily become more complex because of failures of communication and record keeping. Anyone can make a mistake, and missing a bath is not the end of the world, but if the issues relate to a more serious matter, such as a client refusing to take prescribed medication, or the sharing of important information related to the person's health and well-being, the consequences could be much more serious.

The Audit Commission made a series of recommendations related to record keeping. For more information visit http://www.audit-commission.gov.uk/. The main recommendations, given in Table 4.1, represent good practice for all healthcare professionals.

Table 4.1 Audit Commission recommendations on record keeping

Recommendations	Comments
Records should be actual, consistent and accurate	Write what you know or what you observed. For example, detail the exact temperature that was recorded, not that the patient's temperature was 'normal'.
Records should be written contemporaneously	Records should be written at the time, for example, during a period of clinical practice.
Records should be written clearly and in such a manner that the writing cannot be erased.	Handwritten notes should be in black pen. Computer-generated notes are usually designed so that once completed and saved they cannot be changed.
Alterations or additions should be dated, timed and signed.	It is common practice that changes to written notes are scored through in red or black pen so that what is crossed out can be seen, and the alteration signed. You will need to ask what the local policy is for changes to computer-generated records.
Records should be signed and dated by an accepted/recognised signatory.	Most NHS trusts, social services and independent sector organisations keep records of all staff signatures (including bank staff) for comparison so as to confirm authenticity.
Nonaccepted abbreviations, jargon, meaningless phrases, irrelevant speculation and offensive subjective statements should not be included in either written or computer-generated documents.	Abbreviations can have more than one meaning, for example DOA might mean 'dead on arrival' or 'direct occipital anterior'. Irrelevant phrases and speculation: an example is 'Had a good day.' ... compared with what? Offensive, subjective statements: an example is 'Remained continent all day, what a change.' (This comment could be seen as unprofessional at the very least.)

From a legal and healthcare professional perspective, healthcare records should:

- give a clear and full account of any assessment, planned care and the outcome of the care given
- give clear and objective information, including any action taken in the light of observations or changes
- demonstrate a healthcare professional's duty of care.

The law tends to adopt the approach that if an assessment, interaction or intervention is not recorded, it is considered not to have taken place.

The Access to Health Records Act 1990 is clear that only health professionals or qualified practitioners allied to medicine and healthcare are eligible to sign documents. Therefore others (such as students, unqualified or nonprofessional members of a healthcare team) should have their input into records and documents countersigned by a suitable professional. This ensures that the documents are legal, and protects both students and practitioners.

Record keeping as a very important part of healthcare interventions, and the NMC succinctly addresses this point by stating that good record keeping helps protect the welfare of clients by promoting high standards of clinical care and continuity of care. It improves communication and dissemination of information to benefit both service users and those providing the care.

Conclusion

This chapter has considered ethical principles and the relationship between law and professional practice. It has reviewed four areas of practice from a legal and professional perspective so that students and unqualified members of healthcare teams can consider their actions and activities in relation to accountability, consent and capacity to consent, confidentiality and record keeping. By examining these areas and reflecting on the activities set out in this chapter, you will be able to develop and enhance your practice, knowledge and skills, and move towards becoming a knowledgeable, competent practitioner.

References

Beauchamp, T. L. and Childress, J. F. (2004) *Principles and Practice of Medical Ethics*, Oxford, Oxford University Press.

British Medical Association (BMA) (2007) Guidance for Health Professionals [online] http://www.bma.org.uk/health_promotion_ethics/consent_and_capacity/mencapact05.jsp (accessed 23 December 2008).

BMA and Law Society (2003) *Code of Medical Ethics*, London, BMJ books.

Collins Dictionary (2000) London, Harper Collins.

Crisp, R. and Slote, M. (1997) *Virtue Ethics*, Oxford, Oxford University Press.

Department of Health (1991) *The Patients Charter*, London, DH.

DH (1997) *The New NHS: Modern, dependable*, London, HMSO.

DH (2001a) *The Essence of Care: Patient focused benchmarks for health practitioners*, London, DH.

DH (2001b) *Guidelines to Consent for Examination or Treatment*, London, DH.

DH (2004) *National Service Framework for Children, Young People and Maternity Services*, London, DH.

Dimond, B. (2005) *Legal Aspects of Nursing*, Harlow, Pearson Education.

Gillick competence: RE L Medical Treatment: Gillick Competence (1999) Review 58.

Gillon, R. *Philosophical Medical Ethics*, Chichester, Wiley.

Hawley, G. (2007) *Ethics in Clinical Practice: An interprofessional approach*, Harlow, Pearson Education.

Hendrick, J. (2004) *Law and Ethics*, Foundations in Nursing and Healthcare Series, Cheltenham, Nelson Thornes.

DH (1999) *For the Record: Managing records in the NHS health trusts and health authorities*, London, DH.

International Code of Medical Ethics (2003) [online] http://www.wma.net/e/policy/c8.htm (accessed 23 December 2008).

Jackson, N. and Rogers, L. (2008) 'Ethically managed self, people and resources to improve the health and wellbeing of patients and clients in the community', ch. 16 in Coles, L. and Porter, E. (eds), *Public Health Skills: A practical guide for nurses and public health practitioners*, Oxford, Blackwell.

Kitson, A. (2007) cited in Brown, J. and Libberton, P. (eds), *Principles of Professional Studies in Nursing*, Basingstoke, Palgrave-Macmillan.

Kolb, A. (1984) *Experiential Learning: Experience as the source of learning and development*, Englewood Cliffs, N. J., Prentice-Hall.

Melia, K. M. (2000) in Thompson, I. E., Kelia, K. M. and Boyd, K. M. (eds), *Nursing Ethics*, 4th edn, Ediburgh, Churchill Livingstone.

Nursing and Midwifery Council (NMC) (2004) *Guidelines for Records and Record Keeping*, London, NMC.

NMC (2008) *The Code: Standards of conduct, performance and ethics for nurses and midwives*, London, NMC.

Seedhouse, D. (1998, 2nd edn 2001) *Ethics: The heart of health care*, Chichester, Wiley.

Thompson and colleagues (1999) reference to follow

Thompson, I. E., Melia, K. M., Boyd, K. M. and Horsburgh, D. (2006) *Nursing Ethics*, 5th edn, Edinburgh, Churchill Livingstone.

Tschudin, V. (ed.) (2006) *Essentials of Teaching and Learning in Nursing Ethics: Perspectives and methods*, Edinburgh, Churchill Livingstone.

Whitney, S. N., McGuire, A. L. and McCullough, L. B. (2004) 'A typology of shared decision making, informed consent and simple consent', *Annals of Internal Medicine* **140**(1), 54–9.

Legislation

Access to Health Records Act 1990

Children Act 1989

Human Rights Act 1998

Mental Health Act 1983

Mental Capacity Act 2005

Chapter

5

Communication

WITHDRAWN
FROM STOCK

Alan Glasper and
Jennie Quiddington

Links to other chapters in *Foundation Studies for Caring*

Links to other chapters in *Foundation Skills for Caring*

W Don't forget to visit www.palgrave.com/glasper for additional
online resources relating to this chapter.

Introduction

It is important that by the end of your foundation programme you have a good working knowledge of how to communicate with clients and each other within cultural contexts. Crucially healthcare students should see communication skills as part of the toolkit of essential life skills that you will need for future professional practice irrespective of your discipline. Additionally it is important to have a basic understanding of how to integrate the theory of communication with other subject areas, and to reflect on how this informs practice in the delivery of holistic care.

Learning outcomes

This chapter will enable you to:

- gain a basic understanding of concepts, definitions and categories associated with communication, considering how values, attitudes and beliefs influence communication processes
- develop an awareness of a range of communication frameworks and counselling models and how they might be utilised in healthcare practice
- reflect on practice and learn to critically analyse and identify personal strengths and limitations in communicating with other professionals and with clients
- identify role limitations and the nature of referral within a multidisciplinary team with clients in need of special-ised communication, recognising that different client groups will need differing strategies of communication

- appreciate those factors that enhance or detract from effective communication
- identify strategies of breaking significant news to clients in distress, and offer support where required
- understand the role of Heron's work and its application in practice
- recognise the pivotal role of nurses as client advocates especially for those who are too weak or because of developmental age are unable to 'speak' for themselves
- appreciate the use of the telephone as a medium of communication
- explore the use of written patient information leaflets, the internet and voice mail as methods of client communication.

Concepts

- Active listening
- Client-centred communication

- Nonverbal communication
- Email etiquette

- Information giving

The basics of communication

Successful communication requires:

- a sender: that is, the person initiating the exchange
- a message: the information that person wants to convey
- a medium: a way of passing the message from one person to another, such as an email or a face to face conversation
- a receiver: someone who receives the message from the sender.

Factors influencing communication

Developmental age/social interaction

A baby's only communication tool in the early part of life is the cry. The cry is used to signify hunger or discomfort, and is used effectively by all human infants to attract the care giver's attention. Bell and Salter-Ainsworth (1972) suggest that crying becomes a mode of communication in infants specifically directed at the mother, and as the mother learns to interpret the cry through early responses there is a decline by the baby in its use. During the second six months of life, as the infant develops it can begin to discriminate words spoken by the mother. Although normal speech development occurs in most infants, you need to be aware that an early period of hospitalisation or factors such as depression in the mother might mean that speech does not develop as quickly as it might otherwise have done.

Communication noise

This is the term for anything that interferes with communication channels. It does not just mean a 'buzz' on a telephone line: in our context it includes for example pain, discomfort, fear and fatigue, all of which make it more difficult to convey or receive a message. All healthcare professionals need to be aware of communication noise and how it might adversely impact on the communication episode with a client. Ask yourself how many times you have been distracted in a conversation because of discomfort, for example, and have missed an important message. Chant and colleagues (2002) lament the lack of communication skills teaching in a nurse education, and reinforce the need for better communication strategies between healthcare professionals and patients.

Nonverbal communication

This is a very important aspect of overall communication, and can aid or detract from effective communication. Chambers (2003) identifies a number of important factors that healthcare professionals need to take note of when using nonverbal communication techniques. Physical appearance, including issues such as what you wear, is particularly important in certain client specialities such as mental health. Clearly the way we look is important in professional/client relationships, and that is why uniform code is strictly adhered to by universities offering healthcare education. Most schools have policies on hair code, body piercing, tattoos and footwear. As well as for reasons of hygiene, these are often set down to ensure that people 'look the part', which helps in communicating with clients.

Facial expressions are another element of nonverbal communication, with the smile being probably the only international language shared by people everywhere. You will find that a smile is appreciated by all clients. There are other elements of nonverbal communication which professionals can use in their dealing with healthcare clients. Caris-Verhallen, Kerkstra and Bensing (1999) have identified a number of nonverbal behaviours in a study of how nurses communicate nonverbally with the elderly. In addition to smiling these included patient-directed eye gazing, positive head nodding, leaning forward when talking and emotional touch. They believe that these aspects of nonverbal behaviour are helpful in establishing a positive relationship with a patient. Physical proximity and posture are important, but can however be misconstrued: you need to balance a friendly attitude with respect.

Many practitioners use the SOLER stance, which is nonthreatening and helps with active listening.

Using the SOLER stance

The SOLER stance has been described by Egan (1990). This is an acronym for:
- **S**it squarely in relation to the client/patient.
- Maintain an **O**pen body posture.
- **L**ean slightly forward towards the client/patient.
- Use and maintain appropriate **E**ye contact.
- Try to look **R**elaxed.

Effective communication with patients is critical to effective nursing practice. Surprisingly, there is little information on nurses' experiences in caring for patients who are unable to speak.

> **a** Learning activity
>
> In your learning group and using role play, practise the SOLER stance and other communication strategies with each other.

Encoding and decoding

Encoding and *encryption* are the (synonymous) terms for the way in which a communication is embodied. They cover both verbal and nonverbal aspects: the words used (if any), and also expressions, gestures and the like.

In both verbal and nonverbal communication, two key factors are crucial to the overall effectiveness and efficiency of the exercise. The first is the accurate encryption of the message. All aspects of it need to be in sync, or there will be an *encryption error*, and the recipient will find it difficult or impossible to work out what is being conveyed.

Imagine for example that someone says 'Have a nice day' but does not smile and uses a tone of voice that comes across as uninterested or even slightly threatening. Not all elements of the message here convey the same meaning. The recipient might pick up on one of the possible meanings (for instance, that the tone means the words are not genuinely meant) and ignore or discount the other(s), or they might find it impossible to decipher the message at all. This type of encryption error, deliberate or not, can potentially ruin the whole point of communication with the healthcare client.

The second is the clarity of communication. Issues such as the use of regional dialects and/or the use of slang can impact on the success of the communication. It is important to speak clearly, and in a way that will be as understandable as possible to clients who might for example have hearing problems or not be native English speakers.

You should also be aware of the work of Miller (1987), who has described how clients/ parents may actively monitor health information messages/communications as a tangible way of confronting the threats of ill health, or conversely psychologically blunt the communication to avoid the impending threat of ill health. Both monitors and blunters bring their own problems for the healthcare professional who wants to successfully deliver a health message, with some clients wanting more than the professional can perhaps deliver, and some failing to or not wanting to 'hear' the message. Sadly clients do not have this information emblazoned across their chests, and you need to explore this potential foil to communication, and find out for yourself which people fall into which category.

The communication loop

The *communication loop* (see Figure 5.1) is a model of a simple two-way communication process. An encoded message (such as a verbal or written message) is sent via a *medium* (such as face to face conversation, a tape recording or a publication) to a *recipient* (in our context, typically a patient/client). The recipient decodes the message and gives *feedback* (verbal, nonverbal or both) to the sender.

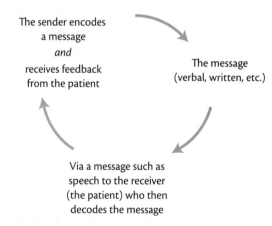

The sender encodes
a message
and
receives feedback
from the patient

The message
(verbal, written, etc.)

Via a message such as
speech to the receiver
(the patient) who then
decodes the message

Figure 5.1 The communication loop

This simple process is fraught with difficulties. The types of problem we have outlined briefly above mean that inaccuracies can creep in at every stage. They can be summarised by the statement:

I know you believe you understand what you think I have just said to you, but I am not sure you realise that what you heard is not actually what I meant.

Developing good communication skills

(C) Professional conversation

Michael, a first-year nursing student, is on placement with his mentor Gary. He comments,

'I have been on placement on an endocrine unit for three weeks and my mentor Gary and I had a very difficult meeting with a patient who quite rudely told me that I never spent sufficient time listening to what he had to say. The patient was very anxious about returning home, having recently been diagnosed with diabetes.

'After discussing this with my mentor I now understand that communication and understanding how to use different communication strategies in dealing with anxious clients is an essential skill for all healthcare professionals.'

Good communication depends on a number of interrelated factors. It is built on respect for the individual client or patient. Importantly all healthcare professionals need to recognise that there are no short cuts in communicating with those individuals receiving care.

Allow enough time

Temporal issues always impinge on healthcare professionals. We often feel we are short of time, and sometimes we unintentionally (or indeed intentionally) convey that feeling to our clients.

Pollock and Grime (2002), in a qualitative study, found that patients perceived that time constraints were a significant factor in their meetings with general practitioners. The patients believed that this anxiety about time prevented them from fully discussing their problems with the doctor. Although this research did not cover other healthcare professionals, much the same is true of them. All healthcare professionals should endeavour to bear in mind that patients perceive time entitlement to be problematic. Of course they are not always wrong, but when you have important information to give to someone and/or obtain from them, it is essential to allow the time needed to do so. At the start of your conversation, it is helpful to consciously convey to the other person that you have as much time as is needed.

Ask open-ended questions

Particularly at the initial stage of a dialogue with patients, it is helpful to use open-ended questions: that is, questions such as 'Can you describe the pain?' which invite a detailed answer, instead of closed questions such as 'Are you in pain?' which invite a short yes/no answer. This helps you to identify precisely what the patient's concerns are, which makes it easier to select an appropriate intervention.

Develop client-centred styles of communication

'Client-centred' or 'person-centred' styles can be contrasted with 'position centred' styles: in the former, you are focused on the person you are talking to, while in the latter, there is an emphasis on your own role in the relationship (that is, as the professional talking to a lay person). Much modern research has emphasised the advantages of developing a client-centred style. Instead of talking *at* the other person, you need to talk *with* them, obtaining information as well as conveying it.

What does this mean in practice? Munson and Wilcox (2007) describe the Calgary-Cambridge model of communication, which details the stages necessary for an optimum patient/client communication encounter. They include preparing the environment, forming a relationship with the client and clarifying the reason for the conversation.

The core of the conversation is of course the exchange of information, and you will often want to gain objective physiological or anatomical information: to find out how they feel, or to take their temperature, for example. But you also need to set this information in context, exploring with the client their problems as they appear from their perspective.

Build a relationship by developing a rapport and by involving the client

Structure the encounter by sharing with the client summaries of what has been discussed or elicited. You can provide signposts: directing the client to other sources of information such as kitemarked internet sites, which will give them more information to back up and expand on what you are able to tell them. It is also important to check with the client that all their concerns have been addressed.

Ensure that the right type and amount of information has been given

You must ensure that the client has fully understood the information you have given them. Equally, you need to ensure that your understanding of the client's problem matches their own understanding. (Repeating to them what you believe they have told you is an useful technique here.) Once you both understand each other's position, you are in a position to agree in partnership a plan of action.

Conclude with forward planning

There is a skill too to closing the encounter. You need to reach a mutual end point when you are both satisfied that enough has been shared. You can then conclude with some forward planning as necessary.

Overcoming communication barriers

Remember that successful communication involves the exchange of information between one person and another. In turn this communication is embellished and expressed with nuances such as tone, inflection, feelings and clarity. All of this must be received and understood by the client.

Active listening (based on Quilter Wheeler and Windt, 1993)

Good communication depends on respecting the client and importantly using active listening skills. 'Active listening' is a specific technique that has been developed: it means more than simply being there and letting people's words reach you. You need to be sincerely attentive, and also to find ways to demonstrate that you have taken in what has been told to you, and that you value the speaker and their opinions. We all like to receive attention from a good listener, and healthcare clients are no exception.

Active listening:
- helps you to decode accurately the messages that are sent to you
- demonstrates to the client that you have understood their views, thoughts and feelings
- helps establish good relationships at an early stage in the communication episode
- fosters a good, honest and productive dialogue.

How do you achieve this? There are a number of simple techniques that you can use.

Reflecting

This technique resembles holding a mirror to the other person. You consciously pick up on some of the key words or phrases they have used, and introduce them into your own side of the conversation. (So for example, if they use 'tummy' when you would say 'stomach', you use 'tummy' sometimes too.) This acts as a validation of the other person's vocabulary as well as of their message. Of course, you need to take care to understand that you *do* know what their wording means, by putting it in context and also using your own words (see the next section).

Using paraphrasing and summarising

In this technique you consciously repeat back to someone in *your own* words what they have told you. (For instance, they say, 'I've got a tummy ache' and you say, 'So your stomach is painful.') This both confirms to them that you have taken in the message, and acts as a check that you are both talking about the same thing.

Reflecting nonverbal signals

One way of conveying empathy to people is by reflecting the nonverbal signals they give you. You need to get in tune with the 'rhythm and beat' of the message. Then you echo it in the way you act and speak in turn. To some extent you will find yourself doing this unconsciously, but if you also consciously do it, it acts as a kind of check on the accuracy of your perceptions.

Le May (2007) makes the useful point that the very problems that make people clients of healthcare services can affect their ability to communicate. The problems of old age in particular can cause communication difficulties. Most older people see and hear less well than they did when younger. Someone who has suffered a stroke, for instance, may be left with speech and language difficulties. Strokes and neurological disorders such as Parkinson's disease can also affect the ability to use facial expressions and make gestures. Patients may have a limited choice of posture, body position and clothing, and all this restricts the messages they are able to convey.

Use praise

This not only makes people feel good, it also encourages them to talk about their needs and problems. Praising specific behaviours or accomplishments is worthwhile with clients of all ages, and especially children.

The main benefits of active listening are that:

- clients feel more understood
- clients feel liberated to express their thoughts more clearly and concisely
- importantly clients have an opportunity to correct any misunderstandings.

The three Rs of listening

- **Readying**: this is the process of preparing to actively listen to someone.
- **Reaching**: this is what you do in encouraging the client to articulate their needs.
- **Reflecting**: this is the process of ensuring that you understand, and conveying this to the other person.

> **a Learning activity**
>
> Read Le May's (2007) article on communicating care. In your learning group, role play clients with a variety of communication disorders. Discuss what strategies you could use to overcome these and communicate with the individuals.

Areas of communication difficulty

Quilter Wheeler and Windt (1993) identified a number of areas of communication difficulty of which you should be aware.

Perceptual

We all need to be aware of how perceptions can alter our feelings about people. The way they look, dress and their manner all convey messages to us, and these messages are not always positive ones. It is very easy to give in to bias, discrimination and stereotyping, but as professionals we must all make efforts to overcome any negative perceptions and to treat everyone fairly and pleasantly. A young person who wears a 'hoodie' might not be – probably is not – a thug. You need to be aware of your feelings and prejudices, and make a continual effort to be open-minded and avoid prejudging people. Perceptions can work both ways, of course: just as you take in a host of nonverbal messages from patients, they take in messages from your appearance and manner. This is one reason that it is important to observe dress and professional behaviour codes rigorously, so that you come across as the competent professional clients expect and hope to deal with.

Emotional

Emotions can run high in people with healthcare issues, and it is easy for them to become a barrier to communication. There is a particular problem in complex cases where clients whose problems are not easily (if at all) overcome may come to lose trust in the practitioner. Emotional overload and denial only add to the difficulties. In these circumstances you may have to work very hard to establish a trusting relationship and keep communication going.

Informational

Active listening is the ideal, but it is not one that we always achieve. Sometimes practitioners do not actively listen and ask leading rather than open questions. This much reduces the chances of a client conveying their needs. The remedies are the ones we outlined above: use active listening techniques, take time, and ask open questions.

Time constraints

As was mentioned above, there is a risk that if you give clients insufficient time or convey to them that you are in a hurry, you will fail to take in vital information.

Linguistic

By this is meant both the use of medical jargon, and difficulties when the two people conversing do not have the same first language. Although you need to learn the jargon of healthcare for your professional role, you also need to remember that patients have not undergone the same training, and it will not be familiar to them. It is important to speak to people using words that they will understand.

If the difficulties are caused by the lack of a common language, you will need to find a translator. All hospitals keep a directory of local interpreters. When you know this problem is likely to arise with a client, it is good practice to book one in advance. However, on occasions you might need to communicate urgently with someone when no translator is available. Panesar and Sheikh (2006) have suggested a number of strategies for talking to clients from other backgrounds. In particular, they recommend using language resources such as Language Line.

S Scenario: Michael's experiences

Michael, the first year student nurse, is on placement in a busy surgical day care unit. One of the patient's theatre slots is postponed to the following week. The patient had been psyched up for the operation, and becomes quite angry when he is told this. Michael's mentor deals with the angry patient and his relatives, and this is an opportunity for Michael to observe professional communication skills being used in a difficult context.

---

a Learning activity   **W**

With your learning group, find out which hospitals/healthcare facilities in your area keep a dossier of interpreters, List the languages covered and discuss how a practitioner might access the service. Go to www.languageline.co.uk/ and critically review how effective it is in providing language services to the NHS.

Read Panesar and Sheikh's (2006) article on 'How to talk with people from other backgrounds'. Discuss how practitioners can respond to the challenges of communicating with people with whom they do not share a common language.

Communication techniques for special client groups

You can read more about very special techniques for dealing with young people with communication difficulties in the companion skills book.

Heron's six-category intervention analysis

John Heron (1976, 1990) has developed an analytic training tool which can help in developing practical therapeutic interacting skills that you can use in communicating with clients. Burnard and Morrison (2005) believe that this model of therapeutic communication can be used in a wide variety of clinical and other communication situations. In essence Heron divides types of communication into six intervention categories which apply in one to one, one to group and intergroup communication situations. 'Intervention' in this context means that they are all focused on offering an enabling service to the client.

Three basic values underpin the everyday use of these categories. They are:

- hierarchical: one person acts as the professional, the other as the client
- cooperative: the aim is to use consultation and discussion and to come to an agreement
- based on autonomy: ways of facilitating clients so that they can act and make decisions for themselves.

The first three intervention categories are authoritative categories: that is, their basic stance is 'I tell you'. Here the practitioner takes a dominant role, taking responsibility, guiding behaviour and giving instructions.

Prescriptive

The aim here is to direct the client's behaviour, and the focus is on giving straightforward advice and information about a particular problem. This is used, for instance, when a client makes a simple request (like 'How do I get an appointment?'). Nurses working for NHS Direct and other national telephone helplines use this form of communication. Although the aim is to influence and direct, clients are still free to make their own decisions. They are given the advice they requested, and can decide whether they wish to follow it.

Informative

The emphasis here is on giving knowledge or information to a client: there is not the same overtone of directing as in the first category. This might be intended to help people care for themselves more easily, and the focus is on sharing knowledge in a way that fosters independence. The information provided should be seen by clients as relevant to their healthcare needs and interests. It could be either general knowledge about healthcare, or specific information about the individual's condition and circumstances. You can use this type of intervention to interpret information about health and illness for the client.

Confronting

Here the aim is to raise the client's awareness of a limiting behaviour. Perhaps they have an attitude or habit of which they are not fully aware, that is affecting their recovery, and you need to draw it more fully to their attention, to encourage them to change. This is a difficult form of communication, and confronting interventions are only effective when the client feels you are acting in their best interests.

The other three categories are facilitative: their basic stance is 'You tell me'. The role of the practitioner is to listen and to respond in a way that is enabling. Your aim is to encourage the client to be autonomous and to support them by affirming their uniqueness. This form of communication is often used in rehabilitation work: for example, in stroke recovery.

Cathartic

The aim here is to enable the release of pent-up emotions such as grief, fear or anger. This can be very therapeutic but the skill is to manage the release at a level of distress which the client is comfortable dealing with.

Catalytic

Here the aim is to enable self-discovery, self-directed living, learning or problem solving for example.

Supportive

In supportive communication your aim is to affirm the worth and value of a client's qualities, actions and attitudes. In other words, you provide a 'feel-good factor'. This skill is essential for successful therapeutic communication with a range of clients.

All six categories:
- are fundamentally supportive of the client
- have an implicit aim of increasing the capacity of the client for creative self-direction
- are value free, in that no one category is of greater or lesser value than the others.

Application of the categories

In practice, no conversation will fall neatly into just one of these categories. The six categories will be woven together, so that for example a catalytic intervention also has an informative element. You should used them as appropriate, in a way that reflects the:
- client/practitioner relationship
- current state and potential of the client
- creativity and insight of the practitioner
- context of the communication encounter.

Once you have developed your intervention communication skills, you should be:
- equally proficient in each of the six types of intervention
- able to move seamlessly from one type of intervention to other, as the encounter develops
- conscious during the communication episode of what type of intervention you are using and why.

> **a Learning activity**
>
> In your interprofessional leaning group, role play all six categories. You will need to work up a variety of scenarios to illuminate them. Your group facilitator will help you in this task.

Communicating by telephone

Telephone triage or consultation has developed considerably over the first few years of the twenty-first century. This has included the establishment of NHS Direct in England, and similar services elsewhere. This might seem strange at first, because the telephone is hardly a new technology: it was first patented in 1876 by Alexander Graham Bell, and it has been used since the nineteenth century (Glasper et al, 2000) as a way of advising patients and diagnosing illnesses.

Telephone consultation today involves nurses and other healthcare professionals listening to the problems of people who are often fraught and emotional, and giving them appropriate advice. In an acute episode a caller might be very anxious about themselves, or someone close to them: for example, a mother might call about the problems of her child. Glasper and colleagues (2000) have discussed how professionals are helped in this task by decision-making telephone advice software. Even with this help, communicating with clients on the telephone can be very difficult. Most of us have some negative experiences of telephone helplines, even when the topic is something much less emotional like a broken washing machine, and obviously the problems are multiplied when it is people's health and wellbeing at stake.

Bowing (2000) has described telephone consultation as communicating in the dark, without any of the visual clues that help a face to face conversation. A telephone conversation does not depend just on words, however: nonverbal elements such as tone of voice play a large part.

Because people telephoning a healthcare professional are often tense and emotional, and may be ill at ease discussing sensitive issues, your first priority in this situation is to help them relax and feel comfortable in talking freely (Quilter Wheeler and Windt ,1993). Learning to deal effectively with clients on the telephone is a skill that has to be acquired: it does not come naturally to most of us. It is important to convey a calm and reassuring manner, and not to reflect the caller's anxiety. The words you use are just as important as your tone. You can use the active listening skills discussed earlier in the chapter, coupled with reflection, to get all the necessary information from the client, and just as importantly, make sure that they hear and understand the advice they are given in return. Bowing (2000) believes that even in the absence of visual cues, good communication skills can help us achieve an accurate assessment of client needs by telephone.

Developing a repertoire of skills to handle a wide variety of telephone client encounters is particularly important for NHS Direct telephone consultants, but other healthcare professionals too need to develop skills in this area.

Car and Sheikh (2003) suggested that a successful telephone consultation calls for:
- active listening and detailed history taking
- frequent clarifying and paraphrasing (to ensure that the messages have got across in both directions)
- picking up cues (such as pace, pauses, change in voice intonation)
- offering opportunities to ask questions
- offering patient education.

Using the internet, voicemail, texting and email

Newer technologies also have a role to play today in professional communications. The advent of the mobile phone, and quick and easy access to the internet from for example cyber cafés and home computers, are changing the way in which people in every field communicate with each other.

Internet services

NHS Direct Online (http://www.nhsdirect.nhs.uk/) was launched in December 1999. The service offers clients a range of databases covering health topics. They are available 24 hours a day, and receive more than 450,000 visitors each month. Clients using the service have access to an online encyclopaedia of some 400 conditions which also gives details of appropriate support groups (Eaton, 2002). Users can also browse a number of databases to obtain information about health and health services and contemporary health news items.

Huntington and colleagues (2002) are among the researchers who have discussed the wider implications of this for health care. Is it true that providing people with healthcare information leads to better health outcomes? It is certainly leading to changes in the relationship between healthcare professionals and their clients. Increasingly people use the internet to get information related to their problem or condition before they contact a doctor or healthcare professional. This means that they are better prepared, and in modern jargon 'empowered': they have information independently of their adviser, and can make requests or even demands, rather than wait to see what is recommended.

NHS Direct Online now has a facility for people who cannot find what they want from the website to email an enquiry, which should answered within five working days.

Voicemail

Prerecorded voice messages (voice mail) are useful for communicating health promotion

a Learning activity

As part of your learning group activities, visit the NHS Direct Online website. Consider how the information available might be of use to a range of clients in your discipline. Critically review the information provided. Do you think it is useful or not, and why? What do you think about the way it is presented?

Find out about the policy on internet usage in your placement organisation. Are there any issues to be resolved if you want to use the internet to get information for your clients?

messages, and to give people basic information on topics. They are not much used now as a standalone communication system, since the internet has superseded some of these functions, but they are still embedded in systems such as NHS Direct Online. Interactive voice response systems (IVRS) are a development of this technology. This was described by Haeok and colleagues (2003) as a telephone attached to a talking computer which communicates health messages to a client caller. The services are available 24 hours a day, seven days per week and can be activated in both directions: so clients can call for information, or their healthcare professional can trigger the system to call them, for example to give guidance on post-discharge management. The level of information provided varies. At the simplest, clients can make a limited range of choices via a touchtone telephone; in more complex set-ups, they might receive individual information related for example to management of hypertension.

Texting

SMS (text messaging) is such a predominant form of communication now that it is no wonder healthcare professionals are looking at how best to use it. In particular it has been suggested as a way of improving outpatient appointments. Downer, Mears and Da Costa (2005) looked at its pros and cons, and concluded that its main advantage is the ease with which large numbers of texts can be customised and sent. Because of this, they suggest that its use will grow in healthcare settings.

Email

Much the same is true of email. Car and Sheikh (2004) looked at patient satisfaction with email communications, which not surprisingly depends on how rapidly they get a reply. Bauchner, Adams and Burstin (2002) are cautious about the use of email in healthcare, because of the increased workload it could lead to. In addition they raise a number of legal and ethical issues, not least that email correspondence should be part of the patient record.

Another issue is the potential for misunderstanding and conflict. Bruner (2003) made some telling points in this context:

- Emails are read in isolation, without visual or verbal cues from the sender, and this increases the risk of misunderstanding.
- It is easy to forget the courtesy and humanness which normally accompanies a communication. What is intended as quick and informal can come across as aggressive and impolite.
- Emails can be read and reread by the recipient, and hurtful or unwise phrasing that might be forgotten in a conversation can be built up into a major cause of grudge and resentment.

Cleary and Freeman (2005) make some useful points about email etiquette (or netiquette):

- Be aware that some perceived insults may be totally unintended. People sometimes write emails quickly without giving full thought to every word, and this exaggerates the possibilities of misunderstanding that exist in every form of communication.
- Watch for enhanced aggressiveness, and check how you respond to an email that annoys or upsets you.
- As well as taking offence at messages you receive, you can cause offence by messages you send. Always reread your message before sending, and

a Learning activity

Read Cleary and Freeman (2005) and in your learning group, critically appraise their list of do's and don'ts.

Michael gets an email from his mentor which he perceives to be unfriendly. He discusses it with his learning group. How should he respond?

try to gauge the reaction of the person who will be reading it. It is too late once you have clicked the 'send' button.

- Be aware of your relationship with the reader of your message. Take care to observe courtesies such as sending best wishes.

Communicating through written material

Healthcare professionals have become increasingly aware that they need to improve the way they communicate with patients and the public. The policy today is to move towards a patient-led NHS, empowering people to choose their treatment and decide how to live their lives, and written information (for instance, leaflets on specific health-related topics) plays a sizeable role in this.

Designing and writing this kind of material is a job for specialists, and information resources need to be developed with input from both users of services and appropriate members of the interprofessional healthcare team, to ensure they reach the highest standards.

Written communication has major advantages over verbal information. Not least, it registers for longer: people forget what they are told verbally very quickly, particularly when they are under stress (Glasper and Burge, 1992), and it is a good idea to give them written information on things they need to recall. However written instructions are not suitable for everyone: some people cannot read, many others read poorly, and others still do not read the languages in which material is available. According to the Literacy Trust (http://www.literacytrust.org. uk/Database/stats/adultstats.html), nearly four out of ten adults in some parts of England cannot read or write properly, and many find difficulty with complex material. So although written material is an useful communication tool, it needs to be used with care and thought.

Jacobson and colleagues (1999) have shown how specially designed low-literacy-level information sheets can improve patient compliance to health messages. You will not always be able to find the right ready-produced information, though, and you may find reason to try to write something yourself to give to your clients. This might not sound too difficult, but it is not a breeze either. Few people can put together a patient information leaflet in a lunch break on their laptop. It takes a little skill to lay it out acceptably (although desktop publishing software has made that much easier), and rather more skill to convey the right information at the right level.

The Write Stuff is a newsletter produced by Brunner three times a year (http://www. brunerbiz.com/page4o.htm) dedicated to the art of communicating through the written word. It has offered some useful rules for writing for patients. Much of this advice derives from Robert Gunning (1968), who recognised that writers must always allow for the literacy level of their readers. Griffin, McKenna and Tooth (2003) discuss the use of readability formulae which allow writers to pitch their leaflets at the right level.

Ten principles of clear writing (Gunning, 1968) are:

- Keep sentences short.
- Use simple rather than complex explanations.
- Use familiar words where possible.
- Avoid unnecessary words.
- Put action into verbs used.
- Write like you talk.
- Use terms your readers can picture.
- Link in with your readers' experience.
- Use a wide variety of writing techniques.
- Write to express, not impress.

Writing patient information leaflets

Some of the advice here is based on Lang (nd). Information leaflets should be:

- comprehensible: does the reader understand the text?
- usable/readable: can the reader apply the information?
- accessible: can the reader find the information easily (or is it lost in a sea of ambiguous text)?

Before rushing to your computer to produce your patient information leaflet:

- Know your purpose. What is it you want to achieve?
- Know your target audience. Who are you writing for (for instance, the child, carer or both)?
- Know your subject. Do you have the knowledge to write the material?
- Know the setting under which the target audience will read the leaflet.

When writing information leaflets ensure that they contain:

- awareness information which allows the reader to relate to the contents
- 'how to' information which allows the reader to do what is intended
- 'principles' information which gives real concrete information on why for example certain drugs actually work.

If you are not confident of producing a leaflet to the standard you feel is needed, you may be able to get help from an information professional at your place of work, such as a librarian.

Style

- Use informative, not descriptive headings. For example 'Mobile phone disease' is not very inspiring. 'What is mobile phone disease?' is better; 'Living with mobile phone disease' is the best of all.
- Try to personalise the leaflet by using personal pronouns such as I, we, us and you.
- Use decisive language which is clear and unambiguous.
- Describe actions positively, not negatively. Avoid for example 'Do not administer unless the client is developing a fever' and prefer 'Give only when the patient has a temperature above 38 degrees centigrade.'
- Use familiar words: not 'Your partner has fractured his tibia' but 'Your partner has broken his lower leg.' Medical jargon is poorly understood by the general public.
- Use short paragraphs with strong topic sentences.
- Use simple visual images.
- Use at least 12 point type, and larger still for younger and older readers.

Note that most hospitals have systems in place for validating and approving patient information leaflets.

---

a Learning activity

In your interprofessional learning group, source appropriate examples of client information leaflets and critically appraise their usefulness.

Conclusion

This chapter aimed to help you appreciate every aspect of using strategies of communication efficiently and effectively in your day to day work. Being able to communicate positively with clients lies at the very heart of healthcare professionalism. You need to become adept at using the full repertoire of communication methods. Because information giving is the very key to client empowerment, you may wish to read this chapter several times over.

References

Bauchner, H., Adams, W. and Burstin, H. (2002) 'You've got mail: issues in communicating with patients and their families by email', *Pediatrics* **109**(5), 954–6.

Bell, S. M. and Salter Ainsworth, M.D. (1972) 'Infant crying and maternal responsiveness', *Child Development* **43**(4), 1171–90.

Bowing, T. (2000) 'Communication in the dark', *Practice Nursing* **11**(8), 17–20.

Bruner (2003) The Write Stuff, winter [online] http://www.brunerbiz. com/page4o.htm (accessed 23 December 2008).

Burnard, P. and Morrison, P. (2005) 'Nurses' perceptions of their interpersonal skills: a descriptive study using six category intervention analysis', *Nurse Education Today* **25**(8), 612–17.

Chant, S., Jenkinson, T., Randle, J. and Russell, G. (2002) 'Communication skills; some problems in nurse education and practice', *Journal of Clinical Nursing* 11, 12–21.

Car, J. and Sheikh, A. (2003) 'Telephone consultations', *British Medical Journal* 326, 966–9.

Car, J. and Sheikh, A. (2004) 'Email consultations in healthcare 2: acceptability and safe application', *British Medical Journal* 329, 439–42.

Caris-Verhallen, W. M. C. M., Kerkstra, A. and Bensing, J. M.(1999) 'Non-verbal behaviour in nurse–elderly patient communication', *Journal of Advanced Nursing* 29(4), 808–18.

Chambers, S. (2003) 'Use of non -verbal communication skills to improve nursing care', *British Journal of Nursing* 129(14), 874–8.

Cleary, M. and Freeman, A. (2005) 'Email etiquette: guidelines for mental health nurses', *International Journal of Mental Health Nursing* 14, 62--5.

Downer, S. R., Mears, J. G. and Da Costa, A. C. (2005) 'Use of SMS text messaging to improve outpatient attendance', *Medical Journal of Australia* **183**(7), 366–8.

Eaton, L. (2002) 'NHS Direct Online explores partnership with other health organisations', *British Medical Journal* 324, 568.

Egan, G. (1990) *The Skilled Helper*, 4th edn, Pacific Grove, Calif., Brooks/Cole.

Glasper, A. and Burge, D. (1992) 'Developing family information leaflets', *Nursing Standard* 6(25), 24–7.

Glasper, E. A., Lattimer, V. A., Thompson, F. and Wray, D. (2000) 'NHS Direct; examining the challenges for nursing practice', *British Journal of Nursing* 9(17), 1173–8.

Giffin, J., McKenna, K. and Tooth, L. (2003) 'Written health education materials: making them more effective', *Australian Occupational Therapy Journal* 50, 170–7.

Gunning, R. (1968) *The Technique of Clear Writing*, Philadelphia, Pa., McGraw-Hill.

Haeok, L., Friedman, M. E., Cukor, P. and Ahern, D. (2003) 'Interactive voice response system (IVRS) in health services', *Nursing Outlook* **51**(6), 227–83.

Heron, J. (1976) 'A six-category intervention analysis', *British Journal of Guidance and Counselling* 4920,143–55.

Heron, J. (1990) *Helping the Client: A creative practical guide*, London, Sage.

Huntington, P., Nicholas, D., Williams, P. and Gunter, B. (2002) 'Characterising the health information consumer: an examination of digital television users', *Libri* 52,16–27.

Huntington, P., Williams, P. and Blackburn, P. (2001) 'Digital health information provision and health outcomes', *Journal of Information Science* 27(4), 265–76.

Jacobson, T. A., Thomas, D. M., James Morton, F., Offutt, G., Shevlin, J. and Ray, S. (1999) 'Use of a low literacy patient education tool to enhance pneumococcal vaccination rates: a randomised controlled trial', JAMA 282, 646–50.

Lang, T. A. (nd) 'How to write patient education handouts', Cleveland Clinic Foundation Department of Scientific Publications (unpublished).

Le May, A. (2007) 'Communicating care', *Nursing and Residential Care* 9(8),363–6.

Miller, S. M. (1987) 'Monitoring and blunting: validation of a questionnaire to assess styles of information seeking under threat', *Journal of Personality and Social Psychology* 52, 345–53.

Munson, E. and Willcox, A. (2007) 'Applying the Calgary-Cambridge Model', *Practice Nursing* 18(9), 464–8.

Panesar, S. S. and Sheikh, S. (2006) 'How to talk with people from other backgrounds', *Practice Nursing* 17(2), 93--6.

Pollock, K. and Grime, J. (2002) 'Patients' perceptions of entitlement to time in general practice consultations for depression: qualitative study', *British Medical Journal* 325, 687.

Quilter Wheeler, S. and Windt, J. H. (1993) *Telephone Triage: Theory, practice and protocol development*, New York, Delmar.

Chapter

6

Culture

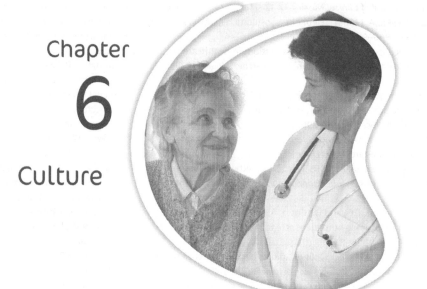

Jim Richardson

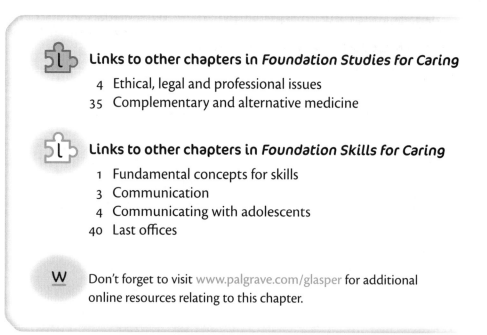

Links to other chapters in *Foundation Studies for Caring*

Links to other chapters in *Foundation Skills for Caring*

W   Don't forget to visit www.palgrave.com/glasper for additional online resources relating to this chapter.

Introduction

By the end of your foundation programme you will need a good working knowledge of the role of culture in your relationships with clients and each other. Culture affects how we relate to each other, what we expect of each other and how we interpret the communication we receive from others. This chapter explains how you can use ideas of culture to ensure that the therapeutic encounter is safe, effective and mutually satisfying.

Learning outcomes

This chapter will enable you to:

- recognise the role of the family in a child's life and well-being, and propose strategies to work collaboratively with children and families

- recognise the significance of culture and ethnicity in healthcare, and formulate principles for ensuring that care is delivered in a culturally safe way.

Concepts

- Childhood
- The family – structure and function
- Ethnicity, race and culture
- Stereotyping, prejudice and racism
- Social support
- Acute children's healthcare and the professional's role
- Chronic illness in childhood
- Family-centered care

The chapter explores the care issues of a 7-year-old boy, Deepak, who has asthma. He is the child of a single-parent family of Gujarati origin. His story will help us examine aspects of family-centred care, and ethnic and cultural issues. The focus on a young family also illustrates ideas of relevance to other healthcare sectors.

[S] Scenario: Introducing Deepak Patel

Deepak's mother has been a single parent since her husband died four years ago. She has relatives in the United Kingdom but the nearest lives in a town some three hours away by public transport from the hospital where Deepak is being treated. She has some friends locally but none that she would describe as close. Deepak and his mother are dependent on social welfare payments for their basic income. They live in a small rented flat in which dampness is a problem.

(a) Learning activity

From this account, can you identify issues which might pose a challenge for Deepak and his mother in their daily lives?

Some issues you might consider in connection with the learning activity are:

- **Social support**: Who provides Deepak and his mother with support, help and encouragement? With whom can Deepak's mother discuss her anxieties? Might Deepak's mother want more social interaction, and if so, whom might she ask to mind Deepak? This is particularly significant because given the unpredictable nature of asthma, she cannot be certain when Deepak might have a sudden attack and whether the minder might be able to cope appropriately with such a situation. Without social support, Deepak and his mother might feel lonely, isolated and uncertain.

- **Financial**: living on a low income can constitute a chronic stressor for families like Deepak's. Many families who receive social welfare support do not receive the full range of benefits to which they are entitled simply because they are not aware of their entitlement.
- **Housing**: poor living conditions can cause stress, and the damp state of the flat might contribute to Deepak's asthma problems if house dust mites and fungal spores act as trigger factors in his case.

In order to ascertain whether these factors are indeed issues for this family, you would find it useful to assess the situation from the family's viewpoint. It is all too easy to make assumptions about people's position: for example, that a single-parent family suffers from lack of social support and interaction. This might not be the case.

Tools for assessing families

An useful tool in carrying out an assessment is an ecomap which you can construct to illustrate a family's social position. Figure 6.1 shows an example. The ecomap graphically illustrates relationships within the family, and between a family and other individuals such as the wider family, friends and neighbours, and with agencies such as the school, the workplace and healthcare bodies. It is also possible to show the nature of these relationships: whether they are close, over-close or conflictual.

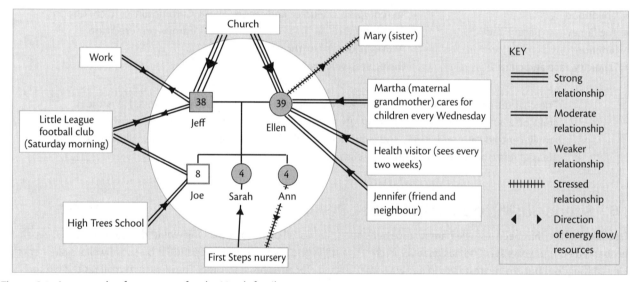

Figure 6.1   An example of an ecomap for the Marsh family

To practise the technique and explore its possibilities, you might find it useful to construct an ecomap of your own family, or of a family in your care at the moment.

Learning activity

To supplement your understanding of families' experience of caring for an ill child, the papers by Smith and Daughtry (2000), Smith, Coleman and Bradshaw (2002) and Neill (2000) offer many insights derived from research work involving such families. You might also find useful views of the child's experience in the work of Sartain, Clarke and Heyman (2000).

While you read these papers, consider whether, based on the quality and nature of the research they describe, you are prepared to accept the findings of these researchers. In other words, is this good-quality research which provides results that are valid and reliable? You might find it useful to make notes about the issues you find in the article which convince you that it describes good-quality research – or not!

Make a list of the observations in these papers that you might want to bear in mind as potential issues when working with families such as Deepak's.

It will be important to use your observations from the research above critically. Not all families respond in the same ways to difficulties relating to child health. It is unhelpful to assume that there are difficulties when they do not exist, but equally unhelpful to fail to recognise difficulties that are present. A respect for family individuality, and careful information gathering and sharing, can help to avoid these pitfalls in planning and delivering care for families such as Deepak's.

Among others, your list in response to the learning activity might include:

- social worker
- welfare benefits adviser
- local authority housing officer
- community groups
- self-help groups such as Action Asthma
- link families with a child with a similar health issue.

> **a Learning activity**
>
> Can you suggest which agencies, individuals and professionals might be able to offer help and support to Deepak and his mother if they have any of the potential problems you have identified?

Cultural issues

> **S Scenario continued**
>
> Mrs Patel came to the United Kingdom in the late 1970s with her husband from India. Their families are of Gujarati origin and Gujarati remains their home language. Mrs. Patel speaks English but naturally prefers her mother tongue to receive and express complex ideas. Deepak has a native command of both Gujarati and English appropriate to a 7-year-old.

> **a Learning activity**
>
> Given Mrs Patel's Indian background and upbringing, can you propose any cultural issues which it might be helpful to take into account when caring for her and her son?

You need to pay attention to cultural issues in healthcare in order to avoid discrimination. If you are aware of the cultural aspects of children's (and other people's) needs, that should help to ensure equality. One issue you should bear in mind when dealing with members of a cultural minority is that you are identifying them as belonging to a group, within which their beliefs, values and customs are shared in just the same way as members of the majority cultural group share their beliefs, values and customs. This emphasis on the group can be helpful, but it can also be problematic, especially if it leads you to stereotype the individuals. You need to avoid making assumptions about someone's culture based on your perception of the group they belong to, rather than asking them directly. An emphasis on individuality remains the key to working with all consumers of health services.

There can be no doubt that people from cultural minority groups will have encountered attitudes which are less favourable than those met by people from the majority cultural group. This difference might be based on ignorance of cultural needs or on prejudicial attitudes. Whatever the reasons, you must avoid giving different treatment (Nursing and Midwifery Council, 2008). In order to treat people fairly and appropriately, you need to understand how culture affects the interactions between patients and healthcare professionals.

Culture has been defined by Helman (2001) as an inherited 'lens' through which a person perceives the world they live in. This can be interpreted as the beliefs, values and ideas about what is right and wrong which guide a person's behaviour or customs, and which allow the person to make sense of the world. These beliefs and values are derived from a person's

> **a Learning activity**
>
> Can you define the terms 'cultural', 'ethnic' and 'race'?

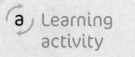

upbringing, and help to identify that person as belonging to a group. Of particular interest in our context are people's beliefs about what health is, how it is preserved and what action should be taken when there is a health problem. Often these beliefs are deeply embedded in our consciousness and they can be quite difficult to articulate.

Suman Fernando (2001) offers an interesting discussion on race, culture and ethnicity. He argues that *culture* is characterised by behaviour and attitudes which are determined by upbringing and choice, and that these as perceived as changeable through, for example, acculturation (that is, the process of adapting to a different culture). *Ethnicity*, he proposes, is characterised by a sense of belonging and group identity, which are determined by social pressures and psychological need. He makes a case that ethnicity is a partially changeable phenomenon. Finally, Fernando suggests that *race* is characterised by physical appearance dictated by genetic ancestry, and that this is perceived as permanent. It could be argued that 'race' is not a relevant issue in today's society; many people claim that it is an outmoded concept, and that someone's 'race' is no more significant than their eye or hair colour.

> ### ⓐ Learning activity
>
> Take some time to consider how you explain a minor ailment such as a cold or chill. How do you treat yourself when you have such a problem? How do other members of your family respond when they have the same problem? Your beliefs in this area are affected by culturally determined health beliefs as well as your education.
>
> Have you heard the expression, 'feed a cold and starve a fever'? What would you say is the basis for this prescription?

> ### ⓐ Learning activity
>
> Take a few minutes to consider Fernando's definitions. Can you think of any grounds on which you might challenge the validity of these ideas?

If we accept Fernando's definition of culture, it should be clear to you that it is possible to define certain groups in any society by their culture, independent of their members' race or ethnicity.

> ### ⓐ Learning activity
>
> Could you make a case for the elderly or those in a certain social class or professional group as constituting a cultural group? In what ways might it be useful to use definitions this way?

The impact of cultural issues on attitudes to healthcare

In Mrs Patel's case her culture and ethnicity might have an influence on how she explains Deepak's ill health. This might or might not differ from the Western biomedical explanation for asthma, which is likely to form the basis of his treatment. For example, perhaps she was brought up to understand that breathlessness can be caused by a dietary imbalance. In that case she could well struggle to understand why Deepak is being given medication but no attempt is being made to modify his diet.

> ### ⓐ Learning activity
>
> If there is a mismatch between the treatment that Mrs Patel feels her son should receive and that which is actually being given, how might Mrs Patel feel about this?

If Mrs Patel is bewildered by her son's treatment, she could be less supportive of it, and it should be clear to you that this could lead to problems. Consider the situation of the parent who visits a GP with her child who has an upper respiratory tract infection. She might well expect her child to be prescribed an antibiotic. Perhaps the GP does not agree to do this, because she knows that this infection is viral in origin, and an antibiotic would be ineffective. Moreover, over-prescription of antibiotics when they are not necessary can lead to bacterial resistance to antibiotics, and store up problems for the future.

However, the mother might believe that all chest infections are treatable with antibiotics, and that her child is not being given the best treatment if this does not happen. The mother's and the GP's perceptions of what should be done differ, and unless the GP gives, and the mother takes in, a careful explanation, it is possible that they will not reach common ground. The mother's faith in the GP's advice might be shaken, and as a result she might see no usefulness in the GP's suggestion that she give symptomatic care of hydration, rest and antipyretic medicine. In that case she might follow these suggestions half-heartedly, if at all.

The role of communication

In the learning activity above, did you suggest a careful exploration of what the parent and child understand the problem to be and what they expect should be done to treat the problem? Devoting time to this enquiry can sometimes yield surprising results from the healthcare professional's perspective.

Another option is to offer the parent and child information about the biomedical explanation for the child's problem. This kind of information can be quite difficult for the parent and child to assimilate, and they might require time to think about what they have been told and then have the opportunity to ask questions to clarify some of the issues.

Now consider the Learning Activity on the right. Your list might include:

- The parent and child can read the leaflet at their own pace and retain it for later reference.
- These leaflets often contain diagrams that illustrate features of the disorders. For example, the characteristic bronchospasm of asthma can be explained by a drawing.
- The leaflet offers information in one form, which might not be understood, or could indeed be misunderstood. It will still be important for the nurse to be available to discuss questions which arise from the parent and child's reading of this material
- Many adults and children have difficulty in reading the sometimes rather sophisticated language contained in explanatory leaflets. This difficulty might be heightened if the parent's native language is not English. In this case, alternative means of information giving such as audio or videotapes might be explored.

Whatever mode of information giving is employed, it will be important for the practitioner to take time to check on the parent's and child's understanding of the information which has been given.

Broader cultural needs

Other aspects of family life that might be culturally determined include dietary requirements and preferences, spiritual expression and pastoral care needs, hygiene practices, clothing, language use and child-rearing practices. For all families, it will be important to establish the

> **a Learning activity**
>
> Can you propose a strategy for resolving the situation where parent/child and healthcare professional differ in their understanding of an appropriate course of action to deal with a health problem?

> **a Learning activity**
>
> List what you think might be the potential benefits and limitations of using the written word for information giving.

family's requirements regarding such daily living practices. Failure to do so might alarm or alienate the parent and child.

Differences between people in cultural or ethnic beliefs have the potential to escalate to form the basis of discrimination, prejudice or even racism. Many people in cultural and ethnic minority groups have experienced this, and they will naturally be sensitive and anxious about being exposed to such responses again. It is one of the primary values of the nursing professions that discriminatory attitudes and behaviour are not tolerable and that all are approached with respect.

Important principles which might be reflected in your guidelines may include:

- Maintain a respectful attitude towards the beliefs and customs of others so long as these do not lead to harmful effects.
- Remain committed to achieving an understanding of what parents and children expect of their treatment and why.
- Take time and patience to explore the parent's and the child's explanation for and understanding of the child's health problem.
- Ensure that the child and family receive a full explanation of the child's problem. This should be in a format that both the child and parent can assimilate.
- Negotiate with the child and parent to achieve a consensus about what should be done to alleviate the child's problem and how this should be done. It could be argued that taking the child and parent's resources and preferences into account will improve the chances of successful collaboration.

If you adopt these strategies it will help you to work successful with not only families with ethnic backgrounds different from your own, but also those with other cultural orientations.

The role of family-centred care

Taking these principles of working together and translating them into action in planning and delivering healthcare will help to ensure that family-centred care is instituted.

Family-centred care has been evolving in the United Kingdom since the 1950s (Smith, Coleman and Bradshaw, 2002). Practitioners working in healthcare have continued to move from making care decisions and delivering that care to negotiating with families about the patient's care needs and who should satisfy them. Darbyshire's research (1994) demonstrates that this move is part of a continuing evolution in care philosophy.

> **a) Learning activity**
>
> Try to define what family-centred care could involve. How can it help to address cultural issues?

Family-centred care is particularly useful when dealing with children. Some issues that characterise family-centred care include:

- recognition that parents or primary carers satisfy the child's important basic care needs in the normal situation, until children have developed the ability to do this themselves
- appreciation that parents can usually learn to care for the child's enhanced needs brought about by a change in health status, but that they may need help, support and guidance to learn these skills
- acceptance that if parents are to care for their child's need they may require supportive care themselves
- recognition that the nurse's role in this form of care may move from that of care deliverer to that of care facilitator
- acceptance that the child is an integral part of the family unit and to improve the child's health involves addressing that family unit as a whole.

> **a) Learning activity**
>
> Can you suggest potential advantages and disadvantages to this form of care delivery?

Facilitating parents' ability to satisfy their child's care needs involves helping them to acquire new knowledge and skills which can be transferred to the home setting. This means that the parent is enabled to develop their ability to undertake their child's care.

When we assist parents to become independent in their child's care, it improves the family's ability to function autonomously. Parents can and do learn to delivery complex care in their own homes. Examples of this are the administration of intravenous antibiotics and the care of the child with a tracheostomy.

Working together means that all of the nurse's and parent's resources and energy are directed in a complementary fashion towards satisfying the child's care need. If communication and negotiation between nurse and parent are less than ideal, parents can be left uncertain what is expected of them. This can leave them bewildered and anxious. If they do not get sufficient support, parents can quickly become tired and stressed. They may feel isolated and left to get on with it themselves if the supportive care offered by the nurse is incomplete.

> **a) Learning activity**
>
> Make notes on what supportive care you think a parent may need while resident on the children's ward and involved in their child's care.

The parent needs the knowledge and skills necessary to care for the child. It is one thing to be responsible for satisfying the child's hygiene needs with a daily bath at home, but it is quite a different situation if the child is on a ward and has an intravenous cannula in their hand. Parents may need help to adapt their usual care practices to meet such changed conditions.

In order to meet the demands of satisfying their child's care needs, the parents' own care needs need to be attended to. This might include:

- facilities where the parent can rest and sleep
- facilities where the parent can wash and change their clothes
- access to adequate and appropriate food and drink
- the means to communicate with the wider family back home.

For many parents, it is equally important that they receive validation that what they are doing is a positive help to their child.

It could be argued that these conditions are best achieved by the nurse working side-by-side with the parent, not simply leaving them to get on with their child's care.

The role of collaborative care

Many of these ideas were combined in a model of collaborative care delivery proposed by Casey in the late 1980s (1993: 183) which has gained wide currency in the United Kingdom: see Figure 6.2. This model and explanation offer a picture of care delivery that is family-centred. Its operation, however, is based on a continuous assessment of family need, and care delivery that is negotiated and collaborative.

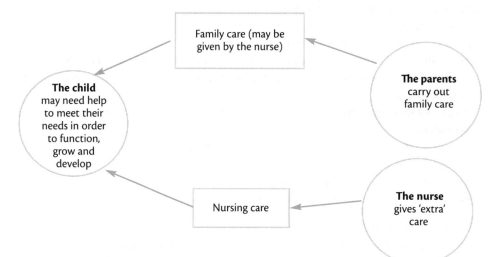

Figure 6.2 Casey's collaborative model

There are a number of benefits to collaborative care:
- The parent might be stressed and tired, and collaborative care gives them a chance to rest so that they are able to continue to care for the child in the longer term.
- The child's situation might require adaptation to the parent's normal care practices. For example, if the child has a plaster cast on a leg, helping the child to bathe or go to the toilet will become more complicated. The parent might need to see this adapted procedure demonstrated, and have the opportunity to practise it while being supported by the healthcare practitioner.
- The parent might have competing responsibilities, such as a need to go to work or to care for other children at home, which means they cannot stay in hospital to participate in the child's care. The nurse will then have to explore other methods of ensuring that the parent's participation continues as far as conditions allow.
- On rare occasions, the parent's actions are not in the child's best interests.

Family-centred care occurs in dynamic, ever-changing situations, and it is important to continually assess the situation and make necessary adjustments to the care approach. The cornerstone of collaborative work between parent, child and healthcare professional is effective communication in the form of appraisal and negotiation. The research undertaken by Swallow and Jacoby (2001) illustrates this well. Equally, Darbyshire (1994) was able to show that poor communication makes collaborative family-centred work difficult or impossible.

In response to the learning activity, you could suggest that in the acute phase, Mrs Patel might be helped and supported to deliver care that satisfies Deepak's basic needs. She can help Deepak to drink

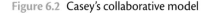

a Learning activity

You will note that in this model 'family' care might be delivered by the professional. Suggest why this could become necessary.

a Learning activity

In the case of Deepak and his mother, what might be the components of family-centred care?

a Learning activity

Now you have considered the themes introduced in this chapter, can you suggest the principles that should be observed to ensure that family-centred care occurs satisfactorily?

small amounts of fluids, she can help him to wash, and she can help to reassure and comfort him. As Mrs Patel's understanding of the tasks of management improve, she can begin to take responsibility for monitoring Deepak's condition using observation and peak flow measurement. She can ensure that his medication is administered effectively. In the longer term she can work to ensure the normality of their everyday experience by, for example, minimising the effect of trigger factors that provoke Deepak's asthma. Over time Deepak and his mother will learn to be flexible, to adapt these care practices to integrate them into family life, and to make the changes necessary to meet new situations.

The Millennium Charter

Action for Sick Children (ASC) (2000), a consumer organisation which represents the views of parents whose children need the services of healthcare professionals, has summarised the important principles of child healthcare from their perspective in the Millennium Charter. These ideas might be seen as prerequisites for, and underpinning of, family-centred healthcare:

1   All children shall have equal access to the best clinical care within a network of services that collaborate with each other.
2   Health services for children and young people should be provided in a child-centred environment separately from adults so that they are made to feel welcome, safe and secure at all times.
3   Parents should be empowered to participate in decisions regarding the treatment and care of their child through a process of clear communication and adequate support.
4   Children should be informed and involved to an extent appropriate to their development and understanding.
5   Children should be cared for at home with the support and practical assistance of community children's nursing services, unless the care that they require can only be provided in hospital.
6   All staff caring for children shall be specifically trained to understand and respond to their clinical, emotional, developmental and cultural needs.
7   Every hospital admitting children should provide overnight accommodation for parents, free of charge.
8   Parents should be encouraged and supported to participate in the care of their child when they are sick.
9   Every child in hospital shall have full opportunity for play, recreation and education.
10   Adolescents will be recognised as having different needs to those of younger children and adults. Health services should therefore be readily available to meet their particular needs.

Conclusion

This chapter has presented a range of ideas and themes in relation to ways of integrating cultural and ethnic issues in healthcare, in order to help assure effective and sensitive care delivery. It also stressed the importance of family-centred care as a mechanism to achieve this, and ensure all care provided is appropriate to the patient's needs and background.

References

Action for Sick Children (2000) *Millennium Charter for Children's Health Services*, London, ASC.

Carter, B. and Dearmun, A. K. (1995) *Child Healthcare Nursing: Concepts, theory and practice*, Oxford, Blackwell Science.

Casey, A. (1993) 'Development and use of the partnership model of nursing care', In: Glasper, E. A. and Tucker, A. (eds), *Advances in Child Health Nursing*, London, Scutari Press.

Culley, L. and Dyson, S. (eds) (2001) *Ethnicity and Nursing Practice*, Basingstoke, Palgrave.

Darbyshire, P. (1994) *Living with a Sick Child in Hospital: The experience of parents and nurses*, London, Chapman and Hall.

Fernando, S. (2001) *Mental Health, Race and Culture*, Basingstoke, Palgrave.

Helman, C. (2007) *Culture, Health and Illness*, 5th edn, London, Hodder Arnold.

Holland, K. and Hogg, C. (2001) Cultural Awareness in Nursing and

Healthcare, London, Arnold.

Neill, S. (2000) 'Acute childhood illness at home: the parents' perspective', *Journal of Advanced Nursing* **31**(4), 821–32.

Nursing and Midwifery Council (NMC) (2008) *The Code: Standards for conduct, performance and ethics for nurses and midwives*, London, NMC.

Panesar, S. S. and Sheikh, S. (2006) 'How to talk with people from other backgrounds', *Practice Nursing* **17** (2), 93–6.

Sartain, S. A., Clarke, C. L. and Heyman, R. (2000) 'Hearing the voices of children with chronic illness', *Journal of Advanced Nursing* **32**(4), 913–21.

Smith, L. and Daughtrey, H. (2000) 'Weaving the seamless web of care: an analysis of parents' perceptions of their needs following discharge of their child from hospital', *Journal of Advanced Nursing* **31**(4), 812–20.

Smith, S., Coleman, V. and Bradshaw, M. (2002) *Family-Centred Care: Concept, theory and practice*, Basingstoke, Palgrave.

Swallow, V. M. and Jacoby, A. (2001) 'Mothers' evolving relationships with doctors and nurses during the chronic childhood illness trajectory', *Journal of Advanced Nursing* **36**(6), 755–64.

Further reading

Bernardes, J. (1997) *Family Studies: An introduction*, London, Routledge. A wide-ranging introduction to the family; what it constitutes; what it is for and how it works. Good coverage of family diversity. Provides many thought-provoking exercises.

Bradford, R. (1997) *Children, Families and Chronic Disease: Psychological models and methods of care*, London, Routledge. An accessible guide to the psychosocial issues for families with a child with a chronic illness. Offers a challenging critique of how care services can help families to adjust to their difficulties.

Carter, B. and Dearmun, A. K. (1995) *Child Healthcare Nursing: Concepts, theory and practice*, Oxford, Blackwell Science. A clear and comprehensive review of child health nursing principles and practice.

Culley, L. and Dyson, S. (eds) (2001) *Ethnicity and Nursing Practice*, Basingstoke, Palgrave. A new, fresh exploration of aspects of race and ethnicity in healthcare delivery in our society. Challenges many of the past assumptions of transcultural nursing.

Darbyshire, P. (1994) *Living with a Sick Child in Hospital: The experience of parents and nurses*, London, Chapman and Hall. A key text in the arena of children's nursing. Exposes factors that promote and inhibit the constructive development of child and family-centered care.

Holland, K. and Hogg, C. (2001) *Cultural Awareness in Nursing and Healthcare*, London, Arnold. A very readable book which helps translate some of the complex, abstract ideas of culture, race and ethnicity into practical, everyday nursing activity.

Hubband, S. and Trigg, E. (2001) *Practices in Children's Nursing*, Edinburgh, Churchill Livingstone. A practical text giving a description and rationale for skills employed in child health nursing. Addresses not just secondary healthcare settings but also skills used in primary healthcare.

Smith, L., Coleman, V. and Bradshaw, M. (2002) *Family-Centered Care: Concept, theory and practice*, Basingstoke, Palgrave. A fundamentally important book exploring the development of family-centred nursing care. Contains a wealth of references to assist in further study.

Chapter

7

Public health and health promotion

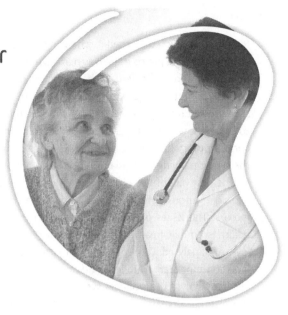

Geraldine Clay

 Links to other chapters in *Foundation Studies for Caring*

2 Interprofessional learning
3 Evidence-based practice and research
8 Healthcare governance
10 Nutritional assessment and needs
13 Infection prevention and control
18 Maternity
25 Care of the older adult – community
26 Mental health
27 Learning disability
34 Primary care

 Links to other chapters in *Foundation Skills for Caring*

1 Fundamental concepts for skills
2 IT skills
3 Communication
23 Diabetic foot assessment
27 Preparation of infant feeds

W Don't forget to visit www.palgrave.com/glasper for additional online resources relating to this chapter.

Introduction

Public health is concerned with using policy to create healthy environments and with empowering people to improve their own health. This chapter aims to develop your political awareness and equip you with the knowledge, skills and attitudes required to fulfil your health promotion role with patients, clients and communities. Throughout the chapter, a scenario addressing the needs of a young family with overweight and obesity issues is used to show how current policy, public health and health promotion theory are applied to contemporary healthcare practice. Because some policies relate only to England, please visit the accompanying website for information relating to other countries in the United Kingdom.

The first half of the chapter briefly discusses the historical context of public health, then explores various definitions to demonstrate that people's health is influenced by a range of factors. The issues of social status, poverty and culture are acknowledged determinants of health, so public health strategies to address inequalities in health at both local and national level are analysed. Current policy initiatives are then considered to demonstrate that obesity is a contemporary public health concern. A 'systems theory' model of policy making is used to analyse the political system, demonstrating the external environmental drivers, and the internal demands and supports that influence the policy process. Then the political decisions made, in the shape of policy outputs, are examined and the consequences, or policy outcomes, of those decisions are discussed. This section concludes with analysis of the ways in which healthcare practitioners can influence the policy process.

The second part of the chapter begins by introducing epidemiology, defined as the study of health events in human populations. The concept is applied in a discussion of obesity to demonstrate how it contributes to the process of health needs assessment, the starting point of any health promotion activity. A range of models and approaches are then used to distinguish the activities of health education, prevention and protection, which are combined under the broad umbrella of health promotion. In particular, discussion focuses on attitudes to health and the strategies that can be used to bring about behaviour change with individuals and families affected by obesity. Finally, ethical frameworks are introduced and critically applied to address the ethical considerations underpinning public health and health promotion practice.

Learning outcomes

This chapter will enable you to:

- discuss the historical context of public health, explore a range of definitions and examine current public health priorities relating to overweight and obesity
- consider the impact of determinants such as social status, poverty and culture on health, and discuss health inequalities relating to obesity
- explore the policy process, the factors that influence policy development and the impact of policy on healthcare provision
- describe the use of epidemiology to assess health needs
- analyse health promotion models and approaches to select appropriate health education interventions for practice
- analyse ethical issues in health promotion practice.

Concepts

- Public health: definition and history
- Contemporary public health policy and government obesity strategy
- Public health workforce
- Health inequalities, links between inequality and obesity
- Definitions of policy
- Policy-making process and systems theory
- Policy and professional roles
- Epidemiology

- Health needs assessment
- Health promotion definitions and approaches
- Models of health promotion
- Attitudes to health
- Overweight and obesity issues in children
- NICE care pathways for overweight and obese individuals
- Ethical issues in health promotion

[S] Scenario: introducing Charlotte and her family

Charlotte, 34 years old, is married to Damien who is the same age. The couple have one child, Lola aged 11. As Charlotte is a healthcare assistant and Damien works as a lorry driver, the couple live on a modest budget and cannot afford luxuries although they regularly treat themselves to takeaway meals while watching their favourite films on DVD. Charlotte's body mass index (BMI) is 25, just within normal BMI limits of 20–25, but Damien has gained weight rapidly in recent years and with a BMI of 35 he is obese. Like her father, Lola is fond of fatty foods and Charlotte struggles to get her to eat fruit or vegetables as she prefers biscuits and chips. The family has been contacted by the school nurse who has carried out routine screening of year 6 pupils and found Lola to be overweight. Charlotte has decided to address these issues. She has persuaded Damien to consult the family's general practitioner, and is now in contact with the school nurse.

Public health: historical perspective

Public health has been defined as 'the science and art of preventing disease, prolonging life and promoting health through the organised efforts and informed choices of society, organisations, public and private, communities and individuals' (Wanless, 2004).

Throughout the nineteenth century the major threats to public health came from diseases such as cholera and typhoid which thrived in urban homes and factories affected by poor ventilation and inadequate hygiene. In 1848, the first ever Public Health Act for England and Wales acknowledged the need for environmental change, and public health boards were formed to tackle issues such as poor sanitation through improved water supply and sewage removal (Gormley, 1999).

By the end of the nineteenth century, increased bacteriological understanding and the emerging germ theory of disease led to a more individualistic approach to disease prevention. According to Ashton and Seymour (1988), there began to be a shift in public health from a largely environmental focus on housing and sanitation, to an emphasis on individual responsibility for health and personal preventive services.

The establishment of the World Health Organization (WHO) in 1948 began a further shift in notions of health from the purely biological to the recognition that all sectors of government and society have a part to play in promoting and maintaining health (Douglas et al, 2007). There followed a number of important WHO landmarks in the health promotion phase of public health:

- Alma Ata Declaration (WHO, 1974)
- Global Strategy for Health for All by the year 2000 (WHO, 1985)
- Ottawa Charter for Health Promotion (WHO, 1986).

In each of these strategies, health promotion deliberately tried to address issues of policy, power, social and economic structures (Bunton, 1992, cited in Adams, Amos and Munro, 2002). Wanless (2004) in *Securing Good Health for the Whole Population* provided an update of the challenges involved in implementing this fully engaged scenario, which resulted in the declaration that we still have a national sickness service, not a national health service.

[a] Learning activity

In your interprofessional learning group make a list of the contemporary public health issues that you are aware of, and identify any current UK public health policies that you have encountered in practice.

Public health: contemporary perspective and policies

The essential elements of modern public health can be seen as:

- a population perspective
- an emphasis on prevention and on collective responsibility for health
- a concern for the underlying socioeconomic determinants of health as well as disease
- a multidisciplinary basis and emphasis on partnership with the population (DH, 2001).

This emphasises that health status is influenced by a range of factors, and that in addition to the lifestyle choices of individuals, there is a need for action at a broader social and political level to promote health and well-being. As Last (1987:6) observes, 'Public health activities change with changing technology and social values, but the goals remain the same – to reduce the amount of disease, premature death and disease-produced discomfort and disability in the population.'

The current overarching priorities for public health in England and Wales are identified by the Department of Health in *Choosing Health: Making healthy choices easier* (DH, 2004b) as:

- reducing the numbers of people who smoke because it leads to heart disease, strokes, cancer and many other fatal diseases
- reducing obesity and improving diet and nutrition because the rapid increase in child and adult obesity over the past decade is storing up very serious health problems for the future if it is not addressed now
- increasing exercise because it reduces the risk of major chronic diseases and premature death: over a third of people are not active enough to benefit their health
- encouraging and supporting sensible drinking because alcohol misuse is associated with deaths from stroke, cancer, liver disease, injury and suicide as well as being related to absenteeism, domestic violence and violent crime
- improving sexual health because risk-taking sexual behaviour is increasing; diagnoses of HIV, chlamydia, genital warts and syphilis have also increased in recent years, and sexually transmitted infections can lead to cancer, infertility and death
- improving mental health because mental well-being is crucial to good physical health, stress is the commonest cause of sickness absence and mental ill-health can lead to suicide.

This demonstrates that obesity, diet, nutrition and exercise are among the government's current public health priorities for England and Wales.

The increasing problem of childhood obesity is also recognised in the recent *National Service Framework (NSF) for Children, Young People and Maternity Services* (DH, 2004a). Health promotion is the first core standard of the NSF, and strategies relating to diet and activity are proposed. The importance of prevention and early intervention is recognised, and the aim is to enable children and young people to make informed choices about healthy lifestyles, thus empowering them to improve their own health. The framework highlights the responsibility of the health sector, schools and other agencies dealing with children's health in helping them achieve this.

More recently, the Department of Health launched *Healthy Weight, Healthy Lives: A cross-government strategy for England*, with this Foreword by Gordon Brown, prime minister:

> In England alone, nearly a quarter of men and women are now obese. The trends for children are even more cause for concern. Almost a fifth of 2 to 5 year-olds are obese, while a further 14 per cent are overweight. The Foresight report indicated that on current trends nearly 60 per cent of the UK population will be obese by 2050: that is almost two out of three in the population defined as severely overweight. If we do not reverse this, millions of adults and children will inevitably face deteriorating health and a lower quality of life and we face spiralling health and social care costs .... Our ambition is that by 2020 we will not only have reversed the trend in rising obesity and overweight among children but also reduced it back to the 2000 levels.

(DH, 2008, iii)

Clearly then, obesity is one of the major contemporary public health concerns in the United Kingdom, and this trend is reflected at a global level. The latest WHO estimates are that approximately 1.2 billion people in the world are overweight, of whom at least 300 million are obese. In some countries, including the United States and the United Kingdom, the rates of obesity have more than doubled in the last 25 years, and being overweight has become the norm for adults. The rate of increase in the United Kingdom is greater than most comparable countries in Europe. Globally, most experts agree that the United States has the greatest problem, with the United Kingdom and Australia not far behind (Foresight, 2007).

The public health workforce

The Department of Health (2001) has identified a broad range of professionals who can and should be involved in promoting health and well-being (see Figure 7.1). At a strategic level, specialists such as public health consultants with a high level of associated knowledge and skills are responsible for developing and leading public health programmes across organisational boundaries. Then there are public health practitioners such as specialist community public health nurses who spend a major part of their time undertaking public health activities, working with individuals, groups and communities to promote and protect their health. Finally, there is a wider workforce of people who have a role in improving health and helping to reduce health inequalities but who might not recognise or fully appreciate their potential contribution. This group includes a wide range of individuals, such as hospital nurses, teachers, community workers, police, local business leaders and health service managers, whose practice should be informed by health improvement principles.

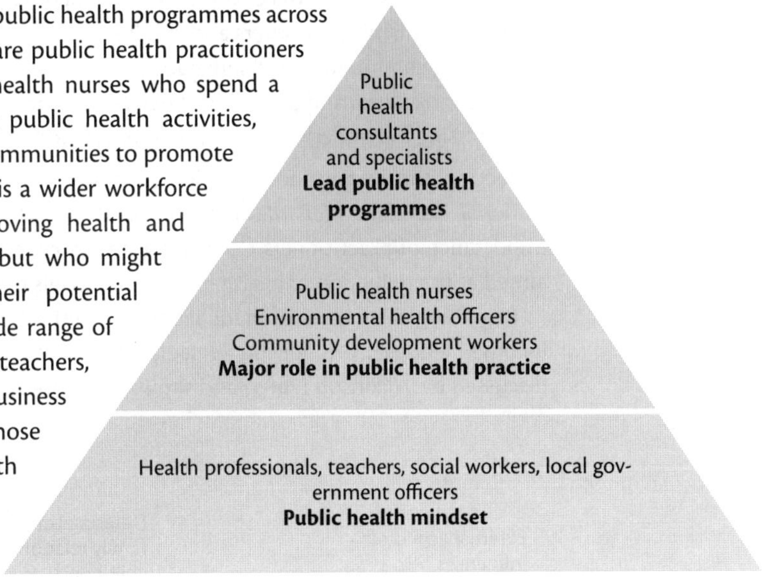

> **(a) Learning activity**
>
> Access the WHO website on www.who.int to explore the global picture relating to overweight and obesity and the WHO's public health response to the issue.

Public health consultants and specialists
Lead public health programmes

Public health nurses
Environmental health officers
Community development workers
Major role in public health practice

Health professionals, teachers, social workers, local government officers
Public health mindset

Figure 7.1 Public health roles

Health inequalities

The term 'health inequalities' refers to the variation in indicators of health, such as incidence of disease, associated with economic status (Ewles, 2005). As far back as 1842, Edwin Chadwick's *General Report on the Sanitary Conditions of the Labouring Population of Great Britain* showed that high rates of disease among the labouring classes were caused by squalid living conditions, and that on average, male heads of these households would not survive to 45 years old, living almost 13 years less than should have been expected.

By 1977, in a report on health inequalities commissioned by the outgoing Labour government, the chairman Sir Douglas Black controversially claimed that:

> The crude differences in mortality rates between the various social classes are worrying. To take the extreme example, in 1971 the death rate for adult men in social class V (unskilled workers) was nearly twice that of adult men in social class I (professional workers) .... Social class differences in mortality begin at birth. In 1971 neo-natal death rates (deaths within the first month of life) were twice as high for the children of fathers in social class V as they were in social class I. Death rates for the post-neo-natal period (from one month up to one year) were nearly 5 times higher in social class V than in

social class I .... it is a major challenge for the next 10 or more years to try to narrow the gap in health standards between different social classes.

(quoted in Ennals, 1977 cited in Aggleton, 1990)

However, following Labour's 1979 election defeat, it was clear that the report's calls for taxation, increased public expenditure and redistribution of wealth would not find favour with the new Conservative government. In fact, the publication of the Black Report over a bank holiday weekend in 1980 by the Thatcher administration, a deliberate attempt to suppress it, signalled the end of political commitment to public health for the next two decades.

Almost 20 years later, following their return to political power, the New Labour government commissioned Sir Donald Acheson to chair a further independent inquiry into health inequalities. Acheson reported that the health inequalities identified by Black had not only persisted, in many areas they had actually increased: 'The gap in health between those at the top and bottom of the social scale has widened, particularly between the mid-1970s and the mid-1990s. This is significantly avoidable and fundamentally unfair' (DH, 1998). As a result, *Tackling Health Inequalities: A programme for action* (DH, 2003) addressed concerns that health and life expectancy continue to be linked to socioeconomic circumstances, and identified four themes for action:

- supporting families, mothers and children
- engaging communities and individuals
- preventing illness and providing effective treatment and care
- addressing the underlying determinants of health.

Reflecting the importance of addressing determinants of health, the *National Standards for the Practice of Public Health* emphasise the importance of practitioners developing health programmes and services aimed at the reduction of health inequalities (Skills for Health, 2004).

Regarding the causes of inequalities in health, the complex effects of income inequality on individuals' social and psychological well-being are discussed by Wilkinson (2005) and shown in Figure 7.2.

> **a) Learning activity**
>
> In your learning group consider the links in Figure 7.2 between economic factors, quality of family life, physical, psychological and social problems. Suggest some possible explanations for them.

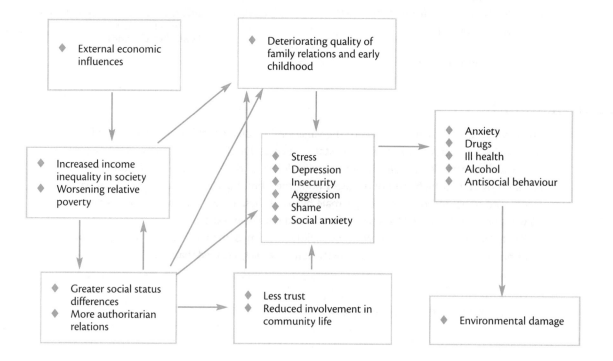

Figure 7.2 The effects of income inequality on social and psychological well-being

Inequality and obesity

There are considerable differences in the levels of obesity experienced according to socioeconomic group. McPherson, Marsh and Brown (2007) highlight the greater prevalence of overweight and obesity in some regions of Britain, including Scotland and the North-East of England, and predict that these will continue rise in the coming decades.

The Department of Health (2004b) identified that obese children, especially girls, are more likely to come from lower social groups. In addition, children who are obese are more likely to become obese adults. This likelihood increases the more obese a child is, as well as increasing if the child's parents are obese. Hence, obesity is a disease associated with deprivation which is likely to perpetuate a cycle of health inequality. There are associated practical constraints since barriers to eating healthy foods, such as fruit and vegetables, include lack of availability, low income, poor transport and lack of cooking knowledge and skills (White, 2003).

Clearly, overweight and obese individuals have much to gain by consulting with healthcare practitioners regarding health concerns. However, social background also appears to have a significant influence on whether or not an individual is likely to consult a doctor. Among women, for example, the ratio of medical consultations to rates of illness in social class 1 is 2.0 compared with 0.7 in social class 5. In other words, women from professional backgrounds are more than twice as likely to consult their GPs (Martin and Henderson, 2001). This may mean that those individuals from lower social classes whose health is most affected by overweight and obesity issues are least likely to seek professional help.

Wall and Owen (1999) are critical that much health promotion rests on the assumption that people are both able and willing to change their behaviour in the interests of promoting health. This, they argue, ignores the limited control people have over housing, income and working conditions, and the way these shape the personal choices they make about lifestyle. In other words, while change is possible, it involves more than willpower to adopt healthy lifestyles.

a Learning activity

Compare the following two sets of guidelines for healthy living. The first is from the government's chief medical officer and the second is a slightly tongue-in-cheek response to it from a public health expert. What message is Gordon trying to convey in his response to Donaldson's 'Ten tips'?

Ten tips for better health (Donaldson, 1999)

1 Don't smoke. If you can, stop; if you can't, cut down.
2 Follow a balanced diet with plenty of fruit and vegetables.
3 Keep physically active.
4 Manage stress, for example, talking things through and making time to relax.
5 If you drink alcohol, do so in moderation.
6 Cover up in the sun and protect children from sunburn.
7 Practise safe sex.
8 Take up cancer screening opportunities.
9 Be safe on the roads: follow the highway code.
10 Learn the First Aid ABC: airways, breathing, circulation.

Alternative ten tips for better health (Gordon, 1999, quoted in Tones and Green, 2004)

1 Don't be poor. If you can, stop. If you can't, don't be poor for long.
2 Don't have poor parents.
3 Own a car.
4 Don't work in stressful, low-paid manual work.
5 Don't live in damp, low-quality housing.
6 Be able to afford to go on a foreign holiday and sunbathe.
7 Practise not losing your job and don't become unemployed.
8 Take up all the benefits you are entitled to if you are unemployed, retired, sick or disabled.
9 Don't live near a busy road or near a polluting factory.
10 Learn how to fill in the complicated housing benefit application forms before you become homeless.

There is considerable variation in many health outcomes between local authorities, and much of this variation is linked with deprivation. Consider the following evidence of links between regional deprivation and obesity taken from the Association of Public Health Observatories (July 2004):

- Between 1994–96 and 2000–02 the national increase in obesity prevalence for males was 5.6 percentage points (36 per cent increase from 1994–96 level) and for women was 4.4 percentage points (25 per cent increase from 1994–96 level).
- In 2000–02, the prevalence of obesity in men was high in the North-East, and low in London.
- In 2000–02, the prevalence of obesity in women was high in the East Midlands and West Midlands and low in the South-East and South-West.

> **Ⓐ Learning activity** ⩁
>
> Access the Department of Health website on www. dh.gov.uk and search for more information about health inequalities and regional differences relating to obesity.

Defining policy

Perhaps the first question that arises is, 'Why do healthcare practitioners need to learn about policy?' The answer is clear. As healthcare practitioners, our working lives and the lives of our clients are defined and controlled by legislation, so studying the policy process can provide a better understanding of the organisations and systems in which we work. According to Abrahamsson (1993), the National Health Service (NHS) is a system, existing to fulfil the needs of a range of stakeholders such as clients, patients, healthcare professionals and the state, which constantly adjusts to environmental pressures and to forces within the system. Hence, the provision of healthcare is an inherently political activity. This means that health and social care professionals need to have a critical awareness of the ways in which legislation influences, and is influenced by, the broader professional, socioeconomic and cultural environment.

The next question might be, 'What exactly is meant by the word policy?' According to the context in which it is used, a policy may refer to different things, including (Palfrey, 2000):

- a piece of legislation
- a formally authorised action
- a process
- a mission statement
- a proposal or protocol
- a statement of intended action.

Using Palfrey's fairly broad definition, it can be seen that healthcare practice could be influenced by policy at a national or 'macro' level through government legislation in the form of white papers, at a middle or 'meso' level by a strategic health authority's formally authorised action plans, and at a local or 'micro' level by mission statements and protocols in the practice area. In this way, a national policy such as *Healthy Weight, Healthy Lives* (DH, 2008) addresses the issue of overweight and obesity at macro level by implementing a Healthy Food Code of Good Practice in partnership with the food and drink industry, at meso level with policies for primary care trusts (PCTs) to submit child measurement data to the NHS Information Centre, and at micro level through schools developing healthy lunchbox policies (FSA, 2003).

> **Ⓐ Learning activity**
>
> It is important that healthcare practitioners understand how macro-level policies influence practice at micro level. In your learning group choose a mission statement or protocol from your practice area and explore the Department of Health website to identify how this local or micro level policy is linked to legislation at national or macro level.

The policy process

Titmuss (1958, cited in Alcock et al, 2001) describes social policy as the study of the social sciences whose object is the improvement of the conditions of life of the individual in the setting of family and group relations. It incorporates the study of health, employment, social services, housing, education and transport policies to name but a few!

Major sectors that play a role in tackling excess weight are (DH, 2008):

- employers
- educational establishments
- local strategic partnerships
- voluntary sector
- institutions (such as prisons)
- the health service
- local government
- media
- public transport
- town planners

- leisure industry
- in-home entertainment
- hospitality industry
- gyms/sports facilities and so on
- food producers
- food retailers
- food manufacturers
- restaurants
- school/work canteens.

The study of social policy further involves the exploration of the values that lie behind policy decisions. This is acknowledged by Easton (1953, cited in Ham, 1999), who states that a policy consists of a web of decisions and actions that allocate values, and in turn, these have an effect on the way in which health and social care is developed and provided. So political activity can be analysed in terms of a system affected by external drivers and containing a number of processes which must remain in balance if the activity is to survive. Easton's (1965, cited in Ham, 1999) model of systems theory (Figure 7.3) is valuable in emphasising the interdependence of the various processes that comprise political activity and showing how they fit together to form a whole. Each element of the model is now analysed in turn.

a Learning activity

It is recognised that policy responds to a range of forces or 'drivers' in the external environment. What drivers can you identify for the current government policies on overweight and obesity?

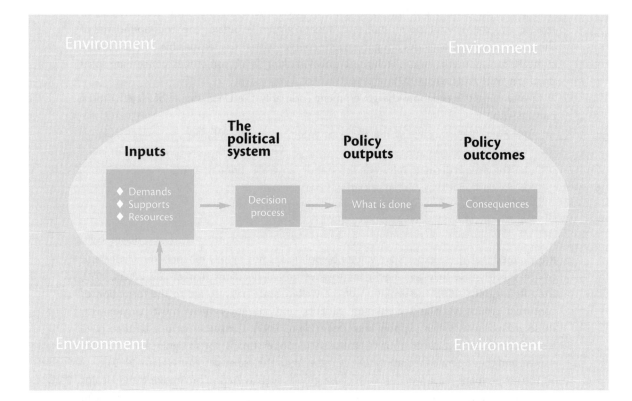

Figure 7.3 Systems theory

Environment

According to Easton's model (Figure 7.3), factors in the external environment that act as drivers for health policy include epidemiological issues such as rising incidence of specific diseases, demographic factors such as shifts in the age of the population with more elderly people requiring healthcare, and technological developments meaning new possibilities for potentially expensive treatment.

To illustrate how the rising incidence of obesity can be an environmental factor that acts as a driver for policy making, consider this epidemiological evidence:

> The government commissioned the Foresight project (2007) which predicted that by the year 2050, around 60 per cent of men and 50 per cent of women could be clinically obese. The cost of overweight and obesity to the NHS is projected to reach £10 billion per year by 2050 and unless there is political intervention, the wider costs to society and business of obesity-related diseases are by then estimated to reach £49.9 billion per year at today's prices.

Clearly, policy makers will respond to such predicted epidemiological changes or drivers in the environment by developing strategies aimed at reducing the rising incidence of obesity as a health problem.

Inputs

Demands involve actions by groups seeking decisive allocation of values from the authorities. It is argued that a group's success depends on its resources and ability to make a political noise (Ham, 1999). Therefore power is not equally dispersed and some groups are able to affect policy more than others. *Pluralism* is the concept in which power is dispersed within society and whereby the activities of the state are checked by the counter-effect of groups. According to Crick (1972), this entails the working of a pluralist system in advanced societies which seeks to maximise the freedom and power of all social groups. No group is without power and no group is dominant, so power is fragmented and diffused. In pluralist societies, pressure groups have grown alongside the formal institutions of government and play an important part in representing the views of specific interests. Pressure groups lie outside the strict boundaries of the system, and their activities bring them into contact with those responsible for the delivery of healthcare, sometimes at the highest policy-making level, sometimes concerning local provision (Wall and Owen, 1999).

In managing the economy the government (primarily the Department of Health) must bargain with:

> Producer Groups such as the National Union of Teachers lobby, the Department of Education and Science, or the British Medical Association .... They are brought together by:
> 1 The group's desire to influence the authoritative allocation of values.
> 2 Government's need for information from groups.
> 3 Government seeking co-operation in implementing policy.
> 4 Group endorsement of policy is important.
>
> (Ham, 1999)

It is claimed that these experts are valued by politicians not merely for their knowledge and advice, but because they give legitimacy to government decisions (Barker and Peters, 1993, cited in Baggott, 2000). The evolution of the welfare state has also led to the formation of consumer groups, such as tenants and patients, and the government must bargain with these groups to win their support and votes (Ham, 1999). Consumer groups tend to have less influence than producer groups because their cooperation is not so significant for policy makers and they operate through influence rather than the use of sanctions (Ham, 1999).

The government must also deal with cause groups such as Action on Smoking and Health (ASH), which campaigns for controls on smoking, and may also have backing from powerful producer groups such as the Royal College of Physicians (Ham, 1999).

Clearly it is difficult to distinguish the complex web of relationships surrounding pressure groups (Popham, 1981, cited in Ham, 1999).

To illustrate the impact of two pressure groups, a producer group which markets infant formula and a cause group which promotes breast feeding, consider this evidence:

> New EU restrictions on the labelling and promotion of infant formula, aimed at improving breastfeeding rates, were due to come into force in January 2008 but were suspended after a legal challenge by infant formula manufacturers. Pressure group 'Baby Milk Action', who back a total ban on advertising of infant formula, issued a counter-challenge stating that parents should be offered unbiased information and support to help them to make healthy choices but that work on breastfeeding is being undermined by commercial promotion.
>
> (Duffy, 2008)

As a result of the dispute, the issue is being scrutinised again by government and a decision has not yet been reached. This demonstrates that the government faces demands from pressure groups with competing political interests, and that in attempting to respond to demands from one group it might provoke demands from another group with a different agenda.

Supports comprise actions such as voting, obeying the law and paying taxes. In turn, payment of direct and indirect taxation provides governments with resources to finance their policy implementation. However, governments must consider the financial implications of their policies and apply taxation with caution, as the public are unlikely to provide support by voting for political parties if they believe that they will be taxed excessively.

The political system

Political decision making is influenced by the inputs mentioned, but the process is shrouded in secrecy, to the point that the conversion of inputs to outputs is often referred to as the black box of decision making.

Policy outputs

Policy outputs are the result of decisions made by the authorities. Generally, they are concerned with what the system does, so services are the most tangible outputs. Outputs may come in the form of white papers such as *Healthy Weight, Healthy Lives* (DH, 2008) which discuss the services to be provided to the population:

> Schools and children's centres will continue to be critical to supporting parents in raising their children. That is why we are both committed to going further. On top of the £1.3 billion of extra investment in school food, schools PE and sport, and play announced both in The Children's Plan and the Comprehensive Spending Review, this strategy sets out plans to introduce compulsory cooking for all 11 to 14 year olds by 2011. This will give all young people the understanding and skills to eat more healthily, skills that will serve them well throughout their life.
>
> (DH, 2008)

Policy outcomes

Policy outcomes are the consequences, intended or unintended, resulting from political action or inaction (Easton, 1965, cited in Ham,1999). Given the impact of policy on people's lives, there is a clear need for critical evaluation of its effects. Critics analyse current policies to comment on whether or not they are likely to achieve their goals, and also evaluate the outcomes of previous policies and highlight their shortcomings. In turn, criticism of policy outputs may feed back into the systems model of policy process as a new demand. As an example, in spring 2004 a report on obesity from the House of Commons Select Health Committee criticised the government for failing to acknowledge the complexity of addressing obesity in the population, and argued that obesity prevention and treatment has not been sufficiently high priority to PCTs. It suggested establishing a strategic framework for prevention and treatment of obesity in the NHS, and in particular recommended screening and increased access to services for children (Magnusson, 2005b). Following this, the government introduced *Supporting Healthy Lifestyles: The National Child Measurement Programme* (DH 2005).

> **a** Learning activity
>
> Consider a recent health policy:
> * What were the outputs or intended consequences of this policy?
> * What were the outcomes or unintended consequences of this policy?

Tackling obesity: a whole systems approach

The Foresight project (2007), commissioned by the government, has taken a strategic 40-year forward look at how society could respond to the obesity epidemic:

> Most adults in the UK are already overweight and modern living ensures that every generation is heavier than the last. Foresight's work indicates that a bold whole system approach is critical – from production and promotion of healthy diets to redesigning the built environment to promote walking, together with wider cultural changes to shift societal values around food and activity. This will require a broad set of integrated policies including both population and targeted measures and must necessarily include action not only by government, both central and local, but also action by industry, communities, families and society as a whole.
>
> (Foresight, 2007)

Policy and professional roles

Policy agendas determine those issues to be addressed by governments and policy makers. Kingdon (1995) argues that agendas are forged through the interaction of problems, politics and participants. In turn, it is suggested that policy agendas are relatively fluid, so participants such as healthcare practitioners can draw attention to the issues that affect them most, and should not be deterred from doing so because the agendas for discussion are often defined according to the needs of politicians. Scott and West (2001) support this view, suggesting that since there is a close relationship between healthcare provision and health policy, healthcare practitioners are well placed to contribute to health policy development, implementation and evaluation.

To do so, all healthcare practitioners must participate in the debates that influence health policy and engage with the policy process, which means they need the skills to analyse health policy and translate it into healthcare practice (Toofany, 2005). As Toofany (2005) observes, healthcare practitioners have ideas about how care can be improved but they need to understand that policy drivers are required to put these ideas into practice; only when ideas are linked to policy are they likely to work. In accordance with this view, Geese (1991) suggests that by attaining a high level of education and belonging to professional organisations, healthcare practitioners will increase their political involvement, and that practitioners with degrees are more likely to be politically active than those without.

Epidemiology

The word 'epidemiology' originates from ancient Greek, with its roots in
epi (upon),
demos (people) and
logos (science). The study of epidemiology can be traced back to the Greek physician Hippocrates, who commented:

> Whoever would study medicine aright must learn of the following subjects. First he must consider the effect of each of the seasons of the year and the differences between

them. Secondly he must study the warm and the cold winds, both those which are common to every country and those peculiar to a particular locality. The effect of water on the health must not be forgotten …

When, therefore, a physician comes to a district previously unknown to him, he should consider both its situation and its aspect to the winds …. Similarly, the nature of the water supply must be considered …. Then think of the soil, whether it be bare and waterless or thickly covered with vegetation and well-watered; whether in a hollow and stifling, or exposed and cold. Lastly consider the life of the inhabitants themselves; are they heavy drinkers and eaters and consequently unable to stand fatigue or, being fond of work and exercise, eat wisely but drink sparely?

(Hippocrates, c. 400 BC cited in Lloyd, 1978:148)

Despite its early origins in ancient Greece, John Snow (1813–1858) is the physician considered the founder of epidemiology in Britain following his work identifying the source of cholera. In August 1854, after investigating an outbreak that occurred in Soho and plotting cases of cholera on a map of the area, Snow was able to identify a water pump as the source of the disease. He had the handle of the pump removed and cases of cholera immediately began to diminish. Sadly, he died before his 'germ' theory of disease became widely accepted in the 1860s.

More recently, epidemiology has been defined as a science concerned with health events in human populations. It studies how states of health are distributed in the population, and examines the environmental conditions, lifestyles or other circumstances associated with the presence or absence of disease (Valanis, 1992). In this way, epidemiologists can be seen as medical detectives concerned with the who, what, where, when and how of disease causation. Last (1987) emphasises that epidemiology studies the distribution and determinants of health-related states and events in defined populations, and the application of this study to the control of health problems.

Determinants refer to the causes and enabling factors of any health-related state. They include:

- **Agent factors** – the presence of infection and toxic agents or the absence of essential nutrients may lead to disease causation.
- **Host factors** – age, sex, ethnicity, genetic make-up, physiological state and nutritional condition determine the susceptibility of the individual to developing disease.
- **Environmental factors** – family size and composition, crowding, hygiene, occupation, geographic and climatic conditions, as well as lifestyle factors such as diet and use of alcohol, drugs or tobacco determine the host's exposure to the specific agent, and in turn their susceptibility. Environmental influences on diet often involve physical ease of access to food and drink, for example, from supermarkets for home consumption, from takeaways and from restaurants. As eating habits become more unstructured, the availability of and access to 'food on the go' is an important consideration.

A range of host and lifestyle determinants, or factors affecting health, are illustrated in Figure 7.4.

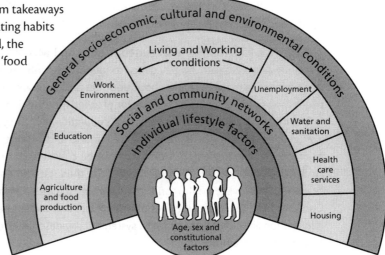

Figure 7.4 Factors impacting on health

Source: Dahlgren and Whitehead (1991).

> **a   Learning activity**
>
> In your interprofessional learning group construct a list of lifestyle factors, or determinants of health, that could predispose individuals to problems of overweight and obesity.

Ultimately, the goals of epidemiology are to prevent or limit the consequences of illness and disability in humans and maximise their state of health (Watterson, 2003). To this end, epidemiological data is collected and used to (Coggon, Rose and Barker, 1997):

- describe the distribution and determinants of health states
- plan and evaluate strategies to prevent illness
- provide a guide to the management of patients with a disease
- measure disease outcomes in a population at risk.

Epidemiological data have identified that in the first half of the twentieth century it was uncommon for individuals to be overweight or obese. Since then it demonstrates that the number of people with persistent, severe weight problems affecting their health has risen steadily, with obesity rates accelerating in the late 1980s and early 1990s. Recent years have seen dramatic changes in the way people live: food is cheaper, more abundant and more convenient than ever; working lives are physically far less demanding; and technological change has given individuals a wealth of new, passive ways to entertain themselves.

Alan Johnson, secretary of state for health as this book went to press, summed up the determinants of obesity succinctly:

> The core of the problem is simple – we eat too much and undertake too little physical activity. The solution is more complex. From the nature of the food that we eat to the built environment through to the way our children lead their lives, it is harder to avoid obesity in the modern environment.
>
> (DH, 2008: vii)

Overall, the epidemiological evidence indicates that the determinants of obesity are complex, encompassing biology and behaviour, but set within a cultural, environmental and social framework. Although personal responsibility plays a crucial part in weight gain, it is acknowledged that human biology is being overwhelmed by the effects of today's 'obesogenic' environment, with its abundance of energy-dense food, motorised transport and sedentary lifestyles. As a result, the people of the United Kingdom are becoming heavier simply by living in the environment of today, a process known as 'passive obesity', and some members of the population, including the most disadvantaged, are especially vulnerable to these conditions (Foresight, 2007).

Health needs assessment

A *need* is the gap between what currently exists and what people could benefit from. *Needs assessment* involves gathering evidence to identify, describe and analyse these gaps and using this evidence to make decisions about priorities and programmes. In health promotion, health needs assessment is the starting point for planned interventions at all levels (Wright, 1999).

Health needs assessment starts with a *population*, which might be defined by geography, age, gender, ethnicity or issue. It is a systematic and explicit process, which identifies the health issues affecting a population that can be changed. Health needs assessment results in clear health priorities for the population. It is then used to create programmes for tackling priorities, improving health and reducing inequalities (Hooper and Longworth, 2002). Choosing health priorities involves using explicit criteria identified from a systematic review of information about the population to systematically describe (Hooper and Longworth, 2002):

- what the problem is

- what can be done about it
- how this can be done.

Each of the following public health strategies or policies has incorporated the process of health needs assessment:

- *Health Survey for England: The health of children and young people* (DH, 2002)
- *National Service Framework for Children, Young People and Maternity Services* (DH, 2004a)
- *Supporting Healthy Lifestyles: The National Child Measurement Programme* (DH, 2005)
- *Forecasting Obesity to 2010* (DH, 2006)
- *Healthy Weight, Healthy Lives: A cross-government strategy for England* (DH, 2008).

In the year 2000, to assist the process of health needs assessment, the government established regional public health observatories (PHOs) to provide information for directors of public health. At the same time the Association of Public Health Observatories (APHO) was established as a network of 12 PHOs working across the five nations of England, Scotland, Wales, Northern Ireland and the Republic of Ireland to provide coordination of PHOs' activities. The regional PHOs and APHO are funded by the Department of Health to deliver the functions of:

- promoting and delivering health intelligence to decision makers to improve health and reduce health inequalities
- acting as advocates for population health information, ensuring that high-quality, relevant information is available to a range of stakeholders
- developing a skilled health intelligence workforce.

In addition to participating in health needs assessment at a population level, healthcare practitioners are also required to assess the health needs of individuals and families. Bradshaw (1972, cited in Perkins, Simnett and Wright, 1999) proposed a four-part typology of needs assessment:

- **Normative need**: defined by professionals, based on judgements about normal levels or values, measured against set standards such as percentile charts or BMI.
- **Felt need**: the individual's own perception of what they want, which is shaped by experience, and depends on the insight that an individual or population has regarding a particular problem.
- **Expressed need**: people say what they need. Clients' expectations or demands are reflected by the use of services, required access and motivation.
- **Comparative need**: some individuals or groups are seen to lack resources others have, or experience greater levels of need or deprivation than the general population.

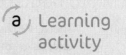

> **Learning activity**
>
> Access the Department of Health website on www. dh.gov.uk to read the executive summary of one of the policy documents mentioned.

> **Learning activity**
>
> Search online to locate your regional PHO and obtain information about the issues of overweight and obesity in your region.
>
> How do levels of overweight and obesity your region compare with national trends?

Part

I

> **Learning activity**
>
> In your learning group use the scenario from the start of the chapter to consider how concepts of need apply to practice:
>
> - Damien has been concerned that he is gaining weight although he is unsure what he should do about it. What type of need is this?
> - Lola's school is in an area of deprivation where many of the children have significant health issues. What type of need is this?
>
> - The school nurse has contacted the family to make them aware that Lola is overweight. What type of need is this?
> - Charlotte has visited the health centre to discuss her concerns about Lola with the general practitioner. What type of need is this?

Health promotion definitions, approaches and models

The WHO has moved the definition of health promotion away from prevention of specific diseases or the detection of risk groups, towards a focus on the health and well-being of whole populations. In this context, health promotion incorporates all measures deliberately designed to promote health and minimise the impact of disease. A major feature of such health promotion, addressed in the first half of this chapter, is the importance of public policy on health, with its potential to achieve social change. A set of guiding principles for health promotion were issued as part of the WHO's commitment to Health for All (WHO, 1985):

- equity
- empowerment
- community participation
- multisectoral collaboration
- emphasis on primary healthcare.

These principles emphasise the WHO's view that health is everybody's business and that public health should involve healthcare practitioners working in partnership with individuals and communities as well as statutory (government) and nonstatutory (independent) organisations working collaboratively. In addition, the principles reflect the WHO's commitment to equity and the reduction of health inequalities.

Ewles and Simnett (1999) highlight the ambiguity that surrounds the terms 'health education' and 'health promotion', an issue confusing to those who are new to this field. Health education has a longer history than health promotion, as it grew out of the public health movement in the nineteenth century, and it has only been overtaken by health promotion in recent decades. Health education is traditionally epidemiologically based, as it focuses mainly on prevention of disease and achieving mortality or morbidity targets. Most health education programmes endeavour to reduce the lifestyle and environmental risk factors responsible for specific diseases, so this approach emphasises narrow medical definitions of health as the absence of disease. Individuals are exposed to information and they are expected to act rationally by changing their lifestyles accordingly. This approach therefore emphasises personal responsibility and the belief that providing information on risky health behaviour may be all that is required.

Since the mid-1970s, however, the health education focus on bringing about individual attitude and behaviour change has been criticised for being too narrow and victim-blaming, so work was done on wider issues such as social policies. This went beyond the scope of traditional health education, and as a result, health promotion became the umbrella term to encompass a broader range of activities: education, prevention and protection. Thus, health promotion comprises efforts at all levels of society to enhance positive health and prevent ill-health. As a result, health promotion features prominently in current policy and is one of the core standards of the *National Service Framework for Children, Young People and Maternity Services* (DH, 2004a). The NSF aims to empower young people to make informed healthy choices about their lifestyle, and emphasises the responsibility of the health service, education and other agencies to work collaboratively.

There are a variety of ways in which health promotion interventions or strategies can be planned, implemented and evaluated. Naidoo and Wills (2000) discuss the five approaches outlined in Table 7.1, which reflect differences in the way that health promotion is conceptualised and practised. In turn, various health promotion models can be analysed to discuss the approaches underpinning them. These approaches are valuable as they enable practitioners to compare and contrast a range of models, evaluating their similarities and differences, strengths and weaknesses.

> **a Learning activity**
>
> Can you identify three key differences between health education and health promotion?

Table 7.1 Approaches to health promotion interventions and strategies

Approach	Aim	Method	Evaluation
Medical or preventive approach	Increase medical interventions aimed at preventing illness and premature death.	Immunisation or screening based on sound epidemiological evidence.	Short-term uptake of screening. Long-term reduction in morbidity and mortality.
Behaviour change or lifestyles approach	Encourage individuals to adopt healthier behaviours.	Expert-led, uses mass media, group or one-to-one communication.	Immediate behaviour change (impact) or longer term (outcome).
Educational approach	Provide information so people can make informed choices.	Develop knowledge, attitudes and skills using media, one-to-one or group techniques.	Measure increases in knowledge, no guarantee that change will take place.
Empowerment and community development approach	Enable people to identify their concerns and gain confidence to act on them.	Client-centred, facilitates identification of concerns, raises self-esteem.	Feelings of empowerment (process). Project aims being met (outcome).
Social change or radical approach	Focus on policy to change physical, social or economic environment.	Top-down approach with consultation and public support.	Legislative change to promote health, for instance a ban on smoking in public.

(a) Learning activity

What health promotion approaches are used in the Counterweight programme described below?

W

Counterweight (http://www.counterweight.org/) is a primary care weight management programme that aims to achieve and maintain medically valuable weight loss of 5–10 per cent in adults aged between 18 and 75. It incorporates a structured pathway and guidance for the management of obesity in primary care settings, and includes training for GPs and practice nurses. The programme recommends initial changes in lifestyle to individuals or groups, and secondary interventions may include the use of anti-obesity medications, referral to a dietician, psychologist and/or a secondary care service. Patients are followed up at least quarterly for 12 months after the programme, and reviewed annually thereafter.

Models of health promotion

Models of health promotion draw upon a diverse range of theories about health, education, psychology, sociology, policy and healthcare practice. Naidoo and Wills (1998) advise that models of health promotion help practitioners to stand back and make sense of the complexity and reality of practice by mapping the strategic choices they face. In their view, different models may:

- map the field of health promotion
- analyse existing practice
- chart the possibilities for interventions.

Hence, it is useful for healthcare practitioners to be aware of a variety of health promotion models as they may provide a framework for planning interventions.

Downie, Tannahill and Tannahill's (1990) model

Downie, Tannahill and Tannahill (1990) propose a model comprising three areas of activity: health education, prevention and protection, which relate to each other in an overall process of health promotion (see Figure 7.5). The model enables practitioners to locate their efforts within the overall schema of health promotion and to consider their potential for overlap with other areas of activity.

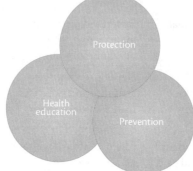

Figure 7.5 Downie and colleagues' model

- **Health education**: communication activity aimed at enhancing well-being and preventing ill health by influencing knowledge and attitudes.
- **Prevention**: comprises medical interventions for primary prevention of the onset of a disease process through risk reduction, secondary prevention of progression of a disease process or other unwanted state through early detection when this favourably affects outcome, and tertiary prevention of avoidable complications of an irreversible, manifest disease or some other unwanted state.
- **Protection**: emphasises legal or fiscal controls, other regulations and policies, and voluntary codes of practice, aimed at the enhancement of positive health and the prevention of ill-health.

Table 7.2 Applications of Downie and colleagues' model

Area of activity	Application to management of overweight and obesity
Health education	'Why weight matters' booklets circulated by the Department of Health to GP surgeries.
Primary prevention	Measuring children in schools
Secondary prevention	Care pathway for management of overweight and obesity in adults
Tertiary prevention	Intra-gastric balloon insertion for the treatment of morbid obesity
Protection	Policies such as *Healthy Weight, Healthy Lives* (DH, 2008) to ensure all schools make cooking a compulsory part of the 11–14 year-old curriculum by 2011

Beattie's (1991) model

Beattie's model (Figure 7.6) comprises four approaches set within two paradigms
- mode of intervention – authoritative or negotiated
- focus of intervention – individual or collective.

The advantage of the Beattie model is that it allows the healthcare practitioner to explore which actions are likely to prove useful in delivering change, and where a particular initiative fits into the overall local and national strategies. It also demonstrates that a coordinated approach is needed to achieve health gains since activities are unlikely to succeed if they do not occur across each of the four approaches. Placing those whose health is affected at the heart of policy is increasingly seen as the best way to ensure sustainable health promotion. Hence, the Beattie model fits well with contemporary government health promotion policy as it emphasises the importance of sound partnership working, with government setting the legislative, resource and policy framework, and with individuals and communities experiencing the most acute health inequalities also playing an active role.

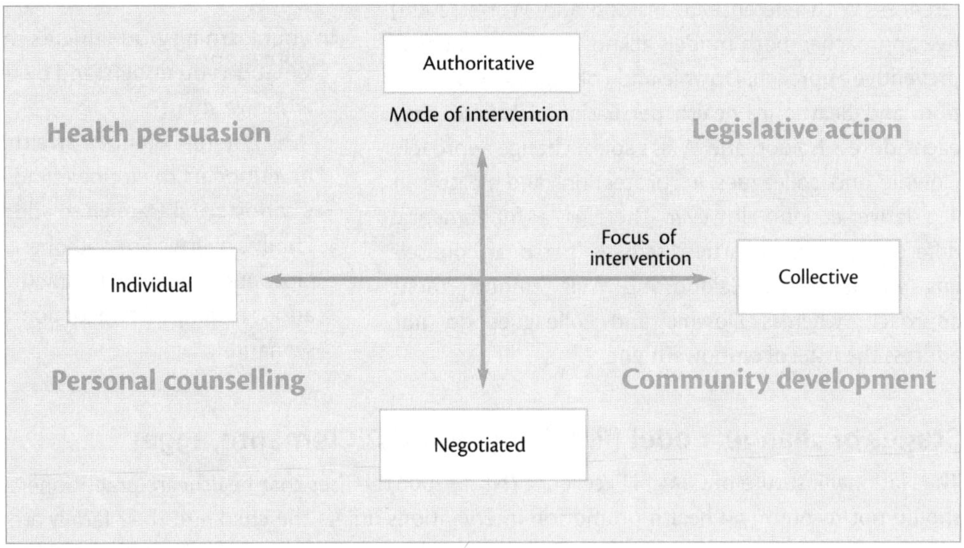

Figure 7.6 Beattie's model

- **Health persuasion**: led by healthcare practitioners and directed at individuals. Deals with evidence-based risk factors and requires the user to change from damaging to safe health behaviours. This approach is useful in the short term, but by itself is unlikely to be effective in the longer term as it is necessary to understand the reasons people engage in unhealthy behaviour before developing effective health promotion strategies.
- **Legislative action**: a top-down approach, with government setting the legislative, resource and policy framework, and healthcare practitioners, individuals and communities also playing an active role. It attempts to redirect behaviour towards healthiness at a macro level but is unlikely to work without wider consultation and support.
- **Personal counselling**: a process of active listening and reflection to empower the individual, based on their current knowledge and behaviour, to become more capable of making genuine choices. Again, this is unlikely to be successful unless there is political commitment to addressing structural or socioeconomic factors affecting the health issue.
- **Community development**: Enables those in similar need to work together to seek changes in their environment as part of a bottom-up rather than top-down approach to regeneration. Empowerment at a community level and community-based action are the goals.

Table 7.3 Applications of Beattie's model

Area of activity	Application to management of overweight and obesity
Health persuasion	General practitioner weighing patient and advising 1000 calorie diet to reduce weight
Legislative action	Policies such as *Healthy Weight, Healthy Lives* (DH, 2008) with resources of £1.3 billion extra investment in school food, school PE, sport and play
Personal counselling	School nurse working with a pupil's concerns on issues of self-esteem and overeating as a coping mechanism
Community development	Community worker supporting local people with the establishment of a food cooperative in a deprived neighbourhood

Analysing the areas of activity and the application to management of overweight and obesity for both the Downie and colleagues (1990) and Beattie (1991) models, it is evident that the models share some common underlying approaches to health promotion as well as having some distinct differences. With reference to Naidoo and Wills's (2000) five approaches, both models acknowledge the medical preventive approach, Downie and colleagues in 'prevention' and Beattie in 'health persuasion'. Likewise, they each address Naidoo and Wills's social change approach, Downie and colleagues in 'protection' and Beattie in 'legislative action'. However, there is a fundamental difference in that Beattie discusses 'personal counselling' which reflects Naidoo and Wills' empowerment approach, whereas Downie and colleagues do not address the issue of empowerment.

ⓐ Learning activity

In your learning group discuss the following:
- What do you understand by the concept of empowerment?
- Why is it important for healthcare practitioners to empower individuals like Charlotte and Damien to address their family's overweight and obesity issues?
- How might healthcare practitioners adopt an empowerment approach in this scenario?

Stages of change model (Prochashka and DiClemente, 1992)

The National Institute of Clinical Excellence (NICE, 2006) advises that healthcare practitioners should not recommend health promotion interventions unless the child and their family are ready to change. They caution that ineffective and ill-timed interventions should be avoided as they may diminish the child's self-esteem and impair future weight loss efforts. Instead, individuals or families who are not yet ready to change should be offered the chance to return for further consultations when they are ready to discuss their weight again, and willing or able to make lifestyle changes. They should also be given information on the benefits of losing weight, healthy eating and increased physical activity (NICE, 2006). This indicates that the timing of health promotion interventions is an important consideration for healthcare practitioners. The significance of readiness for change is acknowledged within the stages of change model (Prochashka and DiClemente, 1992).

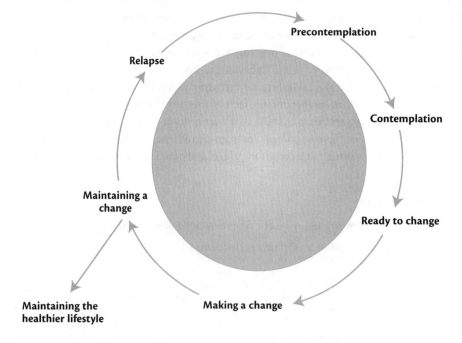

Figure 7.7 Stages of change model

The aim of the model is to encourage changes in health behaviour which would benefit the client. The underpinning assumption is that people go through stages when trying to change or acquire behaviours, but do not go through each in an orderly way. The key to successful interventions is for clients to be motivated, although healthcare practitioners must recognise that clients may not share their views about the benefits of change. Where clients are not ready for change they may consider modification.

The stages are:

- Pre-contemplation: the person has not considered changing their lifestyle or become aware of a risk.
- Contemplation: the individual is aware of the benefits of change but not yet ready to change. They may seek help.
- Ready to change: the individual accepts that the perceived benefits outweigh the costs, and the change seems possible and worthwhile.
- Making the change: the early days of change require a positive decision to behave differently, so clear goals, a realistic plan, support and rewards are features of this stage.
- Maintenance: new behaviour is sustained and the person adopts a healthier lifestyle.
- Relapse: this does not mean failure. A client may go both backwards and forwards through cycles of change.

The Foresight Project (2007:10) claimed that 'Behaviour change is an important component of any response to obesity' and that preventing obesity requires changes in individual, family and group behaviour. NICE (2006) advises that people's ability or willingness to change can be diminished by surprise, anger, denial or disbelief regarding their diagnosis of overweight or obesity. Stressing that obesity is a clinical term with specific health implications, rather than a question of how the individual looks, may help to avoid this reaction. Regarding the effectiveness of change, literature reviews indicate that targeting parents and children together, and involving one parent in a programme, are effective in treating overweight and obese children (Mulvihill and Quigley, 2003). Indeed, Lake (2007) found that more than half the parents involved in a weight-loss programme for children changed their own lifestyle and acted as role models to their offspring.

(C) Professional conversation

Viv, a school nurse comments, 'I find that behavioural techniques such as gradually reshaping food preferences can be used to promote healthier eating. Parents in Charlotte's position tend to believe that their children's food preferences are fixed on unhealthy items like biscuits and chips and that they will be totally resistant to change. In fact, there is research evidence (Robinson, 1999) demonstrating that with greater exposure to certain healthy tastes and lots of encouragement from parents, children such as Lola will eventually increase their liking for fruits and vegetables.'

Attitudes to health

> In Glasgow, death is viewed as imminent, in Canada as inevitable and in California as optional.
>
> (Lewis et al, 2001)

This humorous quote illustrates that individuals may perceive their health status in different ways according to circumstances such as their geographical location, education or social class. Glasgow has some of the most socioeconomically deprived areas in the United Kingdom, and death rates are high, with male life expectancy at birth estimated to be 68.1 years (Glasgow Centre for Population Health, 2008). Contrast this with Canada, where male life expectancy at birth is ten years longer (CIA, 2008). Clearly, these stark differences in life expectancy may cause individuals living in deprived areas to be fatalistic about their health. In the field of health education, sociocognitive theory was used to attempt to predict or explain how individuals respond regarding health issues, and this gave rise to the development of the 'locus of control' concept (Rotter, 1954, cited in Naidoo and Wills, 2000).

Locus of control

Locus of control is concerned with how individuals perceive their ability to control their lives. The underpinning assumption is that people who feel in control are more likely both to care for themselves and to respond positively to health education than those who feel powerless. Locus of control identifies three main categories and the type of responses typically made by people in each category (Rotter, 1954):

- **Internal locus of control**: 'The main thing that affects my health is what I myself do.'
- **Powerful others locus of control**: 'When I recover from an illness it's usually because other people have been taking good care of me.'
- **Chance locus of control**: 'No matter what I do, if I'm going to get sick I will get sick.'

> **a** Learning activity
>
> In your learning group identify how healthcare practitioners might adapt their health promotion approach according to their client's locus of control.

The health beliefs model (Becker, 1974)

The health beliefs model seeks to explain what motivates individuals to engage in disease-prevention activity. Individuals must first perceive that they are susceptible to disease and the condition will have serious consequences. The likelihood of engagement will be modified by a number of factors:

- age, sex, ethnicity, personality, socioeconomic status, knowledge
- perceived threat of disease
- cues to action such as education, symptoms and media information.

The likelihood of action will be further influenced by perceived benefits balanced against perceived barriers to behavioural change. The outcome is the likelihood that individuals will engage in behavioural change (Becker, 1974).

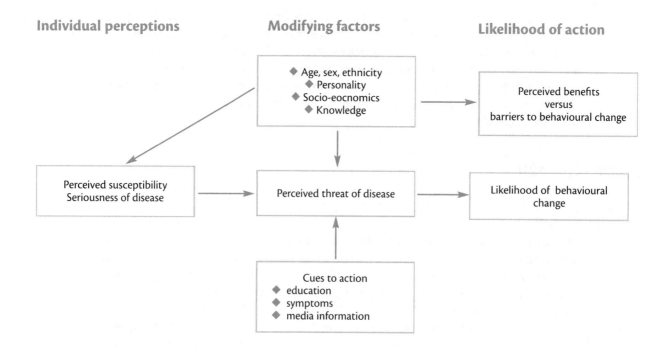

Figure 7.8 The health beliefs model

Men's attitudes to health

As the health beliefs model identifies, attitudes to health are influenced by factors such as age, education, social class, ethnicity and gender. Regarding gender, the Department of Health (2006) predicts that three in four men will be obese by 2010. Abdominal fat is the type most harmful to health, and is linked to increased risk of heart disease, circulatory problems, type 2 diabetes and cancer (Royal College of Physicians, 2004). Excess abdominal adiposity is generally defined as a man's waist measuring over 101.5 cm (Muckle, 2007). Yet it is recognised that men have a distorted view of their own body and therefore tend to grossly underestimate their waist size.

Research undertaken by McCreary and Sadava (2001) indicates that, in comparison with the views expressed by overweight women, overweight men think they are healthier, more attractive and report higher levels of life satisfaction. As a result, they may be at serious risk of overweight and obesity-related problems but lack awareness of the issues. In addition, it is argued that even when they are aware of health concerns, male ego and fear prevent many men from coming forward to utilise health promotion services (Harrison, 2007).

> ### ⟲ a ⟳ Learning activity
>
> In your interprofessional learning group, apply the health beliefs model to Damien's scenario to highlight any modifying factors. Identify how a healthcare practitioner, such as the practice nurse or occupational health nurse, might address his perception of severity and susceptibility to increase the likelihood of his taking action to improve his health.

The Foresight Project (2007) claims that in modern societies there is psychological conflict for individuals between the fatty, sweet foods and alcohol that they want to consume and their desire to be healthy and slim. These mixed feelings and beliefs about healthy lifestyles complicate individual choices, since most people know that eating fatty foods in excess is generally bad for them while taking exercise is generally beneficial. Yet they still tend to enjoy eating foods that are high in calories or contain excessive salt, and find it difficult to make time to exercise.

In accordance with the health beliefs model, the role of the healthcare practitioner is to encourage individuals to consider the benefits of adopting a healthier lifestyle and to support them in overcoming barriers. To do this, healthcare practitioners such as GPs, practice nurses, health visitors, school nurses and occupational health nurses might draw attention to the susceptibility of individuals who are overweight or obese and to the severity of associated diseases. NICE (2006) advice suggests showing parents and young people where their measurements are plotted on a BMI chart so that they can recognise the extent of the problem. A diagnosis of overweight and obesity is not just concerned with weight, it is important to calculate the proportion of body fat and its relative contribution to overall body weight, which can be gauged using BMI, a skinfolds measure and waist circumference (Magnusson, 2005a).

NICE (2006) has developed the pathways shown in Figures 7.9 and 7.10 to identify how staff in GP surgeries and hospitals should assess whether people are overweight or obese, and advise what staff should do to help people lose weight. NICE guidance on public health covers England; for information relating to other countries in the United Kingdom please visit the accompanying website.

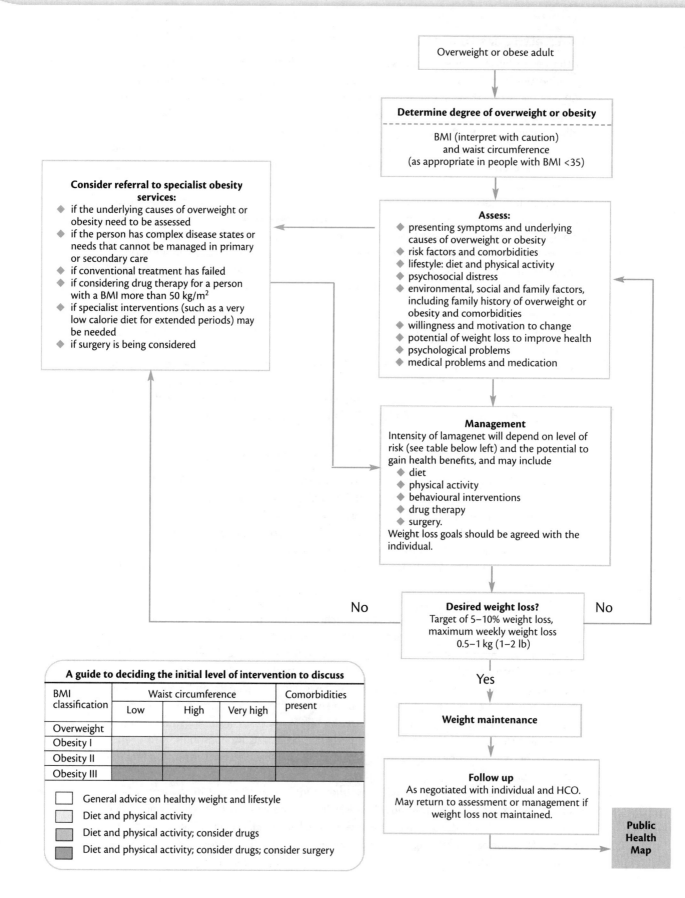

Figure 7.9 Clinical care pathway for adults

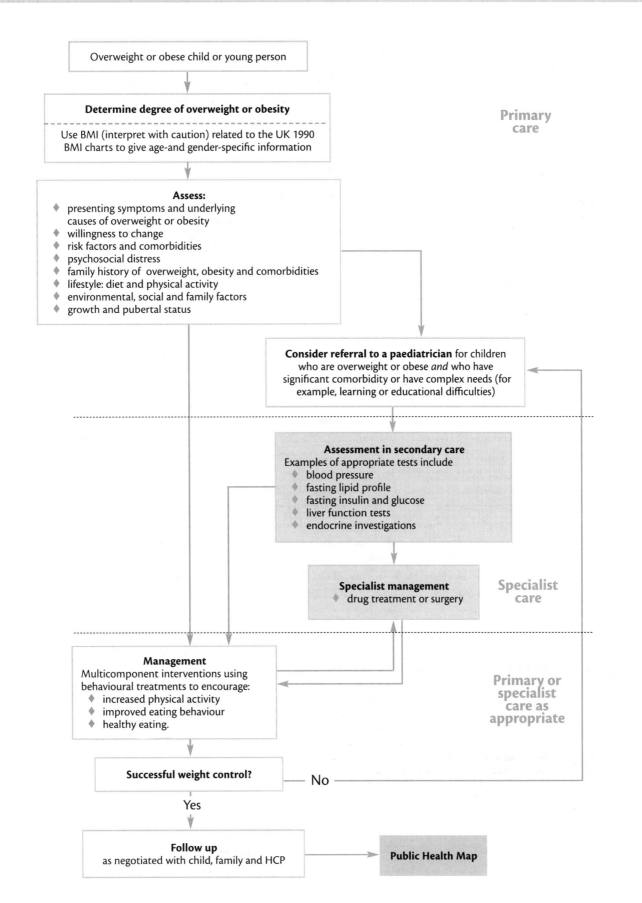

Figure 7.10 Clinical care pathway for children

a Learning activity

Using the NICE (2006) clinical care pathways for adults (Figure 7.9) and for children (Figure 7.10), formulate plans for assessing and managing Damien's obesity problem and Lola's overweight problem.

Overweight and obesity issues in children

The *Health Survey for England* (DH, 2002) reported that 21.8 per cent of boys and 27.5 per cent of girls aged 2–15 years were either overweight or obese, and that the prevalence had increased from 1995 to 2002. Of these obese children and adolescents, 20–25 per cent were found to have impaired glucose tolerance, and evidence suggests that insulin resistance syndrome, previously associated with obesity in adults, is occurring in children (Goran, Ball and Cruz, 2003). Furthermore, it is recognised that obese adolescents are more likely to become obese adults (Freedman et al, 2005).

c Professional conversation

Nadeem, a practice nurse comments, 'I find that measurement for overweight and obesity in children and adults can be confusing. Using centile charts for children, scores over the 85th centile are considered overweight and over the 95th centile obese. In adults, body mass index is most commonly used: a BMI of >25 is overweight and >30 obese. Yet, BMI is criticised for not differentiating between fat and lean mass, so a person with a large amount of muscle may be incorrectly identified as obese. Skinfold callipers can be used to measure the breadth of a fold of skin so subcutaneous fat levels can be compared with standard tables to assess body fat content. Although skinfold is a valid measure of body fat it is used cautiously with children as it can be difficult to do and can be intimidating for the child. Waist measurement is also important, as fat accumulated around the waist is known to have greater implications for health than fat in other areas, and abdominal obesity has been associated with cardiovascular risk factors. Centiles for waist circumference in children have been developed, and together with BMI may be used to establish increased risk. To ensure that I am following correct procedures that use the latest evidence base, I always refer to current NICE guidelines.'

Practice nurses, and specialist community public health nurses such as health visitors and school nurses, are ideally placed to provide evidence-based physical, psychological and emotional support and monitoring to those living with overweight or obesity who want to improve their health and well-being (Muckle, 2007). It is suggested that a loss of 10 per cent of total body weight over a six-month period is an appropriate goal because it is achievable, has health benefits and can be maintained (National Institute for Health, 1998). However, where children are still growing and developing, weight maintenance may be a more appropriate goal than weight loss (Scottish Intercollegiate Guidelines Network, 2003).

Ways to help children achieve the recommended one hour of daily activity

With parents:
- walking or cycling to school
- walking the dog
- trips to the local playground or nature trail.

In the local park:
- football
- cricket
- frisbee
- running
- skipping
- hide and seek.

At the leisure centre:
- swimming
- gymnastics
- badminton or tennis
- climbing walls
- skateboarding.

Source: DH (2007).

W For further information visit: www.playgroundfun.org.uk; www.activeplaces.com

Prejudice and stigmatisation

Negative health outcomes resulting from overweight and obesity may be psychological as well as physical, since it is acknowledged that obesity is a highly stigmatised condition associated with negative stereotypes, prejudice and discrimination (Brown, 2008). Stigmatisation begins early in life. Overweight children are subject to bullying in school and are even perceived by teachers as less intelligent than their peers (Janssen et al, 2004). By early adolescence, obese young people have significantly lower self-esteem than their slimmer peers, with associated feelings of sadness, loneliness and nervousness (Strauss, 2000).

It is argued that obese people suffer prejudice, discrimination and stigmatisation at all levels of social functioning (Sobal and Stunkard, 1989). Negative stereotypes of obese people may portray them as lazy, greedy, unintelligent, lacking in self-discipline and unattractive (Puhl and Brownell, 2001). Research has even demonstrated that overweight and obese individuals face prejudice from healthcare practitioners who have deeply ingrained negative attitudes towards this client group (Brown, 2006). In fact, Puhl and Brownell (2006) found that contact with doctors headed a list of situations in which individuals felt most stigmatised. Clearly, unless healthcare practitioners challenge and address prejudice and stigmatisation against overweight and obese individuals, it is unlikely that they will be seen as the source of support envisaged in current public health policy.

Ethical issues in health promotion

'Ethically managing self, people and resources to improve health and wellbeing' is one of the national occupational standards established for public health practitioners by Skills for Health, the organisation that develops NHS workforce competences (Skills for Health, 2004). Therefore, it is important that healthcare practitioners are aware of ethical concepts and their application to public health practice. You can also read about this in Chapter 4.

Historically, ethics is the formal study of the principles on which moral rules and values are based. The two main forms of ethical reasoning are *deontology* and *consequentialism*. Consequentialism may be concerned primarily with the needs of individuals themselves (egoism) or the needs of other individuals (altruism). *Utilitarianism* is a branch of consequentialism concerned with the needs of the wider society, rather than individuals. The main features of these three forms of ethical decision making are:

Deontology

- Concerned with means rather than ends.
- There are universal moral rules that individuals have a duty to follow.
- Derives the rightness or wrongness of an act from the character of the act itself rather than the outcomes.
- A moral individual must always do their duty regardless of the outcome.
- By obeying the rules, individuals are always doing the right thing irrespective of the consequences.

Consequentialism

- Concerned with ends rather than means.
- The consequences of an act make it ethically right or wrong.
- The rightness or wrongness of an act should be judged on whether it produces more benefits than disadvantages.
- Egoism; consequences for the individual themselves matter more than any other result.
- Altruism; individuals should take actions that have the best consequences for others, not themselves.

Utilitarianism

- Concerned with the effects of an action on the wider society, aimed at producing the most good for the greatest number.

- An act is morally right if, and only if, it maximises social utility.
- The act is right if, given the available alternatives, it is the one that produces the best balance of positive over negative consequences.
- An action is morally right if the consequences are more favourable than unfavourable to everyone.
- Takes account of results not motives, considering both long-term and short-term consequences.

Beauchamp and Childress (2001) highlight the limitations of applying past ethical reasoning to complex modern healthcare settings, and have developed four principles to show how ethical theory can illuminate problems in contemporary healthcare:

- Autonomy: respect the decisions of autonomous individuals.
- Beneficence: provide benefits, and balance benefits against risks.
- Nonmaleficence: Avoid causing harm.
- Justice: show fairness in the distribution of benefits and risks.

Autonomy

This concept derives from the Greek term 'autonomous' meaning self-rule, and refers to a person's capacity to choose freely and be able to direct their own life. Clearly, individuals do not live in isolation so there will be restrictions on individual freedom. The autonomous person must have a sense of responsibility regarding the effects of their actions upon others.

According to Naidoo and Wills (2000), autonomy is constrained by:

- reason and the ability to make rational choices
- the ability to understand one's environment
- the ability to act on one's environment.

Hence, autonomy is not absolute but is attainable to a greater or lesser extent.

> **(a) Learning activity**
>
> In your learning group discuss which individuals or groups in society might experience difficulty in exercising autonomy and why.

Seedhouse (1998) identifies that autonomy is a central consideration when working for health, and distinguishes between creating autonomy and respecting autonomy. *Creating autonomy* is making efforts to improve the quality of people's autonomy by enhancing what they are able to do and enabling them to make informed choices. To make informed choices, individuals must fully understand the potential consequences of their actions, for both themselves and others. In order to create autonomy, the healthcare practitioner may need to educate individuals about health issues and the potential implications of their lifestyle choices.

Respecting autonomy involves agreeing to the wishes of the individual and respecting their choice whether or not you approve of it, unless it is against the interests of others. Respecting autonomy involves recognising people's rights and dignity. In the context of health promotion, this means that the relationship with clients is based on respect for them as unique individuals with freedom to make informed choices.

These two concepts are closely linked, as individuals cannot express free wishes if they are not aware of the possibilities open to them. In this instance it may be ethically justifiable not to respond to clients' initial expressed wishes, but to attempt to create autonomy by offering health education and opening up other options (Naidoo and Wills, 2000). In order to avoid victim blaming, or seeing individuals as solely responsible for their own health, health promoters must also recognise factors, such as social or economic circumstances, which limit clients' autonomy.

Beneficence

Beneficence concerns the fact that healthcare professionals should act to benefit the patient. This principle may clash with the principle of respect for autonomy when the patient makes a decision that you think will not be beneficial and is not in the patient's best interests.

Nonmaleficence

Nonmaleficence refers to avoiding or preventing harm. Healthcare practitioners avoid harm by observing the principle of informed consent as part of their duty to care. You should ensure that clients are informed of and understand the implications of their behaviour, as well as having information about action that would be beneficial.

Justice

Justice is traditionally seen to incorporate:
- the fair distribution of scarce resources
- respect for individual and group rights
- following morally acceptable laws.

Justice requires that people are treated equally, but the concept is elusive. Equal treatment may mean allocating resources according to (Naidoo and Wills, 2000):
- equal need
- equal ability
- equal contribution.

The NHS was established to provide free medical care to those who need it, but demand far outweighs available resources. Need is an obvious criterion for distributing care, yet it is difficult to apply objective measurement in the assessment of care needs, and the process invariably involves making subjective value judgements (Naidoo and Wills, 2000). Sir Douglas Black (1994, cited by Robinson and Elkan, 1996) argued that:

> We need a balance between what should be done in terms of need; what can be done at a practical level; and what can be afforded … meeting health needs is a moral or ethical question, what we as a society value and what goals or outcomes we desire to bring about.

Clearly, there may be tension between the basic ethical principles when they are to be applied in practice. Seedhouse (1998) has attempted to address the complexity of practice situations by developing an ethical grid, a theoretical framework divided into four levels in order to assist healthcare practitioners consider all aspects of their ethical decision making (see Figure 7.11).

- The innermost box (respect persons equally/respect autonomy/serve needs first/create autonomy, which Seedhouse refers to as the blue layer) represents central conditions in working for health, with core foundations such as creating and respecting autonomy. At least one of the four core elements should be used in any healthcare deliberation.
- The next box (Seedhouse's red layer, keep promises/tell the truth/minimise harm; do most positive good) addresses the duties and motives of the healthcare worker. By incorporating key principles such as telling the truth and keeping promises, it corresponds with the deontological perspective.
- The third box (Seedhouse's green layer) divides consequentialism into four key areas (most beneficial outcomes for the individual/most beneficial outcomes for oneself/most beneficial outcomes for a particular group/most beneficial outcomes for society) and helps practitioners to prioritise by considering the outcome to be achieved for self, the individual, others or society. The needs of an individual or group may need to be sacrificed for the good of the wider society.
- The fourth, outer box (Seedhouse's black layer) represents the influence of external considerations such as evidence base, codes of practice and the law. In reality, legal considerations may define the course of action and take decision making away from the practitioner.

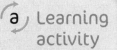

Learning activity

With a colleague, debate the following ethical issues:
- Should an obese boy be removed from the care of his parents if they refuse to restrict his dietary intake?
- Should healthcare practitioners place an obese long-term mental health patient on a restricted diet against her wishes?

Learning activity

With a colleague, debate the following ethical issues:
- Is it ethical to refuse IVF to a woman because she is overweight?
- An obese man fails to stick to a reducing diet. Is it justifiable to refuse surgery until he loses weight?

Part

I

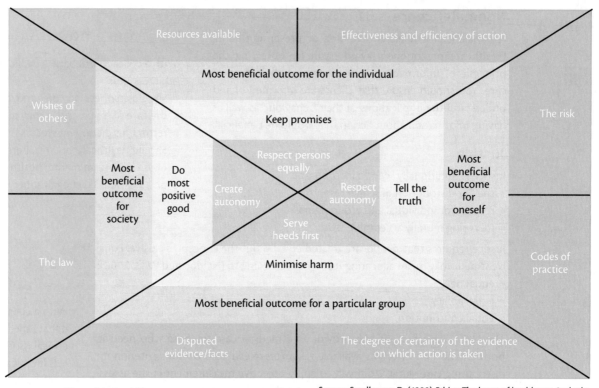

Figure 7.11 **The ethical grid**   Source: Seedhouse, D. (1998) *Ethics: The heart of healthcare*, 2nd edn, Chichester, John Wiley. Reprinted with kind permission of Wiley Blackwell

The intention is not for healthcare practitioners to work through the ethical grid in any systematic way, but for it to be used to stimulate the questioning of values and encourage analysis of complex clinical scenarios from a variety of perspectives.

> **ⓐ Learning activity**
>
> Apply the Seedhouse grid to analyse a clinical scenario from your practice and try to identify any ethical issues.

Conclusion

In summary, this chapter has demonstrated that public health uses policy to create healthy environments and empower people to improve their health. In the nineteenth century, the major threats to public health came from diseases related to deprivation and poor sanitary conditions. Today, despite increased overall wealth, public health problems remain closely linked to inequality, so public health practice is still focused on addressing the socioeconomic determinants of health.

Obesity has emerged as a global threat to public health, and is therefore the target of recent UK government policy. After identifying that policy affects healthcare at all levels, the chapter used systems theory to analyse environmental drivers and inputs to the political system and demonstrate that policy outputs may have outcomes, or consequences, that do not reflect the original intentions. Therefore, a whole systems approach, incorporating the efforts of individuals, families, communities, voluntary groups, industry and government, will be needed to address the predicted obesity epidemic.

Epidemiology, the study of health events, was explored to demonstrate the determinants leading to increased incidence of overweight and obesity. The process of health needs assessment was used to demonstrate how agencies such as public health observatories provide information for healthcare practitioners who are involved in making decisions about priorities and needs.

Discussion then focused on a range of health promotion models and their underpinning approaches. The Downie and colleagues and Beattie models were contrasted to highlight the former's emphasis on medical prevention and the latter's concern with individual and community empowerment. Behaviour change models, in the form of stages of change and health beliefs, were then analysed to suggest strategies for managing overweight and obesity.

Finally, current NICE care pathways were introduced and ethical frameworks were analysed to emphasise the importance of concepts such as autonomy and justice in the promotion of health with overweight and obese individuals.

References

Abrahamsson. A (1993) *The Logic of Organisations*, London, Sage.

Adams, L., Amos, M. and Munro, J. (eds) (2002) *Promoting Health: Politics and practice*, London, Sage.

Aggleton, P. (1990) *Health*, London, Routledge.

Alcock, P., Glennerster, H., Oakley, A. and Sinfield. A. (2001) *Welfare and Wellbeing: Richard Titmuss's contribution to social policy*, London, Polity Press.

Ashton, J. and Seymour, H. (1988) *The New Public Health*, Milton Keynes, Open University Press.

Association of Public Health Observatories (2004) *Indications of Public Health in the English Revions*, Vol. 1, No. 2 [online] www.apho.org.uk/resource/item.aspx?RID=39362 (accessed 8 January 2009).

Baggott, R. (2000) *Public Health: Policy and politics*, Basingstoke, Macmillan.

Beattie. A. (1991) 'Knowledge and control in health promotion: a test case for social policy and social theory', in Gabe, J., Calnan, M. and Bury, M. (eds), *The Sociology of the Health Service*, London, Routledge.

Beauchamp, T. and Childress, J. (2001) *Principles of Biomedical Ethics*, 5th edn, Oxford, Oxford University Press.

Becker (1974) *The Health Belief Model and Personal Health Behaviour*, New Jersey, Thorofare.

Brown. I. (2006) 'Nurses' attitudes towards adult patients who are obese: literature review', *Journal of Advanced Nursing* **53**(2), 221–32.

Brown. I. (2008) 'Images of obesity', *Community Practitioner* **81**(3), 14–15.

Central Intelligence Agency (CIA) (2008) *The World Factbook* [online] https://www.cia.gov/library/publications/download/ (accessed 8 January 2009)

Coggon, D., Rose, G. and Barker, D. (1997) *Epidemiology for the Uninitiated*, 4th edn, London, BMJ Publications.

Crick, B. (1972) *In Defence of Politics*, 2nd edn, Chicago, University of Chicago Press.

Dahlgren, G. and Whitehead, M. (1991) *Policies and Strategies to Promote Social Equity in Health*, Stockholm, Institute of Futures Studies.

Department of Health (DH) (1998) *Independent Inquiry into Inequalities in Health* (The Acheson Report), London, DH.

DH (2001) *The Report of the Chief Medical Officer's Project to Strengthen the Public Health Function*, London, DH.

DH (2002) *Health Survey for England: The health of children and young people*, London, DH.

DH (2003) *Tackling Health Inequalities: A programme for action*, London, DH.

DH (2004a) *National Service Framework for Children, Young People and Maternity Services*, London, DH.

DH (2004b) *Choosing Health: Making healthy choices easier*, London, DH.

DH (2005) *Supporting Healthy Lifestyles: The National Child Measurement Programme*, London, DH.

DH (2006) *Forecasting Obesity to 2010*, London, DH.

DH (2007) 'Why your child's weight matters', London, DH.

DH (2008) *Healthy Weight, Healthy Lives: A cross-government strategy for England*, London, DH.

Department of Health and Social Security (DHSS) (1980) *Inequalities in Health: Report of a research working party* (The Black Report), London, DHSS.

Donaldson, L. (1999) 'Ten tips for better health' in DH, *Our Healthier Nation*, London, DH.

Douglas, J., Earle, S., Handsley, S., Lloyd, C. and Spurr, S. (2007) *A Reader in Promoting Public Health: Challenge and controversy*, London, Sage /Open University.

Downie, R., Tannahill, C. and Tannahill, A. (1990) *Health Promotion: Models and values*, Oxford, Oxford University Press.

Duffy. J. (2008) 'Legal challenge to baby-milk law', *Sunday Herald*, 20 January.

Ewles, L. (ed.) (2005) *Key Topics in Public Health: Essential briefings on prevention and health promotion*, Edinburgh, Elsevier Churchill Livingstone.

Ewles, L. and Simnett, I. (1999) *Promoting Health: A practical guide*, London, Bailliere Tindall.

Food Standards Agency (2003) *School Lunchbox Survey* [online] www.foodstandards-gov-uk/news/newsarchive/lunchboxes (accessed 8 January 2009).

Foresight (2007) *Tackling Obesities: Future choices*, Project Report, 2nd edn, London, Government Office for Science.

Freedman, D., Khan, L., Serdula, M., Dietz, W., Scrinivasan, S. and Bereson, G. (2005) 'The relation of childhood BMI to adult adiposity: the Bogalusa Heart Study', *Paediatrics* **115**, 22–7.

Geese, T. (1991) 'Political participation behaviours of nurse-midwives', *Journal of Nurse Midwifery* **36**(3), 184–91.

Glasgow Centre for Population Health (GCPH) (2008) *A Community Health and Wellbeing Profile for East Glasgow*, Glasgow, GCPH.

Goran, M., Ball, G. and Cruz, M. (2003) 'Obesity and risk of type 2 diabetes and cardiovascular disease in children and adolescents', *Journal of Clinical Endocrinology and Metabolism* **88**(4), 1417–27.

Gormley, K. (ed.) (1999) *Social Policy and Healthcare*, London, Churchill Livingstone.

Ham, C. (1999) *Health Policy in Britain*, 4th edn, Basingstoke, Palgrave.

Harrison, A. (2007) 'Health of men – weight management partnership', *Community Practitioner* **80**(9), 31–4.

Hooper, J. and Longworth, P. (2002) *Health Needs Assessment Workbook*, London, Health Development Agency [online] www.hda.nhs.uk (accessed 8 January 2009).

House of Commons Select Health Committee on Obesity (2004) *Third Report of Session 2003–04*, London, The Stationery Office.

Janssen, I., Craig, W., Boyce, W. and Pickett, W. (2004) 'Associations between overweight and obesity with bullying behaviours in school-aged children', *Paediatrics* **113**(5), 1187–94.

Kingdon, J. (1995) *Agendas, Alternatives and Public Policies*, 2nd edn, London. Harper Collins.

Lake, K. (2007) 'Family intervention and therapy for overweight and obese kids', *Community Practitioner* **80**(6), 10–12.

Last, J. (1987) *Public Health and Human Ecology*, London, Prentice-Hall.

Lewis, S., Donaldson, C., Mitton, C. and Currie, G. (2001) 'The future of healthcare in Canada', *British Medical Journal* **323**: 926–9.

Lloyd, G. E. R. (1978) *Hippocratic Writings*, Oxford, Blackwell.

Magnusson, J. (2005a) 'Childhood obesity: diagnosis, prevalence and implications for health', *Community Practitioner* **78**(2), 66–8.

Magnusson, J. (2005b) 'Childhood obesity: prevention, treatment and recommendations for health', *Community Practitioner* **78**(4), 147–9.

Martin, V. and Henderson, E. (2001) *Managing in Health and Social Care*, London, Routledge.

McCreary, D. and Sadava, S. (2001) 'Gender differences in relationships among perceived attractiveness, life satisfaction and health in adults as a function of body mass index and perceived weight', *Psychology of Men and Masculinity*, **2**, 108–16.

McPherson, K. Marsh, T. and Brown, M. (2007) 'Modelling future trends in obesity and the impact on health', in Foresight, *Tackling Obesities: Future Choices* [online] http://www.foresight.gov.uk (accessed 8 January 2009).

Muckle, S. (2007) 'An evaluation of a primary care-based weight management initiative', *Community Practitioner* **80**(7), 20–3.

Mulvihill, C. and Quigley, R. (2003) 'The management of obesity and overweight: an analysis of reviews of diet, physical activity and behavioural approaches', Evidence briefing 1st edn, London, Health Development Agency.

Naidoo, J. and Wills, J. (1998) *Practising Health Promotion*, London, Bailliere Tindall.

Naidoo, J. and Wills, J. (2000) *Health Promotion: Foundations for practice*, 2nd edn, London, Bailliere Tindall.

Naidoo, J. and Wills, J. (2005) *Public Health and Health Promotion: Developing practice*, 2nd edn, London, Bailliere Tindall.

National Audit Office (NAO) (2001) *Tackling Obesity in England*, London, NAO.

National Institute of Clinical Excellence (NICE) (2006) 'Obesity: the prevention, identification, assessment and management of overweight and obesity in adults and children' [online] http://guidance.nice.org.uk/CG43/?c=296726 (accessed 8 January 2009).

National Institute for Health (1998) *National Heart, Lung and Blood Institute Clinical Guidelines on the Identification, Evaluation and Treatment of Overweight and Obesity in Adults* [online] www.nhlbi.nih.gov/publications (accessed 8 January 2009).

Palfrey, C. (2002) *Key Concepts in Healthcare Policy and Planning*, Basingstoke, Macmillan.

Perkins, R., Simnett, I. and Wright, L. (eds) (1999) *Evidence-Based Health Promotion*, Chichester, John Wiley.

Prochaska, J. and DiClemente, C (1992) *Stages of Change in the Modification of Problem Behaviors*, Thousand Oaks, Calif., Sage.

Puhl, R. and Brownell, K. (2001) 'Bias, discrimination and obesity', *Obesity Research* **9**, 788–805.

Puhl, R. and Brownell, K. (2006) 'Confronting and coping with weight stigma: an investigation of overweight and obese adults', *Obesity* **14**(10), 1802–15.

Robinson, J. and Elkan, R. (1996) *Health Needs Assessment*, London, Churchill Livingstone.

Robinson, T. (1999) 'Behavioural treatment of childhood and adolescent obesity', *International Journal of Obesity* **23**(2), 52–7.

Rotter, J. (1954) *Social Learning and Clinical Psychology*, New York, Prentice Hall.

Royal College of Physicians (RCP) (2004) *Storing Up Problems: The medical case for a slimmer nation*, London. RCP.

Scott, C. and West, E. (2001) 'Nursing in the public sphere: health policy research in a changing world', *Journal of Advanced Nursing* **33**(3), 387–95.

Scottish Intercollegiate Guidelines Network (2003) Management of Obesity in Children and Young People, Edinburgh, Scottish Intercollegiate Guidelines Network.

Seedhouse, D. (1998) *Ethics: The heart of healthcare*, 2nd edn, Chichester, John Wiley.

Skills for Health (2004) *National Occupational Standards for the Practice of Public Health Guide*, Bristol, Skills for Health.

Sobal, J. and Stunkard, A. (1989) 'Socioeconomic status and obesity: a review of the literature', *Psychological Bulletin* **105**, 260–75.

Strauss, R. (2000) 'Childhood obesity and self-esteem', *Paediatrics* **105**(1),15.

Tones, K. and Green, G. (2004) *Health Promotion: Planning and strategies*, London, Sage.

Toofany, S. (2005) 'Nurses and health policy', *Nursing Management* **12**(3), 26–30.

Valanis, B. (1992) *Epidemiology in Nursing and Healthcare*, 2nd edn, Connecticut, Appleton and Lange.

Wall, A. and Owen, B. (1999) *Health Policy*, East Sussex, Gildredge Press.

Wanless , D. (2004) *Securing Good Health for the Whole Population (Wanless Report)*, London, HMSO.

White, J. (2003) 'Barriers to eating five-a-day fruit and vegetables', *Community Practitioner* **76**(10), 377–80.

Wilkinson, R. (2005) *The Impact of Inequality*, London, Routledge.

World Health Organisation (WHO) (1974) *Alma Ata Declaration*, Geneva, WHO.

WHO (1985) *Targets for Health for All*, Copenhagen, WHO Regional Office for Europe.

WHO (1986) *Ottawa Charter for Health Promotion*, Geneva, WHO.

Wright, L. (1999) 'Health Promotion Needs Assessment', in Perkins, R., Simnett, I. and Wright, L. (eds), *Evidence-Based Health Promotion*, Chichester, John Wiley.

Websites

www.dh.gov.uk/PolicyAndGuidance/HealthAndSocialCareTopics/Obesity/

www.fatmanslim.com

www.wiredforhealth.comed

Chapter

8

Healthcare governance

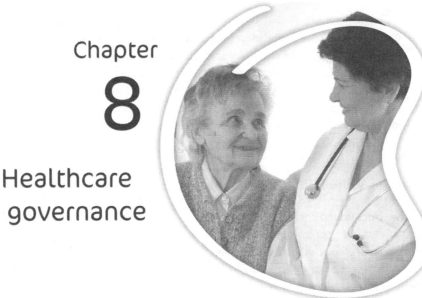

Alan Glasper and Rory Farrelly

 Links to other chapters in *Foundation Studies for Caring*

- 2 Interprofessional learning
- 3 Evidence-based practice and research
- 4 Ethical, legal and professional issues
- 16 Safeguarding children
- 17 Safeguarding adults
- 35 Complementary and alternative medicines

 Links to other chapters in *Foundation Skills for Caring*

- 1 Fundamental concepts for skills
- 3 Communication

 Don't forget to visit www.palgrave.com/glasper for additional online resources relating to this chapter.

Introduction

By the end of your foundation programme you need a good working knowledge of how healthcare is regulated and how it deals with quality assurance matters. You should see governance activities as part of the toolkit of essential life skills you will need for future professional practice, irrespective of your discipline. It is important to have a basic understanding of how to integrate the theory of governance with other subject areas, and reflect on how this informs practice in the delivery of holistic care in a patient-led National Health Service (NHS).

Learning outcomes

This chapter will enable you to:

- appreciate the structure and operation of the NHS
- gain a basic understanding of concepts, definitions and categories associated with healthcare governance
- develop an awareness of a range of regulatory healthcare bodies and how they ensure that healthcare professionals are fit for practice and purpose fit for public protection
- reflect on practice and learn to critically analyse how healthcare organisations deal with and respond to complaints from the public and service users
- appreciate the factors that enhance or detract from effective governance

- understand the role of the ombudsman and its application in practice
- recognise the pivotal role of healthcare professionals in designing and implementing audit tools to facilitate benchmarking.
- understand the role of external auditors such as the Healthcare Commission in England
- appreciate the role of healthcare professionals in promoting public and patient involvement in healthcare.

Concepts

- Healthcare governance
- Healthcare audit
- Patient involvement
- Regulatory control of the healthcare professions
- iatrogenic illness

S **Scenario: Introducing Sri**

Sri is a first-year student nurse on placement in a rehabilitation medical ward in an old hospital built in the 1930s. One of the older patients who remembers the founding of the health service asks her about the current configuration of the NHS. Sri, who has a learning group meeting the following day, is determined to find out how the contemporary health service operates.

The structure of the NHS

Rivett (1998) tells the story of the founding of the NHS by the then health minister Aneurin Bevan in 1948. For the first time, after the Second World War the new NHS promised universal access to free healthcare. Since that time the service has continued to evolve. There are now some differences between healthcare structures in the four countries of the United Kingdom, but throughout the United Kingdom we can analyse the structure in terms of primary, secondary and tertiary healthcare.

- **Primary care** is front-line care centred around health services in the local community. It is spearheaded by the family practitioner service, and involves many healthcare professionals including general practitioners (GPs), practice nurses, dentists and pharmacists. These front-line services, including the new nurse-led walk-in centres, are usually the first and sometimes the only link between patients and the NHS. The NHS places much store in the efficiency of primary care, and many professionals regard primary care as the backbone

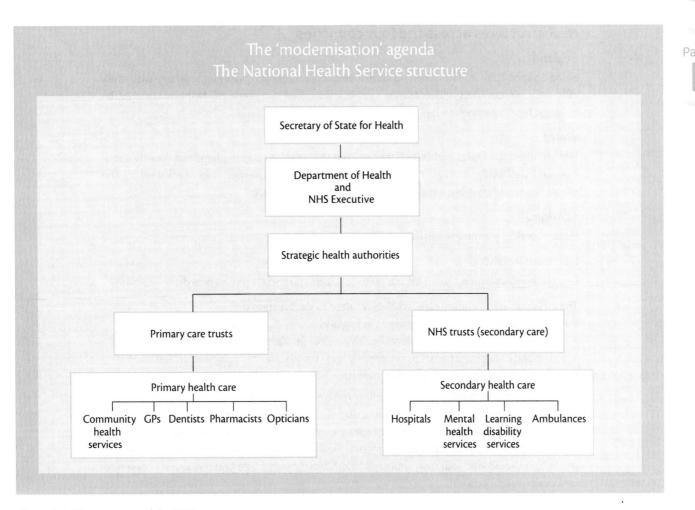

The 'modernisation' agenda
The National Health Service structure

Secretary of State for Health

Department of Health
and
NHS Executive

Strategic health authorities

Primary care trusts

NHS trusts (secondary care)

Primary health care

Community health services | GPs | Dentists | Pharmacists | Opticians

Secondary health care

Hospitals | Mental health services | Learning disability services | Ambulances

Figure 8.1 The structure of the NHS

W
to the whole service (http://www.dh.gov.uk/en/Policyandguidance/Organisationpolicy/ Primarycare/index.htm).

- **Secondary care** comprises specialised healthcare services and hospital care (outpatient and inpatient services) provided by healthcare specialists who generally have not been the patient's first point of contact. Much secondary care provision can be classed as ambulatory care, a term to describe treatment often conducted through an outpatient visit to a hospital, which does not always involve an overnight hospital stay. Secondary care services are usually accessed through a referral from one of the members of the primary healthcare services – often a GP. Recently there has been an explosion of secondary care service provision in the NHS, with the introduction of treatment centres that can give safe, fast, pre-booked day and short-stay surgery and diagnostic procedures in a range of medical specialties such as orthopaedics. These centres may be hosted by NHS hospitals, or (as in the case in England) commissioned by primary care trusts (PCTs) from the independent healthcare sector.

- **Tertiary healthcare** services are usually located in general hospitals which also provide secondary care. Tertiary healthcare is in effect specialised care provided by consultants in a range of medical disciplines. Access to these specialised services is arranged through referral from a primary or secondary care practitioner. The tertiary services are thus provided by specialists, working usually in a hospital setting, where facilities and staff are available for the provision of special investigations and treatment. Tertiary care can be part of a general hospital or a regional hospital, ands sometimes for very specialist services it is located in a super-regional hospital, when it is sometimes referred to as **quadreniary care**.

NHS structures across the four countries

England

Since 1 April 2002 PCTs in England have been responsible for planning services, with their efficiency, effectiveness and economy (sometimes called the three Es) being monitored by strategic health authorities (SHAs).

Wales

Health boards and local authorities are required to formulate and implement a 'health, social care and well being strategy' for their local area, which is governed and monitored by the Welsh National Assembly, which issues regulations and guidance.

Scotland

Health services planning is carried out by NHS boards.

Northern Ireland

Health services planning is carried out by four health and social services boards.

The emphasis on a primary care-led NHS resulted in the creation of:
- PCTs (previously primary care groups) in England
- local health boards (previously local health groups) in Wales
- community health partnerships (previously local healthcare co-operatives) in Scotland
- local health and social care groups in Northern Ireland.

These have various levels of responsibility in planning and commissioning health services. NHS trusts or their equivalents continue to provide services, although their number has diminished. A variety of trust configurations exist across the United Kingdom, including primary care, foundation, and acute, mental health and combined acute and community trusts. You should visit your own country's health service website to find out about changes to service configurations.

What is healthcare governance?

Clinical governance, as healthcare governance is commonly known in the United Kingdom, lies at the heart of the NHS's mission, since the Bristol Inquiry, to develop a modern, patient-led health service which delivers high-quality and safe client/patient care. The report of the Bristol Inquiry (DH, 2001), which was perhaps the most in-depth analysis of a modern health service and systems, made a number of key recommendations for improving communication, and subsequently many national initiatives have emerged.

Scally and Donaldson (1998) describe the antecedents to clinical governance, which were partly based on concerns about the quality of care being delivered to patients and their families. Politicians of all parties have been at pains to stress that the NHS takes quality issues seriously. Scally and Donaldson (1998) define clinical governance as:

> A framework through which NHS organisations are accountable for continuously improving the quality of their services and safeguarding high standards of care by creating an environment in which excellence in clinical care will flourish.

Healthcare services should therefore be efficient, effective and economic.

Halligan and Donaldson (2001) point out that this is the responsibility of all who work in health services, not just doctors and nurses. This means that all staff need to feel valued and part of the bigger picture. Governance is not a top-down edict but a shared philosophy in which all can contribute as they deliver the best standard of care they can, while continually seeking improvement. Clinical governance is part of the NHS drive to ensure safe, high-quality care from all involved in the patient's journey, and ensure that the client remains at the centre of the activities that support governance.

The clinical governance support team at the English Department of Health was developed to oversee the governance activities of the NHS, but its role ceased in March 2008 and the function was transferred to the individual SHAs, which are now responsible for clinical governance in their health environments.

There are a number of components to clinical governance, some of which are covered in more depth later in this chapter: These include

- patient, public and carer involvement
- risk management – incident reporting, infection control, prevention and control of risk
- staff management and performance – recruitment, workforce planning, appraisals
- education, training and continuous professional development – professional revalidation, management development, confidentiality and data protection
- clinical effectiveness – clinical audit management, planning and monitoring, learning through research and audit
- information management (of patient records, and so on)
- communication – with the patient and public, external partners, internal, board and organisation-wide
- leadership – throughout the organisation, including board, chair and non-executive directors, chief executive and executive directors, managers and clinicians
- team working – within the service, senior managers, clinical and multidisciplinary teams, and across organisations.

At the heart of clinical governance lies a mission to ensure patient safety, provide the highest quality of care, and promote lifelong learning among healthcare staff. Clinical governance belongs to everybody who works for the NHS. It can be argued that the care patients and clients receive is only ever as good as the healthcare professional who delivers it. Healthcare staff are usually the first point of contact with patients, and that is why communication studies features so strongly in healthcare curricula. It is important for you to be aware that simple nonverbal communication such as a smile can have major positive effects on worried patients or relatives. Clinical governance therefore encompasses a range of issues, from the simple to the complex, but at its heart lies a mission to deliver patient-focused care in which the culture of the healthcare setting is effectiveness, efficiency and importantly economy. However, governance is not just about saving money.

The world of healthcare is regularly scrutinised by both the media and politicians. It is crucial that those who work in this highly visible environment have a full understanding of what governance is and how to use it for better patient care. It is also a mandatory requirement for healthcare staff to have a full understanding of governance.

The seven pillars of clinical governance

The seven pillars of clinical governance model (see Figure 8.2) was first articulated by the NHS Clinical Governance Support Team in 1999, and has been adopted by many clinical environments ever since to coordinate their governance activities. The pillars are still perceived to be relevant, and the pinnacle of sound governance is the 'partnership' between the patient and the healthcare professional as they each strive to achieve optimum healthcare. The personal traits of the healthcare professional and how they act cements or demolishes trust. It affects the patient's perspectives not only on the care given by that professional, but on the organisation as a whole. If partnership is to be truly embraced by staff, as part of its governance activities the organisation must embrace notions of patient and public involvement with all aspects of healthcare planning and delivery.

The seven pillars are:
- clinical effectiveness
- risk management
- patient experience

- communication effectiveness
- resource effectiveness
- strategic effectiveness
- learning effectiveness.

You will see from the figure that they are supported by five foundation stones:

- systems awareness
- team work
- communication
- ownership
- leadership.

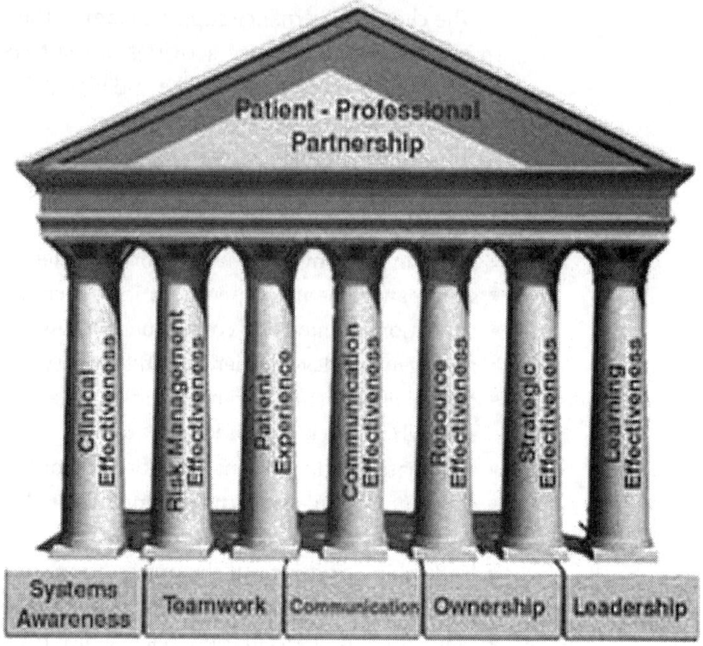

Figure 8.2 The seven pillars of clinical governance

Reproduced with permission of NHS Clinical Governance support team, 1999.

These foundation principles underpin the whole edifice of governance, and need to be regularly inspected to ensure that the pillars remain secure. Each of the pillars is dependent on the others, and if one pillar does not deliver its commitment to the principles enshrined in governance, the whole structure collapses. In short, healthcare governance activity cannot be cherry picked. Investigations carried out by the Healthcare Commission (2005), and the reports of the Bristol Inquiry (DH, 2001) and the Victoria Climbié Inquiry (DH, 2003) remind us of the consequences when governance pillars such as communication, and foundation stones such as are team work and leadership, come crashing down.

The SfBH standards

Standards for Better Health (SfBH) (DH, 2004) is now seen as the policy vehicle for the continued application of clinical governance to the health service in England. Clearly for clinical governance to work, practitioners need to make sure that the foundations are secure. Imagine SfBH as the expensive curtains at the window that is your healthcare environment. Clinical governance is the sound, clean and draught proof window by which the curtains can be hung to their best advantage. Stained, faded and mildewed curtains soon expose the reality of the state of the building – on in this case the institution.

The publication of the SfBH policy recommendations was not intended to replace or succeed the concept of clinical governance. In fact, clinical governance has a vital role to play in ensuring that healthcare organisations can satisfy the demands of the healthcare watchdogs such as the Healthcare Commission in England. These bodies monitor how institutions comply with these benchmarked standards, on which future organisational performance measurement is estimated.

The standards set out in SfBH cover seven 'domains':

- safety
- clinical and cost effectiveness
- governance
- patient focus
- accessible and responsive care
- care environment and amenities
- public health.

SfBH standards are presented in two groups linked to the seven domains, of 24 core standards and 13 developmental standards.

The 24 core standards

These are designated to ensure that all current care is safe, based upon the best available evidence, and is patient centred. Managers of every of every NHS organisation in England must take steps to provide evidence that the care provided meets all the stated aspects of these core standards. (The other countries of the United Kingdom have similar policy documents.) For the clinical elements, the evidence to underpin this is derived from the organisation's clinical governance systems, processes and outcomes. (For the nonclinical elements, the board will look to the other elements of its 'assurance framework'.) The Clinical Governance Committee has a vital role in ensuring that the organisation's systems, processes and outcomes are mapped to the standards, and that they generate a robust body of evidence on the basis of which the board can complete the 'self-assessment of core standard compliance'.

Where the Clinical Governance Committee uncovers any significant lapse, or any absence of assurance, they have a duty to make this known to the board and to initiate steps to remedy the situation. An organisation's internal audit processes should test and comment upon the effectiveness of this relationship, the robustness and validity of the evidence that is generated and the extent of the board's corporate ownership of the clinical governance agenda.

The 13 developmental standards

The second aim is a continuous improvement in services to patients and to local communities, so that care is effectively managed across intra-organisational interfaces (such as between Accident and Emergency (A&E) and theatre staff), interorganisational boundaries (such as between primary and secondary care) and (where appropriate) sectoral frontiers (such as between health and social care). The aspiration to achieve the 13 developmental standards is a key component of the clinical governance drive for continuous improvement and more effective integration of care.

In pursuing the developmental standards therefore, a trust's board should look to the Clinical Governance Committee to work in effective collaborative partnerships with other trusts (and other care providers) in the local health community, to identify concrete local developmental priorities, to benchmark the current position, and to develop robust evidence of improvement in patient experience and in clinical outcomes. Clinical governance has a vital role to play in generating trust board assurance in relation to both core and developmental standards, and the leading role in ensuring that NHS organisations fulfil their statutory duty of quality.

User involvement in healthcare

The Commission for Patient and Public Involvement in Health (CPPIH) which was established in January 2003 was abolished on 31 March 2008 and replaced by local involvement networks (LINks).These networks are intended to give everyone a voice in shaping their local health and social services. The new networks will be developed by all local authorities, to be in place by September 2008. The end of CPPIH and the introduction of LINks was instigated to give more power to local communities, to help them have a greater say in the design of service configurations.

It is therefore useful to reflect on how successful the whole initiative of patient and public involvement has been in reflecting the views of, for example, young users of health services. Wicke and colleagues (2007) point out that children and young people are still not as fully involved in decisions about their healthcare, as is mandated in a range of government policies. Healthcare polices such as standard 7 of the *National Service Framework for Children, Young People and Maternity Services* (DH, 2003b) and *Standards for Better Health* (DH, 2006) are quite explicit in emphasising the need for NHS trusts to engage with patients and members of the public in developing services. Despite this Coles and colleagues (2007), in an audit of compliance to this standard, found that involvement of children and their families in service planning was at a low level of development. Hill and colleagues (2004) point out the reality that children are some of the highest users of state services, and yet their voice is rarely sought and many initiatives are designed, delivered and evaluated by adults.

Children are not just involved as patients: many of them act as carers for their sick parents. Doran, Drever and Whitehead (2003), in analysing the data from the 2003 census, confirmed that the previous estimates of young carers (of between 10,000 and 50,000) were very wide of the mark, and that the real figure was closer to 114,000. Recent press reports put it as high as 175,000 or more. Clearly the young are both in receipt of care and major deliverers of care to others. It is therefore crucial that healthcare professionals begin to take a more proactive stance in seeking this silent group's view. They should have a say on not only what a really good hospital for children and young people should be like, but also what services they need to function effectively.

As part of its ongoing commitment to reconfiguration of children's services, one English hospital has made contact with a city youth parliament (see http://www.ukyouthparliament. org.uk/) and conducted focus group consultation exercises with its members. Youth parliaments aim to give young people around the United Kingdom a voice which is heard and listened to by local and national government, and importantly by providers of services for young people. This particular youth parliament is hosted by Connexions (http://www. connexions-direct.com/), which is a support service for 13 to 19-year-olds (and people aged up to 24 who have additional needs).The service acts as a one-stop shop, providing referral to other services for helping with the transition to adult life. There is support for all with planning their next stage from pre-16 education into work, training or further learning, and additional services support or refer young people who have problems with relationships, housing or health issues. The Connexion service is provided with government funding given to local authorities from April 2008, and either delivered as a service directly by the authorities, or subcontracted to other organisations.

Participants were asked at one meeting to consider what a child about to be admitted to hospital might be thinking about, and at a subsequent meeting what a child actually in hospital might be thinking about. In analysing the data it became clear that a number of factors are perceived by young people as inhibiting or enhancing childhood hospital admission. Among the inhibiting factors were fear of the unknown, being frightened and fears of hospital-acquired infection, not surprising perhaps given the media coverage of the subject. Things that enhanced a child's admission to hospital included age-appropriate wards, friendly staff and having a named nurse they can turn to. Many of the young people's comments were related to the environment of care, and the child's personal and individual needs or requirements, including being able to use mobile phones.

Although there are undoubtedly many important areas of existing consultation with children and young people, and with other service users, LINks are being introduced to help strengthen the system that enables sections of the community such as the 11 million children which live in England to influence the care they receive.

a **Learning activity**

In your learning groups consider how different groups in society are consulted about the configuration of health services.

Developing an audit tool to measure compliance to policy

Implementing governance to ensure that policy standards are met usually involves audit. This plays a key role in assessing how well an organisation meets set standards. Cooper and Benjamin (2004) believe that audit exists to improve the quality of patient care and clinical practice. It does this through a number of steps:

W

- Select a topic (for example, management of patients' pain).
- Decide on criteria and standards (using for example the various policies related to pain management) (see www.rcn.org.uk/development/practice/clinicalguidelines/pain).
- Design and pilot the audit tool.
- Determine how the data or information will be collected. (For example, how many patients' records will be surveyed?)
- Collect the data within a strict time frame.
- Analyse the information and see whether the results tally with the standard(s). Identify where compliance to the standard(s) falls short.
- Design and implement an action plan to address the areas of concern.
- Repeat the audit according to your action plan, to monitor progress using the same audit tool.

Developing a local audit topic

Coles and colleagues (2007) reported measuring compliance to one of the standards of the *Children's National Service Framework* in an English SHA. They designed a tool which used a five-point scale, with 1 indicating the lowest level of compliance and 5 the highest. The results demonstrated that a number of areas required further work before all the criteria of the standard were fully met within the time period specified by the Department of Health.

Before setting out on the audit trail, someone needs to be appointed as the audit lead. This person liaises with the multidisciplinary team where necessary to ensure that the audit tool design is suitable for the topic under investigation. For maximum effect and to prevent noncooperation the auditing team should be peers rather than managers. This method ensures maximum enthusiasm for the task ahead. The writers of policy and other similar documents usually phrase the standards so they can easily be converted into audit tools.

S   Scenario continued

As part of her interprofessional learning group activity, Sri has been asked to collect a range of policy documents that are applicable to healthcare practice (for example, a national service framework). She and her fellow students, who include a physiotherapist, an occupational therapist, a student taking a foundation degree in health care and a medical student, have been instructed to design a project with an appropriate measurement tool that will successfully complete the audit cycle.

Part of a sample audit tool

Benchmarks

1.1   Individualised pain assessment tool

No pain assessment tool is available.	Assessment tools are used and documented in less than 25% of records.	Assessment tools are used and documented in 25–50% of records.	Assessment tools are used and documented in 50–75% of records.	Assessment tools are used and documented in 75–100% of records.	If not applicable, please state why.
Score 1	Score 2	Score 3	Score 4	Score 5	

Evidence

Please indicate the presence or lack of evidence. For example:

- Pain assessment tool (state type) ....
- Completed pain assessment tools in patient records.
- Pain audit results.

Other (please state) ....

Remember that audit is designed eventually to produce an outcome for a patient or service user group. It is important to make reference to benchmarks in designing audit tools.

Benchmarking

Benchmarking is simply comparing your practice against others offering similar services. For example you might wish to compare your hand washing audit results with those of another hospital. This tells you whether, as a practitioner or group of practitioners, you are doing as well as, less well than or better than people in similar organisations, and gives an indication of whether you need to improve your service.

The origins of benchmarking are lost in history, but we can trace its use for centuries in different contexts. For example, in the middle of the nineteenth century standard measurements for screw length were agreed in developed countries. This was needed to enable products or product components built in different parts of the country to be interchangeable. For instance, interchangeable gun parts allowed repairs to be made on the battlefield. A mark on the craftsman's bench indicated the agreed sizes for the components such as metal bolts.

Ellis (2000) has described how clinical benchmarking can help practitioners determine the evidence base on which the benchmarks for practice are agreed. Important aspects are accepting the status of a benchmark to allow both measurement (in the form of scores often using a 10 cm visual analogue scale) and comparison, and the sharing of best practice with other similar institutions. Benchmarked standards are now a key feature of many policy documents. The standards are drawn up on the basis of evidence from a number of sources.

One key policy which is relevant to all healthcare practitioners is *Essence of Care* (DH, 2003a). This policy now details 11 sets of benchmarks. They are intended to stimulate healthcare practitioners to look at how the service they provide compares with similar services elsewhere, and on that basis, to work to improve it.

> **(a) Learning activity**   W
>
> Go to: http://www.dh.gov.uk/en/Publicationsandstatistics/Publications/
> PublicationsPolicyAndGuidance/DH _4005475 and examine each of the 11
> benchmarked *Essence of Care* standards. In your learning group debate how you could
> compare your current practice with each one.

The role of healthcare regulators

UK regulators of healthcare professionals include the:

- General Chiropractic Council
- General Dental Council
- General Medical Council
- General Optical Council
- General Osteopathic Council

- Nursing and Midwifery Council
- Pharmaceutical Society of NI
- Royal Pharmaceutical Society of Great Britain.

All healthcare regulators are committed to protecting the public through maintaining professional standards. They achieve this through:

- setting standards for the professionals in their field
- approving courses such as pre-registration nursing programmes
- keeping and maintaining a register of qualified professionals
- taking action against registrants when necessary.

> **[S] Scenario continued**
>
> Sri is working with her mentor, who explains that she has just received a letter from the Nursing and Midwifery Council asking for her annual registration fee. Sri is interested to know about the activities of her future regulator.

From time to time however even this thorough regulation process fails to protect patients. Among the cases of professional misbehaviour which have shocked both healthcare professionals and the public are those of Dr Harold Shipman, who was convicted of 15 murders but is thought to have killed 236 patients (Horton, 2001), and enrolled nurse Beverley Allitt, who was convicted of murdering four children and injuring nine others while she was employed on a six-month fixed-term contract on the children's ward at Grantham and Kesteven District General Hospital. Both of these terrible crimes were exposed, and MacDonald (1996) shows how the mystery of the unexplained deaths of children at Kesteven was solved with the help of other nurses who had become suspicious of Allitt. Investigations into the (fortunately rare) cases such as these help to suggest steps that can be taken to ensure there is no repetition of them.

The Nursing and Midwifery Council (NMC): an example of a regulatory body

The NMC was established under the Nursing and Midwifery Order (2001) and came into being on 1 April 2002 as the successor to the UK Central Council (UKCC, itself the successor to the original General Nursing Council), and four national boards. New rules for education, registration and registration appeals, midwifery and fitness to practise were developed, and came into force in August 2004.

The NMC's remit now includes dealing with allegations made against nurses. A nurse's fitness to practise might be brought into question because of their:

- misconduct
- lack of competence
- conviction or caution for a criminal offence
- physical or mental health problems
- fitness to practise being judged to be impaired by another regulatory body
- incorrect or fraudulent entry in the professional register.

The NMC and other regulatory bodies can exercise a number of sanctions against registrants who fail to comply or adhere to the professional code of conduct:

- interim suspension
- imposing interim conditions of practice
- removal from the register for at least five years
- a caution, which remains in force for between one and five years
- suspension from the register
- imposing (more permanent) conditions of practice.

Note that it is your responsibility monitor changes in healthcare regulations, for example by periodically reviewing the appropriate websites. The government has agreed that the non-medical professional regulatory bodies such as the NMC should continue to be responsible for the educational standards of the professionals they regulate (HM Government, 2007).

The *NMC Code of Professional Conduct: Standards for conduct, performance and ethics* (NMC, 2004) states that:

> As a registered nurse, midwife or specialist community public health nurse, you are personally accountable for your practice. In caring for patients and clients you must:
> - Respect the patient or client as an individual
> - Obtain consent before you give any treatment or care
> - Protect confidential information
> - Co-operate with others in the team.
> - Maintain your professional knowledge and competence.
> - Be trustworthy.
> - Act to identify and minimise risk to patients and clients.

These are the shared values of all the United Kingdom healthcare regulatory bodies.

Dealing with complaints and adverse incidents within the health service

The role of the NHS Litigation Authority (NHSLA)

The NHSLA is a special health authority whose primary mission is to administer strategies which help English trusts deal with clinical negligence claims. It does this through promoting good risk management and healthcare governance (http://www.nhsla.com/). The NHSLA auditors gather information from acute trusts in England on five specific risk areas, each with ten separate criteria (see Table 8.1). Trusts are assessed at four specific levels, which are categorised from 0 to 3. Level 0 trusts are assessed annually until they reach level 1, where they are offered a 10 per cent discount on their indemnity contributions. Trusts achieving level 3 scores are those with the strongest risk management and governance strategies, and they are entitled to a 30 per cent discount on their contributions, so there are clearly financial advantages for trust that have good risk management and governance strategies.

All healthcare professionals are committed to safeguarding their patients or clients. Healthcare institutions are inherently dangerous places, especially for those too sick, young or weak to protect themselves. It is important to recognise that all healthcare professionals have a duty of care, and must work in such a way that all reasonable steps are taken to prevent harm from happening to patients. It is now more than 30 years since Illich (1974) first defined iatrogenic illness. Clinical iatrogenesis is the harm caused to patients by treatments or healthcare interventions which result in a negative outcome (for example when a patient receives the wrong drug or drug dose). All healthcare professionals aim to avoid adverse incidents happening to patients or clients, but despite this things do go wrong, and patients and their families feel aggrieved. Sometimes an adverse incident results in an official complaint.

Dealing with a complaint

An *adverse incident* can be defined as any healthcare occurrence that has led to an unintended or unexplained harm to a patient. A *near miss* is defined as an occurrence that could have led to a patient being harmed, but either the mistake was aborted before harm occurred, or fortunately no harm actually resulted.

To ensure that complaints are resolved as quickly and fully as possible, the government has produced a framework and targets for responding to complaints. These are detailed on the NHS Direct website (http://www.nhsdirect.nhs.uk/articles/article.aspx?articleId=1084).

Table 8.1 Overview of NHSLA risk areas

Standard → Criterion ↓	1 Governance	2 Competent and capable workforce	3 Safe environment	4 Clinical care	5 Learning from experience
1	Risk management strategy	Corporate induction	Secure environment	Patient identification	Incident reporting
2	Policy on procedural documents	Local induction of permanent staff	Safeguarding children	Patient information	Raising concerns
3	Risk management committee(s)	Local induction of temporary staff	Safeguarding adults	Consent	Complaints
4	Risk awareness training for senior management	Supervision of medical staff in training	Moving and handling	Clinical record-keeping standards	Claims
5	Risk management process	Risk management training	Slips, trips and falls	Transfer of patients	Investigations
6	Risk register	Training needs analysis	Inoculation incidents	Medicines management	Analysis
7	Responding to external recommendations specific to the organisation	Medical devices training	Maintenance of medical devices and equipment	Blood transfusion	Improvement
8	Clinical records management	Hand hygiene training	Harassment and bullying	Resuscitation	Best practice – NICE, NCEs and national guidance
9	Professional clinical registration	Moving and handling training	Violence and aggression	Infection control	Best practice – NSFs and high-level enquiries
10	Employment checks	Supporting staff involved in an incident, complaint or claim	Stress	Discharge of patients	Being open

Reproduced with permission of the NHSLA.

There are three stages to dealing with a healthcare complaint.

Local resolution

This first stage of the NHS complaints procedure is called 'local resolution', and aims to resolve complaints quickly and appropriately. This is activated after a complaint or a letter of complaint has been received. The organisation attempts to resolve the complaint as directly and quickly as possible. The person in charge of the complaints procedure obtains informal responses from front-line staff. If necessary a formal investigation is conducted, and a written response is sent to the patient or family. Often the Patient Advice and Liaison Service (PALS) is involved with helping patients or families articulate their concerns. Although PALS was introduced as part of a range of measures to make the NHS more patient-centred, South (2007) argues that in its current configuration it can never fully be successful in closing the gap between the NHS and its users. It is weighted to inherently support the interests of the healthcare provider rather that its clients.

Independent review by the Healthcare Commission

If after local resolution a patient is still not happy, they have the right to an independent review. This is handled by the Healthcare Commission, which acts as convener in assessing the case and all correspondence. If residual concerns remain, the Healthcare Commission can either refer the case back for local resolution, agree to undertake an independent review, or fast-track the complaint to the Office of the Healthcare Ombudsman (Glasper and Lowson, 2006).

The Health Service Ombudsman

The ombudsman is completely independent of the NHS and government, and will investigate whether correct protocols were followed at the local resolution stage. In particular they are interested in the communication between the client and the healthcare professionals. Glasper and Lowson (2006) believe this to be a major issue in any complaint.

> **(a) Learning activity**
>
> What is your role in dealing with complaints?
>
> Obtain a copy of your local complaints policy and ascertain how your ward/department deals with complaints.

Responding to an adverse incident

Reason (1990) has indicated that 10 per cent of patients in hospital suffer an adverse incident during their period of care. The elderly, people with mental health problems or learning difficulties and children are especially vulnerable, and healthcare professionals working in these environments must consider the context in which they work and deliver care. The biggest proportion of incidents in acute care settings consists of patient accidents, such as falls especially in the elderly, incidents arising from treatments and procedures, drug errors, and case note or other documentation incidents. Mathews (2007) summarises the causes as:

- medication delivery
- mismatching patients and their treatment
- equipment error
- working beyond competency
- failure or delay to make an accurate diagnosis
- suboptimal handover
- suboptimal continuity of care
- failure to ensure follow-up of investigations
- lack of awareness of local procedures and policies.

This is a high incidence of procedures leading to an adverse incident, and it emphasises the importance of healthcare professionals keeping closely to local policies and guidelines, which are formulated to reduce the chance of things going wrong. Clinical protocols must be established on best evidence and importantly be updated regularly. Crucially the staff who provide care must be educated to do so, and their competency assessed through annual monitoring, coordinated through personal development plans.

Practices to minimise adverse incidents

Among the good practice that has been suggested to minimise the risk of things going wrong is:

- Develop a healthcare governance forum where risk issues are discussed monthly.
- Establish a local lead for risk management activities.
- Undertake a regular review of adverse event reporting.
- Make a full investigation (root cause analysis) of all 'red' National Patient Safety Agency graded incidents.
- Provide evidence of lessons learned and practice change, such as NG tube checking and cannula dressings.
- Link these activities to the audit programme.

The different countries of the United Kingdom differ in the way that they deal with patient safety. Although it is beyond the scope of this book to cover all the differences in detail, below is an example of how Scotland deals with such issues. If you work in another part of the United Kingdom you should consult the appropriate health service website.

The Scottish Patient Safety Programme

The objective of the Scottish Patient Safety Programme is to steadily improve the safety of hospital care right across the country. This will be achieved by using evidence-based tools and techniques to improve the reliability and safety of everyday healthcare systems and processes.

It is intended that real-time data will be gathered ward/unit-by-ward/unit, and the staff caring directly for patients will lead the changes required to achieve the aims of the Programme.

Aims of the Scottish Patient Safety Programme

The Scottish Patient Safety Programme recognises the complexities involved in delivering modern healthcare, and so it has been designed to standardise approaches to care. There is good research to show which interventions make a difference when it comes to protecting patient safety, and these will be implemented uniformly in acute hospitals across the country.

Over the coming years, steps will be taken to:

- ensure early interventions for deteriorating patients
- deliver evidence-based care to prevent deaths from heart attack
- prevent adverse drug events
- prevent central line infections
- prevent surgical site infections
- prevent ventilator associated pneumonia
- prevent pressure ulcers
- reduce staphylococcus aureus (MRSA plus MSSA) infection
- prevent harm from high alert medications
- reduce surgical complications
- deliver evidence-based care for congestive heart failure
- drive a change in the safety culture in NHS organisations.

Scottish Patient Safety Programme evidence base

UK and international evidence indicates that one in ten patients experience an adverse event in hospital.

Adverse events are defined as unintended consequences of care, and may include contracting an infection such as MRSA, experiencing a drug error or a post-surgical complication, or developing a pressure sore. Research shows that 50 per cent of adverse events can be avoided if rigorous patient safety processes are routinely followed.

Quite apart from the personal impact on patients, adverse events are estimated to cost NHS Scotland around £200 million each year in extra treatment and lost bed days.

As the Scottish Patient Safety Programme develops, NHS Scotland will be gathering data to monitor prevalence and impact.

(a) Learning activity

Go to the companion website to access some links to recent studies and reports that highlight aspects of the challenge, and describe some responses:

- Health Protection Scotland hand hygiene campaign
- Safer Healthcare ventilator care improvement report
- The Health Foundation
- The Institute for Healthcare Improvement.

Scottish Patient Safety Programme facts

In its first phase, which is scheduled to run for five years, the Scottish Patient Safety Programme will be implemented in acute hospitals in each of Scotland's 14 Health Board areas and the Golden Jubilee National Hospital in Clydebank near Glasgow, which is a special Health Board. Each NHS Scotland Health Board has a Patient Safety Programme manager, and multidisciplinary teams have been formed to drive local improvements in:

- Intensive Care Units
- Medicines management
- General wards
- Perioperative care
- Safety leadership.

Initially, the Scottish Patient Safety Programme will be introduced in all acute hospitals across Scotland. However, as many patient safety improvements, such as medicines management and infection control, also involve community-based healthcare, the Programme will roll out to include Community Health Partnerships and Primary Care services.

Ultimately, every member of NHS Scotland's staff has an important part to play in promoting patient safety, and each can make a valuable contribution to the national drive for safety excellence.

> **(a) Learning activity**
>
> In your learning group, consider how patient safety is addressed in your own country.

Conclusion

Although the configuration of health services in the four countries of the United Kingdom varies, all are committed to providing first-class care based on best evidence. They all endeavour to reduce risk to patients, and all take steps to audit compliance by health institutions to national policy.

References

Coles, L., Glasper, E. A., Fitzgerald, C., LeFluffy, T., Turner, S. and Wilkes-Holmes, C. (2007) 'Measuring compliance to the NSF for children and young people in one English strategic health', *Journal of Children's and Young People's Nursing* 1(1), 7–15.

Cooper, J. and Benjamin, M. (2004) 'Clinical audit in practice', *Nursing Standard* 18(28), 47–53.

Department of Health (DH) (2001) *Final Report of the Bristol Royal Infirmary Inquiry* [online] http://www.bristol-inquiry.org.uk/final_report/index.htm (accessed 2 December 2007).

DH (2003a) *Essence of Care*, London, DH.

DH (2003b) *National Service Framework for Children, Young People and Maternity services: Standard for children and young people in hospital*, London, DH.

DH (2003c) *The Victoria Climbié Inquiry*, London, DH.

DH (2004) *Standards for Better Health*, London, DH.

DH (2006) *Standards for Better Health*, London, DH.

Doran, T., Drever, F. and Whitehead, M. (2003) 'Health of young and elderly informal carers: analysis of UK census data', *British Medical Journal* 327, 1388.

Ellis, J. (2000) 'Sharing the evidence: clinical practice benchmarking to improve continuously the quality of care', *Journal of Advanced Nursing* 32(1), 215–25.

Glasper, E. A. and Lowson, S. (2006) 'Contemporary child health policy: the implications for children's nurses', in Glasper, E. A. and Richardson, J. A. (eds), *Textbook of Children's and Young People's Nursing*, Edinburgh, Churchill Livingstone.

Halligan, A. and Donaldson, L. (20001) 'Implementing clinical governance: turning vision into reality', *British Medical Journal* 322, 1413–17.

Healthcare Commission (2005) *Patient Survey Report 2004: Young patients*, London, Healthcare Commission.

Hill, M., Davis, J., Prout, A. and Tisdall, K. (2004) 'Moving the participation agenda forward', *Children and Society* 18, 77–96.

HM Government (2007) *Trust, Assurance and Safety: The regulation of the health professionals in the 21st century*, London, HMSO.

Horton, R. (2001) 'The real lessons from Harold Frederick Shipman', *The Lancet* 357(25), 82–3.

Illich, I. (1974) *Limits to Medicine: Medical nemesis, the expropriation of health*, London, Marion Boyars.

MacDonald, A. (1996) 'Response to the results of the Beverly Allitt inquiry', *Nursing Times* 292, 23–5.

Mathews, P. (2007) 'Adverse incident reporting', in Glasper, E. A., McEwing, G. and Richardson, J. (eds), *Oxford Handbook of Children's and Young People's Nursing*, Oxford, Oxford University Press.

Nursing and Midwifery Council (NMC) (2004) *The NMC Code of Professional Conduct: Standards for conduct, performance and ethics*, London, NMC.

Reason, J. (1990) *Human Error*, Cambridge, Cambridge University Press.

Rivett, G. (1998) *From the Cradle to Grave: Fifty years of the NHS*, Kings Fund [online] www.nhshistory.net (accessed 15 December 2008).

Scally, G. and Donaldson, L. (1998) 'Clinical governance and the driver for quality improvement in the new NHS', *British Medical Journal* 317, 61–5.

South, J. (2007) 'Bridging the gap? A critical analysis of the development of the Patient Advice and Liaison Service (PALS)', *Journal of Health, Organisation and Management* 21(2), 149–65.

Wicke, D., Coppin, R., Doorbar, P. and Le May, A. (2007) 'Every child matters, but what matters to them? Using teenager's views to shape health services', *Journal of Children's and Young People's Nursing* 1(3),129–36.

Legislation

Nursing and Midwifery Order 2001.

Insights into essential care issues

Chapters

Chapter

9

Moving and handling

Part

II

Marion Aylott

Links to other chapters in *Foundation Studies for Caring*

Links to other chapters in *Foundation Skills for Caring*

W Don't forget to visit www.palgrave.com/glasper for additional online resources relating to this chapter.

Introduction

Manual handling is 'any activity that involves the use of bodily force in lifting, lowering, pushing, pulling, carrying, supporting or otherwise moving a person or object.' (HSE, 1998a: 6). Patient handling and movement activities are an essential part of fundamental nursing care. However, healthcare providers are gradually accepting the reality that manually lifting and transferring dependent patients are high-risk activities, for both the healthcare worker and the patient being transferred.

Nurses as a group of professionals, irrespective of their age and experience, are at high risk of musculoskeletal injury while performing tasks such as helping to get patients out of bed and transferring them from bed to chair (Smith, 2005). Symptoms of musculoskeletal injury include pain, numbness, fatigue and weakness. In the early stage of injury, the pain or altered/ loss of sensation might disappear after a rest away from work, but later these symptoms do not disappear even after several days rest (HSE, 2004). The principal risk factor for these types of injuries is frequent or forceful manual lifting. Reducing the risk of injury lies in nurses first assessing what is needed to accomplish a patient moving and handling task safely and then carrying out the task appropriately. Many tasks require the use of mechanical equipment for patient handling and movement aids. This is called an *ergonomic intervention*.

Opportunities to improve quality of patient care through an ergonomic approach also exist in relation to increased patient comfort, independence, security and dignity during patient handling and moving episodes. The safe and compassionate handling of patients is an integral aspect of effective nursing practice (NMC, 2008).

This chapter aims to equip you with knowledge and understanding of safe working principles and practices during moving and handling procedures, and awareness of your legal responsibilities regarding moving and handling.

Learning outcomes

This chapter will enable you to:

- define manual handling
- explain the importance of posture and back care
- list the four curves of the vertebral column
- state the possible consequences of a prolapsed disc
- cite the relevant pieces of legislation relating to manual handling

- outline your rights and responsibilities as an employee according to the manual handling operations regulations (HSE, 1998a)
- recognise high-risk patient care activities
- discuss environmental, load, individual, task and equipment aspects of the risk assessment procedure.

Concepts

- Manual handling
- Health and safety
- Hazard

- Risk assessment
- Injury

- Back care
- Normal movement

Why is back care important?

Research has shown that nurses and nursing assistants have high rates of low back pain. This is especially true of those working in long-term care (Nelson and Baptiste, 2004). There is no doubt that the higher rates of low back pain are related to manual patient transfers. Other risk factors include continuous standing and walking and static postures in awkward positions. Think about the roof on your home: if you don't maintain and protect it, it might spring a leak. Once it's sprung a leak, you can take steps to limit the damage (like fetching a bucket) but if you cared for the roof in the first place, the problem would never have arisen.

The same applies to back care. It is more important and smarter to stop or prevent a back injury before it occurs. Once you have an injury (leaky roof), damage has already occurred. Be proactive! It's your back.

The 'S' curve and stabilisation

The spine is divided into four natural curves, two forward and two (balancing) backward. Throughout a lift or patient-handling manoeuvre, maintain the natural hollow S curve of your back/spine by locking your back muscles to minimise your risk. The muscles brace the spine and protect motion segments. In doing so, you stabilise your spine, which reduces low back strain.

[S] Scenario: Introducing Farid

Farid, who is 58 years of age, 5 ft 10 ins tall and weighs 11 stone, is a patient on a general medical ward. Farid has Parkinson's disease, a progressive neurological disorder caused by the loss of dopamine-producing cells in the basal ganglia in the brain. He was admitted to the ward following a fall at home. He fell in his bathroom, and his home carer who found him thinks he might have been on lying on the floor of his bathroom for up to 48 hours. He was admitted with hypothermia and confusion, and has sustained a fracture to his right clavicle. His right arm is in a sling and his cardiovascular condition is being stabilised while he awaits an orthopaedic surgical review.

(a) Learning activity   W

To gain some understanding of Parkinson's disease and the difficulties it causes for patients in controlling their movements, watch the following video on YouTube; http://uk.youtube.com/watch?v=q458IgW-ILk&feature=related

(c) Professional conversation

During patient handover, your colleague Louise comments, 'This morning I had to get Farid up because he was lying in a wet bed and I was concerned about his skin integrity. I was so busy, and I was worried about being late giving out my patients' medicines. I know I'm supposed to use a hoist to do things like that, but I couldn't see it nearby, so I just got him up by myself. While I was lifting him, I was thinking, "I'm not supposed to be doing this." I guess I was lucky that I didn't hurt myself.'

(a) Learning activity

What should have happened in this situation?

⚠ Professional alert!

Statistics show that the highest number of injuries caused by handling occur within the health and social care sector.

The spine coordinates whole body power via proper execution of movements. Good posture pays dividends by reducing stress and loads. Stress and loads can lead to tension in the antigravity musculature, degeneration of weight-bearing structures, less efficient movement, misalignment, and create the risk of injury (Nelson, Fragala and Menzel, 2003). More specifically:

- the cervical spine gives your head freedom of movement
- the thoracic allows rotation of your torso
- the lumbar spines provides stability

Part
II

- the sacrum provides the base for your spine to sit on
- the sacroiliac joints act as a pivotal axes allowing movement integration between your legs, pelvis and spine.

How your back works

Knowing how your back works, along with its allied components, will help you understand why things go wrong with it. The back is a powerful but delicate machine upon which much of your body depends. It supports the skull, ribs, pelvis and shoulder bones. The back houses the spinal column, which contains 33 vertebrae, of which 24 are separated by *intervertebral discs* of cartilage which house and protects the spinal cord (see Figure 9.1). Each disc forms a cartilaginous joint to allow slight movement of the vertebrae, and acts as a ligament to hold the vertebrae together.

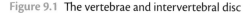
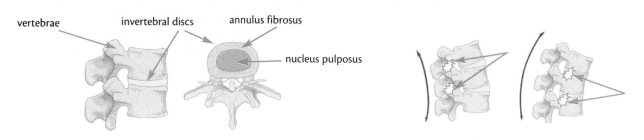
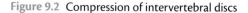

Figure 9.1 The vertebrae and intervertebral disc   Figure 9.2 Compression of intervertebral discs

The *annulus fibrosus* consists of numerous strong layers of fibrocartilage, a bit like the insides of a sliced onion, which contain the *nucleus pulposus* and distribute pressure evenly across the disc. The nucleus pulposus contains loose fibres suspended in a gel (Marieb, 2004). The nucleus of the disc acts as a shock absorber, absorbing the impact of the body's daily activities and keeping each two vertebrae separated. The design of these discs is equipped to accommodate the spine when it moves in several directions smoothly and 'spring-like' (see Figure 9.2).

There is a limit to how much compression these discs are designed to handle. If the spine becomes compressed, the pressure on one or more of the discs is increased. If the pressure becomes too great or is unevenly applied, the discs will begin to bulge; eventually, one might even burst (what is known as a herniated disc) (see Figure 9.3). The pain associated with either condition is usually severe. The outer layer of the discs is well supplied with nerves, and as a result, pain is often caused by mechanical distension or stretching of the outer wall. In addition to this, the herniated disc will often exert pressure on the nerves that branch off the spine (Nelson, Owen et al, 2003).

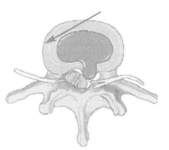

Figure 9.3 Invertebral disc prolapse

Easy ways to harm your back include:
- repetitive or heavy lifting
- bending and twisting
- exerting too much force
- not recognising symptoms and taking action.

The legal and professional requirements for manual handling

Under the Health and Safety at Work Act (HSAWA) 1974, the employer has an obligation to ensure the safety of all employees involved in manual handling activities. The subsequent introduction of the Manual Handling Operations Regulations (MHOR) in 1992 defined this legal obligation to both employees and employers with regard to tasks involving moving and handling. The emphasis is always on the avoidance of manual handling activities unless an adequate risk assessment has been carried out and employees have had suitable training.

HSAWA and associated regulations are supported by the Health and Safety Executive (HSE), which provides guidance and codes of practice. Among those relevant are the:

- MHOR 1992 (see HSE, 1998a)
- Management of Health and Safety at Work Regulations (MHSWR) 1999 (see HSC, 2000b)
- Reporting of Injuries Diseases and Dangerous Occurrences Regulations (RIDDOR) 1995
- Lifting Operations and Lifting Equipment Regulations (LOLER)1998 (see HSC, 2000a)
- Provision and Use of Workplace Equipment Regulations (PUWER) 1998 (see HSE, 1998b).

Many cared-for people have mobility problems and require assistance to move. There is a legal requirement to conduct a risk assessment before doing so (Nazarko, 2005). A risk assessment is nothing more than careful examination of what could cause harm to a patient or staff. The aim is to make sure that no one gets hurt (Griffin, 2004). The important things to decide are whether manual handling is appropriate, and whether satisfactory precautions can be taken so that the risk is reduced. The HSE (2004) puts forward a simple hierarchy that can be followed to ensure that the risk level is reduced to the lowest practicable level (see Figure 9.4).

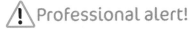

- **Avoid**: MHOR states that manual handling operations that involve a risk of injury should be avoided if possible. This means where reasonably practicable: for example, if the cost of providing a piece of equipment is grossly disproportionate to the benefit, the employer does not have an absolute duty to provide it. Avoiding the task eliminates the risk, but the majority of care is unavoidable, so we need to implement the next stage.
- **Assess**: The goal of the assessment is to reduce the level of risk that cannot be avoided to the lowest practicable level.
- **Reduce**: Recommendations made as a result of the assessment findings are put into effect. For example, it might be decided that an additional member of staff is necessary, or the use of a hoist or transfer belt, or this could involve for example training or sharing of information.
- **Review**: It is essential that assessments are reviewed periodically to ensure they are still relevant and effective, or if the mobility of the patient changes.

Figure 9.4
Hierarchy of control measures

⚠ Professional alert!

Moving and handling training is mandatory for all staff working within the health and social care industry.

Developing safe manual handling practices is linked to risk assessment.

⟳ Learning activity

Who is *responsible* for safety?
Who is *accountable* for safety performance?
Go to the NHS Confederation website (http://www.nhsconfed.org/) for help with answering these questions.

The HSE (1998c) has set out five steps to risk assessment;

Step 1   Look for hazards.
Step 2   Decide who might be harmed and how.
Step 3   Evaluate the risks and decide whether the existing precautions are adequate or whether more should be done. Consider using equipment to reduce risk.
Step 4   Record your findings.
Step 5   Review your assessments and revise if necessary in response to patient need.

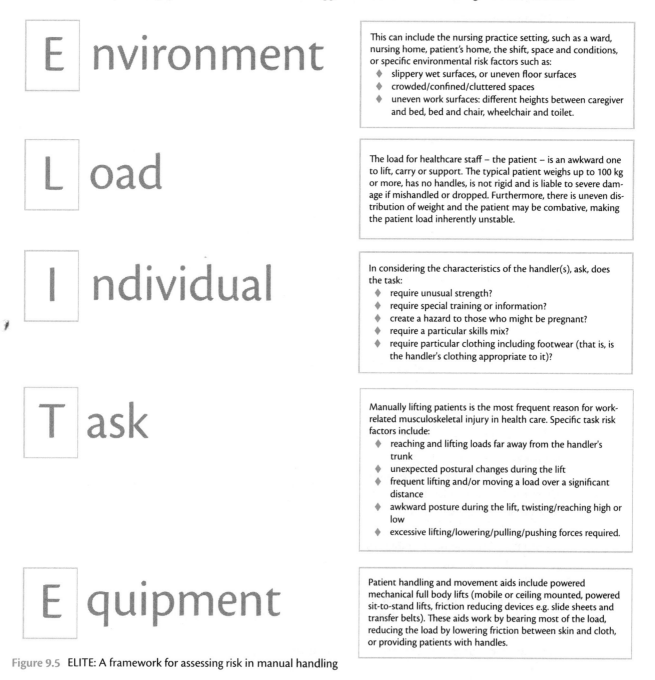

Learning activity

Refer to HSE (1998c: a web address is in the references) and answer the following questions:

- What is a hazard?
- What is a risk?
- What is a control measure?
- How are handlers affected by risk assessments?

Risk factors

The key to safe nursing work is careful analysis of the factors that that explain the risk involved in providing patient care. ELITE is the suggested format for recording risk assessments.

E nvironment

This can include the nursing practice setting, such as a ward, nursing home, patient's home, the shift, space and conditions, or specific environmental risk factors such as:

- slippery wet surfaces, or uneven floor surfaces
- crowded/confined/cluttered spaces
- uneven work surfaces: different heights between caregiver and bed, bed and chair, wheelchair and toilet.

L oad

The load for healthcare staff – the patient – is an awkward one to lift, carry or support. The typical patient weighs up to 100 kg or more, has no handles, is not rigid and is liable to severe damage if mishandled or dropped. Furthermore, there is uneven distribution of weight and the patient may be combative, making the patient load inherently unstable.

I ndividual

In considering the characteristics of the handler(s), ask, does the task:

- require unusual strength?
- require special training or information?
- create a hazard to those who might be pregnant?
- require a particular skills mix?
- require particular clothing including footwear (that is, is the handler's clothing appropriate to it)?

T ask

Manually lifting patients is the most frequent reason for work-related musculoskeletal injury in health care. Specific task risk factors include:

- reaching and lifting loads far away from the handler's trunk
- unexpected postural changes during the lift
- frequent lifting and/or moving a load over a significant distance
- awkward posture during the lift, twisting/reaching high or low
- excessive lifting/lowering/pulling/pushing forces required.

E quipment

Patient handling and movement aids include powered mechanical full body lifts (mobile or ceiling mounted, powered sit-to-stand lifts, friction reducing devices e.g. slide sheets and transfer belts). These aids work by bearing most of the load, reducing the load by lowering friction between skin and cloth, or providing patients with handles.

Figure 9.5 ELITE: A framework for assessing risk in manual handling

It focuses on ergonomic assessments of the characteristics of five key factors: **e**nvironment, **l**oad, **i**ndividual, **t**ask and **e**quipment (see Figure 9.5). Risk assessment is an extremely useful tool, and employed correctly it is the single most effective way of reducing workplace injuries (RCN, 2003).

Maximum weights that can be lifted

The most common guidelines for lifting were created for lifting objects, not people. However, they give a rough idea about acceptable weights (HSE, 2004). The guidelines do not account for lifting in a constrained work space or lifting during unexpected conditions, such as a patient moving unexpectedly during a lift. Using these guidelines, the most a male can lift with minimal risk of injury under ideal conditions is 20 kg, and for a female it is 15 kg. Among the factors that reduce the weight that can be handled safely are:

- increased horizontal distance between the body and the load
- a load positioned below the knees or above the shoulders at the beginning or end of the lift
- increased vertical distance covered by the lift
- increased frequency of lifting
- increased twisting
- poor handle quality.

The variables that lower the acceptable weight reduce the amount that can be lifted safely in any situation, including patient handling. Each box in Figure 9.6 shows guideline weights for lifting and lowering. There is no such thing as a completely 'safe' manual handling operation, but working within the guidelines will cut the risk and reduce the need for a more detailed assessment.

> **t☆**
> **Practice tip**
> Key to effective back injury prevention is the use of ergonomic-based approaches that analyse job tasks and identify risk factors with the purpose of changing unacceptable job demands.

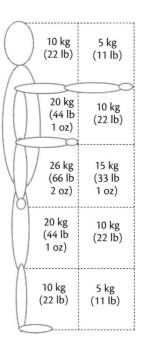

Figure 9.6 Guidance on lifting (the filter system)

Left figure weights:
3 kg (8 lb 9 oz) | 7 kg (16 lb 8 oz)
7 kg (16 lb 8 oz) | 13 kg (28 lb 10 oz)
10 kg (22 lb) | 16 kg (36 lb 4 oz)
7 kg (16 lb 8 oz) | 13 kg (28 lb 10 oz)
3 kg (8 lb 9 oz) | 7 kg (16 lb 8 oz)

Right figure weights:
10 kg (22 lb) | 5 kg (11 lb)
20 kg (44 lb 1 oz) | 10 kg (22 lb)
26 kg (66 lb 2 oz) | 15 kg (33 lb 1 oz)
20 kg (44 lb 1 oz) | 10 kg (22 lb)
10 kg (22 lb) | 5 kg (11 lb)

(e) Evidence-based practice   W

A court case in February 2003 highlighted the conflict between the rights of disabled people and the rights of paid carers – an issue that often introduces confusion into moving and handling considerations (Mandelstam, 2003). East Sussex County Council was sued over its refusal to instruct carers to lift two disabled sisters. It seems clear that blanket 'no-lift' policies cannot be imposed, and this may raise the question of whether lifting should be used if hoisting is an alternative but is refused. The judgment does seem to seriously question the Royal College of Nursing (RCN) guidance which advises that 'the manual lifting of patients is eliminated in all but exceptional or life threatening situations' (1996).

View the report on http://www.channel4.com/news/2003/02/week_3/18_disabled.html and http://news.bbc.co.uk/1/hi/england/2782083.stm

Biomechanical principles of safe movement

Body mechanics describes body positions that are thought to provide some protection from the force associated with lifting and moving patients. You should adopt the following biomechanical principles when moving and handling:

- Secure the pelvis and stabilise the scapulae; avoid twisting your body.
- When providing care, put the bed at hip-to-waist level.
- Position the head and face in the direction of your movement.
- Keep the patient as close to your body as possible.
- Set the feet/foundation to maintain a wide stable base.

Use these principles in conjunction with patient handling and movement aids when handling and moving patients, because body mechanics alone are not sufficient to protect you from the heavy weight, awkward postures and repetition involved in manual handling.

Keeping your spine in neutral

A neutral alignment optimises the spine's natural curves, with each part adding to whole body movement (see Figure 9.7). It is the posture or position of greatest efficiency, around your centre of gravity, with muscles on all sides exerting pull. Additionally, in this position, the balanced lumbar curve is the position in which the lumbar spine and the pelvis are best aligned to receive the weight of the trunk with minimal joint stress. When the lumbar curve is balanced you transfer forces between your upper and lower body with ease. Powerful movements depend on every part of the spine being strong (Hignett and McAtmney, 2000).

The centre of gravity

The body has a centre of gravity (COG) that is constantly altering. In standing the COG is found 'inside' the pelvis, so control of the pelvis is paramount for standing, walking and sitting. The intricate arrangement and forces of muscles allow smooth coordinated movement at the hip. Control centres are the head, shoulders, hips and knees.

Remember that your back and spine is your power foundation. It is a stacked framework from your feet through your legs, hips, spine and shoulders to your head (Parore, 2001). The COG is where most of the weight is concentrated, which is the centre of the pelvis (see Figure 9.8). A low COG gives a more stable base of support: as an analogy, putting heavy books on the top shelf of a heavy bookcase will make it top-heavy and more likely to tip over, while putting heavy books on the bottom shelf is more stable. Bending your knees during lifting lowers your pelvis (and COG), making you much more stable. This in turn protects you from any loss of balance which will increase the stress (load) on your spine (Hignett et al, 2003).

The upper body can be thought of as a lever arm, and the low back as the fulcrum point around which the trunk rotates. For this reason, the compressive forces on the spine are the greatest in this region, and consequently can cause the most damage to the discs that sit between each vertebra. For instance, lifting a 5 kg weight at arms' length away from the body produces approximately 50 kg of compressive force on the disc at the fulcrum point (Nelson and Owen, 2003). This is ten times the weight of

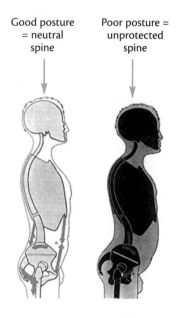

Good posture = neutral spine   Poor posture = unprotected spine

Figure 9.7   Neutral spine

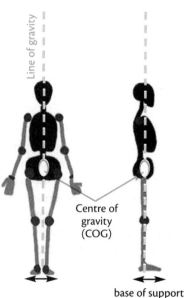

Line of gravity

Centre of gravity (COG)

base of support

Figure 9.8   Centre of gravity

the actual object lifted! In this case it is not only the distance of the weight from the body that contributes to the large compressive force, but also the weight of the trunk as it is bent forward. The muscles in the back have to work to support not only the weight being lifted, but also the weight of the upper body. For this reason, even if a person is not lifting an object, large compressive forces are produced just to maintain the trunk in a forward bent posture. Therefore, moving and handling tasks should ideally be carried out close, with elbows at waist height to reduce spinal loading and stress (Nelson, Owen et al, 2003).

Near lift   **Far lift**

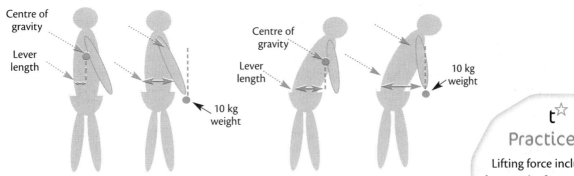

Figure 9.9 The lever effect: 'lifting' force = distance x weight

The advantages of a wide split stance

All objects and people have a platform or surface which is in contact with the floor or another surface: for instance a bed, or the soles of the feet. This platform is known as a base of support (BOS). The larger the BOS, the more stable the object will be, so for example, a tricycle is harder to tip over than a bicycle, which is in turn harder to push over than a unicycle. The area between your feet is your platform. If you spread your feet apart, side by side, hip-width distance apart, the BOS becomes wider or larger, like the bicycle. If you stand with your feet hip-width apart with one just in front of the other, your BOS is wider still and you have greater stability (see Figure 9.10).

Good foot position allows you to keep your balance and bring into play the full power of your leg muscles (Alexander et al, 2002). Leg muscles are more powerful and more durable than back muscles. Let your leg muscles do the work. Again, footwork is important once you avoid twisting your upper body. Use your feet to change direction. Do not twist your body. Twisting compounds the stress of the lift on your back and affects your balance.

This principle is important for the handler to consider. A good BOS enables manual handling manoeuvres to be carried out with greater ease and safety. If the handler stands with their feet together while using a slide sheet or helping a patient to stand, the BOS is very small. Any unexpected movements from the patient might throw the handler off balance and cause an injury.

Manual handling questions

Brooks (2008) presents a logical and hierarchical tool consisting of five manual handling questions which provide a principles-based approach to assessment and decision making before moving or handling a person.

t ☆
Practice tip

Lifting force includes two factors: the force required to move the upper torso (body), and the force required to move the load.

Part

II

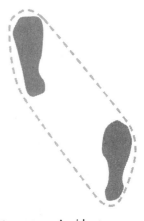

Figure 9.10 A wide stance = a greater BOS = greater stability

These questions, answered in sequence, prompt the handler to think systematically through a moving and handling problem. They should result in an intervention at an appropriate level;

1 What is normal movement for this task?
2 Can I teach the patient to do this unaided? If yes, how? If no, move to Q3.
3 If they could not do it completely unaided, is there any equipment available that could mean the patient could do this for themselves? If yes, what? If no, move to Q4.
4 If they are unable to perform the task themself, what is the minimum of assistance one and then two people can give (a) without equipment and (b) with equipment?
5 Are there any unsafe ways of doing this that must be avoided? If so what are they?

> **S** Scenario continued
>
> Farid now has a normal body temperature, is well hydrated and much less confused. You have been asked to help Farid transfer from his bed to a chair. This involves facilitating sit-to-stand activities which have been identified as a major cause of back pain in nurses (Hignett et al, 2002).

For solving the problem posed by the scenario, we shall use the framework known as APIE: **a**ssess, **p**lan, **i**mplement and **e**valuate (NMC, 2008). Patient assessment must start with first considering the nursing aim in the task. In this case it could be:

> To safely assist Farid to transfer himself from bed to chair in a manner that respects his autonomy, maintains his dignity, promotes his independence and therefore his rehabilitation without injury to Farid or myself.

Now let's apply the moving and handling questions above to plan this task. The first task is to consider the normal movement for getting out of bed:

- The head is lifted from the pillows.
- The person rolls onto their side. They do this by:
  - making a space so that they do not roll out of bed
  - turning their head in the direction of the roll
  - moving their arm across their body in the direction of the roll
  - bending their knee(s).
- The hand that crosses the body pushes down on the bed, or the elbow on the side that is rolled onto is pushed into the mattress.
- Both legs swing over the edge of the bed together.
- Standing from the bed:
  - the head moves forward
  - the feet go back under the bed slightly
  - the person shuffles their bottom to the edge of the bed
  - they lean forward at the hips
  - they propel themselves forward.
- To stand and turn:
  - they take one step forward
  - they pivot on their toe
  - they step forward.
- To sit in the chair:
  - they walk backwards
  - they feel for the chair with their arms and back of legs
  - their head comes forward so they bend at the hips
  - their knees bend so that their bottom can reach the seat
  - they push on the armrests on the chair while lowering themselves and repositioning to the rear of the chair seat.

This long outline emphasises that everyday activities involve complex movement patterns that have been learned in our development from birth. Knowing what the common patterns are and understanding how we normally move helps us in dealing with people who have some movement dysfunction or some psychological factors that are limiting their movement. But what is the normal movement for Farid?

(a) Learning activity

How is this normal movement altered for Farid who has Parkinson's disease? Go to the following YouTube websites;

http://uk.youtube.com/watch?v=wuDq4jgwbuQ and http://uk.youtube.com/watch?v=y1dkh2crci4&feature=related

- Study the movement of the people in the video clips. Note their altered body movements. In the second video, note how a change in flooring impedes the sufferer.

- What are the implications of this movement when assisting Farid to get out of bed and sit in his chair? Now view this video on the effects of music on movement:

http://uk.youtube.com/watch?v=qxDmP8c4QUI&feature=related

Clearly not all movement interventions are medically orientated!

(S) Scenario

Farid's designated carer, Geeta, asks him, 'Farid, I know that you have Parkinson's and I have some details in your care plan. But can you explain to me how your movement is affected?'

Farid explains that he is almost fully independent at home but sometimes requires the assistance and patient encouragement of his wife Anna, who is well informed about his condition. He goes on to describe how his muscles can become tight and rigid as they fail to receive messages from the brain to relax. Thus the resulting muscle spasm further slows movement. This causes muscle aches, a stooped posture and slow movement. Walking may be limited to short, shuffling steps. Getting out of bed often takes extra effort.

Sometimes he becomes 'frozen', unable to continue movement at all (McChance and Heuther, 2006). In this case, he might need help to enable him to resume movement. Anna helps him at home by 'putting her foot in front of him to step over.' Sometimes he has problems with balance, causing him to fall.

Maintaining posture requires rapid adjustments in response to changing forces on the body, which is not possible in someone with the slowed movement and stiffened muscles of Parkinson's. In the scenario Farid has described the typical characteristics associated with Parkinson's (McChance and Heuther, 2007);

- hand tremor
- a stooped posture (see Figure 9.11)
- a short, shuffling gait with no associated arm movements
- a tendency to fall over, either forwards or backwards
- difficulty both in starting to walk and in stopping
- difficulty rolling over in bed and in getting in and out of a car or chair
- poorly coordinated hand use.

The decline in mobility in Parkinson's is sometimes called a TRAP:

- **t**remor
- **r**igidity
- **a**kinesia/bradykinesia
- **p**ostural reflexes.

Let's go on to manual handling question 2: can you teach Farid to do the movements needed to get out of bed and into the chair unaided?

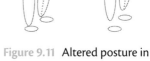

Figure 9.11 Altered posture in Parkinson's disease

Yes, you can coach him to do this manoeuvre and maintain his independence. He is no longer confused and is able to follow instructions, but he is still very weak. Although he may not be able to walk far, he can bear his own weight sufficiently to stand, turn and sit again immediately: you will know that if you have observed him moving himself up the bed. As he is still fatigued and has lost some confidence in his abilities as a result of his fall, you will want to build his confidence through a positive experience of beginning to mobilise again. Break this task down into a number of simple steps, keep it simple and avoid exerting him too much (see a checklist of factors considered in Table 9.1).

Table 9.1   Patient assessment considerations for movement

Physical function	Mental status and cognition	Medical condition	Communication
→ Height → Weight → Balance → Sensation → Vision → Hearing → Body awareness → Limb control → Subluxed shoulder (CVA)	→ Aggressive → Unpredictable → Focus/good concentration → Confused → Agitated → Memory	→ Pain → Medication → Fatigue → Fractures → Delicate skin → Changing condition → Wounds	→ Ability to speak → Language → Confidence

In helping Farid and considering his movement deficits because of his Parkinson's, help him to get out of bed by instructing him to follow a normal pattern of movement by first, turning on to his side bending and his knees. Then ask him to move his feet off the bed and use his arms to push himself up (see Figure 9.12).

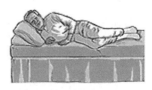

Figure 9.12 Positioning at the edge of the bed

You can help him to keep his balance by encouraging him to keep his feet apart and take long steps while swinging his arms when walking. If he becomes 'frozen', you should as his wife does and encourage him to imagine that he is stepping over a series of lines (see Figure 9.13). Farid is unlikely to accomplish a pivot turn associated with normal movement, so you should encourage him to walk in an arc to turn, and give him sufficient time to accomplish this in his own time.

Question 3 asks, is there any equipment available that could mean the patient could do this for themselves? Or in this scenario more specifically, is there any equipment available that he could use to reduce the workload involved in this task?

In order to reduce the risk of injury to Farid and to yourself, a bed lever may be used. This is a grab rail which can be slotted between the bed mattress and base, which Farid can use to help him roll over in bed (Figure 9.14). You should also place a slide sheet under his legs when he swings them off the bed to propel himself into a sitting position. This will lessen the friction on the surface of the bed once he is positioned at the edge (see Figure 9.15).

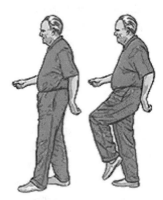

Figure 9.13 Imagine stepping over a series of lines

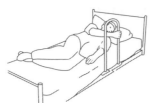

Figure 9.14 Bed lever

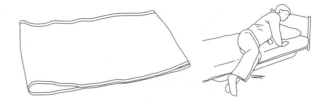

Figure 9.15 Slide sheet

Question 4 asks, what is the minimum of assistance the person needs, either without equipment or with equipment? With or without equipment, Farid will need the assistance of one handler, which is how he manages at home. Any handling will be simply supportive and comforting to reduce his anxiety. When assisting a patient like Farid to move, mechanical principles are used in the following ways:

- putting effort through the centre of gravity: that is, the pelvic area
- using contact points on the trunk, preferably the shoulder and pelvis
- making use of low-friction devices to reduce the effort in horizontal movement
- ensuring that both feet are in contact with the floor during the effort to provide a stable base
- making use of head movement to initiate body movement
- avoiding too much muscular tension and using smooth movement by playing background music
- keeping levers short by getting as close to the weight as possible
- keeping vertical effort to a minimum; raising the height of the bed to allow the legs to swing in a pendulum motion off the bed and then lower as the patient moves into a sitting position at the edge of the bed
- encouraging the patient to use the major muscle groups in their legs for effort
- ensuring that the patient stands and walks through the turn before sitting in the chair.

The final question asks, are there any unsafe ways of doing this that you must avoid? And if so, what are they?

Nurses have a pivotal role to play in clinical risk management and promoting patient safety. Indeed as we have seen above, they have a legal obligation to their patients, their employer and themselves. Injuries to both carers and patients happen when a patient is helped to move because either the carer manually lifts or manoeuvres the patient or for example, supports them to remain standing, or the patient cannot stay upright and collapses back, and the carer attempts to hold them up.

Clearly, there is a relationship between safe patient handling and quality of care measures. Research repeatedly demonstrates that safe patient-handling approaches result in fewer and less severe injuries to patients and caregivers (Nelson, Collins et al, 2008).

Patient-handling tasks, including transferring, are physically demanding and unpredictable, as they are often performed when a patient is not functioning at their usual level of ability. Therefore, it must be accepted that this is a high-risk activity for the patient and the care giver, because they impose potentially significant biomechanical and postural stresses on the handler.

Patient safety in this procedure is reliant on a thorough nursing assessment and timely reassessment and evaluation of patient ability during the task. Breaking the task down into a number of subtasks signposts appropriate times to pause and reassess the patient's ability and the plan. If at any time the patient appears to be losing balance, or struggling to bear their weight, for example, the task must be stopped and reevaluated, negating the risk of injury to both the patient and the handler.

To reduce the risk to yourself you should be mindful to maintain the proper alignment of your head and neck with your spine, maintain the natural curve of your spine, not bend at your waist, and avoid twisting your body. Most importantly you should not attempt to support the patient's weight at any point in the procedure.

More specifically, there is also danger associated with the misuse of a slide sheet (Geoff, 2001). While the device is used because of its friction-free advantages, it can become a hazard if it is used inappropriately. Be mindful to use it at the appropriate time and remove it from the vicinity of the patient at other times during the procedure when it could pose a slip/fall hazard.

Part

II

Overview of the whole procedure

1   Assess the patient and the environment, using the assessment criteria (ELITE), care plan and professional discussion with the patient. It is essential before a sit-to-stand procedure to ensure that the patient is able to stand and bear their own weight.

2   Organise the physical environment and the equipment to ensure safe completion of the task. This includes locking the wheels of the bed, putting the bed at the correct height, removing clutter, and making sure any mobile equipment is charged (if being used). Ensure the patient and you are suitably clothed, with good footwear especially (Graveling, Melrose and Hansson, 2003).

3   Position the chair in relation to the bed (and patient) angled at about 45–90° to minimise the turning area for the patient. Ensure that the bed brakes are 'on'.

4   Gather the appropriate equipment and take responsibility for knowing how equipment works and teaching this to the patient.

5   Moving and handling procedures require communication and coordination. Make sure the patient knows their and your role. Rehearse if necessary.

6   Coach the patient. Tell them what action you plan and expect from them. Show them what to do, and then help them move through the activity with prompts.

7   Position yourself throughout using the principles of body mechanics (as above).

8   When giving instructions it is important to always start with the head as this initiates movement for the rest of the body. Clear commands must be given for each movement to avoid confusion.

9   Adjust the bed height so you are comfortable while instructing the patient.

10   Break the procedure down into sections. *Notes for you as carer, below, are in italics.*

11   Sitting on the edge of the bed (from lying supine), instruct the patient as follows:
   - Turn your head to face the way you are going to turn (left) (Hignett, 2003).
   - Put one arm (right) across your chest in the direction you are to going turn. Pull on the bed lever to help you if needed.
   - Put the other hand (left) near to your face.
   - Bend your knee (right) keeping your foot flat on the bed.
   - Push through the heel of your bent leg and roll onto your side.
   - With your hand (right) flat on the bed, push up onto your other elbow.
   - *Place the slide sheet in position to reduce friction and shearing (Battles and Reyes, 2002).*

- Dangle your feet over the side of the bed.
- Bring both your legs over the edge of the bed (the slide sheet will help you) and come up into a sitting position all in one movement (the lower heavy half of your body will help the upper body to swing up rather like a pendulum) (Keir and MacDonell, 2004).
- *Stand in front of the patient face-to-face while you lower the bed so their feet will now touch the floor easily. Use this time to check that they have independent balance. Keep your feet shoulder-width apart, your knees bent toward the patient's knees and your back is in a natural, straight position.*

12   From sitting to standing at the side of the bed, continue to instruct the patient as follows:
   - Bring your head forward over your knees.
   - Put your hands on the edge of the bed.
   - Shuffle your bottom forward to the edge of the bed or (if the patient cannot manage this) lean forward and raise first one buttock and then the other to rock yourself to the edge of the bed.
   - Put one foot forward and one foot back a little under the bed base, about hip-width apart so that one foot is slightly in front of the other on the floor.
   - *Stand to the side of the patient facing the direction of their movement. Keep your feet shoulder-width apart, your knees bent toward the patient's knees and your back in a natural, straight position.*
   - Lean forward so your nose is over your toes and lift your head, looking forward.
   - *Place the palm of your inside hand on the front of the patient's near shoulder to help right their trunk and stabilise them if necessary.*
   - *Place the palm of your outside hand at the base of the patient's spine to help them bring their upper body over their feet ready to move (see Figure 9.16).*

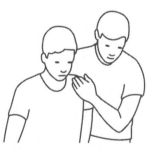

Figure 9.16   Reassuring hand positions

- Push forward from the bed onto your feet and bring your head up as you stand.
- *The patient may find it useful to gently rock back and*

forth to build up momentum to help them stand. Say clearly, 'Ready (rock), steady (rock), stand' (stand) to lead them through the manoeuvre.

13   Walking the turn in an arc, instruct the patient as follows:

- *Offer the patient your nearest hand to hold – palm-to-palm so they can grab your hand should they feel they are going to fall.*
- *Walk in unison with the patient, walking to one side, and in step with them, facing the direction in which they and you are to walk. Take care not to impede their natural stepping/shuffling. Place your furthest hand lightly on their far hip (Graveling et al, 2003).*
- *Keep your feet shoulder-width apart, your knees bent toward the patient's knees and your back is in a natural, straight position.*
- *Reassure the patient that they should move in their own time.*

14   Sitting down: instruct the patient as follows:

- *Keep your feet shoulder-width apart, your knees bent toward the patient's knees and your back in a natural, straight position (see Figure 9.17).*
- Stand with your back to the chair and shuffle backwards until you can feel the back of the chair behind your knees.
- Place one foot behind the other.
- Position yourself with your hands as before when you stood up from the edge of the bed.
- Flex your hips and grasp one or both armrests.

- Push your bottom out as you bend nose over toes once again.
- Lower your body into the back of the chair (see Figure 9.18).
- Raise your shoulders and then relax them for greater comfort.
- Release the skin tension under your thighs.
- *Congratulate the patient on their achievement and ensure they are comfortable, with the nurse call bell and everything else they require to hand.*
- *Document their progress.*

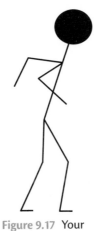

Figure 9.17 Your working posture

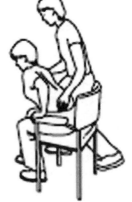

Figure 9.18 Lowering into a chair

Conclusion

Providing care and treatment for patients usually requires moving and handling activities associated with high rates of back injuries. The personal and financial cost of back pain and injuries to health staff mean there is an urgent need to improve practice in this area. This chapter provides information and guidance about safe patient handling, but it must be stressed that there are no completely safe techniques for handling people as loads, as all techniques involve some risk. 'Inherent limitation of human memory, effects of stress and fatigue, the risks associated with distraction and interruptions and limited ability to multitask ENSURE that even skilled, experienced providers WILL make mistakes' (Leonard, Graham and Bonacum, 2004: 85). However, applying the right risk management strategies can reduce injury and increase employee satisfaction. Rinds (2007) explains the importance of valuing staff and using appropriate training, and equipment.

Manual handling is about safe movement of people and objects; it is not just about lifting, or just about patient handling. Back care does not stop when you leave work, it is a 24-hour-a-day activity. The changing manual handling needs of staff must be reflected in their training. In order to allow for professional development, it is essential that those involved in health and social care have dedicated time to attend educational sessions on manual handling, where problem solving is encouraged (Alexander, 2008). All those involved in health and social care need to be informed and involved in risk management: that is, the process for identification, assessment, and reduction and control of manual handling risks.

References

Alexander, P. (2008) 'The changing face of manual handling in the community', *British Journal of Community Nursing* **13**(7), 316–22.

Alexander, P., Crumpton, E., Fletcher, B., Fray, F., Hignett, S. and Ruszala, S. (2002) *Evidence-Based Patient Handling: Techniques and equipment*, London, Routledge.

Battles, J. B. and Reyes, M. A. (2002). 'Technology and patient safety: a two-edged sword', *Biomedical Instrument Technology* **36**(2), 84–8.

Brooks, A. S. (2008) 'Manual handling questions', *The Column* **20**(1), 11–13.

Geoff A. (2001). 'Using manual handling equipment safely', *Professional Nurse* **16**(6), 1153–6.

Graveling, R. A., Melrose, A. S. and Hansson, M. A. (2003) *The Principles of Good Manual Handling: Achieving a consensus*, Norwich, HSE Books.

Griffin, M. (2004) *Study Notes: Moving and handling legislation* [online] http://www.otdirect.co.uk/mov_law.html (accessed 28 January 2009).

Health and Safety Commission (HSC) (2000a) *Management of Health and Safety at Work Regulations 1999: Approved code of practice and guidance*, 2nd edn, London, HSC.

HSC (2000b) *Lifting Operations and Lifting Equipment Regulations (LOLER) 1998: Approved code of practice and guidance*, London, HSC [online] http://www.hse.gov.uk/lau/lacs/90-4.htm (accessed 28 January 2009).

Health and Safety Executive (HSE) (1998a) *Manual Handling Operations Regulations 1992: Guidance on regulations*, London, HSE [online] http://www.opsi.gov.uk/si/si1992/Uksi_19922793_en_1.htm (accessed 28 January 2009).

HSE (1998b) *Manual Handling in the Health Service*, Health and Safety Commission's Health Service Advisory Committee, London, HSE Books.

HSE (1998c) *Five Steps to Risk Assessment*, London, HSE Books [online] www.hse.gov.uk/pubns/indg163.pdf (accessed 28 January 2009).

HSE (2004) *Getting to Grips with Manual Handling*, London, HSE [online] http://www.hse.gov.uk/pubns/indg143.pdf (accessed 28 January 2009).

Hignett, S. (2003) 'Systematic review of patient handling activities starting in lying, sitting, and standing positions', *Journal of Advanced Nursing* **41**(6), 545–52.

Hignett, S., Crumpton, E., Ruszala, S., Alexander, P., Fray, M. and Fletcher, B. (2003) 'Evidence-based patient handling: Systemic review', *Nursing Standard* **17**(33), 33–6.

Hignett, S. and McAtmney, L. (2000) 'Rapid Entire Body Assessment (REBA)', *Applied Ergonomics* 31, 201–5.

Keir, P. J. and MacDonell, C. W. (2004) 'Muscle activity during patient transfers: a preliminary study on the influence of lift assists and experience', *Ergonomics* **47**(3), 296–306.

Leonard, M., Graham, S. and Bonacum, D. (2004) 'The human factor: the critical importance of effective teamwork and communication in providing safe care', *Quality and Safety in Health Care* **13**(supp. 1), 85–90.

Mandelstam, M. (2002) *Manual Handling in Health and Social Care*, London, Jessica Kingsley.

Mandelstam, M. (2003) 'Disabled people, manual handling and human rights', *British Journal of Occupational Therapy* **66**(11), 528–30.

Marieb, E. N. (2004) *Human Anatomy and Physiology*, 6th edn, San Francisco, Calif., Addison-Wesley

McChance, K. L. and Heuther, S. E. (2006) *Pathophysiology: The biologic basis for disease in adults and children*, 5th edition, St Louis, Miss., Elsevier Mosby.

Nazarko, L. (2005) 'Safe moving and handling: a guide to hoists', *Nursing and Residential Care* **7**(12), 551–3.

Nelson, A. and Baptiste, A. S. (2004) 'Evidence-based practices for safe patient handling and movement', *Online Journal of Issues in Nursing* **9**(3), 1–26.

Nelson, A., Collins, J., Siddharthen, K., Matz, M. and Waters, T. (2008) 'Links between safe patient handling and patient outcomes in long-term care', *Rehabilitation Nursing* **33**(1), 32–43.

Nelson, A., Fragala, G. and Menzel, N. (2003). 'Myths and facts about back injuries in nursing', *American Journal of Nursing* **103**(2), 32–41.

Nelson, A., Lloyd, J., Menzel, N. and Gross, C. (2003a) 'Preventing nursing back injuries: redesigning patient handling tasks', *American Association of Health Nurses Journal* **51**(3), 126–34.

Nelson, A. and Owen, B. (2003) 'Safe patient handling movement'. *American Journal of Nursing* **103**(3), 32–44.

Nelson, A., Owen, B., Lloyd, J. D., Fragala, G., Matz, M. W., Amato, M., Bowers, J., Moss-Cureton, S., Ramser, G. and Lentz, K. (2003b) 'Safe patient handling and movement: preventing back injury among nurses requires careful selection of the safest equipment and techniques', *American Journal of Nursing* **103**(3), 32–44.

Nursing and Midwifery Council (NMC) (2008) *The Code: Standards of conduct performance and ethics for nurses and midwives*, London, NMC [online] http://www.nmc-uk.org/aFrameDisplay.aspx?DocumentID=3954 (accessed 28 January 2009).

Parore, P. (2001) *Power Posture: The foundation of strength*, New York, Apple Tree.

Royal College of Nursing (RCN) (1996) *Code of Practice for Patient Handling*, London, RCN.

RCN (2003) *Manual Handling Risk Assessments in Hospitals and the Community: A guide* [online] http://www.rcn.org.uk/__data/assets/pdf_file/0008/78488/000605.pdf (accessed 28 January 2009).

Rinds, G. (2007) 'Moving and handling, Part 2: risk assessment', *Nursing and Residential Care* **9**(7), 306–9.

Smith, J. (ed.) (2005) *The Guide to the Handling of People*, 5th edn, Teddington, Middlesex, ARJO, RCN and National Back Exchange.

Legislation

Health and Safety at Work Act (HSAWA) 1974
Lifting Operations and Lifting Equipment Regulations (LOLER) 1998
Manual Handling Operations Regulations (MHOR) 1992
Management of Health and Safety at Work Regulations (MHSWR) 1999
Provision and Use of Workplace Equipment Regulations (PUWER) 1998
Reporting of Injuries Diseases and Dangerous Occurrences Regulations (RIDDOR) 1995

Chapter

10

Nutritional assessment and needs

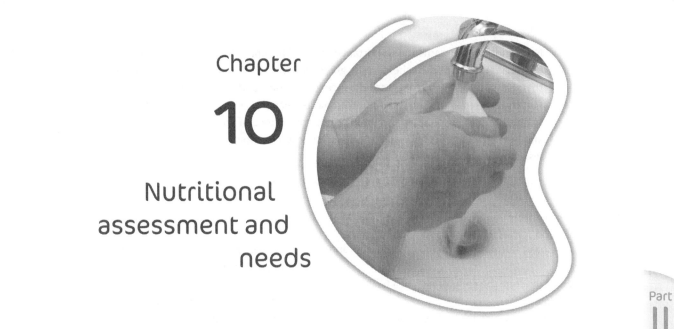

Pam Jackson

Part

II

Links to other chapters in *Foundation Studies for Caring*

Links to other chapters in *Foundation Skills for Caring*

W   Don't forget to visit www.palgrave.com/glasper for additional online resources relating to this chapter.

Introduction

Nutrition is of fundamental importance to life. This chapter explores a number of aspects of nutrition. It considers the current guidelines for healthy eating and how to implement them. It looks at the factors that influence food choice and food consumption, and provides guidelines on how to undertake a nutritional assessment, and policies to identify and prevent malnutrition in hospitals. It also looks at the importance of good nutrition in the prevention and management of other health problems, such as constipation and pressure ulcers. Finally, it discusses methods of nutritional support.

Learning outcomes

This chapter will enable you to:

- discuss the basic nutritional principles of nutrients and energy
- explore and describe the components of a healthy, balanced diet
- outline the factors which may influence food choices in the elderly, in both hospital and community settings
- recognise the need for assessment of nutritional status, and know how to carry out a simple nutritional screening test
- outline six strategies for promoting appetite and suggest ways of optimising oral nutritional intake
- discuss the consequences of malnutrition
- list ten factors that can contribute to constipation, and discuss its management
- suggest five strategies that could be used to improve nutrition in hospitals
- list three methods of providing enteral nutrition and discuss their use.

Concepts

- Nutrition
- Screening
- Balanced diet
- Assessment
- Malnutrition
- Health education
- Dehydration
- Healthy eating
- Constipation
- Food choices
- Ageing
- Nutrition in different ethnic groups
- Bereavement
- Adjustment
- Loneliness
- Community support
- Pressure ulcers
- Motivation
- Nutritional support
- Enteral nutrition

> **S** Scenario: Introducing Jack
>
> Jack is an 82-year-old man, living alone in a house in the old part of town. He does not eat well and has recently lost weight. Jack's wife Hetty died six months ago, less than a year after the couple had celebrated their diamond wedding anniversary.

> **a** Learning activity
>
> Consider the factors that affect your food choice and food consumption. Then think about those factors that might affect what Jack eats.
>
> In your practice placement, find out what factors interfere with normal eating and drinking. Consider how Jack might be feeling after his wife's death. How might this affect his health?

Factors that affect food choices

We shall consider these with specific relation to Jack.

- **Physiological changes.** Jack is 82 years old. There is physiological deterioration in most body systems with increasing age, and slower structural repair. In the gastrointestinal system there are reductions in secretion, absorption and motility, and impaired ability to metabolise and synthesise. Other systems have similar deterioration, such as reduced senses, muscle weakness, reflexes and so on. Jack's loss of appetite might partly be a result of these effects of ageing. (For a more detailed discussion of the effects of ageing, see Chapter 25 on older people.)
- **Psychological factors.** Jack is feeling very low following the death of his wife. This can affect appetite and lead to anorexia. (For a more detailed discussion of the effects of bereavement and depression, see Chapter 29 on loss, grief, bereavement and palliative care.)
- **Socioeconomic factors.** Jack feels lonely and isolated. He has no one to eat meals with. He only has his pension to live on.
- **Cultural factors.** His wife has always done the shopping and cooking. Jack is used to very traditional English cooking.
- **Cognitive factors.** Jack does not know what constitutes a healthy, balanced diet and has little awareness of the links between nutrition and illness.
- **Psychomotor ability.** Jack is physically able to care for himself, but lacks experience of such things as shopping and cooking, and his motivation is low. He finds carrying shopping any distance a problem.
- **Resources available.** Jack has a kitchen with a hob, an oven and a fridge, but has difficulty getting to a supermarket and the local shops do not sell much fresh produce.
- **Health and disease.** Jack has enjoyed quite good health, but has suffered from indigestion for several months and has recurrent back pain. He is currently suffering from constipation and a sore mouth.
- **Convenience.** Jack is likely to choose foods that require little preparation or cooking.
- **Drug–nutrient interactions.** Some drugs, including alcohol, interfere with normal digestion. Jack takes regular antacids for his indigestion and ibuprofen for his back pain. He drinks alcohol most days.

In hospital there may be other factors:

- **environmental factors** such as unfamiliar food, strange surroundings and smells, and reduced access to food and drinks
- **loss of independence**, with reduced choice over types of meal and timing
- **effects of treatment** which can reduce appetite
- **institutional factors** such as change in routine and mealtimes
- **increased nutritional requirements** as a result of illness, surgery or trauma.

S Scenario continued

Jack became a publican after the Second World War, and only retired ten years ago. Hetty had always looked after him, doing all the shopping and cooking, as he was so busy running the pub. Jack still enjoys a drink, and smokes 20 cigarettes a day. He has one son who lives abroad. Although he has enjoyed reasonably good health, he suffers from indigestion, for which he takes regular antacids, and back strain, which he puts down to handling heavy barrels of beer over the years. Since his wife died, he has tended to neglect his health, and has been suffering from constipation for the past few months.

---

a Learning activity

Why might Jack be suffering from constipation? Think about this before moving on to the next section.

Causes of constipation

Normal defecation can be defined as the regular and easy passage of a soft, well-formed and complete stool. There is a wide range of normal frequency, from three times a day to three times a week (Brocklehurst, 1990). If a person has difficulty with evacuation of faeces, they are said to be suffering from constipation.

Constipation can be caused by a wide range of factors. It can be:

* **self-induced**, by for example a diet that is poor in fibre, eating too little, not drinking enough, lack of exercise/immobility, ignoring the call to defecate, or unnecessary use of laxatives
* **environmentally induced**, by issues such as poor toilet facilities, travel or admission to hospital
* **drug-induced**: many analgesics, anticholinergics, aluminium-based antacids and antidepressants have this side-effect
* **disease-related**, the result of for example neurological disorders, muscular deficiencies, obstruction, endocrine or metabolic disorders or psychiatric problems
* **psychological,** caused by a disorder such as depression
* related to **local tissue factors** such as haemorrhoids, or weak pelvic floor muscles.

See Winney (1998) for further information.

> **a) Learning activity**
>
> Think about people who were constipated that you have met in your practice placements. What specific factors might have contributed to their constipation?

> **S** Scenario continued
>
> Jack went to the chemist to buy a laxative, to try to alleviate his constipation. The pharmacist overheard him asking for a laxative. He advised senna, 1–2 tablets, but also suggested that Jack might find it helpful to see the practice nurse at his local surgery.

> **a) Learning activity**
>
> * How do laxatives work?
> * What is the role of the pharmacist at a chemist's shop?
> * How might the practice nurse help Jack manage his constipation? You might wish to review your answer to this question once you have read the following paragraphs.

Management of constipation

Sufferers from constipation could be advised to;

* **Increase their fibre intake.** This could come from cereals, especially porridge and bran types, grains and wholemeal bread, fruit and vegetables, pulses and beans. Stools that are high in fibre are bulkier and have a higher water content, and are therefore softer in consistency, and easier to expel. The fibre also provides a more acidic environment which is conducive to normal gut flora activity.

  It is often difficult to effect a change of diet, as many people are resistant to changing lifetime habits. However, this can be done by suggesting the gradual introduction of high-fibre cereals, encouraging brown/granary/wholemeal bread instead of white, and trying to increase the number of servings of fruit and vegetables.

* **Increase their fluid intake.** They should aim for a minimum intake of 1–1.5 litres a day. Inadequate fluid intake reduces the stimulus for intestinal activity and triggers a greater absorptive response in the colon, leaving the stool hard and dry. Some fluids stimulate bowel activity, for instance fruit juices, real ale and tea. (As Jack enjoys a drink, the mention of real ale might encourage him.)

- **Increase their activity level.** Exercise and general mobility help prevent constipation, by stimulating smooth muscle activity in the gut, and aiding the process of defecation.
- **Re-establish regular bowel emptying.** Ignoring the call to stool leads to increased water absorption from the stool as a result of the prolonged transit time, and reduced response to gut activity.
- **Avoid unnecessary use of laxatives.** Stimulant laxatives such as bisocodyl should only be used short-term, as the large bowel becomes insensitive to their action, and then stronger laxatives will be needed to effect the same result. Ideally, suppositories or micro-enemas should be used in preference to laxatives, as they will only have a local action of irritating the mucosa and lubricating the passage.

For further reading on the effectiveness of laxatives in the elderly, see Centre for Research and Dissemination (2001).

S Scenario continued

Jack still misses his wife and finds it hard to cope without her.

He never did visit the practice nurse, but because he is feeling lonely, he decides to write to his son. Part of his letter reads:

I still miss your mother very much and sometimes I find the silence almost unbearable. I can picture her in the kitchen with her apron on, busy baking an apple pie for dinner. I can smell it even now! I don't seem to have much of an appetite these days and there doesn't seem much point in getting a meal when there's just me. Anyway, your mother never let me in the kitchen, so I wouldn't know how to cook dinner. I get by mainly on soup and sandwiches. I still go down the King's Head most evenings for a couple of pints and my pack of cigarettes. If I don't go there, I can go for days without seeing anyone.

a Learning activity

Consider what effect his bereavement might have had on Jack's appetite and nutritional status, before reviewing the next few paragraphs.

Do you know what constitutes a healthy, balanced diet? You might also like to think about what you know before reading on.

Part II

A healthy, balanced diet

The following recommendations for healthy eating are based on *The Balance of Good Health* (BNF, 2005), which is consistent with the government's eight tips for eating well.

- **Base your meals on starchy foods.** About a third of your food intake should consist of complex carbohydrates, as they are rich in fibre, vitamins and minerals, and a good energy source. These include pasta, rice, potatoes and bread, especially wholemeal varieties.
- **Eat lots of vegetables and fruit.** These too should make up about a third of your food intake. Aim to eat at least five servings of vegetables and fruit a day, as they are rich in fibre and vitamins, especially dark green and orange fruit and vegetables. (Did you know there is a DH five a day website (DH, 2003), with details of research related to fruit and vegetable intake?)
- **Eat more fish.** Eat fish at least twice a week, especially oily fish, such as salmon, tuna, mackerel and sardines, as these are rich in Omega-3 fatty acids, which help reduce the risk of heart disease.
- **Cut down on saturated fat and sugar.** Eat in small amounts and not too often. Fat is a good source of energy and fat-soluble vitamins. Sugar can increase the risk of dental caries.
- **Try to eat less salt.** Aim to consume no more than 6 g a day. Avoid adding salt at the table and reduce salt in cooking (microwave cooking avoids the need for salt), as salt increases the risk of hypertension.
- **Get active and try to be a healthy weight.** Activity can take a variety of forms such as regular exercise through sport or work, and everyday activities.

- **Drink plenty of water.** Good hydration can help prevent pressure ulcers, urinary tract infections, cardiovascular disease, confusion, falls and many other health problems.
- **Don't skip breakfast.** A healthy meal at the start of the day can reduce feelings of hunger and maintain energy levels.
- In addition, eat moderate amounts of **meat, fish and alternatives**, as they are a good source of protein, vitamins and minerals. Choose lean meats. This group includes eggs, pulses, soya and nuts. Also eat moderate amounts of milk and dairy foods, as they are all good sources of protein and calcium. Choose low-fat alternatives if possible, except for children under 5 years of age.

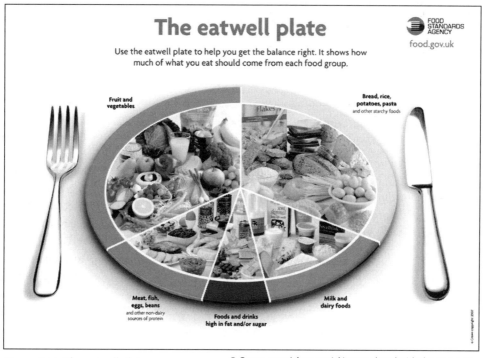

Figure 10.1 The eatwell plate

© Crown copyright material is reproduced with the permission of the controller of HMSO and Queen's Printer for Scotland.

Learning activity

What is the current level of obesity in the United Kingdom? Find out the *Health of the Nation* targets (DH, 1992) linked to nutrition. What factors have contributed to the large increase in obesity over the past 10–15 years? What are the key risks associated with obesity? Look at the World Health Organization (WHO) website report on *Diet, Nutrition and the Prevention of Chronic Diseases* (2003).

Work out a balanced healthy menu for Jack over two or three days, taking into account his age and lifestyle.

Find out what facilities related to nutrition are available for the elderly in your community: for example Meals on Wheels, luncheon clubs or help with shopping (see also Chapter 25 on older people).

S Scenario continued

Jack lacks any appetite and finds it hard to motivate himself to eat.

Learning activity

Why is food important? Consider your response before moving on.

Why is food important? Nutrition science

Food is absolutely essential for life. Human metabolism is a complex process which is constantly active, and which relies on a supply of specific chemicals, or nutrients. These provide energy, and maintain structure and function. Many of these chemicals can be synthesised by the body, but some cannot. These are called *essential nutrients*, and we have to ingest them as we cannot synthesise them. Broadly, there are three categories of essential nutrients:

- **Minerals.** These are usually only required in small amounts (for example, iron and calcium) or very small amounts (trace elements such as iodine).
- **Organic compounds.** These are synthesised in the food chain, but not by humans. They include essential fatty acids, vitamins and essential amino acids.
- **Organic precursors.** These are necessary as the substrates for synthesis of organic compounds needed by humans. If the diet does not provide sufficient precursors, the body is unable to synthesise the compounds needed for maintaining structure and function.

The chemical compounds present in food fit into one or more of the following categories:

- **nutrients**: carbohydrates, fats, proteins, vitamins, minerals and water
- **energy sources**: carbohydrates, fats, proteins and alcohol
- **other compounds**: additives and toxins for example.

As can be seen, several food groups appear in more than one category. They can be used for a variety of purposes, depending on the individual requirements. Maintenance of a stable metabolic state requires sufficient energy and nutrients to satisfy metabolic demand. If food intake is restricted, the body's energy requirements to maintain metabolism will take priority over other activities such as maintaining structure and function.

For more detailed explanations and further reading about major food groups and metabolism, see either Barasi (2003) or Garrow, James and Ralph (2000).

Part II

> **S Scenario continued**
>
> Jack's lack of motivation and poor appetite are contributed to by his feeling constipated, suffering from indigestion, and by a sore mouth, caused partly by his dentures no longer fitting properly, and possible vitamin B deficiency, as a result of an inadequate food intake.
>
> Jack has lost 12 kg in weight since his wife died. Six months ago he weighed 71 kg. He is 1.75 m tall.

> **a Learning activity**
>
> What effect can a sore mouth have? (See Holmes, 1996, for information on oral care in older patients.)
>
> How would you describe Jack's current weight?
>
> What is body mass index (BMI)? Calculate Jack's BMI. Is it in the normal range? (See Table 10.1 for an explanation.)
>
> Work out Jack's percentage weight loss. Is this significant? If so, in what way? (See Bond, 1997, chs 3 and 4.)

Body mass index

BMI measures height and weight, and is used as an estimate of fatness. It is calculated by the equation:

$$\text{BMI} = \frac{\text{Weight (kg)}}{\text{Height}^2 \text{ (m)}}$$

BMI is a better indicator of fatness than weight alone, and is commonly used in nutritional assessment tools. It is considered to be a stable, easily performed and sensitive measure of malnutrition, including for the hospitalised and frail elderly. However, the figures should be interpreted with caution in this age group, as the published norms are based on young adults. In the elderly, there is often reduced muscle mass as well as fat, and therefore ranges are slightly higher than published norms.

The suggested classification of BMI in the United Kingdom is shown in Table 10.1.

Research shows that there is a relationship between BMI and health outcome, with the greatest risks of ill-health associated with the higher and lowest BMI (Bray, 2003).

In cases where height is difficult to measure, there are other parameters that can be used instead, such as the demispan (see Bond, 1997: 68, for details). If both height and weight are difficult to obtain, the mid-upper arm circumference (MUAC) can be used (see the MUST tool on the BAPEN website: www.bapen.org.uk).

Table 10.1 Classification of BMI

19 or less	underweight
20-25	normal weight
26-30	overweight
31-40	obese
40 +	severely obese

W

a) Learning activity

Where does the responsibility lie to survey health needs of the elderly? Which health professionals might be involved? A National Diet and Nutrition Survey is conducted in the United Kingdom at regular intervals. The latest one for people aged 65 years and older was in 1998 (Finch et al, 1998). Find out whether their diet was adequate, and whether it was deficient in any nutrients.

S) Scenario continued

Jack walks down to his local pub most evenings, for a couple of pints and a pack of cigarettes. This is his only regular social contact.

The publican became concerned for Jack's welfare after he had not been in for a few days. He contacted social services, and a caller found Jack at home, disoriented and lying on the floor. There was very little food in the house, and a half-empty carton of stale milk sat on the kitchen table.

Jack was admitted to the Elderly Care Unit of the local community hospital for investigations. The paramedic's assessment notes state that Jack appeared malnourished, dehydrated and confused, and was complaining of soreness over his hip. He was found on the floor, where he had remained immobile for several hours.

a) Learning activity

What are the signs of dehydration? (See Chapters 11 and 12 on Fluid balance, and Bond, 1997, section 6.9).

As Jack's named nurse, you would undertake an initial nutritional screening on his admission to hospital. What would you need to find out and why? (See below for more information.)

Nutritional screening and assessment

Nutritional screening should be carried out with all patients coming into hospital, to identify those with, or at risk of, malnutrition. Factors included in a screening tool may include weight and height (BMI), unintentional weight loss, recent changes to appetite and diet, ability to eat, drink and swallow, gastrointestinal function (such as constipation or diarrhoea), mental condition and medical problems.

W

Learning activity

Find out whether a nutritional assessment tool is used in your practice area, and carry out an assessment, using that tool. Reflect on how easy it was to carry out and how valid and reliable the tool might be.

Find out what percentage of patients are at risk of malnutrition (see www.ageconcern.org.uk).What strategies are in place in your practice area to deal with malnutrition (for example, dietician referral, access to nutritional supplements, protected mealtimes)? Look at the BAPEN website (www.bapen.org.uk) to find details of the Council of Europe UK Alliance '10 key characteristics of good nutritional care in hospitals' which provides a checklist for hospitals and hospital staff to ensure that effective nutritional care is provided..

The National Patient Safety Agency carried out a review in 2007 of the protected mealtimes initiative (NPSA, 2007). Reflect on the benefits and limitations of restricting visitors and ward activities during mealtimes.

The Department of Health published patient-focused benchmarking for healthcare professionals in 2003, and food and nutrition are one of the eight identified areas (DH, 2003). This document, *The Essence of Care*, encourages trusts to be active in improving and raising the profile of nutritional screening and assessment, as a means of reducing malnutrition. It is a valuable resource, which can be used to help improve quality of care as it focuses on fundamental elements of care that matter most to patients.

A number of nutritional screening or assessment tools have been developed to try to identify patients at risk of malnutrition, but very few have been evaluated (Green and Watson, 2005). One that has been validated is the Malnutrition Universal Screening Tool (MUST) developed by Elia (2003) for use in adults. See Figure 10.2.

Learning activity

Visit the DH web pages at http://www.doh.gov.uk/ essenceofcare/intro.htm and see whether any of the other seven identified areas are pertinent to this scenario.

Part II

Learning activity

Work out Jack's nutrition score, using the nutritional risk assessment tool steps given. What are the implications of using unvalidated tools? (See Pattison et al, 1995: 54–5.)

MUST: a nutritional risk assessment tool

MUST (see also Figure 10.2) comprises five steps:

Step 1:   Measure the subject's height and weight to get a BMI score.

Step 2:   Note the percentage of unplanned weight loss, and score it using the tables provided.

Step 3:   Establish the acute disease effect and score it.

Step 4:   Add the scores from steps 1, 2 and 3 to obtain the overall risk of malnutrition.

Step 5:   Use management guidelines and/or local policy to develop a plan of care.

S Scenario continued

Using MUST, Jack scored 3 out of a possible 6 on admission. This placed him in the at-risk category, and he was referred to the dietician.

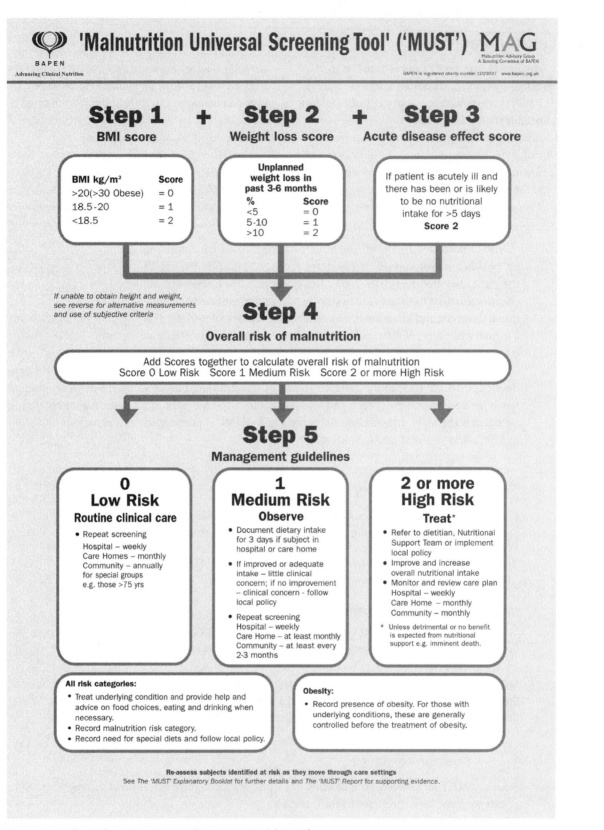

Figure 10.2 The Malnutrition Universal Screening Tool (MUST)

Reproduced here with the kind permission of BAPEN (British Association for Parenteral and Enteral Nutrition). For further information on 'MUST' see www.bapen.org.uk.

C Professional conversation

Jane, a hospital dietician, comments, 'Nurses and dieticians do not have the same role in the management of patient nutrition, but have complementary skills that can be used together in a useful partnership. Many people think dieticians are only interested in patients who need special diets, such as patients with liver or renal disease, but dieticians want to be involved in the management of any patient who is at high risk of malnutrition, so that we can make a full nutritional assessment. We can then try to calculate the exact nutritional needs of an individual. We work closely with occupational therapists and speech and language therapists, especially in the management of patients with swallowing or other eating difficulties, to ensure that the patient receives the optimum nutrition. There is also a dietician in the nutrition support team, where her role is particularly with patients requiring enteral feeding.

'We spend a lot of time talking to patients about their diet and giving information and advice, especially if the nutrition problems are multiple or complex. This could be teaching a group of newly diagnosed diabetic patients the importance of healthy eating, or helping the parents of children with coeliac disease to explore the world of gluten-free diets, or giving one-to-one advice to a patient with diabetes mellitus who has just been diagnosed with coronary heart disease. We see a lot of our patients in outpatient clinics as well as on the wards. We also consider that teaching nurses and other health professionals is important, so that consistent messages are given to patients. It is important that they understand our role, so that they can make appropriate referrals to us.

'We rely on nurses to identify the patients at risk and deal with straightforward nutrition-related problems, reinforcing the nutritional advice given by a dietician. There are only a few dieticians working in each trust, so it's vital that our expertise is used as effectively as possible. Ideally, we should be involved in all cases where the diagnosis or the nutritional advice is complicated, and where nutritional support is required. We are also happy to see anyone who does not seem to be making progress.

'In Jack's case, we were asked to advise after he had been in hospital for a few days. The nurses had carried out an initial nutritional screening and identified him as at risk. We carried out a more detailed assessment and were then able to give them advice about increasing the calories of Jack's food, and help to work out what nutritional advice he needed before going home. It's important that dietary advice is given as practical guidance and not just theoretical principles, with the patient involved in the decisions about his eating patterns and habits.'

a Learning activity

What strategies can be used to increase Jack's nutrient intake and reduce his level of risk? Discuss your ideas with your mentor or other students, then read the section below.

Nutritional support

S Scenario continued

Jack's food and fluid intake was monitored for several days using a food chart to record it, and his nutrition score was reassessed using MUST after one week. Jack is underweight and malnourished. He is therefore in need of building up, and this is the priority rather than trying to make him adhere to healthy eating principles. However, he is elderly and has a small appetite. He does not have any problems associated with swallowing and therefore oral nutrition is appropriate.

Look for ways of fortifying the food a patient like Jack eats, and making every mouthful count. For example:

- encourage the person to drink fluids with calories rather than just water, tea or squash: for example milky drinks with added milk powder, 'sip feeds', high-calorie drinks and thickened soups
- add protein or fat such as grated cheese over potatoes/soup, extra margarine on vegetables, cream/ice-cream with puddings
- add sugar, for example jam or honey in puddings, sugar in drinks
- use neutral or vanilla flavour 'sip feeds' in place of milk on cereals.

> **a Learning activity**
>
> For more ideas, read section 6.1, 'Small is beautiful', in *Eating Matters* (Bond, 1997).
>
> How would you monitor Jack to ensure that he is gaining weight?
>
> What are the potential consequences of malnutrition for Jack?

Consequences of malnutrition

There are a wide variety of complications associated with the development of malnutrition, which may lead to increased mortality:

- reduced mobility, leading to increased risk of deep vein thrombosis and pressure ulcers (see Chapter 28 on rehabilitation for more discussion)
- protein, vitamin and mineral deficiency, leading to increased risk of delayed wound healing
- reduced immunocompetence, leading to increased risk of infection
- muscle atrophy and weakness, causing reduced respiratory function, reduced cardiac function and fatigue, which can lead to a chest infection or heart failure, and can further reduce activity and mobility
- atrophy of the intestinal mucosa, leading to reduced absorption of nutrients and further weight loss
- apathy, lethargy and depression
- increased sensitivity to drugs as a result of drug toxicity.

> **S Scenario continued**
>
> On admission, Jack was also found to have developed a Grade 2 pressure ulcer over his left trocanter.

The pressure ulcer Jack had developed, together with the impact of malnutrition, is likely to result in delayed recovery and a prolonged hospital stay. All these factors have cost implications, for both the individual and the health service.

> **a Learning activity**
>
> What are the factors that would have led to Jack developing a pressure ulcer?

The factors that put people particularly at risk of developing pressure ulcers are malnutrition, dehydration, loss of body weight, age and immobility. See below for factors affecting the development of pressure ulcers. For a more detailed discussion of the importance of nutrition in wound healing, see either Green and McLaren (1998) or Russell (2001).

(e) Evidence-based practice

Assessment and management of pressure ulcers

The critical determinants of pressure ulcers are believed to be the intensity and duration of applied pressure (Cullum and Clark, 1992). There are a number of extrinsic and intrinsic factors that influence tissue tolerance. The intrinsic factors include age, nutritional status, increase or decrease in body weight, immobility, incontinence, neurological factors, vascular factors, and concurrent disease or infection. Extrinsic factors include inadequate support surfaces, poor hygiene, poor positioning, poor moving and handling technique of carers, or prolonged sitting without adequate support.

A pressure ulcer can be defined as an area of localised damage to the skin and underlying tissue caused by pressure, shear, friction and or a combination of these (EPUAP website). Pressure ulcers are unlikely to heal unless the pressure is removed, and as many as possible of the predisposing factors are alleviated. Nutrition is one of the most important factors to address (Green and McLaren, 1998), and specific nutritional guidelines for the prevention and management of pressure ulcers have been developed.

(a) Learning activity   W

Look at the European Pressure Ulcer Advisory Panel website (www.epuap.org) and find the nutritional guidelines developed in 2003. Alternatively, read Clark and colleagues (2004).

Patients like Jack should be assessed on admission for risk of developing further pressure ulcers. A validated risk-assessment tool could be used as part of that assessment.

(a) Learning activity

As the named nurse responsible for Jack's care, how would you select an assessment tool that identifies patients at risk of developing pressure ulcers? What factors are considered? Find out whether a pressure ulcer risk assessment scale is used in the practice area where you are working. Are all patients assessed? If so, how often are they reassessed? Find out whether there is a protocol to follow for patients identified at risk. How suitable would it be for assessing Jack's level of risk? How valid and reliable is it? (See Ratcliffe, 1998.)

(S) Scenario continued

Jack was assessed using the Waterlow pressure ulcer risk assessment scale and scored 13, which put him at moderate risk of developing another pressure ulcer. In addition to the existing Grade 2 pressure ulcer on his trocanter.

(a) Learning activity

See Waterlow (2005) for more details about this particular risk assessment scale. What strategies would you, as the named nurse, use to reduce the risk of Jack developing further pressure ulcers?

There are internationally agreed guidelines for the prevention and treatment of pressure ulcers, based on the best available evidence (EPUAP, 1998).

(a) Learning activity

Look at the EPUAP recommendations and compare them with the strategies you had considered.

Part

II

A high-protein and high-energy diet was ordered for Jack. This included increasing the calorific content of his food, and nutritional supplements. The majority of patients receive their nutrition from the catering department. It is important that all the different agencies that have any responsibility for patient nutrition work together to ensure optimum nutritional care.

(a) Learning activity

Study some hospital menu cards and find out how the needs of different patients are catered for. Consider how flexible you could be over dietary choice if Jack was being cared for in a practice area where you have recently had experience.

Find out whether there are any formal or informal links between the area where you are working and the catering department.

Would it be possible for Jack to receive five small meals/snacks a day, with added butter/cheese to vegetables and added ice cream to puddings? If not, then how else could his dietary needs be met? (See the *Organisation of Food and Nutrition Support in Hospitals* report, BAPEN, 2007; or Millar, 1998.)

In what other ways could Jack's appetite be promoted during his stay in hospital?

Promoting appetite in the elderly

Here are some suggestions for encouraging patients, particularly the elderly, to eat sufficiently:

- **Presentation of food.** Is the portion size appropriate? Does the food look attractive? Is it served at the correct temperature? Are meal times appropriate?
- **Variety and choice of food.** Are familiar foods served? Are they an appropriate type/consistency? Have individual food preferences and the needs of ethnic minority groups been acknowledged?
- **Frequency.** Are smaller or more regular meals/snacks available?
- **Duration.** Are meals rushed?
- **Assistance.** Is help with eating available, if needed? Are there feeding aids to promote independence?
- **Oral hygiene.** Is mouth care offered after meals? Are dentures well fitting? Is the mouth clean, fresh and without infection?
- **Positioning.** Are individuals positioned comfortably, and supported if necessary, to allow them to manage their meal as independently as possible?
- **Exercise.** How active and mobile are individuals? Exercise can improve appetite because it creates an increased demand for energy.
- **Social events.** Do individuals eat alone or do they have company during mealtimes?
- **Distractions.** Are there other activities taking place at mealtimes? Are there any unwanted smells/sounds/sights that might be off-putting?

(a) Learning activity

Reflect on possible ways in which mealtimes in your practice area could be better managed to give a higher priority to patient nutrition. See also the last paragraph of the professional conversation below.

(c) Professional conversation

Anne, sister on an elderly care unit, says, 'Jack is strong enough to feed himself while in hospital, but a number of our patients are not. Various ideas have been promoted in the *Eating Matters* pack (Bond, 1997), such as inviting visitors and friends in at mealtimes to help, or using volunteers. Several trusts have reverted to a bulk food delivery system, so that patients can choose, at the time of each meal, what food they want and how much they wish to eat. Others have employed a unit cook for long-stay wards, so that patients' individual needs and preferences can be met more easily. Another idea is to use red trays to identify patients who need help with eating or whose food intake is being monitored (Bradley and

Rees, 2003). In this unit, we liaise with the catering department to try to ensure patients get the correct diet. We have a responsibility to ensure that our patients receive the food they need, and to monitor their intake (RCN, 1996). I think nutrition should be as much a priority as drugs prescribed to our patients. After all, patients who are malnourished will take longer to recover, and are more likely to develop complications and have their stay extended.

'Nutrition needs to be given the priority it deserves, and the ward organisation needs to reflect this. Nursing staff need to be available to help with mealtimes rather than completing administration, taking our own lunch-break or handing over to nurses on the next shift. Patients need to be on the ward at mealtimes, and investigations, physiotherapy and other essential activities should be planned around mealtimes whenever possible. For patients who are not on the ward when meals are served, there should be provision to ensure that they do not miss their meal. Similarly, there needs to be a procedure for newly admitted patients, or for patients whose surgery has been postponed, to receive a meal. This is especially important now that food can no longer be prepared on the unit, because of the health and safety regulations.

'Mealtimes are not just the main source of nutrition; they are also a social event for most people. We must try to ensure that patients have the opportunity to socialise over meals if their condition allows. Many wards were not designed with communal meals in mind, and nurses need to be imaginative to try to create an atmosphere conducive to eating. This is especially true on long-stay wards and elderly care units such as this one.'

(a) Learning activity   W

Look at *Choosing a Better Diet* (2005b) on the Department of Health website: (www.dh.gov.uk.) and find the *Food and Health Action Plan* (DH, 2007). What actions does it suggest that you could consider implementing?

(s) Scenario

Jack was admitted to a four-bedded bay. In the bed next to him was a rather confused elderly man, Mr Whitehead, who frequently refused to eat. He was already malnourished, and at risk of becoming dehydrated. Nurses tried to persuade him to eat and drink, but often to no avail.

(a) Learning activity

If you were the nurse giving care, what would be your response to Mr Whitehead? You may wish to discuss this with your peers and with practitioners and teachers, in relation to ethical considerations. Read Clibbens (1996: 29–30).

Oral nutritional supplements can be offered to patients whose nutrient intake is insufficient. There are several different types of supplements available, some that can be given to replace a meal and others that supplement a normal diet. They can be given in a variety of different forms, such as freezing to create an ice cream or mousse consistency, or warming and eating as a soup.

(a) Learning activity

Find out what nutritional supplements are available in your clinical area, and discuss the purpose of each of them with your mentor or ward dietician.

Find the NICE reference guide to nutrition support in adults (2006) and discuss the care pathway outlined in it with your mentor or ward dietician. Compare this with the care delivered in your practice placement. For a detailed discussion of enteral nutrition and the care of patients receiving it, read Green and Jackson (2005).

Enteral nutrition is the delivery of nutrients directly into the stomach or small intestines via an enteral tube or percutaneous endoscopic gastrostomy (PEG) feed, and is another option that can be considered in these circumstances

---

S   Scenario continued

The man in the bed opposite was friendly and always keen to come over and talk to Jack. He regaled Jack with stories of his youth in the Punjab region of India. He was a Hindu and a vegetarian, and he found hospital food generally tasteless and unappetising.

The fourth bed in Jack's area was occupied by a recently retired man who had suffered a stroke (see Chapter 25) and was at risk of becoming malnourished as he found it very difficult to swallow. This man had to have his drinks thickened to enable him to swallow them.

---

a   Learning activity   W

Find out about the nutrition provision for ethnic minority groups in the hospital or institution where you are working.

Check out which nutrients are most likely to be deficient in people who are vegetarian or vegan. (See the British Nutrition Foundation briefing paper: vegetarian nutrition on http://www.nutrition.org.uk or read Chappiti, Jean-Marie and Chan, 2000.)

Who in the interprofessional team is likely to be involved in the assessment and care of the man who suffered a stroke? What role can these therapists and others play in nutrition? (See Chapter 28 on rehabilitation and Chapter 25 on older people for more

extensive discussions of the roles of different members of the interprofessional team; see also the professional conversation with a dietician above.) Can you think of any links between nutrition and the risk of having a stroke?

Look at the Bandolier website for a review of research on diet and risk of stroke. You could also explore Barker's research on intrauterine growth retardation and the development of high blood pressure, stroke and diabetes in middle age (Godfrey and Barker, 2000).

Find out why thickening fluids aids swallowing, and practise making up thickened feeds in your skills lab or practice area.

Nutritional assessment

Nutritional assessment is a more in-depth investigation to identify the extent and nature of malnutrition. This may include anthropometric measurements, such as skin-fold thickness and mid-arm circumference, which assess the amount of subcutaneous fat; biochemical measures, such as plasma albumin and plasma transferrin, to measure the level of protein; physical examination, dietary history, and recorded intake of food. A member of the nutrition support team, such as the dietician or nutrition nurse specialist, normally carries this out. (See Bond, 1997, chs3 and 4 for further details of nutritional assessment.)

a   Learning activity

Find out whether there is a nutrition support team, or a nutrition nurse specialist, in the trust where you are working. What are their key responsibilities? How are patients referred to a member of this team?

In summary, what were Jack's problems on admission to hospital? Consider your response before reading on.

Problems on admission to hospital

Jack's problems on admission to hospital, which are common to many elderly patients, were:

- dehydration, leading to fluid and electrolyte imbalance
- malnutrition, leading to increased risk of morbidity (check out the section on the consequences of malnutrition above)
- immobility, leading to pressure ulcer development (have you read the section on development of pressure ulcers above?)
- possible trauma, from his fall

- fear of falling again (see NICE, 2004 and DH, 2001).
- mild confusion, possibly caused by dehydration or vitamin deficiency.

> **a** Learning activity
>
> What nutrition-related actions would you consider to be appropriate on Jack's admission to hospital?

Appropriate nutrition-related actions

Actions that could be taken in these circumstances are:

- **Nutritional support.** This reduces malnutrition and increases the appetite. As Jack is able to swallow and has no known digestive/absorption difficulties, then oral nutrition should be sufficient. (Review the sections above on nutritional support and promoting appetite in the elderly.)
- **Maintenance of fluid and electrolyte balance.** This involves monitoring intake and output, oral/intravenous fluids (if given), and checking the blood levels of electrolytes regularly.
- **Pressure ulcer prevention and management.** This involves pressure relief and regular turning, mobilisation, adequate nutrition and fluids, and wound care. (Revisit the section above on prevention and management of pressure ulcers, and Chapter 28.)
- **Mobilisation.** To reduce muscle atrophy, increase circulation, increase appetite and energy requirements, and increase confidence and independence.

> **S** Scenario continued
>
> Jack is keen to return home as soon as possible.

> **a** Learning activity
>
> What would you include in your discharge planning for Jack?

Discharge planning

In planning the discharge of a patient like Jack, you should consider;

- **health education** on meal planning and healthy eating (review the section above on what constitutes a healthy, balanced diet)
- **community support**: community nutrition, such as Meals on Wheels or luncheon clubs, home help and bereavement counselling
- **investigation of alternative living arrangements**, such as a residential home or warden-assisted flats, or enabling Jack to live more safely in his own home; for example by installing a personal alarm or telephone.

> **a** Learning activity
>
> Who will be responsible for Jack's care when he returns to the community?
> Find out the individual involved in the community where you are placed. What role would they play in maintaining Jack's health?

Part

II

Conclusion

In this chapter you have considered what constitutes a healthy, balanced diet and the factors that might affect it. There have been opportunities to become familiar with a nutrition screening tool, to identify the need for nutritional assessment, and to consider how nutritional needs can be met in both hospital and community settings. Some of the health issues related to poor nutrition, such as constipation and development of pressure ulcers, have been explored and you have examined suitable interventions to prevent and manage these problems. You have also explored other nutrition-related challenges, such as difficulty in swallowing, refusal to eat, alternative diets such as vegetarian and enteral nutrition. You should now be equipped to go out and contribute to meeting your own and your clients' nutritional needs.

References

Age Concern (2007) *Hungry to be Heard*, campaign on malnutrition [online] http://www.ageconcern.org.uk/AgeConcern/hungry2bheard.asp (accessed 23 December 2008).

British Association for Parenteral and Enteral Nutrition (BAPEN) (2003) '10 key characteristics of good nutritional care in hospitals' [online] http://www.bapen.org.uk/pdfs/coe_leaflet.pdf. (accessed 23 December 2008).

BAPEN (2006) MUST tool [online] http://www.bapen.org.uk/musttoolkit.html (accessed 23 December 2008).

BAPEN (2007) *Organisation of Food and Nutrition Support in Hospitals* [online] http://www.bapen.org.uk/res_pub.html (accessed 24 December 2008).

Barasi, M. E. (2003) *Human Nutrition: A health perspective*, London, Arnold.

Bradley, L. and Rees, C. (2003) 'Reducing nutritional risk in hospital: the red tray', *Nursing Standard* **17**(26) , 33–7.

Bray, G. A. (2003) 'Risks of obesity', *Endocrinology Metabolism Clinics of North America* 32, 787–804.

British Nutrition Foundation (BNF) (2007) *Healthy Eating: a whole diet approach* [online] http://www.nutrition.org.uk/home.asp?siteId=43&sectionId=325&subSectionId=320&parentSection=299&which=1 (accessed 3 February 2009).

Brocklehurst, J. (1990) 'Constipation and faecal incontinence', *Nursing the Elderly*, February, 17–18.

Centre for Research and Dissemination (2001) *Guidelines on Laxative Use* [online] http://www.york.ac.uk/inst/crd/EHC/ehc71.pdf (accessed 23 December 2008).

Chappiti, U., Jean-Marie, S. and Chan, W. (2000) 'Cultural and religious influences on adult nutrition in the UK', *Nursing Standard* **14**(29), 47–51.

Clark, M., Schols, J., Benati, G., Jackson, P., Engfer, M., Langer, G., Kerry, B. and Colin, D. (2004) 'Pressure ulcers and nutrition: a new European guideline', *Journal of Wound Care* **13**(7), 267–72.

Clibbens, R. (1996) 'Eating, ethics and Alzheimers', *Nursing Times* **92**(50), 29–30.

Cullum, N. and Clark, M. (1992) 'Matching patient need for pressure sore prevention with the supply of pressure redistributing mattresses', *Journal of Advanced Nursing* 17, 310–16.

Department of Health (DH) (1992) *Health of the Nation: A strategy for health in England*, London, The Stationery Office.

DH (2001) *National Service Framework for Older People: Standard 6–falls* [online] http://www.dh.gov.uk/en/SocialCare/Deliveringadultsocialcare/Olderpeople/OlderpeoplesNSFstandards/DH_4002294 (accessed 23 December 2008).

DH (2003) *Five a Day: Healthy eating advice about fruit and vegetable intake* [online] http://www.dh.gov.uk/en/Policyandguidance/Healthandsocialcaretopics/FiveADay/index.htm (accessed 23 December 2008).

DH (2004) *Choosing Health: Making healthy choices easier*, London, The Stationery Office.

DH (2005a) *Balance of Good Health*, London, The Stationery Office.

DH (2005b) *Choosing a Better Diet: A food and health action plan* [online] http://www.dh.gov.uk/en/Publicationsandstatistics/Publications/PublicationsPolicyAndGuidance/DH_4105356 (accessed 23 December 2008).

DH (2007) *Food and Health Action Plan* [online] http://www.dh.gov.uk/en/Publichealth/Healthimprovement/Healthyliving/Foodandhealthactionplan/index.htm (accessed 3 February 2009).

DH (2008) *The Essence of Care: Patient focused benchmarking for healthcare professionals*, London, DH [online] http://www.dh.gov.uk/en/Publichealth/Patientsafety/Clinicalgovernance/DH_082929 (accessed 23 December 2008).

Elia, M. (2003) *The MUST Report*, Redditch, BAPEN.

Finch, S., Doyle, W., Lowe, S., Bates, C., Prentice, A., Smithers, G. and Clarke, P. (1998) *National Diet and Nutrition Survey: People aged 65 years and older. Volume 1: Report of the diet and nutrition survey*, London, The Stationery Office.

Garrow, J. S., James, W. P. T. and Ralph, A. (2000) *Human Nutrition and Dietetics*, 10th edn, Edinburgh, Churchill Livingstone.

Godfrey, K. M. and Barker, D. J. (2000) 'Fetal nutrition and adult disease', *American Journal of Clinical Nutrition* 71 (suppl 5), SS1344–52.

Green, S. M. and Jackson, P. A. (2005) 'Nutrition', chapter 21 in Alexander, M., Fawcett, J. and Runciman, P. (eds), *Nursing Practice: Hospital and home: the adult*. Edinburgh, Elsevier.

Green, S. M. and McLaren, S. (1998) 'Nutrition and wound healing', *Community Nursing* 4(7), 29–32.

Green, S. M. and Watson, R. (2005) 'Nutritional screening and assessment tools for use by nurses: literature review', *Journal of Advanced Nursing* **50**(1), 69–83.

Holmes, H. S. (1996) 'Nursing management of oral care in older patients', *Nursing Times* **92**(9), 37–9.

Millar, B. (1998) 'Dying for a good meal?' *Health Service Journal*, 23 April, pp. 24–7.

National Institute of Clinical Excellence (NICE) (2004) *Clinical Guideline 21 for the Assessment and Prevention of Falls in Older People* [online] http://www.nice.org.uk (accessed 23 December 2008).

NICE (2006) *Clinical Guideline 32 for Nutrition Support in Adults* [online] http://www.nice.org.uk (accessed 23 December 2008).

National Patient Safety Agency (NPSA) (2007) *Protected Mealtimes Review: Findings and recommendations* [online] http://www.npsa.nhs.uk/nrls/improvingpatientsafety/cleaning-and-nutrition/nutrition/protected-mealtimes/ (accessed 3 December 2008).

NPSA (2008) *Nutritional Screening Project* [online] http://www.npsa.nhs.uk/nrls/improvingpatientsafety/cleaning-and-nutrition/nutrition/nutritional-screening-project/ (accessed 23 December 2008).

Organisation of Food and Nutritional Support in Hospitals Report, BAPEN, 2007 [online] http://www.bapen.org.uk/res_pub.html (accessed 23 December 2008).

Pattison, R., Corr, J., Ogilvie, M., Farquhar, D., Sutherland, D., Davidson, H. I. M. and Richardson, R. A. (1995) Validation of a subjective nutritional scoring system used in the elderly. Clinical Nutrition 14 (Supplement 2), pp. 54-5.

Ratcliffe, P. (1998) 'Under pressure to update research', *Nursing Times* **94**(16), 59–61.

Royal College of Nursing (RCN) (1996) *Statement on Feeding and Nutrition in Hospitals*, London, RCN.

RCN (in conjunction with NICE) (2005) *Clinical Guidelines for Prevention and treatment of Pressure Ulcers* [online] http://www.rcn.org.uk/__data/assets/pdf_file/0007/109843/002444.pdf (accessed 23 December 2008).

Russell, L. (2001) 'The importance of patients' nutritional status in wound healing', *British Journal of Nursing* **10**(6), SS42–S9.

Waterlow, J. (2005) 'From costly treatment to cost-effective prevention: using Waterlow', *British Journal of Community Nursing* **10**(9) SS25–30.

Winney, J. (1998) 'Constipation', *Nursing Standard* **13**(11), 49–53.

World Health Organisation (2003) *Nutrition Programme: Diet, nutrition and the prevention of chronic diseases, WHO Technical Report 916* [online] http://whqlibdoc.who.int/trs/WHO_TRS_916.pdf (accessed 23 December 2008).

Further reading

Bond, S. (ed.) (1997) *Eating Matters*, Newcastle, University of Newcastle-upon-Tyne Centre for Health Service Research. Developed in response to the Association of Community Health Councils' report, *Hungry in Hospital* (1997), this pack brings together the research and expertise of many of the leading nurses in this field. It aims to offer a valuable resource to help nurses provide good nutritional care in hospital. It is full of examples of good practice and advice, as well as including detailed information on topics such as the causes of malnutrition, nutritional assessment and the management of feeding difficulties. It includes suggestions for action and detailed case studies.

Buttriss, J., Wynne, A. and Stanner, S. (2001) *Nutrition: A handbook for community nurses*, London, Whurr. This book provides a wealth of information on various aspects of nutrition for community nurses and others working in public health. The authors are renowned experts in the field of public health nutrition and have written the text in a question and answer format that facilitates ease of access and responds to many of the questions commonly asked by patients. It addresses the issues of nutrition in health and illness, nutrition through the lifespan and nutrition issues in the media. An example question is, 'Are people living alone in the community worse off nutritionally than those being cared for in institutions?' Each answer draws on recent research and directs readers to other resources.

Lennard-Jones, J. E. (1992) *A Positive Approach to Nutrition as Treatment*, London, King's Fund. This is an influential report that identifies a number of ways in which nutritional care could be improved. It recommends that heights and weights should be monitored in adults, and that growth and development be recorded in children. The report emphasises the need for assessing nutritional status, and suggests that this should include recent diet history and changes, as well as physical examination. This report stimulated a number of hospitals to develop their own nutritional assessment tools, for identifying patients at risk of malnutrition.

Sizer, T. (ed.) (1996) *Standards and Guidelines for Nutritional Support of Patients in Hospital*, Maidenhead, British Association for Parenteral and Enteral Nutrition (BAPEN). BAPEN was formed in 1992, following the recommendations made by Lennard-Jones in the King's Fund report. It recommends the development of nutritional guidelines, regular nutritional assessment and records of nutrition intakes. It sets standards for use with hospital patients, and outlines a protocol for nutritional assessment, using the MUST tool.

Useful websites

Bandolier, for critical reviews of research: http://www.jr2.ox.ac.uk/bandolier/booth/booths/eating.html

British Association of Parenteral and Enteral Nutrition, for details of MUST screening tool and nutritional support and ten-point 'Mission Statement' for hospitals to improve nutritional care: www.bapen.org.uk

British Nutrition Foundation, for briefing papers on specific topics: www.nutrition.org.uk

European Pressure Ulcer Advisory Panel, for nutritional and general guidelines on pressure ulcer prevention and treatment: www.epuap.org

National Institute for Health and Clinical Excellence, for clinical guidelines: www.nice.org.uk

Part

II

Chapter

11

Fluid balance
in children

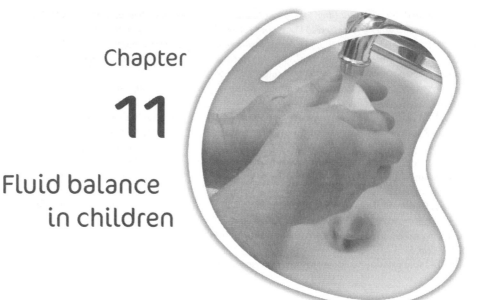

Vanessa Lockyer-Stevens

 Links to other chapters in *Foundation Studies for Caring*

 Links to other chapters in *Foundation Skills for Caring*

W   Don't forget to visit www.palgrave.com/glasper for additional
online resources relating to this chapter.

Introduction

This chapter explores the hydration needs of children using the scenario of a young child who is at risk of hypovolaemic shock from severe vomiting and diarrhoea.

Diarrhoea and vomiting (D&V) in the under-5s is still a leading cause of morbidity and mortality globally. According to Kosek, Bern and Guerrant (2003), diarrhoea kills 2.5 million children every year, accounting for approximately 21 per cent of all-cause mortality for children under five years old in developing countries. This equates to 'one child dying every twelve seconds, or a jumbo jet full of children crashing every 90 minutes' (Kosek, Bern and Guerrant, 2003).

Such staggering statistics make grim reading. While morbidity and mortality rates in developed countries bear little resemblance to those elsewhere in the world, the incidence of D&V from rotavirus in particular remains problematic in the United Kingdom, accounting for seven in 1,000 children aged 5 years and younger who are admitted to hospital each year (McCormick, Fleming and Charlton, 1993). D&V accounts for 16 per cent of medical attendees at Accident and Emergency (A&E) departments and an estimated 526,000 consultations with GPs annually (Armon et al, 2001). In fact, nearly all children are infected by rotavirus by the age of 5 (Health Protection Agency, 2006a). The burden to child and family from this largely preventable illness may be considerable, and it leads to absence from work, disrupted school attendance and hospital admission.

This chapter focuses on how to assess the type and degree of dehydration, calculate resuscitation and maintenance fluid replacement, and discuss the child's care in partnership with their family. Finally, it discusses the role of health professionals in supporting families in the prevention of further infection.

Learning outcomes

This chapter will enable you to:

- identify the population at risk of diarrhoea and vomiting
- examine the nurse's role in the assessment, planning, implementation and evaluation of a child and family with severe D&V
- describe how hypovolaemic shock may arise as a result of severe dehydration
- examine evidence-based literature that supports best practice in the care of the child and family
- discuss the role of the multidisciplinary team in the care of the sick child and family
- list support agencies involved in the child's care following discharge.

Concepts

- Growth and development
- Altered pathophysiology and restoration of homeostasis
- Gastrointestinal infection
- Health education
- Evidence-based practice
- Working in partnership with families
- Assessing hydration
- Record keeping
- Fluid resuscitation
- Multidisciplinary team
- Hypovolaemic shock
- Discharge planning

Learning activity

Have you cared for a child with D&V either in hospital or the community? If so, what do you remember most about their experience? Take a minute to note down key points in the child's care as they will make useful reference points as you read on. Keep a medical dictionary and good anatomy and physiology text with you as well to check your understanding of words, phrases and principles underpinning the altered pathophysiology of the child's illness. Use a pocket-sized address book to start a 'terminology' list for future reference and to add to throughout your course – and beyond!

S Scenario Introducing Sophie

Sophie, a normally fit and healthy 2-year-old girl, is admitted to your ward at 6 am with a history of severe diarrhoea and vomiting. On arrival she has sunken eyes, inelastic skin, dry lips, tongue and mucus membranes, is irritable and listless and complains of a 'tummyache'. She has refused food and fluids for 24 hours. Sophie is accompanied by her parents Paula and Tom. Her older brother and baby sister are being cared for by a neighbour. You are assigned to help with Sophie's care.

a Learning activity

Because children respond to illness differently according to their age it is really important to have explicit understanding of growth and development. In your learning group, brainstorm factors that influence the normal growth and development of a healthy child using the headings physical, environmental, socioeconomic and emotional.

For more detail, use supporting texts such as Hobart and Frankel (2004), Bee (1994) or Whaley and colleagues (1999).

Now, think about those factors that might compromise Sophie's normal growth and development as a result of her illness, and remember, recognition and care of a sick child is best achieved by studying normal growth and development in considerable detail. So, in order for this chapter to be really meaningful you need to reflect back on what you have read on this, with any notes made.

How illness can impact on normal growth and development

In order to evaluate changes in growth and development, we need to take a systematic approach to four main assessment areas: gross motor, fine motor, speech and language, and social development. Each is an important measure of children's well-being (Maill, Rudolf and Levene, 2007). As part of this, you will want to take quantitative measurements, such as the height and weight of the child. Additional measurements include head circumference and body length. These can be plotted on percentile (growth) charts, and give a guide to the rate of growth, and how it compares with the norm, taking account of race and ethnicity. Social and behavioural development, together with language and speech, are in contrast qualitative issues. An example of qualitative research into child development is Swanwick's (1990) seminal work on children's understanding of the 'concept' of illness at various ages.

The normal growth and development of toddlers can be affected in a number of ways by illness:

- **Physical changes.** Growth and development in this age group remains constant, and at the age of 2 a child would be expected to achieve a number of developmental milestones. Their gross and fine motor skills for example will be developing rapidly, enabling them to walk and run, which has important advantages for the enquiring mind of a 2-year-old. As such toddlers need close supervision to reduce the risk of harm particularly from ingestion of unclean items (Whaley and Wong, 1999: 117–97). Other physical changes include increased immunity and a reduction in the percentage of total body water (TBW), which is approximately 10 per cent higher in children than in adulthood, making children less vulnerable to the effects of dehydration, particularly hypovolaemia, as they grow. It is important to their care that illness and starvation are thought to slow down growth, and it is not until recovery begins that the unique phenomenon of catch-up growth takes place (Rudolf and Levene, 2006:4).

- **Psychological factors**. Small children are dependent on their parents and siblings for love, a sense of security and emotional well-being. 'Separation anxiety' is not uncommon in this age group (Whaley and Wong, 1999:572).
- **Socioeconomic factors**. Small children are dependent on their parents to provide sufficient food, warmth, clothing and education (UNICEF, 2001; DH, 2003, 2004).
- **Cultural factors.** Children rely on the daily routines in their lives to feel secure. Admission to hospital may make them feel vulnerable and distressed.
- **Cognitive factors.** Children's language and comprehension develop all the time. Children of this age often use 'horographic' or 'telegraphic' speech, in which key content words are used all the time, for example, 'Daddy gone work' (Campbell and Glasper, 1995: 147). Knowledge of the development of speech and language provides important cues for carers of the unwell child, as toddlers in particular appear sensitive to a change of environment.

Admission to hospital can be particularly stressful for both child and parents. Young children, sensitive to parental stress, may respond by becoming stressed themselves. This phenomenon, which is known as 'social referencing', and described by Lewandowski (1992), takes account of the child's immature coping strategies. In recognising such stresses the nurse is in a unique position to support the child and family at such a vulnerable time (White, 1995). See also Chapter 20 on care of the child and young person.

S Scenario continued

Sophie's current state of development, and the possible impact on it of a hospital stay, are:

- Psychomotor ability: Sophie has reached her expected milestones for running and walking.
- Health and disease: as already mentioned, Sophie is normally a fit, healthy little girl.
- Resources available: the health visitor helps promote the health of children. Together with other community services such as playgroups, Sophie will have access to environments that help to promote normal growth and development.
- Environmental factors: strange surroundings are likely to exacerbate Sophie's distress.

- Disruption of routine: Sophie's sleep pattern and eating habits have been disrupted by her illness and hospital admission.
- Effect on parents: Sophie has become lethargic which will frighten her parents. Paula and Tom now rely on skilled practitioners to provide the care Sophie requires. Information that is clear, understandable and consistent will help reduce their anxiety.
- Institutional factors: the changes to Sophie's routine such as eating and drinking, sleep, noise pollution in the ward, missing siblings and dealing with strangers are likely to heighten her anxiety.
- Increased nutritional requirements: Sophie will probably have lost weight as a result of her illness. Early referral to the dietician may be necessary.

Admission to hospital

On a child's admission to hospital, a child health history is taken. Assessment of care will take account of the child's past and current health status. This requires health professionals to acknowledge the unique knowledge carers often have of their child's needs in health and when they are sick (Sidley, 1995). The context of this view should not be underestimated, as evidence suggests conflict can arise between professional and maternal knowledge. Indeed, a study by Callery (1997) suggests that primary carers sometimes found it difficult to 'convince health professionals that their concerns were justified' about their child's illness.

Practice tip

One way of sharing information about a child's health status is through the use of their personal child health record. This record, which is kept by all families of pre-school children, enables parents and the primary healthcare team to share information about the child's growth and development pattern, and take account of any concerns parents may have about their child.

The personal child health record is used by health visitors when a newborn child is taken onto their caseload. In general these records are kept within the family home, giving parents 'ownership' of important information about their child's progress. They are encouraged to document personal accounts of their child's achievements, or concerns, which can be shared with relevant professionals such the health visitor, general practitioner (GP) or hospital staff. Their use may be of particular value to the admitting nurse, as information such as immunisation dates may prove difficult to recall for anxious parents. So make its request part of your admission plan: it can save you time and parents mental energy (NMC, 2007a).

Learning activity

Look through a copy of a personal child health record and make notes about how growth and development is assessed and monitored. *Do ask permission first.*

Child health records are only one of a number of ways in which families can gain and share advice. Health visitor telephone helplines (Hawley and Howkins 1999), websites (www. Healthvisitors.com) and walk-in children's centres are evolving, with a remit to engage a competent workforce dedicated to identifying children's needs (DH, 2007).

The philosophy embedded in the Children Acts of 1989 and 2004 continues to underpin national policy drivers for the evolution of child and family-centred services, including specialist roles and advanced practice. The twenty-first century will witness unprecedented changes to care strategies for children and families, notably in public health where multidisciplinary teams will form the cornerstone of children's services (NMC, 2007b). Indeed it might be that children in Sophie's situation are cared for within children's centres rather than in secondary care settings. Against this background, it must be remembered that children's health needs are unique and require skilled professionals in this distinct area of practice (Hawley and Howkins, 1999).

Scenario continued

Sophie has been unwell since attending her playmate Melanie's second birthday party the previous afternoon. She vomited once since returning home, but continued to play unperturbed. At 6 pm she asked to go to bed, complaining that she had a tummy ache and was hot and tired. Paula gave her Calpol (children's paracetamol) and telephoned NHS Direct for some help. The nurse suggested that Calpol and clear fluids be given regularly, and that Paula observe for further vomiting.

Sophie continued to vomit accompanied by diarrhoea. The GP was contacted who also suggested regular Calpol, keeping her cool to alleviate a further rise in temperature, and giving clear fluids only to drink. Instructions were left to ring the 'out of hours' doctor service should Sophie remain unwell.

Learning activity

Visit your nearest GP surgery or library and find out what primary health care services are available to Sophie and her family.

Part II

S Scenario continued

Overnight Sophie continued to vomit, with profuse bouts of diarrhoea, and she was admitted to hospital following a visit by the GP at 5 am. Tom and Paula mentioned to their doctor that other children from the party had also been unwell with D&V, which the GP noted in the admission letter.

a Learning activity

What is D&V? Consider what you currently know before reading on.

e Evidence-based practice

Diarrhoea and vomiting: friend or foe?

Diarrhoea is defined by Rudolf and Levene (2006) as 'an increase in the frequency, fluidity and volume of faeces' and they comment that as many as three acute/severe episodes may be experienced by the child before the age of 3. Bacterial or viral pathogens are commonly responsible for infection, although causes extrinsic to the gastrointestinal tract, such as antibiotic-induced diarrhoea, can be a problem in all age groups. Armon and colleagues (2001) state that acute diarrhoea often results from infectious intestinal disease (IID), and describe how as many as one in six children visit their GP with an episode of IID. Care of this group may therefore pose

difficulties for healthcare professionals in terms of identifying children at risk of dehydration, which in severe cases can be a life-threatening consequence of D&V.

Campbell and Glasper (1995) state that vomiting is generally regarded as 'forceful ejection' of stomach contents through the mouth, which arises as a result of stimulation to the vomiting centre in the medulla oblongata (Martini, 2006). Vomiting is not uncommon in infancy and early childhood. The degree and severity of vomiting can vary from a single episode to a precursor of more life-threatening disease such as meningitis or pyloric stenosis (Rudolf and Levene, 2006).

In addition to having an increased percentage of total water in their bodies, babies' immune systems are immature, which results in their being more susceptible to infection and dehydration than older children. The effect of age on physiological processes influences the child's susceptibility to different causes of D&V. Here are some more ideas.

Children of Sophie's age are active and industrious. Regarded as toddlers (age 1–3 years), they rarely rest unless asleep. This period, like infancy, is one of rapid growth during which many developmental milestones are achieved. Among these milestones is a child's insatiable desire to explore the world around them. This potentially leaves them exposed to environments that pose a risk to their health, such as dirty floors, a fascination for toilets, sharing food, sweets and ingesting poisonous substances. It is hardly surprising therefore, that young children are particularly at risk of gastroenteritis.

a Learning activity

What are the common causes of D&V in childhood? Refer to Maill and colleagues (2007: 79).

Now, make a list of the signs and symptoms of each. For a full description of causes of D&V refer to a major child health text such as Hazinski (1999), Rudolf and Levene (2006) or Moules and Ramsey (2008).

Did your answers include looking for causes of D&V in addition to those of the gastrointestinal tract? Examples of possible causes are a common cold, respiratory syncytial virus (RSV) or otitis media or otitis externa (inner or outer ear infection), meningism and febrile convulsion.

S Scenario continued

Following examination Sophie is diagnosed with gastroenteritis probably caused through food contamination. Paula and Tom are clearly anxious about Sophie, and ask whether their other children are at risk of similar infection.

a   Learning activity

Which common organisms give rise to D&V in childhood? See McVerry and Collin (1998: 31–3) for more help.

What help and advice do Sophie's parents require in order to reduce the risk of cross-infection to the family?

What is the role of the infection control nurse at this time?

Find out what types of infective organisms causing diarrhoea require notification to public health services and how this process is undertaken.

Try to create an opportunity to spend some of your time in practice 'shadowing' members of the infection control team. The experience would be invaluable.

Dehydration and its effect on the body

Fluid losses from D&V can result in varying degrees of dehydration, particularly if losses are persistent or the child is unable to tolerate oral fluids.

e   Evidence-based practice

What is dehydration?

Dehydration is a term used when salts and water are lost from the fluid compartments of the body, giving rise to hypovolaemia. It is apparent in clinical conditions in which the total output of fluid exceeds its total intake irrespective of underlying pathophysiology (Campbell and Glasper, 1995). Disturbances to the finely-tuned balance of water and electrolytes disrupt homeostasis, resulting in significant morbidity and in severe cases, mortality.

As early as 1832 a physician called Latta treated patients suffering severe dehydration from cholera with intravenous saline. Yet over a century later, an estimated 3 million children die as a result of dehydration caused by diarrhoea alone, 80 per cent of them in the first two years of life (Rehydration Project, 2002). Chameides and Hazinski (1994) further state that hypovolaemia still remains 'the commonest cause of shock in children worldwide'.

Dehydration is often a common complication of D&V. Babies and young children are more vulnerable, particularly in parts of the developing world where access to clean water, oral and intravenous fluid-replacement therapy is poor.

Charities and organisations across the world play a key role in the delivery and administration of life-saving treatments for children most in need. The World Health Organization (WHO) and National Institute of Clinical Excellence (NICE), for example, provide international national guidance for the promotion, prevention and treatment of illness causing D&V. But even in the developed world, there is a lack of knowledge and training of the use of oral replacement solutions (ORS). Conway and Newport's study in 1994 confirms this by stating that only 29 per cent of children received ORS treatment of this kind at home. Maill, Rudolf and Levene (2007: 79) support the use of oral fluids including continued breastfeeding in babies and young children as a first-line treatment. NICE publishes its recommendations in April 2009. Whether oral or intravenous, fluid and electrolyte replacement therapy are essential to both prevention and reduction of the child's susceptibility to shock and critical illness.

a   Learning activity   W

Find out about oral rehydration therapy. The following resources may be helpful:

- Walker-Smith and colleagues (1997) for recommendations on feeding in childhood gastroenteritis.
- www.rehydrate.org/html/deh010.htm for further reading on the use of ORS.

- The Sleep Tight Video no. 169, *Help for Sleepless Parents*. 'Dehydration in children always happens as a complication of diarrhoea and vomiting, especially if combined with fever – most commonly gastroenteritis'. For further information visit www.drhull.com/Ency/Master/D/dehydration.html.
- Armon and colleagues (2001) for guidelines on acute diarrhoea management: www.archdischild.com.

What do you understand by the term 'fluid compartments' of the body? What is the function of each? Use a text such as Martini (2006) to help you answer.

Name the key electrolytes involved in maintaining normal homeostasis. Explain the function of each, particularly sodium and potassium.

Find out what the normal blood plasma levels of sodium and potassium are. What role does water (H_2O) play in maintaining homeostasis?

Consider what you know about each of these aspects before reading on.

The role of water and electrolytes: pathophysiology perspective

Water and electrolytes are key players in the maintenance of homeostasis, their distribution being dependent on the age of the child. For example, the amount of TBW in a full-term infant is approximately 75 per cent, of which 53 per cent is found in the extracellular compartment (outside the cell, and divided into two further compartments; intravascular and interstitial spaces). Forty-six per cent of water is found in the intracellular ICC (within the cell) compartment (Lam, 1999). As the child grows TBW is replaced by an increase in total body fat (Lam 1998), and by the age of 3 years, the proportion of water is reduced by 10 per cent to about 65 per cent (Rudolf and Levene, 1999).

Any disturbance to the balance between the intake and output mechanisms can cause significant morbidity as the integrity of the meticulous salt and water balance is disrupted. This could derive from:

* sweating
* fluid intake
* urine output
* insensible loss (water vapour in breath and skin)
* stool volume.

Excessive loss of water and electrolytes results in varying degrees of dehydration, with its cause, type and severity depending on the movement and concentration of water and electrolytes during illness. As a complication of D&V, fever may exacerbate the degree of dehydration through increased insensible water loss (IWL) from sweating and mouth-breathing. Normal IWL through the skin and lungs is, for example, 1/2ml/kg/hour which, during fever, increases by 12 per cent for every degree rise in temperature (Lam, 1998). Energy requirements also increase exponentially by 12 per cent for every degree rise above 37 °C (Hazinski, 1992). Thus the younger the child is, the more vulnerable they become because of the differences in total water distribution, which in illness is lost more readily from the extravascular space.

Lastly, the loss of key electrolytes, such as sodium through vomiting and potassium from diarrhoea, disrupts the balance of water in both intracellular and extracellular compartments, causing what is known as a *metabolic acidosis*.

An understanding of the fluid compartments of the body is essential, as fluid replacement therapy depends on this (Lam, 1998).

a Learning activity

Answer the following questions about the causes, types and severity of dehydration, using as sources Maill and colleagues (2007), Rudolf and Levene (2006), Hazinski (1992) or Rehydration Project (2002). Remember to look up unfamiliar words as you read through and add them to your personal glossary.

What is the probable *cause* of Sophie's diarrhoea and vomiting? Refer to McVerry and Collin (1998: 30) for examples of common types of infection.

What *type* of dehydration is it? For example, is it likely to be isotonic, hyponatraemic or hypernatraemic dehydration? See Hazinski (1992: 723–7) for further explanation, and also refer to the section above on the role of water and electrolytes to support your answer.

To find out how the *severity* of Sophie's dehydration is estimated, please see below.

Dehydration: calculating the risk?

The percentage of dehydration is assessed in two ways:

- first, by observation using the criteria of clinical features of dehydration set out below
- second, by measuring the estimated or actual weight loss against the weight of the child pre illness.

Armon and colleagues (2001) argue that this is the 'gold standard' by which treatments are calculated and tested. For example, 1g body weight equals 1 ml of water, therefore a 10 kg child with 10 per cent dehydration would now weigh 9 kg and has suffered a 1000 ml fluid loss. An easy formula (APLS, 2005) to remember for calculating the percentage fluid is:

$$10 \times \text{body weight in kg} \times \text{percentage dehydration} = \text{fluid lost (deficit)}$$

For example: 10×10 kg $\times 10\% = 1000$ ml or 1 kg.

First ask yourself some key questions when assessing any child. Think ABC every time!

- Is this child awake, rousable, irritable, lethargic, conscious?
- Is there any obstruction to their airway?
- Is there any difficulty with breathing?
- Is the pulse rate normal or absent?

Assessing a child's fluid loss

Now you need to think about your assessment of the child using the following headings:

- child's age
- normal physiological parameters for age group
- their current temperature, pulse, respirations and blood pressure if required
- naked weight
- length of illness prior to admission
- advice and treatments given prior to admission
- the normal plasma sodium level.

Clinical features of dehydration

Mild dehydration <5 per cent means 50 ml/kg fluid lost. The child will demonstrate:

- thirst
- may tolerate oral fluids
- urine output normal or slightly reduced: that is, dark yellow but passed at least three times in 24 hours
- a dry mouth
- sleepiness or irritability as dehydration progresses to 5 per cent
- normal capillary refill time <2 seconds (APLS, 2005).

Moderate dehydration means 5–10 per cent: 50–100 ml/kg fluid lost. The child demonstrates all of the above plus:

- cannot tolerate oral fluids
- dry uncomfortable mouth and tongue
- oliguria <1 /2 ml/kg/hour occurs in response to an increased secretion of antidiuretic hormone (ADH) in an attempt to preserve circulating volume, and urine may be dark and offensive
- sunken eyes as a result of loss of intra-occular fat from fluid loss
- tachycardia and corresponding tachypnoea
- crying with few or no tears
- lethargy or confusion
- inelastic skin: for example, when skin is gently lifted, it remains folded for some time.

(a) Learning activity

Sophie is admitted to a side room and as part of your assessment of her you look to see how dehydrated she is. Write down what you need to look for and why.

See Hampton-Evans and Bingham (1998: 188–93) for further information, and Chapter 20 in this volume on care of the child and young person.

Severe dehydration means >10 per cent: 100–150 ml/kg fluid lost. The child will be:

- very confused, semi-conscious or comatose
- have very sunken eyes or fontanelle in children under 18 months old
- have very dry mucous membranes
- acute tachycardia with poor volume (rapid and thready pulse)
- acute tachypnoea caused by lactic acidosis and loss of oxygen carrying circulating volume
- hypotension – a late and very life-threatening sign
- anuric – no urine output
- prolonged capillary refill time > 2 secs.

A child with severe dehydration will be in a 'shocked' state and requires early resuscitation with intravenous fluid therapy.

A history taken from the parents should include:

- Diet and eating habits.
- How many drinks has the child tolerated? If any, how much and what type?
- How many times per day has the child passed urine? Less than three times in 24 hours probably means there is a degree of dehydration (Rudolf and Levene, 2006).
- Vomiting – how often? How much? Colour and characteristics?
- Stools – colour, frequency, smell, consistency?

You should then look at:

- The child's conscious level – are they irritable, lethargic, listless, confused, reluctant to maintain eye contact with close carers (gaze aversion)?
- Their breathing – are they tachypnoeic in an attempt to compensate for any acidosis and adequate oxygen delivery to the tissues?
- Their eyes – are they sunken because of the loss of peri-orbital fat from fluid loss?
- Signs of inelastic skin – for example, does their skin remain in a pinched position if you gently lift together the skin folds over the abdomen? This physiological response occurs when water is lost from within the cells into the extravascular space in order to maintain adequate circulating blood volume, and is called the 'pinch test'. Normal recoil is present in the well child, recoil within 1–2 seconds indicates mild to moderate dehydration and longer than 2 seconds, severe dehydration exists (Armon et al, 2001).
- Moistness of their mucous membranes: mouth and the presence of tears.

> **⌐S⌐ Scenario continued**
>
> Looking at Sophie, you see that she remains lethargic and irritable and that her eyes remain sunken. She has inelastic skin and very dry mucous membranes.

You would complete your assessment of the child by taking their pulse, blood pressure, respirations, temperature and naked weight, and send off a stool and urine specimen for microscopy, culture and sensitivity (M, C&S), then chart and report the observations.

> **⌐S⌐ Scenario continued**
>
> **Sophie's observations**
>
> Temperature 39 °C
> Pulse 130 beats per minute
> Respirations 35 breaths per minute
> Blood pressure 90/60 mmHg
> Naked weight 12.6 kg. Normally weighs 14 kg.
>
> Sophie's urea and electrolyte (U&E) results show plasma sodium result is Na* 125 mmol/L.
> Urine sample (clean catch) report shows no bacterial growth on microscopy. Stool specimen shows heavy growth of Rotavirus.

Part

II

a Learning activity

Find out what the normal temperature, pulse and respirations should be for a 2-year-old child. Are Sophie's observations within normal limits?

Using the following formula, work out what Sophie's approximate systolic blood pressure should be for her age, e.g. 80 + (age in years x 2) (APLS, 2005: 16) and weight:

(kg) = 2 (age + 4) (APLS 2005, p.7) or
(kg) = (age in years x 2) + 8   (Stillwell, 1994: 56)

Using the information about the clinical features of dehydration presented earlier in this chapter, work out what percentage dehydration Sophie is suffering from.

Now let us look at the questions posed in the learning activity on page 197 about the cause, type and severity of Sophie's dehydration.

Cause

Rotavirus is common to ingestion of contaminated food.

Type

Sophie has hyponatraemic dehydration caused by her low sodium levels.

Severity

Sophie is suffering from 10 per cent dehydration which has been calculated in two ways: first, by weight – she has lost 1400 g which is equivalent to 10 per cent of her body weight – and second, by the clinical features she presents with on admission.

S Scenario continued

Sophie's rehydration therapy

Sophie requires intravenous (IV) fluid therapy to replace lost fluid and sodium electrolytes. She is lethargic and experiences 'gaze aversion' when the doctor inserts an intravenous cannula into her left arm. Once the IV site is secured, Sophie receives a bolus of 20 ml/kg (20 ml x 14 kg = 280 ml) of normal saline, followed by a regime of IV fluids that includes sodium. These are written up on the prescription chart and commenced at 108 ml per hour over 24 hours.

Sophie complains of being thirsty and is encouraged to drink 'little' and 'often', with further instructions left to supplement any additional diarrhoea or vomiting with 10 ml/kg oral replacement therapy where possible.

Sophie makes progress over the following 12 hours but has several more watery stools. Paula stays with her and is careful, having been shown how to minimise cross-infection when caring for Sophie. Both later 'cat nap' as they are exhausted.

a Learning activity

Consider how you know that Sophie is receiving the correct amount of intravenous fluids before reading on.

Getting the right balance

When children receive intravenous fluids:
- they must receive the correct type of solution
- the rate per hour must reflect the normal fluid requirements for the weight of the child
- the total amount prescribed must be given.

In general doctors calculate the child's fluid requirements, including volume and rate required. The nurse can confirm the prescription is correct using the fluid requirement formula given in Table 11.1.

Table 11.1 Normal maintenance fluid requirements

Body weight	Fluid requirements per day (ml/kg)	Fluid requirements per hour (ml/kg)
First 10 kg	100	4
Second 10 kg	50	2
Subsequent kg	20	1

Children with dehydration require **two** lots of replacement fluid. The first replaces the percentage of water and salts lost through illness, and the second provides normal maintenance fluid requirements based on the pre-illness weight of the child. Both of these continue until oral fluids are tolerated.

The severity and type of dehydration governs the rate at which replacement fluid is given. For example children with hypernatraemic dehydration can suffer severe cerebral oedema or haemorrhage following rapid infusion of IV replacement fluid (Hazinski, 1992: 729; APLS, 2005: 249), whereas those with severe isotonic dehydration can generally tolerate rapid fluid replacement. Lastly, regular evaluation of plasma sodium levels provides essential information on the child's ongoing recovery.

To check on Sophie's fluid replacements, we know that she has lost 1400 grams in weight. Using the fluid requirement formula above, we can calculate fluid loss as:

10 × 14 kg × 10% = 1400 ml

Sophie's fluid deficit is therefore 1400 ml.

Her maintenance fluid requirements are calculated using the APLS formula:

100 ml/kg for the first 10 kg =1000 ml

50 ml/kg for the second 10 kg which in Sophie's case equals = 4 kg x 50 ml = 200 ml

Sophie's maintenance fluid requirements are therefore 1200 ml per 24 hours. Now add the two together and divide by 24 hours, giving the hourly rate required:

1400 ml + 1200 ml = 2600 ml ÷ 24 hours = 108.3 ml per hour.

a Learning activity

Sophie is receiving 108 ml per hour over 24 hours. Using the formula above, work out whether the amount received is correct. Also, ask yourself why this is such an important question to ask. Do the calculation before reading on.

a Learning activity

How will you ensure Sophie's infusion site remains secure and free from extravasation (fluids that leak into surrounding tissues)? Find out which types of infusion pumps are used for children of different ages, and which types of giving sets are required for different fluids, for example blood products.

Part

II

S Scenario continued

By mid-afternoon Sophie is looking a little brighter. She has not vomited for several hours, feels thirsty and has a very wet nappy. Intravenous fluids have been infusing for seven hours. Sophie has woken up from her nap and points to the television. Her observations are temperature 37.5 °C; respirations 25 breaths per minute; pulse 105 beats per minute.

a Learning activity

List, with reasons, what you would reassess now that Sophie is awake.

Find out what kinds of oral fluids will aid the absorption of water and electrolytes through the bowel wall. Contact your children's dietician to help you.

What would be the normal urine output for a child of this age? Refer to Hazinski (1992) to help you.

In partnership with her family, plan how Sophie might be encouraged to drink.

Find out what types of oral rehydration therapy can be bought over the counter and are also used in your practice areas.

How can the children's dietician help at this time?

The role of the children's dietician

The role of the children's dietician is unique. They often have solutions to the 'fussy eating habits' that most families complain about in their children at some time or another, be it the tantrum 2-year-old or the adolescent with complex eating disorders.

Dieticians also have considerable knowledge in the management of children with a range of complex dietary needs, and work in partnership with families and other specialists such as occupational therapists, health visitors, and speech and language therapists in achieving healthy children in acute and community settings.

The special relationship between the nurse and dietician must not be underestimated either. In hospital settings dieticians rely on the nurse for accurate information about the child's condition, and in particular, comment on the child's progress. Good record keeping is therefore essential not only from a legal perspective, but in enhancing relationships between the dietician, family and nurse.

c Professional conversation

Heather, the children's dietician, says, 'I visited Sophie and her mother soon after admission, having first looked through her medical admission notes, and then I talked to the nurse caring for her. I was asked to advise on the most appropriate kind of oral rehydration therapy and estimate a time when foods could be reintroduced. So, following a detailed assessment of Sophie's likes and dislikes, I was able to give both mum and the nurses some practical guidance relating to Sophie's nutritional needs now, and when she is beginning to feel better.'

a Learning activity

Find out how you would contact the dietician.

Try to arrange to 'shadow' a dietician as part of your clinical placement.

S Scenario continued

Sophie's progress continues, and over the following days she begins to eat and drink. Her diarrhoea subsides and the last specimen sent to the laboratory yields no bacterial growth. Intravenous fluids are discontinued. Sophie is discharged after four days.

a Learning activity

Identify members of the multidisciplinary team who need to be involved in Sophie's discharge planning.

What discharge advice will Tom and Paula require?

In summary, what were Sophie's main problems on admission to hospital? Make your list before reading the review below.

Problems on admission

In Sophie's case, these were:

- D&V leading to dehydration, starvation and weight loss. Review the sections on the effects of illness on growth and development (pages 192–3) and on diarrhoea and vomiting (pp. 195–6).
- Moderate dehydration leading to fluid and electrolyte imbalance. Review the sections on the effects of dehydration on the body (pp. 196–7), and on the role of water and electrolytes from a pathophysiological perspective (p. 197).
- Disruption to activity levels leading to anxiety and fear. Loss of energy to play.

> **Learning activity**
>
> What actions would you consider appropriate at this stage in admission?

Appropriate actions

- Checking for severity of dehydration. Review the section on dehydration and calculating the risk (pp. 198–200).
- Maintenance of fluid in electrolyte balance. Monitor, record and report intake and output of oral and intravenous fluids. Take a blood sample to evaluate serum sodium levels. Review the section on getting the balance right (pp. 200–2).
- Diversion therapy, to help protect against accidental disconnection of Sophie's intravenous fluids. The ways in which illness can impact upon normal growth and development (pp. 192–3) are relevant here: review that section again.
- Preservation of skin integrity: watch out for skin excoriation caused by profuse diarrhoea.
- Be aware of the risk of cross-infection leading to other family members becoming ill.

> **Learning activity**
>
> What would you include in your discharge planning?

Discharge planning

This should include:

- Hospital support from the dietician.
- Community support from the health visitor, community children nurse and practice nurse. Review McVerry and Collin (1998: 31–3).
- Open access arrangements leading to immediate self-referral if required.
- NHS Direct, online or phone. Out of hours GP service.
- Discharge information leaflets regarding cross-infection. The Health Promotion Agency (2006) advocates the 48-hour rule, which is that contact with other children should be avoided for two days following the last episode of diarrhoea or vomiting. Similarly, children should not swim for two weeks following the last episode of diarrhoea.

Conclusion

This chapter has considered the hydration needs of children during a healthcare crisis. Although their relatively small total blood volume exacerbates fluid loss in children, the principles of care and management are common to adults as well. A decrease in circulation blood volume can result in death, and in certain countries this happens frequently with cases of diarrhoea. Fluid resuscitation is therefore key to the management of all patients who, for whatever reason, develop hypovolaemic shock. The role of the nurse in the management of such patients and their families is of paramount importance, and considerable acumen is required to ensure that evidence-based protocols are adhered to during the period when fluid replacement is the major facet of treatment.

References

Armon, K., Stephenson, T., MacFaul, R., Eccleston, P. and Wernerke, U. (2001) 'An evidence-and consensus-based guideline for acute diarrhoea management', *Archives of Diseases in Childhood* 85, 132–42.

Bee, H. (1994) *The Developing Child*, 7th edn, New York, Harper Collins.

Callery, P. (1997) 'Maternal knowledge and professional knowledge: co-operation and conflict in the care of sick children' *International Journal of Nursing Studies* 34(1), 27–34.

Campbell, S. and Glasper, E. A. (1995) *Whaley and Wong's Children's Nursing*, New York, Mosby.

Carter, B. and Dearmun, A. K. (eds) (1995) *Child Health Care Nursing: Concepts, theory and practice*, Oxford, Blackwell Science.

Chameides, L. and Hazinski, M. F. (1994) 'Fluid therapy and medications', sections 6.1–6.18 in *Paediatric Advanced Life Support*, New York, American Heart Association,

Conway, S. P. and Newport, S. P. (1994) 'Are all hospital admissions for acute gastroenteritis necessary?' *Journal of Infection* 29, 5–8.

Dale, J., Crouch, R. and Lloyd, D. (1998) 'Primary care: nurse-led telephone triage and advice out of hours', *Nursing Standard* 12(47), 41–5.

Dearmun, A. K., Campbell, S. and Barlow, J. (1995) 'Nursing support and care: meeting the needs of the child and family with altered gastro-intestinal function', in Carter, B. and Dearmun, A. K. (eds), *Child Health Care Nursing: Concepts, theory and practice*, Oxford, Blackwell Science.

Department of Health (DH) (2003) *Getting the Right Start: National Service Framework for Children*, London, DH.

DH (2004) *Every Child Matters: Next steps*, London, DH.

DH (2007) *Delivering Health Services through Sure Start Children's Centres*, London, DH.

Edwards, N. (1996) 'Temperature rising for paediatrics', *Health Service Journal* (1 February), 24–5.

Glasper, E. A. and Richardson, J. (2006) *A Textbook of Children's and Young People's Nursing*, London, Churchill Livingstone.

Hampton-Evans, D. C. and Bingham, R. M. (1998) 'Paediatric resuscitation: the European resuscitation guidelines (1998)', *Care of the Critically Ill* 14(6), 188–93.

Harms, D. and Scharf, J. (1997) *Memorix: Paediatrics*, Edinburgh, Chapman & Hall Medical.

Hawley, N. and Howkins, E. (1999) 'A health visitor-run helpline: meeting family health needs', *Community Practitioner* 72(7), 208–11.

Hazinski, M. F. (1992) 'Common clinical conditions', pp. 652–9 in *Nursing Care of the Critically Ill Child*, New York, Mosby.

Hazinski, M. F. (ed.) (1999) *Nursing Care of the Critically Ill Child*, 2nd edn, New York, Mosby.

Health Protection Agency. (2006) Rotavirus [online] http://www.hpa.org.uk/infections/topics_az/rotavirus/menu.htm (accessed 26 February 2009).

Health Promotion Agency (2006b) Guidance on Infection Control In Schools and other Child Care Settings [online] http://www.hpa.org.uk/infections/topics_az/schools/schools_guidelines_2006.pdf (accessed 5 February 2009).

Hobart, C. and Frankel, J. (2004) *A Practical Guide to Child Observation and Assessment*, 3rd edn, London, Nelson Thornes.

Kennally, C. and Dale, J. (1998) 'Direct enquiries', *Health Service Journal* (30 July), 24–5.

Kosek, M., Bern, C. and Guerrant, R. L. (2003). 'The global burden of diarrhoeal disease, as estimated from studies published between 1992 and 2000', *Bulletin of the World Health Organization* 81(3), 197–204.

Lam, Hui, W. (1998) 'Fluids in paediatric patients', *Care of the Critically Ill* 14(3), 93–6.

Lam, Hui, W. (1999) 'Mechanism and management of paediatric head injury', *Care of the Critically Ill* 15(3), 95–8.

Lewandowski, L. A. (1992) 'Psychosocial aspects of paediatric critical care', in Hazinski, M. F. (ed.), *Nursing Care of the Critically Ill Child*, New York, Mosby.

Maill, L., Rudolf, M. C. J. and Levene, M. I. (2007) *Paediatrics at a Glance*, 2nd edn, Oxford, Blackwell.

Martini, F. H. (2006) *Fundamentals of Anatomy and Physiology*, 7th edn, Harlow, Pearson International.

McCormick, A., Fleming, D. and Charlton, J. (1993) *Morbidity Statistics from General Practice: Fourth national study 1991/92*, Office of Population Censuses and Surveys Series MB5 No. 3. London, HMSO [online] http://www.statistics.gov.uk/downloads/theme_health/MB5No3.pdf (accessed 5 February 2009).

McVerry, M. and Collin, J. (1998) 'Managing the child with gastroenteritis', *Paediatric Nursing* 10(8), 31–3.

Moules, T and Ramsey, J. (2008) *The Textbook of Children's Nursing*, Oxford, Blackwell.

Nursing and Midwifery Council (NMC) (2007a) *Record Keeping Guidance*, London, NMC.

NMC (2007b) *Nursing: Towards 2015*, London, NMC.

NMC (2008) *Code of Professional Conduct*, London, NMC.

National Institute for Clinical Excellence (NICE) (2009) *Diarrhoea and Vomiting in Children under 5: Management of acute diarrhoea and vomiting due to gastroenteritis in children under 5* (due April), London, NICE.

Rudolf, M. C. J. and Levene, M. I. (2006) *Paediatrics and Child Health*, 2nd edn, Oxford, Blackwell Science.

Sidley, A. (1995) 'Community nursing perspective', in Carter, B. and Dearmun, A. K. (eds), *Child Health Care Nursing: Concepts, theory and practice*, Oxford, Blackwell Science.

Stillwell, S. B. (1994) *Quick Critical Care Reference*, 2nd edn, New York, Mosby.

Swanwick, M. (1990) 'Knowledge and control', *Paediatric Nursing* 2(5), 18–20.

United Nations Children's Fund (UNICEF) (1990) *First Call for Children: World Declaration Plan of Action from the World Summit for Children Convention: The Rights of the Child*, New York, UNICEF.

UNICEF (2001) *Progress since the World Summit for Children: A statistical review* [online] http://www.unicef.org/publications/files/pub_wethechildren_stats_en.pdf (accessed 5 February 2009).

Whaley, D. Hockenberry-Eaton. L., Wilson, D., Winkelstein, M. L., and Ahmann, E. (1999) *Whaley and Wong's Nursing Care of Infants and Children*, 6th edn, New York, Mosby.

Whaley, L. F. and Wong, D. L. (1997) *Essentials of Pediatric Nursing*, 5th edn, New York, Mosby.

White, C. J. (1995) 'Life crisis for children and their families', in Carter, B. and Dearmun, A. K. (eds), *Child Health Care Nursing: Concepts, theory and practice*, Oxford, Blackwell Science.

World Health Organisation (WHO/CDD) (2004) *World Health Report 2004 – Changing history*, Geneva, WHO.

Further reading

Advanced Paediatric Life Support Group (APLS) (2005) *Advanced Paediatric Life Support: The practical approach*, 4th edn, London, BMJ Publishing. This book focuses on the emergency care of children, and is the core text accompanying the APLS (UK) course. The text acknowledges that sick children generate considerable anxiety to those who care for them, thus this easy to read book reflects assessment skills that can be utilised by a range of practitioners.

Rudolf, M. C. J. and Levene, M. I. (1999) *Paediatrics and Child Health*, Oxford, Blackwell Science. This excellent book is easy to read and understand, and examines a range of childhood illnesses including a section on the causes of diarrhoea and dehydration. Rudolf and Levene have published several times, including on neonatal medicine and the causes of diarrhoea in infancy.

Walker-Smith, J. A., Sandhu, B. K., Isolauri, E., Banchini, G., Van Caillie-Bertrand, M., Dias, J. A., Fasano, A., Guandalini, S., Hoekstra, J. H., Juntunen, M., Kolacek, S., Marx, D., Micetic-Turk, D., Razenberg, M. C., Szajewska, H., Taminiau, J., Weizman, Z., Zanacca, C. and

Zetterström, R. (1997) 'Recommendations for feeding in childhood gastroenteritis: medical position paper – guidelines prepared by the ESPGAN working group on acute diarrhoea', *Journal of Pediatric Gastroenterology and Nutrition* 24, 522–7). This work looks at recommendations for feeding children with childhood gastroenteritis. It makes specific reference to the care of children with acute diarrhoea, and has developed guidelines and standards for children of all ages.

World Health Organization (WHO) *Clinical Management of Acute Diarrhoea*, New York, United Nations Childrens Fund/WHO. Geneva, WHO/CDD. This work sets out the guidelines for treatment of diarrhoea and dehydration notably that which arises in the developing world. Its publication is set against powerful evidence that morbidity and mortality can be reduced particularly when ORT is used. Shamsul Hag, minister of health and population control, Government of Bangladesh, comments, 'ORT holds the promise of healthier childhoods and more productive adult lives.' The key role of professionals is also explored.

Websites

Diarrhoeal diseases: www.rehydrate.org/resources
Oral replacement solutions: www.rehydrate.org/html/deh010.htm
Infant and Child advice: www.healthvisitors.com
Professional information: www.rehydrate.org/support_health_professional_health
Rehydration Project (1996–2002) P.O. Box 1, Samara 5235, Costa Rica: www.rehydrate.org.

Treatment plans using oral rehydration therapy to prevent and treat dehydration: www.rehydrate.org.dehydration
http://www.wateraid.org/uk/what_we_do/statistics/default.asp
www.drhull.com/Ency/Master/D/dehydration.html
www.archdischild.com

Videos/DVDs

Sleep Tight, *Help for Sleepless Parents*, Video# no. 169. 'Dehydration in children always happens as a complication of diarrhoea and vomiting, especially if combined with fever – most commonly gastroenteritis.'

Department of Health (2004) *How to Spot a Sick Child*, DVD. This excellent learning resource is designed to aid healthcare practitioners in the recognition of serious illness in children. It's a must have in libraries, child healthcare settings and lecturer resource centres.

Legislation

Children Act 1989
Children Act 2004

Part

1

Chapter

12

Fluid balance in adults

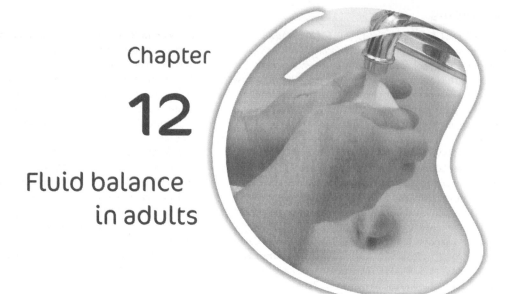

Anne Francis

W   Don't forget to visit www.palgrave.com/glasper for additional online resources relating to this chapter.

Introduction

This chapter looks at fluid balance in adults, using burn injuries as an example. Burn injuries range from minor burns, which can be managed at home or in the community, to the more severe, which need to be treated in a specialist burn centre or unit. A burn can be one of the most devastating injuries that can happen to a person, and it affects them, their family and society. An individual with a significant burn is likely to be critically ill initially, and will possibly need reconstructive surgery. They might experience pain, itching and disfigurement, which can have social and psychological consequences, sometimes for the remainder of their lives.

In many cases the interprofessional team is of paramount importance in caring for a burn-injured individual. Nurses, doctors, physiotherapists, social workers, clinical psychologists, dieticians and others play a vital role in caring for and supporting the individual, their family and significant others. The input of members of the team may vary at different stages of the individual's care episode, from the acute injury through to reintegration in the community and repeated readmissions to hospital for reconstructive surgery.

> Every 90 seconds someone in the UK is burned or scalded in an accident at home and around 112,000 patients are treated in hospital for burns every year. 60 per cent of these are children under 12 years of age. The number of burn victims can only be guessed at, particularly in developing nations.
>
> (http://www.raft.ac.uk/research_burns.htm).

W

A decrease in mortality over the past 40 years has been linked to the introduction of topical silver salts for antibiotic prophylaxis, improved infection control, greater frequency of successful early surgery, and improved intensive care procedures, particularly of renal failure (Lawrence, 1996).

The primary aim of this chapter is to give you an introduction into the needs of an adult with a significant burn injury potentially leading to hypovolaemia. Fluid requirements are different in young children from those in adults and older children, because the content and distribution of water in the human body changes with age (Willcock and Jewkes, 2000). This difference needs to be considered when treating the patient.

Learning outcomes

This chapter will enable you to:

- identify the population at risk of burn injury
- recognise the types and causes of burn injury
- explore the available evidence base to inform the management of the burn-injured individual
- examine the role of the nurse in the multidisciplinary team in the assessment, planning, implementation, evaluation and co-ordination of the care of a burn-injured individual
- identify the factors contributing to maintaining fluid balance in the burn-injured individual
- discuss the ethical and legal aspects of caring for a burn injured individual.

Concepts

- Burn first aid
- Nutrition
- Burn types
- Pain
- Causes of burns
- Wound care
- Fluid resuscitation
- Patient education
- Hypovolaemic and burn shock
- Interprofessional team
- Dehydration
- Evidence based practice
- Assessment
- Split-thickness skin grafts
- Burn management
- Body image
- Inhalation injury
- Disfigurement

First aid

In summary the aims of first aid are to:

1 Maintain the safety of the rescuer, who should not place themself in any danger. For example, if the victim has been electrocuted, the rescuer should ensure that the electricity supply is disabled before attending to the victim, otherwise they could also become a victim.
2 Stop the burning process.
3 Ensure that the victim has a patent airway, is breathing and has a circulatory output.
4 Relieve pain.
5 Cover the burn wound.
6 Seek appropriate medical aid or transport to hospital.

Burn injuries

A burn is an injury resulting in tissue loss or damage. The injury can be caused by exposure to thermal, electrical, chemical or radiation sources. Injury to the tissue is determined by:

- the temperature or causticity of the burning agent
- duration of tissue contact with the source

At a cellular level, the burning produces a dilatation of the capillaries and small vessels, thus increasing cellular permeability. Plasma seeps out into the surrounding tissue, producing blisters and oedema. The type, duration and depth of the burn affect the amount of tissue loss. The tissue loss results in a decrease in circulation blood volume, which if not replaced, can progress. In major burns this can result in death. The primary cause of death from major burns in the past was fluid loss. The fluid loss reduces over time, and is reflected in the amount of fluid replacement that is needed.

The three main stages of a significant burn injury are resuscitation (which refers to fluid resuscitation), the acute phase and the rehabilitative phase. This section of the chapter concentrates on the fluid resuscitation phase.

Some authors suggest that some groups are more susceptible than others to burn injury. These include the very young and the elderly, those suffering from alcohol and substance misuse, those with diabetes, epilepsy or other medical problems such as transient ischaemic attacks, those with mental health problems, and those who are socially deprived (Cason, 1981).

> **a Learning activity**
>
> List the priorities of Peter's primary assessment.

The history of the incident is significant. For example, a person might have had to jump from a building to escape a house fire, therefore they are more likely to have a cervical spine injury than an individual with a scald as a result of spilling boiling water over themself. It is always important to consider the history of the accident when treating a patient.

> **S Scenario continued**
>
> Peter was taken to an accident and emergency department for assessment. Peter is single and has a girlfriend. He lives 250 miles from the burns unit to which he is admitted. He drinks one bottle of wine per day and more at weekends. He has, in the past, been treated for depression with antidepressants and has a medical history of hypertension and mild asthma.

Primary assessment

The main priorities of the primary assessment following a burn injury are ABCDEF: **a**irway, **b**reathing, **c**irculation, **d**isability, **e**xposure and **f**luids.

Airway and cervical spine management

- Clear the patient's airway and open the airway if necessary with a chin lift and/or jaw thrust.
- Ensure that cervical spine movement is kept to a minimum in case a cervical spine injury has occurred.

Breathing

- Expose the patient's chest to ensure that chest expansion is smooth, equal and not compromised. Assist ventilation if necessary.
- Administer oxygen.
- Observe their respiratory rate, use of accessory muscles, rhythm and depth of ventilation.
- Be aware that circumferential burns to the chest could compromise ventilation and require immediate medical attention.

> **a Learning activity**
>
> What signs would you expect to see if there is inhalation injury?
>
> Refer to Settle (1996, chapters 9 and 26), for a more in-depth discussion of the types, signs and symptoms and management of inhalation injuries.

Signs of inhalation injury include:
- burns around the mouth and /or nose
- intraoral burns
- intraoral oedema
- hoarseness of voice
- soot in nostrils, mouth, singed nasal hair
- pharyngeal oedema (visible on examination)
- inspiratory stridor
- laryngeal oedema (visible on examination).

If inspiratory stridor and/or laryngeal oedema are present then intubation will be necessary (Judkins ,1996).

> **S** Scenario continued
>
> On initial assessment, Peter did not have an inhalation injury. It is unlikely that he could have sustained an inhalation injury as his accident did not occur in a confined space. However, he does have mild asthma, which will necessitate careful observation.

An accurate history is vital. This may differ with the individual, therefore it is important to obtain a history from a number of people including witnesses.

Circulation

- Assess the patient's circulation by observing and recording their blood pressure, pulse and temperature (peripheral and core).
- Arrest any bleeding by applying direct pressure.
- Observe peripheral circulation. Where there is a circumferential burn to a limb, a capillary blanch test should be performed. The normal return is 2 seconds. A longer return may indicate circulatory compromise due to a deep burn or hypovolaemia. The doctor should be informed.
- Insert two wide-bore cannulas.
- Pain should be assessed and managed at this stage. Analgesia is best given intravenously at this stage, as it is the most effective route of administration. Intramuscular injections should be avoided as their absorption is erratic because of circulatory changes following a burn injury.

Neurological status

Assess the patient's level of consciousness. Is the patient:

- alert?
- responding to vocal stimuli?
- responding to painful stimuli?
- unresponsive?
- with pupils equal in size and responding to light?

Again, the history might indicate the potential for the patient to have a head injury. This did not indicate a problem in Peter's case.

Extent of burn injury or exposure

Expose the burn wounds, remove any jewellery and observe the depth and percentage total body surface area burned (%TBSA). Once the burn has been assessed, it is important to ensure that the patient does not become hypothermic by keeping the ambient temperature within 28-31°C. This is because skin plays an important role in temperature regulation, and this is altered following a burn injury. When exposing the patient during dressing changes, the room temperature may need to be increased to minimise metabolic requirements. Photography of the wounds by the medical photography department is helpful for future reference and medico-legal proceedings.

> **S** Scenario continued
>
> Peter sustained flame burns to 40 per cent of his body: his face, chest, arms and legs. His burns were mainly partial thickness with deeper areas on his anterior thighs.

t☆
Practice tip

Clingfilm can be applied directly on to the burn tissue once the wound has cooled, and acts as a temporary dressing.

> **ⓐ Learning activity**
>
> How is the percentage burn surface area (%TBSA) estimated? Find out whether there is more than one way to calculate this.

Various charts exist as a guide to assessing the percentage of the body burned, for example, the rule of nines and the Lund and Browder chart shown in Figure 12.1. In all cases, erythema should be disregarded when calculating the percentage BSA, although if the area blisters in the first 16 or so hours, it should be included when assessing percentage BSA. This may mean re-estimating the total burn surface area.

> **ⓔ Evidence-based practice**
>
> **Assessing the percentage of the burn surface area**
>
> It is widely accepted practice that the patient's hand (including fingers, with fingers together) represents approximately 1 per cent TBSA. There is debate as to whether 1 per cent TBSA is the palm minus digits or the whole hand with closed fingers (Perry et al, 1996).
>
> Rossiter, Chapman and Haywood (1996) reviewed the use of the hand when estimating the percentage BSA of adults with burns; they concluded that if the hand alone is used to estimate the percentage TBSA, the burn could be overestimated. They therefore stress the importance of accurately monitoring the burn-injured patient during the shock period of resuscitation.

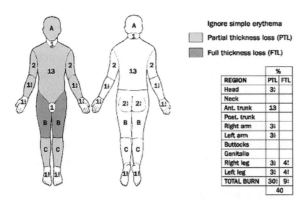

Ignore simple erythema

☐ Partial thickness loss (PTL)

■ Full thickness loss (FTL)

REGION	PTL	FTL
Head	3½	
Neck		
Ant. trunk	13	
Post. trunk		
Right arm	3½	
Left arm	3½	
Buttocks		
Genitalia		
Right leg	3½	4½
Left leg	3½	4½
TOTAL BURN	30½	9½
	40	

Relative percentage of body surface area affected by growth

AREA	AGE 0	1	5	10	15	ADULT
A = ½ of head	9½	8½	6½	5½	4½	3½
B = ½ of one thigh	2½	3½	4	4½	4½	4½
C = ½ of one leg	2½	2½	2½	3	3½	3½

Figure 12.1 Lund and Browder burn assessment chart

> **ⓐ Learning activity**
>
> Why is it important to assess the percentage burn that Peter has sustained?
>   Find out what assessment tool is used to estimate the %TBSA in the hospital where you are currently working.

Adults with greater than 15 per cent burns to their body surface have a reduced circulating blood volume and require intravenous fluid replacement. Body weight is important to assess the normal circulating blood volume.

Fluid assessment

- Assess the amount of fluid replacement necessary and administer that prescribed if the %TBSA is greater than 15 per cent in an adult.
- Assess urinary output by passing a urinary catheter and monitoring hourly.
- Obtain blood for full blood count, urea and electrolytes, coagulation, amylase and carboxyhaemoglobin.

- Assess nutritional status, using a nutritional assessment tool. (See Chapter 10 on nutritional needs for discussion of nutritional assessment tools.) Enteral feeding may be required and should be commenced as soon as possible if indicated.
- Tetanus status should be ascertained. Tetanus is a rare complication following a burn injury, but prophylaxis should be offered.

Mortality can be described as the likelihood of survival or death following an injury or disease.

> **(a) Learning activity**
>
> Revise homeostasis and fluid balance in a physiology textbook. Consider insensible losses.
>
> List the factors that influence the mortality of the burn-injured individual.

Factors affecting survival

Tools exist as a guide to possible mortality rate. It must be remembered they are simply an empirical guide as all patients are individuals and management of burn injury is constantly advancing. The tools consider the age of the patient, an important factor as the old and young have a poorer prognosis than others, but do not consider an individual's past medical history or the involvement of inhalation injury, both of which can affect the individual's outcome. Early excision and grafting of the burn wound can affect the survival of the patient and minimise the risk of infection and sepsis.

Following the primary assessment a secondary assessment needs to be carried out and the primary assessment evaluated.

Shock

> **(a) Learning activity**
>
> What is shock?
>
> What types of shock might result from a significant burn injury? Why?
>
> Define hypovolaemic shock (you may wish search the internet or refer to a critical care text, such as Urden, Lough and Stacey (1996).

Burn shock consists of cellular and hypovolemic shock, and results in decreased cardiac output, extracellular fluid, plasma volume and oliguria. The aim of treating burn shock is to preserve tissue perfusion and avoid ischaemia by restoring circulating volume. Burn shock is complicated by a large fluid volume shift from the intravascular compartments. This is unique to burn shock. The pathophysiology of burn shock is partly because chemical mediators are also involved. These are thought to include histamine, kinins and prostaglandins. See Settle (1996) and Herndon (2001) for more detailed discussion.

Fluid resuscitation

Controversy exists about the type of fluid that is most effective in maintaining the circulatory blood volume with the least harm to the patient. Discussion around this argument can be found in Settle (1996).

Various formulae exist to assist in the calculation of the amount of fluid replacement that a patient requires. They are only guidelines and the patient should be monitored carefully. Care should be taken to ascertain whether the formula is based on crystalloid or colloid fluid replacement.

The Parkland formula

The Parkland formula is widely used in the United States.

Day 1: 4 ml Hartmann solution/Kg/%TBSA in the first 24 hours after the burn. Half is given in the first eight hours after injury and the second half in the next 16 hours.

Day 2: 700-2000ml colloid, to maintain urine output.
no crystalloid and 5 per cent dextrose maintenance fluids.

The time over which the fluid is given is known as a fluid 'period'. The aim is to begin the fluid replacement as soon as possible after the time of injury.

> ### a Learning activity
>
> Consider what factors are included to calculate the amount of fluid that Peter requires. Based on the information presented about Peter, calculate the amount of fluid he will require in each fluid replacement period. Do this before continuing with the text.

In Peter's case:

$$4 \times 70\text{Kg} \times 40\% = \frac{11{,}200 \text{ ml}}{2 \text{ periods}} = 5600 \text{ ml per period.}$$

0–8 hours post-injury = 700 ml Hartmann solution per hour
8–24 hours post-injury = 350 ml Hartmann solution per hour
A maintenance fluid may need to be administered.

Muir and Barclay fluid resuscitation formula

This is another formula, which relies on the administration of colloids. See Herndon (2001, chapter 8) for further discussion.

Colloid resuscitation with plasma

The first 36 hours are divided into time periods of 4, 4, 4, 6, 6 and 12 hours.
Each interval = 0.5 x %BSA x Wt (Kg)
Blood, if needed, following burn injury should be given at the end of the resuscitation phase as haemolysis occurs with a large full-thickness burn, because of the heat of the burning agent. Early excision of the burn wound (within the first 24 hours) can result in the modulation of burn shock and a decrease in the amount of fluid required. The application of a dermal regeneration template can also alter the requirements.

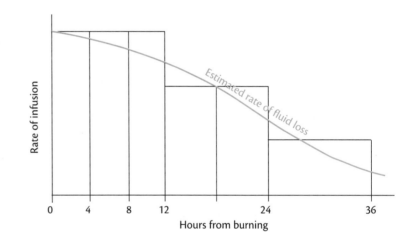

Figure 12.2 Relationship between fluid volume required and fluid lost post burn

> ### a Learning activity
>
> How does this compare with patients receiving intravenous fluids in your clinical area? Suggest reasons if there is a difference.

It must be remembered that the calculated fluid requirements are only a guideline. The quantity and type of fluid required depend on the individual's response, and can be observed by careful monitoring and observation. Peter should be observed for signs of over- and under-transfusion. Under-transfusion can result in under-perfusion and a potential for conversion of a burn wound to a greater depth and renal failure. Too much fluid can result in pulmonary oedema.

a Learning activity

Plan the care that a patient with an intravenous infusion (IVI) requires, giving rationales for your interventions.

Identify what observations should be monitored for Peter for during the resuscitation period. Consider your answer before reading on.

Observations that you could have suggested in response to the learning activity include:

- **Blood pressure and pulse**: the frequency should depend on the clinical condition of patient and be either half-hourly or hourly. Patients may compensate and other factors may affect these, for example pain. Therefore trends in the rate are more important than fluctuations.
- **Respiratory rate**: this is usually raised as a result of an increased metabolic rate, although an increase in the rate and depth could be an indication of shock.
- **Temperature**, both peripheral and core. A difference between the two can indicate the degree of vasoconstriction and thus shock.
- **Skin colour**: perfusion can be demonstrated and is again an indicator of shock. With adequate circulation the patient is pink. A pale appearance could indicate constricted arterioles, and a bluish tinge could indicate stagnation of blood in the capillaries that are dilated.
- **Urine output**: this is an indicator of renal function. The stress response will affect the output. In an adult the expected output is 0.5–1ml/kg body weight per hour. The concentration is also of note. A low urine output with concentrated urine suggests under-transfusion, and a high output with dilute urine over-transfusion, during the resuscitation phase. Urine concentration can be measured with osmolality. The osmolality should decrease after the first 24 hours. A careful record of fluid balance should be kept.
- **Early warning score**: this should be used as an indicator of shock, sepsis and so on.
- **Orientation**: this is of significance as a disoriented patient may be showing signs of sepsis. Other causes are drugs or previous alcohol intake, although these should not be assumed to be the cause without evidence, and the patient should be monitored closely for other causes.
- **Blood samples**: these are usually taken during each 'period' to provide an indication of the adequacy of the fluid replacement. The fluid replacement rate may be altered accordingly.
- **Haematocrit**: this is recorded as a percentage. Haematocrit is the proportion of red blood cells to plasma, and it rises with a low plasma volume. It is a useful adjunct to monitoring, although a normal haematocrit is not an indicator of adequate fluid resuscitation. The patient may require a central venous line to monitor the central venous pressure.
- **Invasive monitoring**: this may be indicated for a more accurate patient assessment.

a Learning activity

How much urine should we expect Peter to produce per hour? (Remember that his weight on admission was 70 kg.)

A fluid challenge may need to be administered. In Peter's case this might be an extra 500 ml of crystalloid given over a one-hour period. He will need to be monitored closely for a rise in blood pressure, tachycardia and increased respiratory rate. The doctor will advise on how much urine volume is expected, usually greater than

50 ml per hour. The nurse needs to communicate the outcome to the doctor.

Consider what steps might be made to correct Peter's fluid balance if it is higher or lower than expected.

Peter's burns were caused by an explosion. List the other main types of burn.

What are the main ways of categorising burn depth?

Burn depth

Categories such as first-degree, second-degree and third-degree burns, though common in lay talk, tend not to be used by healthcare professionals. They are largely replaced by the following descriptions:

- erythema
- partial thickness (superficial or deep dermal)
- full thickness.

See Table 12.1 for a more in-depth classification. For a more thorough discussion of causes and types of burn, see Herndon (2001) or Settle (1996).

Table 12.1   Classification and clinical appearance of burn injury and depth

| | Erythema | Depth of burn | | |
		Partial thickness superficial	Partial thickness deep dermal	Full thickness
Usual history	Sunburn	Scalds of limited duration	Scalds of long duration, contact with high temperature, e.g. hot fat	Contact with high temperature e.g. flame burn, chemicals, electrical injury
Appearance	Red	Red or pink with capillary return	Red without capillary return	Charred, white, dry with thrombosed vessels
Sensation	Painful	Painful	Often painful around the margins with altered pain sensation in deeper areas	Initially insensate but painful at a later stage
Hairs	Present	Present	Present and easily removed or absent	Absent
Blister formation	Absent	Present	Absent	Absent
Results	Heals within days, no dressings needed	Heals within 14 days if infection free	Heals in months therefore surgery indicated	Granulated therefore surgery indicated
Scan formation	No scar	Can remain red and become hypertrophic	Often becomes hypertrophic	Becomes hypertrophic

> **ⓐ Learning activity**
>
> From Table 12.1, identify the possible wound management Peter might require.

Septic shock

Because the burn wound provides an ideal environment for the proliferation of bacteria, and the burn-injured individual is immuno-compromised as a result of a major burn injury, the individual is at risk of developing septic shock.

> **ⓐ Learning activity**
>
> Consider the term 'septic shock'. What signs and symptoms would you expect, and why are they of significance in Peter's case?

There are many signs and symptoms of septic shock, and their discussion is beyond the scope of this chapter. For a more detailed explanation, see Herndon (2001).

Burn wound healing

Partial-thickness burns may heal by regeneration of new skin from epithelial calls at the periphery of the wound, and from adnexal cells such as the hair follicles and sweat glands. This is dependent on, among other things, an adequate nutritional intake and lack of infection. Full thickness burns destroy all the skin structure and can involve muscle and bone.

Wound repair will involve the need for surgery and will result in scar-tissue formation.

S   Scenario continued

Peter's burns were mainly partial thickness with some deeper patches. Peter required surgery to repair the integrity of 50 per cent of his burned skin – that is, 20%TBSA. This surgery was carried out on two separate occasions because of the lack of suitable donor sites. The remainder healed with conservative treatment using dressings. He needed anticoagulant cover as he required a split skin graft on his legs, and needed to be on bed rest for 24 hours to prevent the skin graft from slipping before it had taken.

The first stage of surgery usually involves debridement of the necrotic tissue and harvesting of a split-thickness skin graft. This area is known as the donor site. The harvested skin is then positioned on the recipient site and fixed in position usually with glue or staples. Various processes occur which, it is hoped, will result in the skin 'taking'. Factors affecting the 'non-take' of the skin graft include infection, friction and unsuitable recipient site.

Wound care

The aim of wound care in burns is to maintain a moist, clean environment, protect from infection and further injury, and promote healing and comfort. In the immediate period after burning, the wounds after cooling by applying cold water for 10–20 minutes to reduce pain, and tissue damage can be wrapped in cling film as a temporary dressing.

Most burn wounds are covered with dressings as opposed to being left exposed. The burn wound should be cleansed gently with warmed normal saline before re-dressing. Photographing the wound can give clinicians and the patient an indication of the rate of healing. Care must be taken to comply with the hospital's photography policy.

Dressings should be chosen that allow passage of fluid from the wound bed, are nonadherent and are not painful to remove: for instance, silicone dressings. It is important to keep dressings simple so that if antiseptic dressings are required they can be employed appropriately, and applied as lightly as possible so that mobility is maintained where necessary (for instance, on the hands). The nurse should have a clear rationale for selecting dressing types and for the frequency of changing. Clinical staff often remove dressings more than is necessary, thus causing damage to delicate epithelial tissue of the superficial burn. Silicone dressings can remain in situ for several days without disturbing the wound bed, and the secondary dressing changed as frequently as required.

Debate about the de-roofing of blisters and debridement is ongoing (Flanagan and Graham, 2001; Rockwell and Ehrlich, 1990; Swain, and Azadia, 1987). The nurse should consider the site, size of blisters, stage of healing and depth of the injury when deciding how to manage the wound.

> **ⓐ Learning activity**
>
> Consider what factors you would use to choose the wound care products with which to dress Peter's burn wounds.
>
> For further reading and exploration of cleansing and blister management, see Flanagan and Graham (2001), Hartford (2001), Rockwell and Ehrlich (1990) or Swain and Azadia (1987). For further discussion of wound dressings used in burns, see Fowler (1999).
>
> Review the risks of bed rest and consider the nursing care that Peter would need to prevent complications of bed rest.

The depth, site and rate of healing of the burn wound inform the care options available. If a superficial wound that has been treated in a conservative manner, is not healed by three weeks, referral to a specialist should be considered as surgery may be indicated.

Nutrition

> **ⓐ Learning activity**
>
> Identify how Peter's nutritional needs can be met.
>
> Why is it important to begin feeding Peter as soon as possible? Check out your answer in the information below.

Nutrition is an important factor in wound healing and recovery following a burn injury of more than 15%TBSA in adults. The body enters a catabolic state. Proteins are metabolised leading to a reduction of lean body mass and poor wound healing. Without adequate nutritional support, this can prove to be fatal.

- The patient's nutritional risk should be identified, and various tools have been developed for this. Risk factors include age, size and depth of injury, nutritional status, and drug and alcohol abuse among others (see Chapter 10 on nutritional needs).
- Based on the nutritional risk score, consult with the dietician who will prescribe supplements or enteral feeds to meet the energy requirements of the individual.

> **ⓐ Learning activity**
>
> Work out how many kcals and grams of protein Peter needs per day. Which vitamins and minerals are important for wound healing?

- Metabolic demand for protein and energy will be considerably increased. The patient will need approximately 25 kcal per kg body weight + 40 kcal × % BSA plus 1 g protein per kg body weight, + 3 g × %BSA (Pape, Judkins and Settle, 2001).
- The patient may need to be fed enterally, either via a nasogastric or nasojejunal tube, or if required for more than 30 days, a percutaneous endoscopic gastrostomy (PEG) may need to be considered.
- The patient might develop deficiencies in micronutrients, as well as energy and protein, as losses may be high and demands are higher during wound healing.
- The nurse will have a large part to play in supporting, monitoring and feeding the patient so that the best outcome can be achieved. Eating is a social activity, and patients often have an improved appetite when eating together. However, it should be acknowledged that the odour of the burn wound could affect the appetite.
- Studies have shown that the earlier feeding is started, the better. This protects the gut mucosal lining. Bacterial translocation has been identified as a potential cause of septic shock in patients who are not fed (see Settle, 1996 for a more in-depth explanation).
- It is essential to monitor the patient's nutritional status. This includes recording the nutritional intake, body weight (usually weekly), blood samples for urea, iron, trace elements, electrolyte levels and liver function, in addition to considering and evaluating the rate of healing and need for general anaesthesia.

S Scenario continued

Peter was in quite a lot of pain and he was very anxious.

a Learning activity

How can pain resulting from a burn be assessed, managed and evaluated?

c Professional conversation

Kemal, the staff nurse caring for Peter, says of pain control, 'Peter may not need as much analgesia as expected in the early period, as many of his burns were deep dermal burns, where many of the nerve endings have been destroyed. However, the superficial burns were painful and he was also very anxious. The paramedics at the scene may have given him entonox and small doses of IV morphine once he arrived at the burns unit. IV morphine is not given immediately, as it is not able to be absorbed until the circulation improves an hour or two later.

'When asked, most people would imagine that a burn is one of the most painful injuries that can occur to a person. The cause of the pain is multifactorial and it can differ depending on the time of the day and the treatment being carried out. The burn-injured patient will almost inevitably experience background pain, pain on dressing changes, physiotherapy, and postoperatively after skin grafting. Each cause may require a different form of treatment. The individual's psychological state plays a significant role in the experience of pain; anxiety and depression will also heighten the person's awareness of pain.

'According to Charlton and colleagues (1983), approximately one-third of severely burn-injured patients will exhibit signs of clinical depression. As Peter has already suffered from depression he will be very vulnerable. As a burn wound is rarely uniform in depth, any burn is painful. It is important to assess the patient's pain, administer prescribed analgesia and introduce measures that aim to reduce pain, including listening and believing the patient, giving information, evaluating the treatment and altering the interventions accordingly. The support of a clinical psychologist or psychiatrist may assist the patient.'

a Learning activity

See Chapter 15 on Pain and Chapter 26 on mental health for more detail on many of the aspects mentioned here.

Consider how you perceive yourself: what is your image of yourself? Now imagine you are Peter. In what ways might you perceive yourself differently after the accident? How might this affect your relationships with others?

An individual's body image is personal to them and has been defined in many ways. Inevitably, a badly burned patient will experience a change in their body image, which is often referred to as an altered body image or disfigurement. Price (1990) offers a good introduction to the concept of body image. He suggests that body image has three essential components: body reality, body ideal and body presentation. Following a burn injury, the individual will need to make adjustments to all of them.

Rehabilitation should begin at the time of injury and be supported with explanations to the patient and family. Rehabilitation should involve reintegration into society, and the multidisciplinary team plays a large role. Alcohol dependency may need to be considered, as a person who is dependent on alcohol and abruptly stops drinking can enter a stage of withdrawal.

a Learning activity

Write down your current definition of rehabilitation.

S   Scenario continued

Factors that could adversely affect Peter's psychological recovery include his pre-injury depression, altered body image, a possible negative reaction from his girlfriend and alcohol dependency.

a   Learning activity

Identify the other healthcare professionals that nurses caring for burn injured individuals need to work with.

c   Professional conversation

Chris, a nurse in a burns unit, says of the role of the multidisciplinary team in treating the burn-injured individual, 'As a nurse in a burns unit I really appreciate working in a team with many other healthcare practitioners who are involved in caring for the burn-injured individual. These include burn and plastic surgeons and other doctors, dieticians, physiotherapists, social workers, occupational therapists, clinical psychologists, psychiatrists, specialist nurses, such as the tissue viability nurse, diabetes nurse specialist, palliative care nurse and pain nurse specialist. It is important that the multidisciplinary team work together in a collaborative way, with the joint aim of treating the patient in a holistic manner.'

Communication is a fundamental part of the multidisciplinary team's role. On both an individual basis and group basis, everyone plays a vital role in communicating to other members of the multidisciplinary team. Nurses have a particular role in empowering the patient and acting as patient advocate.

Accountability is an important consideration when treating burn-injured individuals, and healthcare professionals should practice evidence-based care. The clinical governance agenda should inform this process, and nurses should ensure that their practice is supported by life-long learning in order to facilitate best practice for patients.

Accident prevention and health promotion are fundamental parts of the nurse's role. On both an individual basis and a group basis, the nurse is in a prime position to positively influence the health behaviour of patients. The public can be empowered through the attainment of knowledge and information to enable them to make choices and decisions regarding their safety and that of others.

a   Learning activity

If any of the roles mentioned by Chris are unfamiliar to you, check out their main functions and consider what they might contribute to patient care.

Post-burn education

The nurse needs to inform the patient about the following, ensuring that they understands and are therefore likely to follow the advice:

- the importance of cleansing the newly healed skin with unperfumed soap, rinsing it, drying and reapplying moisturising cream and massaging the area twice per day
- the importance of a daily shower/bath when burnt areas are healed
- explanation of cold/heat injury
- information on what to expect regarding scar formation and management, and altered body image
- advice on diet
- advice on sun protection
- advice on managing itching and ongoing pain
- information on follow-up appointments
- information on swimming, exercise and rest.

Part

II

Conclusion

This chapter has considered the hydration needs of adults during a specific healthcare crisis. Peter, a burns victim, reflects one of the commonest forms of accidents in the developing world. Fluid resuscitation is key to the management of all patients who develop hypovolaemic shock for any reason. The role of the nurse in the management of such patients and their families is of paramount importance, and considerable acumen is required to ensure that evidence-based protocols are adhered to during the period when fluid replacement is the major facet of treatment.

References

Cason, J. S. (1981) Treatment of Burns, London, Chapman & Hall.

Charlton, J., Klein, R., Gagliardi, G. and Heimbach, D. M. (1983) 'Factors affecting pain in burned patients - a preliminary report', Post Graduate Medical Journal 59, 604–7.

Flanagan, M. and Graham, J. (2001) 'Should burn blisters be left intact or debrided?' Journal of Wound Care 10(1), 41–5.

Fowler, A. (1999) 'Burns', in Miller, M. and Glover, D. (eds), Wound Management, London, Nursing Times Books.

Hartford, C. (2001) 'Care of out-patient burns', ch. 4 in Herndon, D. (ed.), Total Burn Care, 2nd edn, Philadelphia, Pa., W. B. Saunders.

Herndon, D. (ed.) (2001) Total Burn Care, 2nd edn, Philadelphia, Pa., W. B. Saunders.

Judkins, K. (1996) 'Inhalation injury', in Settle, J. (ed.), Principles and Practice of Burns Management, London, Churchill Livingstone.

Lawrence, J. C. (1996) 'Burns and scalds: aetiology and prevention', in Settle, J. (ed.), Principles and Practice of Burns Management, London, Churchill Livingstone.

Price, B. (1990) Body Image: Nursing concepts and care, London, Prentice Hall.

Rockwell, W. B. and Ehrlich, H. P. (1990) 'Should burn blister fluid be evacuated?' British Journal of Rehabilitation 11, 93–5.

Rossiter, N. D., Chapman, P. and Haywood, I. A. (1996) 'How big is a hand?' Burns 22(3), 230–1.

St John Ambulance Association and British Red Cross (2006) First Aid Manual, 8th edn, London, Dorling Kindersley.

Swain, A. and Azadia, B. (1987) 'Management of blisters in minor burns', British Medical Journal (Clin. Res.) 285, 181.

Urden, L., Lough, M. and Stacey, K. (1996) Critical Care Nursing, London, Mosby.

Willock, J. and Jewkes, F. (2000) 'Making sense of fluid balance in children', Paediatric Nursing 12(7), 37–42.

Further reading

Bosworth, C. (ed.) (1997) Burns Trauma Management and Nursing Care, London, Prentice Hall. An edited book with contributions from healthcare professionals. Of value mainly to nurses who are new to the speciality, it acknowledges the unique nature of burn injury, discusses the pathophysiology of burns, their presentation, management, psychological consequences and reintegration of the patient into society.

Pape, S., Judkins, K. and Settle, J. (2001) Burns: The first five days, 2nd edn, Hull, Smith and Nephew. This slim volume provides concise, readable and practical guidance for those faced with managing and supporting patients following a major burn injury. This booklet is only concerned with major burns in the first few days after injury and does not pretend to be a comprehensive text. It is aimed at all health professionals involved in the care of these patients.

Perry, R. J., Moore, C. A., Morgan, B. D. G. and Plummer, D. L. (1996) 'Determining the approximate area of a burn: an inconsistency investigated and re-evaluated', British Medical Journal 312(25 May), 1338 [online] http://www.bmj.com/cgi/content/full/312/7042/1338 (accessed 5 February 2009).

Settle, J. (1996) Principles and Practice of Burns Management, London, Churchill Livingstone. An edited book written specifically for healthcare professionals, with contributions from experts in burns care. It is separated into principles and practice to divide the underpinning scientific facts from practical management of the burn-injured individual. As an edited book some areas are duplicated, although this often serves to emphasise important points.

Websites

Burn surgery: http://www.burnsurgery.org/ (designed to provide an educational tool for burn care professionals throughout the world).

Changing Faces: http://www.changingfaces.org.uk (a UK charity that supports and represents people with disfigurements of the face or body from any cause, containing links and references for healthcare practitioners).

Department of Health web-page with link to National Burn Care review: http://www.dh.gov.uk/en/PolicyAndGuidance/HealthAndSocialCareTopics/SpecialisedServicesDefinition/DH_4001838

Red Cross: http://www.redcross.org.uk/standard.asp?id=89410 (skin camouflage link to service provided free of charge to individuals with scars or other disfiguring conditions).

St John's Ambulance and Red Cross: http://www.sja.org.uk/sja/first-aid-advice/effects-of-heat-and-cold/burns-and-scalds.aspx (useful information on first aid for burns and scalds).

Site currently being developed for healthcare professionals specifically on burn injury management: http://www.health.nsw.gov.au/public-health/burns/burnsmgt.html

Chapter

13

Infection prevention and control

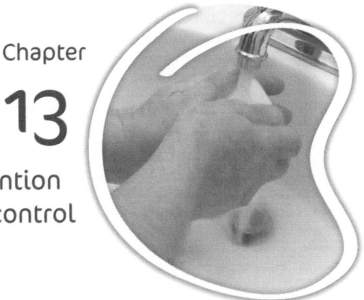

Part

II

Maria Bennallick

Links to other chapters in *Foundation Studies for Caring*

Links to other chapters in *Foundation Skills for Caring*

W   Don't forget to visit www.palgrave.com/glasper for additional
online resources relating to this chapter.

Introduction

Healthcare-associated infections (HCAI) cost the National Health Service (NHS) approximately £1 billion per year (Taylor, Plowman and Roberts, 2000). They are associated with the deaths of approximately 25,000 patients each year, with 5000 patients having their deaths directly linked to HCAI and 20,000 patients having HCAI as a contributory factor towards their deaths. It has been estimated that 15–30 per cent of these infections are preventable (Plowman et al, 1999).

It is important to remember that behind every death there lies a personal and family tragedy, and we therefore have a duty to do everything in our power as practitioners to practise in a way that minimises the risk of HCAI to all patients we care for.

The aim of this chapter is to increase awareness and understanding of the key aspects of infection prevention and control practice which should be implemented at all times when caring for patients. The scenario of a patient with an infected wound is used to help facilitate understanding of the key principles of infection prevention and control.

Learning outcomes

This chapter will enable you to:

- understand the practice of standard precautions
- describe the key points in the National Patient Safety Agency's clean**your**hands campaign
- demonstrate knowledge of how infections are spread
- recognise the main pathogenic organisms that are commonly linked to HCAI
- identify the key steps in carrying out an aseptic technique

- explain the safe procedure for disposal of waste and management of used linen
- understand the importance of the Health Act 2006
- describe why MRSA and clostridium difficile are important in today's NHS
- understand the basic principles of handling food in a safe manner.

Concepts

- Patient safety
- Evidence-based guideline implementation
- Policy and legislation

(C) Professional conversation

Andrew Kingsley, a senior infection control nurse (ICN), comments, 'Healthcare can be so complicated that the fundamentals like infection control, personal hygiene, feeding and pressure care can be forgotten. Infection control needs clinical champions who lead from the front, underpinned by organisations that truly support the concept with hard cash and robust governance systems.'

Fiona Baker, another ICN, adds, 'It is not like other clinical things where you can see the result of bad practice immediately. Cause and effect are divorced, leading to failure to understand the consequences of actions.'

Glossary

Antibiotic: a substance that destroys or inhibits the growth of micro-organisms.

Aseptic: free of micro-organisms.

Cholecystectomy: removal of the gall bladder.

Colonisation: micro-organisms present at a body site without any evidence of symptoms of illness or infection.

Commensal: a micro-organism that is part of the normal flora of the body, such as *E.coli* in the gut.

Decolonisation: removal of micro-organisms which are present at a body site without any evidence of symptoms of illness or infection.

Disinfection: a process which reduces the level of

micro-organisms to a level that is not harmful. Spores may not be removed.

Endogenous infection: an infection caused by micro-organisms originating from the patient's own body.

Exogenous infection: an infection caused by a micro-organism originating in a source other than the patient's own body.

Healthcare-acquired infection: an infection acquired during a period of healthcare.

Healthcare-associated infection: an infection acquired during an episode of clinical care.

Infection: damage of body tissue by micro-organisms or toxins released by micro-organisms.

Micro-organism: an organism that is not visible to the naked eye.

Nosocomial infection: healthcare-acquired infection.

Outbreak: two or more related cases of colonisation or infection, or a rise above the expected level of cases at any given time.

Pathogen: a disease-causing micro-organism.

Pseudomembranous colitis: inflammation of the large intestine related to antibiotic use.

Pyrexia: a body temperature above normal limits. Fever.

Sharps: articles used in the delivery of health care that have the potential to cause a penetrating injury.

Sterilisation: a process that destroys all micro-organisms and spores.

Toxic megacolon: enlarged colon as a result of infection.

Transient organisms: organisms that remain on the hands and other objects for a short while.

Virus: an organism that can only replicate inside another cell.

Part

II

⎡S⎤ Scenario: Introducing Margaret

Margaret Green is 72 years old and lives alone, having been widowed 10 years ago. She is normally quite active, attending weekly tea dance sessions and helping out at the local church with their twice-weekly 'Feeding the Homeless' group.

Health history

Margaret was diagnosed with type 2 diabetes five years ago, and her blood glucose levels are normally well controlled by diet and oral medication. Two years ago, having experienced some discomfort in her upper abdomen, she underwent a cholecystectomy which was carried out using a keyhole surgery technique.

Following surgery, her wound became inflamed and began to discharge offensive-smelling fluid. She was also pyrexial. A specimen of fluid from the wound was found to contain MRSA. Margaret was prescribed antibiotics and her condition improved prior to her being discharged from the surgical ward.

In recent months Margaret has begun to experience pain in her right hip when dancing, and this has become progressively worse. She now has difficulty walking and is awaiting a hip replacement operation.

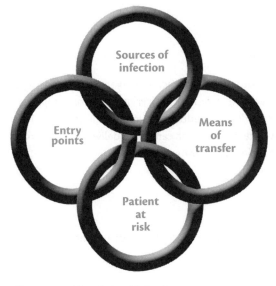

Figure 13.1 The chain of infection

⎡a⎤ Learning activity

Consider each link of the chain of infection shown in Figure 13.1, and note the possible sources of infection, means of organism transfer, groups of patients at risk of infection and entry points for organisms.

C Professional conversation

Andrew comments, 'Infection control is really not that difficult if the principles of transmission of micro-organisms are understood.'

The Health Act 2006

In 2006 the government published *The Health Act 2006: Code of Practice for the Prevention and Control of Health Care Associated Infections* (DH, 2006a), a guidance document issued under the Health Act in order to help NHS organisations reduce the risk of HCAI to patients. Other publications produced by the Department of Health which give guidance on the reduction of HCAI include *Saving Lives: A delivery programme to reduce healthcare associated infection including MRSA* (DH, 2007) and *Essential Steps to Safe Clean Care: Reducing healthcare associated infection* (DH, 2006b).

It is recognised in *The Health Act* that the prevention of HCAI must be embedded into everyday practice by all healthcare workers. If they have a high awareness of the risk of HCAI it is more likely that they will take action to prevent and control HCAI, resulting in better outcomes for patients and staff.

Three main areas of practice are referred to in *The Health Act*:
- management, organisation and the environment
- clinical care protocols
- healthcare workers.

It is stressed throughout *The Health Act* that there is a statutory duty to protect patients, staff and others from HCAI, and to achieve this NHS organisations must have appropriate management systems in place for infection prevention and control.

a Learning activity

Access a copy of the DH's guidance on *The Health Act* (DH, 2006b) and reflect on the duties laid out in that document for NHS organisations. Does the organisation that you are working for have all the relevant clinical protocols in place?

C Professional conversation

Fiona comments, 'Infection control practice may be swayed by the media view and assumptions rather than evidence and expert opinion, leading to confusion and inconsistent practice.'

Saving lives: high-impact interventions

One of the tools that have recently been produced for healthcare workers to assess aspects of their clinical practice is *Saving Lives: Reducing infection, delivering clean and safe care* (DH, 2007). This document and the programme it introduced have been designed to help practitioners in hospital settings to review the standard of care they deliver in relation to specific practices that impact on the risk of patients acquiring HCAI.

C Professional conversation

Andrew comments, 'The *Saving Lives* high-impact interventions should be put into action: no excuses.'

Part
II

> **a Learning activity**   W
>
> Visit the website for the Saving Lives programme (www.clean-safe-care.nhs.uk) and list the high-impact interventions on which guidance is available.

Standard precautions for preventing HCAI

These precautions should be applied by all healthcare practitioners when caring for all hospital in-patients. They include hospital environmental hygiene, hand hygiene, use of personal protective equipment (PPE) and the safe use and disposal of sharps (Pratt et al, 2007).

Hospital environmental hygiene

The hospital environment should be visibly clean, free from dust and spillages. The level of cleanliness should be acceptable to patients being cared for in the area as well as staff working there. It is important that environmental cleaning schedules are adhered to closely, particularly in outbreak situations (Pratt et al, 2007).

As with any aspect of infection prevention and control practice, all healthcare workers should take responsibility for ensuring that the environment in which they are delivering care is cleaned to an acceptable level. Every healthcare worker also needs to ensure that equipment used during the process of care delivery is decontaminated to the appropriate level after use.

If equipment and the environment are kept clean, the opportunities for microbial contamination are reduced.

> **S Scenario continued**
>
> Margaret attends a pre-admission assessment appointment at the local district general hospital in preparation for the hip replacement. Among the investigations carried out is an MRSA screen, which is found to be positive. Margaret is then asked to undertake a decolonisation treatment and be screened again. Three consecutive screens are taken and found to be negative.

> **a Learning activity**
>
> How should the environment in which Margaret is nursed be cleaned?

Hand hygiene

The hands of healthcare workers are the most common route for organisms to be spread from patient to patient (Wilson, 2006). These transient organisms are easily acquired on the surface of the skin of the healthcare worker's hands, and if not removed by hand washing or decontamination can be transmitted to another vulnerable individual. It has been demonstrated that when workers care for patients with a particular organism (such as MRSA), this organism is also frequently found on the hands of those carers (Cookson et al, 1989).

Hands can never be completely free of micro-organisms as resident flora live in the deep crevices of the skin and are impossible to remove. However, it is the transient organisms that are most problematic in the clinical environment.

Preparation of hands

Any cuts on the hands should be covered with a waterproof dressing.

It is necessary to remove hand and wrist jewellery prior to hand decontamination to facilitate the process of effective skin decontamination. Healthcare workers with long fingernails have been shown to be more prone to colonisation with pathogenic organisms

(Moolenaar et al, 2000), therefore nails should be kept short, and false nails and nail extensions should not be worn by staff carrying out clinical procedures (Pratt et al, 2007).

Care of hands

It is important to look after your hands when working in healthcare. Moisturising hands and maintaining skin integrity is necessary outside of working hours. Nails should be kept short and smooth. Any rough edges around the nails and nail beds can provide an environment for microbial growth.

Hand decontamination technique

It has been known for a long time that large areas of the hands are frequently missed when healthcare workers wash their hands (Taylor, 1978). This allows micro-organisms that are left on the unwashed parts of the hands to be transmitted to another patient. Hands should be decontaminated by systematically rubbing all parts of the hands, including the wrists, using either an alcohol-based skin disinfectant or soap and water.

a) Learning activity

Look at your own hands. Do you have any cuts or abrasions on your hands? How long are your fingernails? Are you wearing false nails or nail extensions?

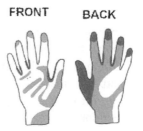

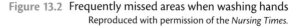

☐ Least frequently missed
▨ Less frequently missed
▨ Most frequently missed

Figure 13.2 Frequently missed areas when washing hands
Reproduced with permission of the *Nursing Times*.

a) Learning activity

Reflect on your own hand decontamination practice when you are in a clinical environment. Are you sure that you wash or decontaminate your hands every time that you are supposed to?

The micro-organisms present on the hands are either resident flora (present most of the time) or transient flora (acquired during the delivery of care and other healthcare activity). These organisms are easy to transmit from person to person when they are deposited on susceptible sites, such as urinary catheters, endotracheal tubes and surgical wounds (Pratt et al, 2007).

Decontamination of the hands is a key aspect of infection prevention and control. It is important that the hands are decontaminated using the correct technique at the appropriate times and using the most suitable decontamination agents. Hands must be decontaminated before and after each episode of patient contact.

Four key factors need to be considered when deciding when it is necessary to decontaminate the hands prior to any clinical activity (Pratt et al, 2007):

- the level of contact that is likely to occur with either the patient or their environment
- the degree of contamination of the hands that would result following the contact
- the activity that is about to be performed with the patient
- the level of susceptibility to infection of the patient.

Alcohol-based hand rub or gel can be used to decontaminate the hands before and after contact with a patient or their environment, after any contact that may result in the hands becoming contaminated, and before handling food. However, if organic matter is present on the hands, liquid soap and water should be used. It is also important to use liquid soap and water when caring for patients with or suspected of having *clostridium difficile*, as alcohol is not active against the spores formed by this organism (Health Care Protection Agency, 2006).

Alcohol-based hand rub or gel, or antimicrobial hand wash products, should be used prior to carrying out an invasive procedure and before putting on a pair of sterile gloves.

The clean**your**hands campaign is designed to significantly improve the rate of hand decontamination in the NHS acute care sector. The campaign is based on improving the availability of alcohol-based hand disinfectants at the patient bedside and on raising staff awareness of the importance of hand decontamination, using posters and other promotional materials. It also aims to involve patients in the improvement process.

Five moments for hand hygiene

The 'Five moments' initiative is being led by the World Health Organization (WHO), and has been designed to rationalise hand hygiene in clinical care delivery. It highlights the 'moments' during a patient's care delivery when hands must be decontaminated to reduce the risk of organism transmission to the patient (Sax et al, 2007).

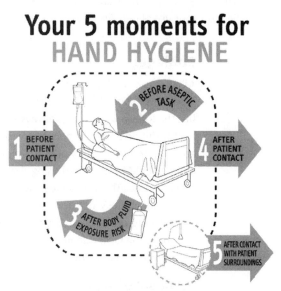

Your 5 moments for HAND HYGIENE

Figure 13.3 Five moments for hand hygiene

Source: www.who.int/gpsc/tools/five_moments/en/index.html
Reproduced with permission of the World Health Organisation.

> **ⓐ Learning activity**
>
> Describe when you should decontaminate your hands during an episode of care with a patient such as Margaret.

Uniforms

As well as being worn to inspire public confidence, uniforms should be worn to facilitate delivery of good patient care. Uniforms or other clothes worn in practice should be changed immediately if they become visibly contaminated or soiled. It is best practice to change into and out of uniforms at work. If this is not possible the uniform should be covered completely when travelling to and from work.

Short sleeves should be worn to facilitate good hand hygiene, and a 'bare below the elbows' policy should be followed at all times: in other words no long sleeves, bracelets, wristwatches, stoned rings or rings other than one gold band should be worn when delivering patient care (DH, 2007).

> **ⓐ Learning activity**
>
> Consider your uniform and how you present yourself in clinical practice. Are your arms bare below the elbows? Is your hair short or tied up? Is your uniform clean?

Use of personal protective equipment (PPE)

The use of PPE provides protection for staff and reduces the opportunity for micro-organism transmission when delivering care (ICNA, 1999). It includes gloves, aprons, mouth and eye protection. The type of PPE required depends on the level of risk associated with the activity about to be undertaken.

When there is no risk of contact with blood and/or body fluids, no PPE is required although hand decontamination should be carried out at all appropriate times. If contact with blood and/or body fluids is expected but there is a low risk of splashing, nonsterile gloves and a disposable apron should be worn. When there is contact with blood and/or body fluids and a high risk of splashing, eye and mouth protection should be worn along with nonsterile disposable gloves and a disposable apron (Pratt et al, 2007).

In addition to these recommendations, PPE should be worn when caring for patients in source and protective isolation. The details of protective clothing required will be dependent on the type of isolation and the organism being isolated (Wilson, 2006).

Part
II

a Learning activity

Consider the type of PPE that you would wear when caring for a patient such as Margaret on a surgical ward when the patient is known to have MRSA.

Reflect on your use of PPE. Are you clear about when you should wear nonsterile gloves? Do you remove them after every episode of care? Do you always wash your hands after you have removed the gloves?

Spillages

All spillages of blood and/or body fluids should be dealt with promptly by an appropriate member of staff. The procedure for dealing with such a spillage varies between organisations but the following principles always apply.

PPE should be worn appropriate to the task. Normally this comprises disposable gloves and apron to reduce the risk of contamination of hands and clothing during the procedure. Any liquid should be absorbed using disposable paper towels or absorbent granules designed for that purpose. The area should be disinfected using a chlorine-based product and following the manufacturer's instructions.

Following disinfection, the area should be thoroughly cleaned using detergent and water and following local cleaning procedures. The PPE should then be removed and disposed of as clinical waste. Hands should then be decontaminated.

Disposal of waste

There are considerable financial and environmental costs involved in waste disposal, which are optimised when the correct procedures are followed. It is important that waste produced during the process of care delivery is disposed of safely and according to current guidelines. The national colour-coding system recommends the segregation of waste into streams linked to the disposal path to be taken (RCN, 2007; DH, 2006):

- yellow stream waste: infectious waste that needs to be disposed of by incineration
- orange stream waste: infectious waste that may be incinerated or treated to ensure safe disposal
- yellow/black stream waste: offensive waste that may be disposed of in licensed landfill sites
- black stream waste: domestic waste that does not contain infectious materials.

It is important that any waste produced in the clinical setting is segregated appropriately at the point of production. This is to ensure that the waste enters the correct waste management stream and therefore poses the minimum of risk to waste handlers (Wilson, 2006):

All healthcare waste must be assessed for its infectious and offensive properties, and colour-coded receptacles should be provided where appropriate to facilitate the correct disposal of waste.

The following questions should be asked to assess healthcare waste (RCN, 2007):

- Has the waste originated from a source that is known or suspected to have an infection or disease caused by a micro-organism or toxin?
- Is the waste a sharp?
- Is the waste offensive?

t Practice tip Disposal of used linen

Used linen that is not soiled should be placed in a clear plastic bag or a fabric linen bag and sent for laundering. The bags must not be overfilled and should be fastened securely to reduce the risk of spillage of linen (Nicol et al, 2004). Used linen in this category is safe to be sorted prior to washing provided that appropriate PPE is worn when it is handled.

Foul and/or infected linen should be placed into a red soluble bag or a bag with a water-soluble seam. This should then be placed directly into a washing machine with a high-temperature wash cycle to eliminate the need for sorting linen that has a high risk of infection.

> **ⓐ Learning activity**
>
> How would you dispose of used linen that has been used during the care of a patient such as Margaret after they have had an episode of diarrhoea?

Use of gloves

You should carry out a risk assessment of the procedure you are about to perform before deciding which type of glove you should wear.

Sterile latex or nitrile gloves should be used when carrying out aseptic procedures, including minor invasive procedures.

Nonsterile latex, vinyl or nitrile gloves should be used when caring for patients and there is a risk of contact with blood or body fluids, or when handling sharps. Gloves that are latex-free should be available to be used by staff if they or their patients have latex sensitisation.

Nonsterile vinyl gloves may be used for tasks which do not involve exposure to blood and body fluids but where protection of the hands is required, such as cleaning with detergent.

Gloves are single-use items. Hands should be decontaminated thoroughly before putting on a pair of well-fitting gloves. They should be put on immediately before carrying out a clinical procedure and be removed immediately after completion of the procedure. They should be disposed of as clinical waste (Pratt et al, 2007), and the hands should then be thoroughly decontaminated (Nicol et al, 2004).

Hands should be washed before and after the wearing of gloves, as hands sweat when in the gloves and this creates a warm, moist environment where microbial growth can flourish. It has been demonstrated that gloves are often punctured during use, and this allows the passage of organisms through the glove (Hampton, 2002).

Use of disposable aprons

Hands should be decontaminated thoroughly before putting on a disposable apron, by placing the apron over the head, avoiding contact with the hair, and tying it loosely around the waist. After use, remove the apron by breaking the neckband, folding the apron down, breaking the waist ties and folding the apron, touching only the side of the apron next to the clothing. The used apron should be disposed of as clinical waste and hands should then be decontaminated thoroughly.

Aprons should be worn when you are in close contact with patients, equipment or the environment which could lead to contamination with blood or body fluids or pathogenic organisms. They should be worn as single-use items, for one episode of patient care or when carrying out one procedure (Pratt et al, 2007).

Use of masks and eye protection

Eye protection and masks should be available for use in clinical settings where there is a risk of splashing of blood and/or body fluids onto the face. Surgical and obstetric procedures are those most commonly requiring this type of PPE (Wilson, 2006).

Use and disposal of sharps

Wilson (2006) defines a 'sharp' as 'any item that may cause a laceration or puncture the skin e.g. needles, scalpel blades, suture removers, glass'. A 'sharps injury' is any injury sustained following contact with a sharp. Clearly, the risk of a healthcare worker acquiring an infection from a sharps injury is related to the degree of contamination of the sharp, the severity of the injury sustained and the presence of a pathogenic organism on the sharp. There have been a number of cases of healthcare workers who have acquired a blood-borne virus such as human immunodeficiency virus (HIV) or hepatitis B (HBV) (Wilson, 2006).

Sharps disposal containers should be made available when carrying out a procedure that results in the production of used sharps. A portable container should be taken to the point of use to facilitate disposal, as this reduces the risk of injury from the used sharp.

Used needles should *never* be resheathed as this increases the risk of sustaining a sharps injury. Sharps should not be passed directly from hand to hand (Pratt et al, 2007).

Used sharps should be disposed of with minimal handling, so needles and syringes should not be separated prior to being placed in a sharps disposal container. The practitioner responsible for disposing of used sharps is the person who used the sharp. Passing used sharps from person to person increases the risk of injury.

Sharps disposal containers should be sealed when no more that two-thirds full. All documentation on the disposal containers must be completed to ensure that tracking of waste is possible if required.

S | Scenario continued

Margaret is admitted for total hip replacement surgery, which is undertaken with apparent lack of complications. However, five days postoperatively she develops a chest infection for which she is prescribed antibiotics. Three days later she develops offensive diarrhoea and abdominal pain. A stool specimen is taken and was found to be positive for the *clostridium difficile* toxin. The antibiotics prescribed for her chest infection are stopped and she is prescribed metronidazole for the treatment of her diarrhoea. This resolves and Margaret is discharged symptom-free to her home a week later.

Isolation of patients with infections

It may be necessary when caring for patients with particular infections to take more precautions to reduce the risk of spread of infection to others. The factors that need to be considered when assessing the need for isolation are (Wilson, 2006):

- the ease of transmission of the organism
- the route of transmission of the organism
- the epidemiological significance of the spread of the organism
- the presence of susceptible individuals.

The purpose of source isolation precautions is to reduce the risk of transmission of infection from the infected source to other individuals (Kilpatrick, Prieto and Wigglesworth, 2008). It is important that isolation of the organism is the main focus of activity rather than isolation of the patient. Unnecessary precautions should not be used as patients may suffer psychological problems when placed in isolation (Wilson, 2006).

It is preferable to nurse patients with infections that are known to be a risk to others in a single room. This is particularly important for organisms that are transmitted via the airborne route such as measles, pulmonary tuberculosis and chickenpox. The room should have a negative pressure for patients where the risk of transmission of airborne organisms is high.

When nursing a patient in isolation, appropriate PPE should be put on outside the room. Following the delivery of care, PPE should be disposed of as clinical waste inside the isolation room and the hands should be decontaminated.

---

a | Learning activity

Reflect on the equipment you would require if you were nursing a patient in isolation. Write down the steps you would take when entering and leaving the room.

Reflect on your practice when you are isolating a patient. Do you understand how infection spreads from person to person? Do you always follow the correct procedures when isolating a patient with an infection? Do you make sure that you spend time talking to patients in isolation to reduce their level of anxiety?

Aseptic technique

The purpose of using an aseptic technique is to prevent transmission of organisms from equipment and hands to susceptible sites such as surgical wounds or intravenous catheter insertion sites. It is important that during the process of the aseptic technique, the susceptible site does not come into contact with any item that is not sterile (Wilson, 2006).

All equipment that is required to carry out the procedure should be collected, and expiry dates and sterility of items should be checked. Hands should then be decontaminated and the sterile pack opened carefully to prevent contamination of the contents. Sterile gloves should be put on to avoid direct skin contact with the susceptible site, without contaminating the outside of the gloves.

During the procedure it is important to ensure that only sterile items come into contact with the susceptible site and that sterile items do not make contact with nonsterile items. Following the completion of the procedure contaminated materials and protective clothing should be disposed of as clinical waste, sharps discarded into a used sharps container and hands decontaminated.

(C) Professional conversation

Andrew comments, 'The term "aseptic technique" is still heard a lot but whether the principles are understood and applied appropriately in the varying settings where healthcare is delivered is questionable.'

MRSA

Meticillin resistant staphylcoccus aureus (MRSA) is a member of the ubiquitous staphylococcus family. Staphylococcus aureus is carried harmlessly on the skin or in the nose of approximately 30 per cent of the population. It can cause infections of the skin, the urinary tract, wounds and even septicaemia. MRSA is a resistant member of that family.

MRSA is resistant to many antibiotics but remains sensitive to vancomycin, which is the antibiotic used when treatment is required for MRSA infection. Although MRSA is often talked about as if it is one organism, there are many strains of MRSA, and these are identifiable according to the resistance patterns they show to a variety of different antibiotics.

Most patients who become positive to MRSA have had some form of healthcare intervention, usually as a hospital in-patient. They have often had some form of clinical intervention and may also have had an invasive device in situ.

Patients colonised but not infected with MRSA may be offered eradication treatment which aims to reduce their bacterial load. The eradication protocol comprises:

- daily skin and hair washes with a chlorhexidine-based skin disinfectant
- hexachlorophene powder applied to axillae and groins
- mupirocin ointment applied to the anterior nares of the nose
- weekly screening for MRSA at all sites.

The purpose of decolonisation is twofold. It attempts to reduce the risk of the positive patient developing an MRSA infection during treatment, and also reduces the risk of transmission to another patient. Although this regime is successful as a long-term clearance solution in no more than 60 per cent of cases, the shedding of MRSA is significantly reduced when it is carried out (DH, 2007).

It is important that standard infection control precautions are followed when caring for patients known to have MRSA. The isolation of patients infected or colonised with MRSA is dependent on the facilities where the patient is being nursed and the associated risk of transmission to others in that environment (Coia et al, 2006).

Part

II

Learning activity

Describe the specific interventions that a patient such as Margaret would experience in relation to their MRSA status.

Look up definitions for these terms:
- commensal organism
- colonisation by organisms
- infection

- endogenous infection
- exogenous infection.

Clostridium difficile

Clostridium difficile infection (CDI) is the most important cause of diarrhoea acquired in hospital. The causative organism is anaerobic and spore forming, and is present in the gut of approximately 3 per cent of healthy adults and 60 per cent of infants. It is very rare for *C.difficile* to cause problems in healthy adults or children, but it can cause severe disease in vulnerable individuals (Kelly and Lamont, 1998).

When the balance of the normal gut flora is compromised because of the use of antibiotics, the *C.difficile* organisms in the gut are able to multiply rapidly, produce toxins which then cause disease. The range of symptoms can vary from mild diarrhoea to severe inflammation of the bowel (pseudomembranous colitis), toxic megacolon and death. Clearly the symptoms can be unpleasant, debilitating and even life threatening (Healthcare Commission, 2007).

The predisposing factors that increase the risk of a patient developing CDI are:
- age
- antibiotic treatment, particularly the use of broad-spectrum antibiotics
- recent surgery or the presence of an underlying disease
- hospital admission
- previous episodes of CDI.

Patients who develop diarrhoea following the use of antibiotics should always have a stool specimen sent for microbiological investigation. The request form should give details of recent antibiotic therapy and the suspicion of CDI. The patient should be nursed in isolation until they have been symptom-free for 48 hours. Hand hygiene is of extreme importance, and because alcohol-based products are ineffective against the *C.difficile* spores, hands should be washed using soap and water when caring for patients with or suspected of having CDI (Heyman, 2004).

The spores formed by the organisms can easily contaminate the environment and thereby present a risk to vulnerable patients being cared for. It is therefore important that particular care is taken in the environmental cleaning when patients are known to have CDI. All horizontal surfaces and other areas should be cleaned well. Chlorine-based products have been shown to be effective against the *C.difficile* spores (Heyman, 2004).

Learning activity

Consider the actions that you need to take when caring for a patient with CDI. Where should the patient be nursed? What PPE would you wear and when would you need to wear it? How long would you need to take these precautions?

Reflect on how it feels to have CDI. What symptoms might you have? How worried do you think you would feel in view of what has been said in the press about this infection?

Food safety

The responsibilities of nurses relating to food handling vary widely depending on their place of work and the system of food production and delivery (Wilson, 2006). The key aspects of food safety can be broken down into

- personal hygiene
- food storage
- food preparation
- cooking food.

Personal hygiene

It is important that staff wash their hands before preparing food to reduce the risk of transmission of organisms to food. Hair should be tied up and no watches or other jewellery should be worn (apart from a plain wedding band). Disposable aprons should be worn over uniforms when dealing with food. Staff should not touch their face or hair when preparing food, nor should they eat, smoke or chew gum.

Cuts and sores should be covered completely with a brightly coloured waterproof dressing.

Staff with any symptoms of vomiting and/or diarrhoea should not come to work and should be monitored carefully to prevent an outbreak of food-borne infection (Food Standards Agency, 2005).

Food storage

Bacteria are able to multiply in most foods kept at room temperature. The process of bacterial multiplication is slowed considerably when the temperature at which the food is stored is reduced. Therefore storing most foods in a refrigerator at 5–8 °C will reduce the risk of transmission of food-borne infection (Sprenger, 2005).

It is also important to store food in a manner that reduces the risk of organism transmission from high-risk food to other food which does not require heating before consumption. For example raw meat should be stored below desserts that are not going to be cooked (Sprenger, 2005). Food stored in the fridge should be covered to reduce the risk of cross-contamination from other foodstuffs.

Meals should not be stored for patients who are not present at mealtimes for longer than an hour (Wilson, 2006). Food that has been stored for longer periods of time may present an increased risk to patients, as reheating the food might not be sufficient to destroy the high level of organisms that can develop.

Food preparation

As much raw food may be contaminated with food-poisoning organisms it is important to ensure that raw food is thoroughly cooked prior to serving. Raw and cooked food should be stored separately to reduce the risk of cross-contamination by organisms from raw food. Food that is eaten raw should be washed under running water to remove harmful organisms (Wilson, 2006).

Separate utensils should be used when preparing cooked and raw food, and preparation surfaces and equipment used in the process of food preparation should be cleaned thoroughly with detergent and water after use.

Learning activity

Review the storage of food in your place of work. Is food that is a risk to your patients stored appropriately?

Learning activity

Identify high-risk food that is stored in your place of work. Is there any risk of contamination of other foodstuffs?

Cooking food

Food that requires cooking should reach temperatures that render it safe to eat by the reduction of harmful bacteria (Sprenger, 2005). Most bacteria are destroyed at temperatures around 60 °C, so it is important to ensure that food is heated to this level. These temperatures must be reached throughout the foodstuff to reduce the risk of viable pathogenic organisms being left in sections of the food. When this is not achieved there is a significant risk of illness: for example, undercooked minced beef in burgers can cause infection with *E.coli* 0157. Thermometers should be used to ensure that food is heated to the correct temperature, with the centre of food needing to be at 70 °C to ensure thorough cooking has occurred.

Food that is to be reheated must also be heated to the correct temperatures as detailed above (Wilson, 2006).

> **(a) Learning activity**
>
> List four common food-poisoning organisms and describe how you would reduce the risk of these infections affecting your patients.

Conclusion

This chapter should have helped you to become aware of the high priority of preventing infections during the care of patients. Many HCAIs are preventable, and your practice can make a significant difference to the clinical outcomes of the patients in your care. Remember to aim to break the chain of infection at all times and you will help save lives. Use the 'five moments' every time you care for patients, and you will know that you are contributing to the provision of safe care.

> **(c) Professional conversation**
>
> Andrew adds, 'Infection control is not an optional extra.'

References

Coia, J. E., Duckworth, G. J., Edwards, D. I., Farrington, M., Fry, C., Humphreys, H., Mallaghan, C. and Tucker, D. R. (2006) 'Guidelines for the control and prevention of meticillin-resistant Staphylococcus aureus (MRSA) in healthcare facilities', *Journal of Hospital Infection*, 1–44.

Cookson, B., Peters, B., Webster, M., Phillips, I., Rahman, M. and Noble, W. (1989) 'Staff carriage of epidemic methicillin-resistant Staphylococcus aureus', *Journal of Clinical Microbiology* 27(7) (July), 1471–6.

Department of Health (DH) (2006a) *Essential Steps to Safe Clean Care: Reducing healthcare associated infection*, London, DH.

DH (2006b) *The Health Act 2006: Code of practice for the prevention and control of health care associated infections*, London, DH.

DH (2007) *Saving Lives: A delivery programme to reduce healthcare associated infection including MRSA*, London, DH.

Food Standards Agency (FSA) (2005) *Safer Food, Better Business*, London, FSA.

Hampton, S. (2002) 'The appropriate use of gloves to reduce allergies and infection'. *British Journal of Nursing* 11, 1120–4.

Healthcare Commission (2007) 'Investigation into outbreaks of Clostridium difficile at Maidstone and Tunbridge Wells NHS Trust', London, Healthcare Commission.

Health Care Protection Agency (HCPA) (2006) *Clostridium difficile: Findings and recommendations from a review of the epidemiology and a survey of Directors of Infection Prevention and Control in England*, London, HCPA.

Heyman, D. L. (2004) *Control of Communicable Diseases Manual*, Atlanta, GA., American Public Health Association.

Infection Control Nurses Asociation (ICNA) (1999) *Glove Usage Guidelines*, London, ICNA and Regent Medical.

Kelly, C.P . and Lamont, J. T. (1998) 'Clostridium difficile infection', *Annual Review of Medicine* 49, 375 –90.

Kilpatrick, C., Prieto, J. and Wigglesworth, N. (2008) 'Single room isolation to prevent the transmission of infection: development of a patine journey tool to support safe practice', *British Journal of Infection Control* 9(6), 19–25.

Moolenaar, R. L., Crutcher, J. M., Venusto, H., San Joaquin, V. H., Sewell, L.V., Hutwagner, C.C., Carson, L.A., Robison, D. A. Smithee, L. M. K. and Jarvis, W. R. (2000) 'A prolonged outbreak of pseudomonas aeruginosa in a neonatal intensive care unit: did staff fingernails play a role in disease transmission?' *Infection Control and Hospital Epidemiology* 21, 80–5.

Nicol, M., Bavin, C., Bedford-Turner, S., Cronin, P., Rawlings-Anderson, K. (2004) *Essential Nursing Skills*, St-Louis, Miss., Mosby.

Plowman, R., Graves, N., Taylor, L. et al (1999) *Socio-economic Burden of Hospital Acquired Infections*, London, DH.

Pratt, R. J, Pellowe, C. M., Wilson, J. A., Loveday, H. P., Harper, P. J., Jones, S. R. L. J., McDougall, C. and Wilcox, M. H. (2007) 'Epic 2: national evidence-based guidelines for preventing healthcare associated infections in NHS hospitals in England', *Journal of Hospital Infection* 65S, S1–S64.

Royal College of Nursing (RCN) (2007) *Safe Management of Health Care Waste*, guidance document, London, RCN.

Sax, H., Allegranzi, B., Uckay, I., Larson, E., Boyce, J. and Pittet, D. (2007) '"My five moments for hand hygiene": a user-centred design approach to understand, train, monitor and report hand hygiene', *Journal of Hospital Infection* **67**(1), 9 –21.

Sprenger, R.A. (2005) *Hygiene for Management*, Doncaster, Highfield.

Taylor, K., Plowman, R. and Roberts, J.A. (2000) *The Challenge of Hospital Acquired Infection*, London, National Audit Office.

Taylor, L. J. (1978) 'An evaluation of handwashing techniques', *Nursing Times* **74**(2) (12 January), 54 –5.

Wilson, J. (2006) *Infection Control in Clinical Practice*, Edinburgh, Balliere Tindall.

Websites

British Infection Society: www.britishinfectionsociety.org

Clean, Safe Care: www.clean-safe-care.nhs.uk (hub for information about reducing healthcare-associated infections)

Department of Health: www.dh.gov.uk

Doctor Fungus: http://www.doctorfungus.org/ (online reference to all mycological matters)

European Antimicrobial Resistance Surveillance System: http://www.earss.rivm.nl/

Evidence based practices in infection control (EPIC): www.epic.tvu.ac.uk

European Commission Public Health information (EUROPA Public Health): http://europa.eu.int/comm/health/ph_overview/overview_en.htm

Faculty of Public Health Medicine of the Royal Colleges of Physicians of the United Kingdom: http://www.fphm.org.uk/

Health Care Standards Unit: www.hcsu.org.uk

Hospital Infection Society: www.his.org.uk

Health Protection Agency: www.hpa.org.uk

Infection Prevention Society: www.ips.uk.net

Infectious Disease Research Network: www.idrn.org

International Scientific Forum on Home Hygiene: http://www.ifh-homehygiene.org/2003/index.html

International Society for Infectious Disease: www.isid.org

Institute for Innovation and Improvement: www.institute.nhs.uk (for knowledge sharing)

Medscape Infectious Diseases: http://www.medscape.com/infectiousdiseaseshome (general information to keep up-to-date about infectious diseases news, new therapies and so on)

National Electronic Library of Infection (NELI): www.neli.org.uk

National Library for Health: www.library.nhs.uk/infections (specialist library)

National Patient Safety Agency: www.npsa.nhs.uk

National Resource for Infection Control: www.nric.org.uk (part of NELI)

Paediatric Infectious Diseases Web (PID Web): www.paediatric-infectious-diseases.com (gateway to resources on paediatric infectious disease)

Royal Institute of Public Health: http://www.riph.org.uk/

Society for General Microbiology: http://www.sgm.ac.uk/

World Health Organization: http://www.who.int

Chapter

14

Pharmacology and medicines

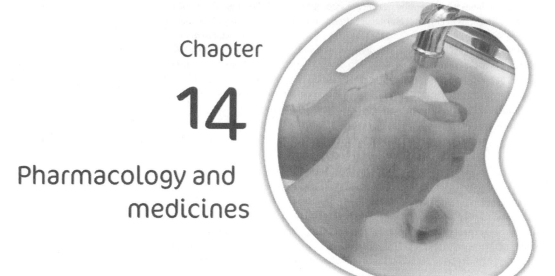

John Bastin and Katie Jackson

Links to other chapters in *Foundation Studies for Caring*

Links to other chapters in *Foundation Skills for Caring*

W   Don't forget to visit www.palgrave.com/glasper for additional
online resources relating to this chapter.

Introduction

This chapter looks at both the history of the use of drugs in medicine and the key aspects of how the body absorbs drugs and utilises them. Drug calculations are directly linked to this body interaction with medication. It offers a glimpse into the future in the form of pharmacogenetics, and how this might change the way in which drugs are prescribed and developed.

The use of drugs is governed by complex legislation, and this is reviewed to help you understand the key issues for the safe administration of medicines, the steps involved in the process and what to do when errors occur.

Learning outcomes

This chapter will enable you to:

- understand the legal and professional implications of administering medications
- administer medications in a safe and effective manner
- perform drug calculations

- know the different types and causes of medication errors
- understand about adverse drug reactions
- understand how to prevent medication errors
- understand incident/drug error reporting.

Concepts

- Pharmacokinetics
- Pharmacodynamics
- Pharmacogenetics

- Drug incompatibility
- Professional requirements
- Legal requirements

- Safety
- Consent
- Documentation

Pharmacology is the study of drugs, and the way in which the body responds to them. The science of pharmacology looks not only at the origin of drugs, their chemical structure, preparation and administration, but also at their mode of action, metabolism and excretion. The application of the action of drugs in the treatment of disease is called *therapeutics*.

History

Drugs have been used for thousands of years, and until the modern era were derived from plants, animal and mineral sources, and administered in the main by a local health expert, a witch doctor. Many of these remedies have been passed down to us, and are known to have beneficial effects, but little was known about how they worked or their chemical structure. Many early medications were mixtures, and their creators might not have realised which was the active ingredient.

With the coming of the Industrial Revolution medical and biosciences changed quite dramatically, and a new science of clinical pharmacology started to evolve. Compounds such as digoxin and morphine, which had been used previously as nonspecific mixtures of plant extracts, could now be isolated, and new compounds could be synthesised from biochemical raw materials. This allowed the development of international standards for drugs, and together with legal changes meant that fraudulent claims and unprofessional practice could now be prevented.

> (a) **Learning activity**   W
>
> If you would like more information on this topic look up www.pharmacy.wsu.edu/history/history15html.

Today the pharmaceutical industry is a complex and influential world with multifaceted research networks.

> ### (a) Learning activity W
>
> Look up www.pfizer.co.uk to view the extent of a large pharmaceutical company.

A medicinal product is defined as:

> Any substance or combination of substances presented for treating or preventing disease in human beings or in animals. Any substance or combination of substances which may be administered to human beings or animals with a view to making a medical diagnosis or to restoring, correcting or modifying physiological functions in human beings or animals is likewise considered a medicinal product.
>
> (EU Council Directive 65/65/EEC)

Pharmacogenetics

Following the decoding of the genome, a new area of pharmacogenetics is emerging, which promises to lead to a new era when drugs can be tailor-made to meet the needs of each individual's genetic make-up. This promises to not only reduce the incidence of side-effects but also reduce the time needed for drugs to gain approval.

This new field in pharmacology has developed following the advances in knowledge regarding an individual's response to drugs, and relies on the identification of genetic variations in a population, which can influence how drugs are metabolised, giving individual responses to the same medication dose.

Screening of a population for genetic variation is now possible because of advances in the sequencing of DNA. The speed and automation that is now possible means that data from many individuals can now be processed at the same time.

Two main strategies are used, phenotyping and genotyping:

- **Phenotyping** determines the presence of a particular group of reactions or receptors from a tissue sample.
- **Genotyping** determines the specific genetic code of an individual, and whether they can successfully metabolise a drug.

Variation in response has been recorded for decades, but with the advent of these new technologies it is hoped to resolve the uncertainties of drug treatment.

> ### (a) Learning activity W
>
> Discuss with a pharmacist the variations in response to some drugs, or look up in www.BNF.org the different responses that occur in individuals to Warfarin.

Legal and professional implications of administering medications

Professional requirements

The Nursing and Midwifery Council (NMC) has produced guidelines for safe practice in the management and administration of medicines, the *Standards for Medicines Management* (2007). There are ten sections :

- methods of supplying and/or administration of medicines
- dispensing
- storage and transportation
- standards for practice of administration of medicines
- delegation
- disposal
- unlicensed medicines

- complementary and alternative therapies
- management of adverse events
- controlled drugs.

It is the duty of a nurse (or any other healthcare practitioner permitted to do so) to administer medication according to standards set by their professional body, and if harm is caused as a result of a breach of the duty of care, they might be considered negligent. In court the performance of a nurse is judged by the standards that would be expected of any respected body of professionals.

The law

A number of pieces of legislation relate to the administration of medicines.

Medicines Act 1968

This Act regulates the licensing, supply and administration of medicines. The Secretary of State has a duty to place on the 'prescription only' list any medicines that may represent a danger, if their use is not supervised by an appropriate practitioner.

It is essential to be aware of the licensed uses of the medication. Those who alter a dose, open capsules or crush medicines are in breach of the 1968 Act as they are not administering the medicines in a licensed form.

> **S** Scenario: Introducing Joy
>
> A patient, Joy Thomas, is due 1 gram of paracetamol at 12 midday. When you go to give her this medication, you learn that she is unable to swallow tablets, the form that has been prescribed for her.

> **a** Learning activity
>
> What should you do when you discover a patient is unable to take medication in the prescribed format? Should you:
> - think about the alternative products that are available?
> - consult the appropriate practitioner about the method of administration?
> - consult the pharmacist?

Paracetamol can be administered via several different routes; oral, rectal and intravenous. If a specific form has been prescribed, an appropriate prescriber must change the prescription chart in order for you to administer via a different route. In the scenario case, the nurse remembers that paracetamol comes in a soluble tablet form which Joy is able to swallow safely.

The law stipulates five requirements in relation to the administration of medicines. Medicines need to be given:

- to the right **person**
- at the right **time**
- in the right **form**
- using the right **dose**
- via the right **route**.

The patient/client has a right to self-determination: in other words, they have the right to accept or decline medical treatment. Therefore the patient's wishes should be respected, and consent must be gained before a medication can be administered.

If the patient does not have the capacity to make the decision to take medication, because of an impairment or disturbance of mental function (for instance, they might be unconscious), they may be treated in what is believed to be their best interests in accordance with the **Mental Capacity Act 2005**. Mental capacity must be formally assessed in these cases. The Mental Capacity Act states that a person with a lasting power of attorney may make the decision on the patient's behalf, so when it is likely that a person's impairment will last permanently or for a considerable time, it is useful for an appropriate person to apply for this power. This person could be a relative, friend or doctor.

Misuse of Drugs Act (MDA) 1971

The MDA sets the statutory requirements for the control and regulation of controlled drugs (CDs). The primary purpose is to prevent misuse of CDs. The specific drugs that are controlled are listed in Schedule 2 of the Act. Additional statutory measures for the management of CDs are laid down in the **Health Act 2006** and its associated regulations.

The legislation states that the prescription should:

- be in ink or such as to be indelible
- be signed and dated by the prescriber
- specify the dose to be taken
- specify the form and possibly the strength of the preparation
- specify either the total quantity (in both words and figures) of the preparation or the number (in both words and figures) of dosage units.

Misuse of Drugs Regulations 2001 (MDR) and Misuse of Drugs Regulations Northern Ireland (NI) 2002

The use of CDs in medicine is permitted by the MDR, which classify the drugs in five schedules according to the different levels of control required. Schedule 1 CDs are subject to the highest level of control, whereas Schedule 5 CDs are subject to a much lower level of control.

Registered nurses should be familiar with Schedule 2 medicines such as opiates (morphine, diamorphine and pethidine), and Schedule 3 drugs such as barbiturates.

Health Act 2006 and Controlled Drugs (Supervision of Management and Use) Regulations 2006

The key points of the Act and regulations are:

- All healthcare organisations and independent hospitals are required to appoint an accountable officer.
- Professional bodies, healthcare organisations and other local and national agencies have a duty to collaborate and to share intelligence on CD issues.
- The police and other nominated people have the power to enter premises to inspect stocks and records of CDs.

Pharmacology

Medical pharmacology looks at the chemicals we refer to as drugs, and how they interact with the human body. These chemical interactions are divided into two areas for consideration:

- pharmacokinetics, or how the body handles a drug
- pharmacodynamics, or how a drug works.

S Scenario: Introducing Mr Watson

Mr Watson is a 50-year-old unemployed man who has had a persistent cough for a week. He presents in the Accident and Emergency Unit (A&E) with severe shortness of breath. He is a known alcoholic.

On triage his oxygen saturation (SpO_2) is 88 per cent, his heart rate (HR) is 120 BPM and his blood pressure (BP) is 90/40 mmHg. Further examination reveals that Mr Watson has a community-acquired pneumonia and requires urgent treatment and high-dependency care in the Intensive Care Unit (ICU).

In the ICU he deteriorates further, and requires invasive ventilation. As with many critically ill patients, Mr Watson now requires a variety of medications – sedation (propofol), analgesia (alfentanyl), inotropes (noradrenaline) and antibiotics (cefradine and rifampicin), all administered via an intravenous (IV) line. Oral/NG analgesia (via a nasogastric tube) is also prescribed.

Pharmacokinetics

If a drug is to have an effect on the cells of the body it must be in the right place, for the right amount of time and at the right concentration, the right concentration being very important if it is to be therapeutic. If the concentration is higher than therapeutic it may well become toxic. In the other extreme, if the concentration of the drug is too low, then it will be nontherapeutic.

Drugs are usually metabolised within the liver by specific enzyme pathways, and the time taken for the plasma level of the drug to be reduced by one half is known as the half life or t½.

Pharmacokinetic data about a drug tells us what dose to give, how often to give it and what other factors to take into consideration. Dosage and body volume are closely linked. For example a tablet containing 100 mg of drug when given to a person with a volume of 100 dm^{-3} will give a concentration of 1 mg dm^{-3}. The same tablet given to a person with a volume of 50 dm^{-3} will result in a concentration of 2 mg dm^{-3}: twice the concentration, and this might pass the toxic threshold. It is important therefore to know the volume mass of the recipient to ensure that a therapeutic dose is maintained.

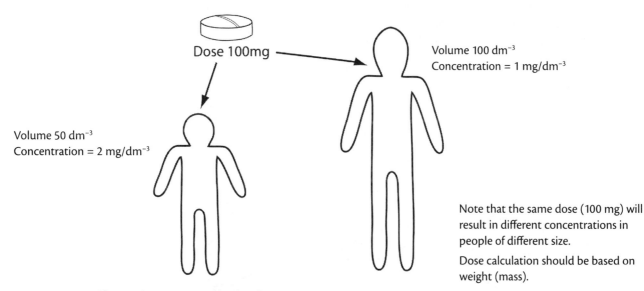

Dose 100mg

Volume 100 dm^{-3}
Concentration = 1 mg/dm^{-3}

Volume 50 dm^{-3}
Concentration = 2 mg/dm^{-3}

Note that the same dose (100 mg) will result in different concentrations in people of different size.

Dose calculation should be based on weight (mass).

Figure 14.1   Dosage and body volume

Pharmacokinetic processes can be divided into four stages: absorption, distribution, metabolism and elimination. Drugs are administered by a variety of routes using a variety of formulations in order to have a desired response. The desired response will only happen if a therapeutic level is maintained, and this in turn relies on bioavailability. The bioavailability of a drug is defined as the proportion of the administered dose that reaches the circulation. For example IV drug administration equals 100 per cent bioavailability. Factors that will affect bioavailability should be considered in any situation where drugs are being used.

Absorption will depend on factors such as whether the drug is water or fat soluble, how it is formulated and what else is in the gut at the same time. Drugs are administered by a variety of routes, often using different formulations, to achieve a desired response.

Following absorption, drugs enter the blood stream and are then carried around the body. This could be in simple solution or attached to protein carriers. **Distribution** will depend on quality of blood flow; poor peripheral circulation can result in the drug not reaching the desired areas. Binding of the drug to protein carriers can be a real issue with polypharmacy because of carrier competition. Some drugs miss the option for transport and do not ever achieve therapeutic levels. Some drugs diffuse out of the circulation pathway into tissue spaces, fat and more rarely cells.

Metabolism in the liver produces new products so called *metabolites*. These are usually waste products but with some formulations the metabolites are the active component of the drug. For example the contraceptive pill when taken contains hormone precursors which are converted to the active hormone in the liver. Liver disease will obviously have an important influence on drug molecule breakdown and the speed at which it occurs. Factors such as blood flow through the liver and the size of the liver are important particularly in neonates.

Elimination or excretion of the drug, usually via the kidney, raises issues of blood flow. Poor kidney function will lead to a serious accumulation in the body of drug or drug metabolites. Other areas of elimination of an administered drug are the gut, sweat glands, and although it is sometimes forgotten, a mother's breast milk, which may contra-indicate with a child's medication.

Physiology

The liver

The liver is the largest organ in the body. It is located in the upper right quadrant of the abdomen and has three basic functions: metabolic, secretory and vascular. The major function however is the excretion of waste products from the blood. From a physiological perspective liver cells contain enzymes which transform poisons into less harmful compounds.

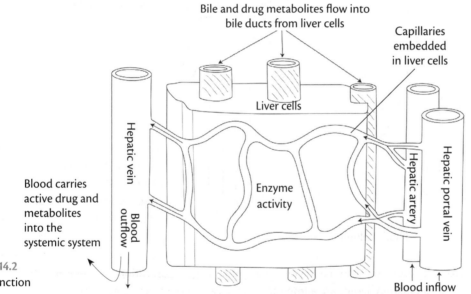

Figure 14.2
Liver function

Specific detoxification enzymes belong to a family called CYP enzymes (Cytochrome P450 due to their ability to absorb light at a frequency of 450 nm), and drugs are either broken down by them or converted into active molecules.

For example CYP2D6 is an enzyme responsible for metabolising a large number of cardiac drugs including beta blockers. People with poor metabolic pathways to deal with these drugs may well have from two to three times the expected plasma concentration, leading to dizziness.

CYP2C9 is involved in Warfarin metabolism, and between 1 and 2 per cent of the population are poor metabolisers, keeping their drug level high much longer than would be expected. Because of this they only require a seventh of the normal dose. They risk overdose and death at normal therapeutic levels.

Rhythmodan (disopyramide), an anti-arrhythmic drug, is also affected by poor metabolism. In this case however it is the metabolite that is active, so although the drug concentration in the blood may be high the actual working molecule level may be below the effective therapeutic level. As a result of this, poor metabolisers will need more drugs to get to the therapeutic level needed. However the side-effects of this increased dosage may well influence other body systems.

CYP enzymes in the liver evolved a long time ago, and enabled animals to metabolise plant toxins ingested in their diet before they entered the systemic circulation and caused damage. Animals that had these enzymes were obviously more advantaged from an evolution perspective than animals that did not have them.

Most early drugs came from plants and resembled plant toxins, and the CYP enzymes were able to metabolise them easily. In reality these enzymes determine what substances can become drugs: if there is no mechanism to eliminate a substance, it cannot be used as a drug.

Although our knowledge of the CYP enzymes is relatively recent we are now in a position to decode the genes for each specific enzyme, and from this their amino acid sequences can be replicated. This has resulted in the production of pure enzymes for all of the human CYP enzymes. As a result considerable advances have been made in our understanding of the effects of specific enzymes on specific drugs, and vice versa.

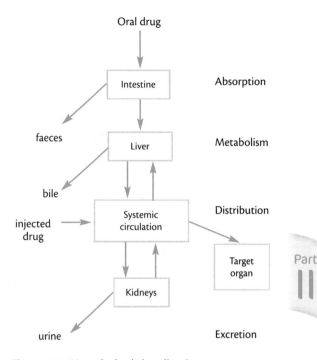

Figure 14.3 How the body handles drugs

Giving paracetamol

> **S Scenario continued**
>
> Mr Watson is prescribed a large number of drugs. Some of these are to be administered intravenously and some orally.
>
> **Drug compatibility**
>
> Paracetamol for oral or via enteral tube to the stomach can come in soluble tablets. These can be given with other oral medications unless specified on that particular medication.
>
> Paracetamol must not be administered with any other IV medications.

> **a Learning activity**
>
> Look up the British National Formulary and make notes regarding the contra-indications of prescribing paracetamol. What are the side-effects of this drug? What is the lethal dose of paracetamol for an adult?

Caution should be taken with oral anticoagulants, as paracetamol may lead to slight variations of International Normalised Ratio (INR) values. In this case, increased monitoring of INR values should be conducted during the period of use as well as for a week after paracetamol treatment has been discontinued.

Precautions for paracetamol use

Paracetamol should be used with caution in cases of:
- reduced liver function
- severe renal impairment
- chronic alcoholism
- chronic malnutrition
- dehydration.

> ### (a) Learning activity
>
> What are INR values? What do they measure and what are normal levels? What might be the result of changes in these levels? Will any aspect of Mr Watson's illness influence the prescription of paracetamol?

Absorption

Absorption of oral/NG medication may be affected in critically ill patients for a number of reasons, including reduced circulation to the gastrointestinal (GI) tract, reduced bowel motility and reduced production of gut secretions. This factor may need to be taken into account when administering oral/NG medications to critically ill patients, and gut motility may need to be monitored by measuring gastric contents. This is achieved by performing an NG aspirate, and calculating the amount of fluid that is withdrawn from the NG tube minus the amount of fluid input to it.

Metabolism

Paracetamol is metabolised mainly in the liver. Some of it is metabolised to a toxic substance (N-acetyl benzoquinone imine) which is normally rapidly detoxified by reduced glutathione and eliminated in the urine. However, during massive overdosing, the quantity of this toxic metabolite is increased.

Elimination

The metabolites of paracetamol are mainly excreted in the urine, and 90 per cent of the dose administered is excreted within 24 hours. Less than 5 per cent is eliminated unchanged. Plasma half-life is 2.7 hours and total body clearance is 18 L/h.

Poly pharmacy

There are many medications that contain paracetamol, and it is important to be aware of this. If paracetamol is administered with a drug such as Co-dydramol this would lead to an overdose as Co-dydramol also contains paracetamol.

> ### (a) Learning activity
>
> Visit a local chemist. Note the different trade names for paracetamol and see how many other preparations contain paracetamol. If they are not too busy, ask the pharmacist to show you some of the drugs that can be bought over the counter that contain paracetamol.
>
> Consider this in relation to accidental overdose, especially when the patient is a child and the total daily dose is much smaller.

Drug continuity and availability

Paracetamol tablets are readily available within the hospital environment. There are no adverse reactions to sudden withdrawal of paracetamol.

IV paracetamol is not administered as a continuous infusion. It has only become available in recent years and it is recommended that it is not used if paracetamol can be administered via the oral route.

It should be noted that other medications can also contain paracetamol and this must be checked prior to administration.

ⓒ Professional conversation

Administering paracetamol to someone with liver cirrhosis

During the drug round Mrs Jefferson, who has been admitted for draining of ascites secondary to liver cirrhosis, complains of abdominal discomfort and asks for some analgesia (pain relief). David, a staff nurse, says, 'We need to check what analgesia Mrs Jefferson can have, because she can't have any containing paracetamol.'

Sandra, a student nurse, asks, 'Why's that, David?'

David explains, 'Paracetamol can be toxic to the liver in large doses, but in the case of liver cirrhosis it can be toxic at much lower doses, so it shouldn't be given unless it's unavoidable. It's sometimes prescribed to people who are suffering from mild to moderate liver disease, but in much smaller doses than normal, and they have to be closely monitored.'

'So what other analgesia might we give Mrs Jefferson?' Sandra asks.

'Liver metabolism is the main route of elimination for drugs,' David says. 'If the liver doesn't work properly, then drugs can accumulate in the body, so that must be taken into account when prescribing medications. There are drawbacks with all analgesics. For instance, care must be taken with opioids as they can accumulate and cause loss of consciousness and respiratory depression. Non-steroidal anti-inflammatory drugs (NSAIDs) such as aspirin and diclofenac increase the risk of gastro-intestinal bleeding. This is a very complex and specialist field, and that's why I need to speak to the doctor, or to a pharmacist or specialist nurse, to get advice on what to give Mrs Jefferson.'

Pharmacodynamics: the study of how drugs work

Most drugs produce their effect by acting on proteins called *receptors*. These receptors are genetic in origin, and allow cells to communicate either with the outside or internally. Receptors usually respond to synaptic transmitters or hormones.

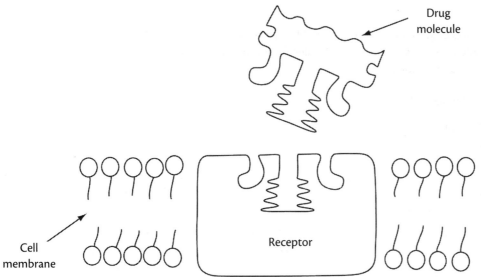

Drug molecule

Cell membrane

Receptor

Drugs have a structural relationship with the receptor molecule in the cell membrane. The closer the fit, the better the cellular response. The drug molecule also needs to be recognised by enzymes in the liver so that it can be broken down or modified. Pharmacogenetics aims to get the drug receptor interface as near perfect as possible.

Figure 14.4 Drugs and receptors

The interaction of the drug and the receptor depends on the fit of the drug molecule to the receptor. The better the fit, the more specific the drug.

Sometimes a drug molecule will affect more than one receptor, and this can be a cause of unwanted side-effects.

Drug action occurs through:

- replacing chemicals that are deficient – hormones, minerals or vitamins
- interfering with cell functions and metabolic pathways by stimulating or inhibiting normal levels of activity – a function that helps with clotting disorders, inflammation, and hormone disorders
- acting against invading or abnormal cells – the action of antibiotics and anticancer drugs
- interfering with the function of receptor sites themselves, enhancing responses (agonists) or preventing normal responses (antagonists).

Agonist drugs bind to the receptor site and improve the response to normal stimulation, producing a reaction that results in improved cell function. For example, metformin hydrochloride increases the receptor sensitivity to insulin in diabetics.

These drugs bind to receptors and enhance cell activity.

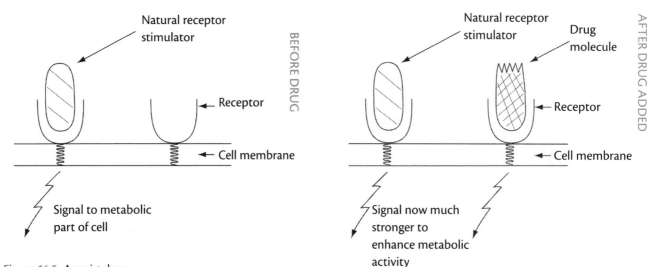

Figure 14.5 Agonist drugs

Antagonist drugs bind to the receptor site and block normal function and cell activity. For example, Tamoxifen prevents oestrogen molecules from docking with a receptor, so it can prevent cell growth stimulation in breast tumours.

These drugs bind to receptors and block cell activity.

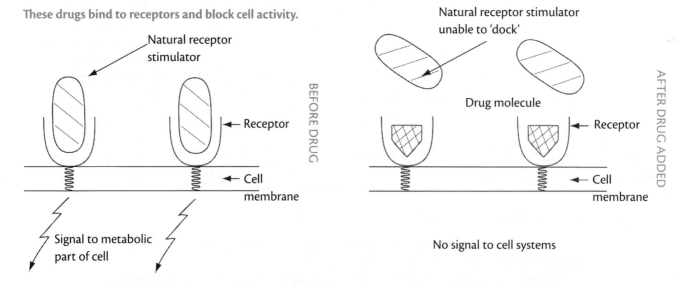

Figure 14.6 Antagonist drugs

Administering drugs to children

Many drugs used for children are in fact not registered for use with children. For a variety of commercial, ethical and practical reasons, the majority of medicines are designed for adults. Recently legislation has encouraged drug companies to conduct more paediatric studies and to seek paediatric marketing authorisations (licences) for new and existing drugs (Grieve et al, 2005). Many children, particularly neonates, are prescribed medicines which are not specifically licensed for use at their age. Many drugs have been trialled and evaluated for adults but have not had a similar pathway to accreditation for children.

There is enormous variation from the neonatal period through to adolescence in the way children absorb, metabolise and excrete drugs (Baber and Pritchard, 2003). The blood brain barrier that filters molecules entering the brain is not well developed in children, and can easily be compromised. For example sulphonamides can cross this barrier in children and cause fits (kerinicterus). Protein-binding sites that are responsible for carrying drug molecules around the body tend to be lower in the first few months of life. Body fat is low in the new born, and fat-soluble drugs may become toxic at adult doses because they are not lost in the fat.

If a product is not specifically marketed for use with children it is usually not available in a suitable formulation for children (Nunn and Williams, 2005). This could mean that capsules and tablets that were designed to be swallowed whole by an adult need to be divided. Doing so could reduce the drug's effect or increase its toxicity, for example if an enteric coating is broken (Baber and Pritchard, 2003). Some tablets are designed to be broken: these tablets are scored across the centre to enable accurate division, and equal amounts of the drug should be available in each half of the tablet. If tablets are not scored there is likely to be uneven distribution of the drug within the tablet, resulting in dosage errors when the tablet is split.

Crushing tablets may alter the therapeutic properties of a medicine, diminishing its effectiveness, and crushing is not covered in product licences. A pharmacist can advise whether the medication is compromised by crushing, and may permit crushing if it has been determined to be in the patient's best interest. However, it not acceptable to disguise the medicine from the recipient as this would be misleading. *Covert administration* is the administration of medicines to a capable adult without their consent. To do this maliciously is a crime under the Offences Against the Person Act 1861. Covert administration must only occur when the recipient lacks the capacity to give consent.

In prescribing for children it is useful to use the following terminology:

* **neonate**: birth to one month
* **infant**: one month to 2 years
* **child**: 2 to 12 years
* **adolescent**: 12 to 18 years.

Children are not 'mini adults'. Paediatric doses should be calculated from paediatric baseline data and not be just a modified adult dose.

Documentation

A number of factors contribute to effective record keeping. Patient and client records should (NMC *Guidelines for Records and Record Keeping*, 2005a – currently under review):

* be factual, consistent and accurate
* be written as soon as possible after an event has occurred
* be written clearly and in such a way that the documentation cannot be erased
* be written with all alterations or additions dated, timed and signed, ensuring that the original entry can still be read
* be accurately dated, timed and signed, with the signature printed alongside the initial entry

- not include abbreviations, jargon or irrelevant and/or offensive information
- be readable on any photocopies.

Local guidelines

A contract of employment will set terms that require employees to perform their duties with due care and skill by meeting legal and professional regulations.

Local guidelines will vary so it is essential that local policies and procedures are read and understood before administering medicines.

The best source of information locally is a pharmacist.

Administration of medicines

The NMC (2007) states that:

> The administration of medicines is an important aspect of the professional practice of persons whose names are on the Council's register. It is not solely a mechanistic task to be performed in strict compliance with the written prescription of a medical practitioner (now independent/supplementary prescriber). It requires thought and the exercise of professional judgement.

Registrants must only supply and administer medicinal products in accordance with one or more of the following processes:

- patient-specific direction (PSD)
- a patient medicines administration chart (which may be called a medicines administration record, MAR)
- patient group direction (PGD)
- Medicines Act exemption
- standing order
- homely remedy protocol
- prescription forms.

Prescription forms

NHS prescription forms are classified as secure stationery. Prescription forms are serially numbered and have anti-counterfeiting and anti-forgery features.

Any qualified and registered independent prescriber may prescribe all prescription-only medicines for all medical conditions. In addition nurse independent prescribers may prescribe some CDs.

Registered nurses are accountable for their actions and omissions. If your role includes administration of medicinal products, always check before administering the product that:

- the substance is not one that the patient is unable to tolerate or is allergic to
- you know the therapeutic uses of the medicine to be administered, its normal dosage, side-effects, precautions and contra-indications
- it is in accordance with the patient's plan of care
- the medicine to be administered has not passed its expiry date
- the patient's condition is acceptable in relation to the medicine being given (for instance, digoxin is not usually to be given if the pulse rate is below 60)
- the patient has given informed consent to administration of the medication and is aware of the purpose of the treatment
- the prescription is legible, unambiguous and indelible
- the prescription is written using the drug's generic or brand name, form, strength, dosage, timing, frequency of administration, start and finish dates, and route of administration
- the prescription is signed and dated by the authorised prescriber
- you have identified the patient for whom the medication is intended.

Remember; before you administer any medications always check that you have:

- the right person
- the right time
- the right route of administration
- the right drug
- the right dose
- checked the expiry date of the drug.

(C) Professional conversation

The five Rs

During a drug round student nurse Sandra asked her mentor why they needed to check the five Rs. Mary, her mentor, replied, 'It's a legal requirement for anyone who is administering medicines. But it's also to ensure that the person we're administering the medicine to comes to no harm, which is a professional requirement. This is just one of the safeguards that have been devised to help reduce the risks to patients. The National Patient Safety Agency is continuously reviewing and updating recommendations to assess risk and take appropriate actions to reduce it. Their recommendations include anything from making sure that different medicines aren't packaged in similar ways to reduce the risk of giving people the wrong drug, to making sure that NG administration tools/sets don't fit into intravenous ports. Then there's no risk of our administering NG drugs via the IV route.'

The process of drug administration

Routes of administration

The possible routes are:

- oral
- enteral (via a nasogastric or gastrostomy tube)
- sublingual (under the tongue)
- subcutaneous injection (injected into the subcutaneous layer of the skin)
- intramuscular injection (injected into a muscle)
- intravenous injection (parenteral – injected into a vein).

(C) Professional conversation

The process of administering medicines

'Why do I need to use the non-touch technique when administering oral medications when I've already washed my hands thoroughly?' student nurse Karim asked his mentor. John, his mentor, replied, 'It's important to prevent cross-infection by all means possible. It's also a precaution to ensure that the medicine doesn't harm you.' 'So what sorts of drugs might harm me?' Karim asked. 'Many different types of drugs can be irritant,' John replied, 'but a common example of harmful drugs we come into contact with is cytotoxic drugs.'

Administration procedures

In a hospital, you can check patients' identification bands before administering medication. In settings such as the community and care homes, you will need to be familiar with your patients and confirm their identity by asking relevant questions.

Hospitals are being encouraged to implement bar-coding or radio frequency identification on wristbands to try to prevent errors in patient identification (NPSA, 2005). However, some mistakes can occur in the actual process of producing and assigning a wristband, and computer systems may have the effect of weakening human vigilance (McDonald, 2006). Wherever possible, you are advised to try to obtain two forms of identification – such as asking the patient their name and date of birth, and checking the wristband – before administering any medicine (McDonald, 2006; NPSA, 2005).

Particular care must be taken to maintain accurate wristbands on patients who are unable to confirm their own identity (NPSA, 2005).

The NMC *Standards for Medicines Management* (2007) state that :

> Where there are difficulties in clarifying an individual's identity e.g. in some areas of learning disabilities, patients with dementia or confusional states, an up-to-date photograph should be attached to the prescription chart/s. For patients with burns where the wearing of a wristband is inappropriate and a photograph would not resemble the patient, local policies should be in place to ensure all staff are familiar with the patients and a system of identification is in place. Registrants are responsible for ensuring the photograph remains up-to-date.

S   Scenario continued

Mr Watson is prescribed a large number of drugs. Some of these are to be administered intravenously and some orally. Paracetamol is prescribed via an enteral tube to the stomach. Sedation (Propofol), analgesia (Alfentanyl), inotropes (Noradrenaline) and antibiotics (Cefradine and Rifampicin) are all administered via an IV line.

Drugs are given via a nasogastric tube when the patient is unable to take the drugs orally, and this is the preferred route of administration. The size of the lumen of the tube needs to be considered. In adults this is usually quite large, but in young children when fine-bore tubes are used, these may be unsuitable for drugs in thick liquid form. It is advisable to seek pharmaceutical advice before administering any solid form medicines via this route. The enteral tube should be flushed with water before and after administering any medicine. Sterile water should be used in neonates (BNF, 2006). Enteral feeds should be interrupted before and after medicine is given, especially if the feed reduces its absorption (for example, for at least an hour before and after administration of phenytoin). In the event of a blockage, flush, using a push-pulling action with at least 10 ml of warm water or soda water in a 50 ml syringe, and gently squeeze the tube along its length to relieve the blockage (NMPDU, 2003). Care must be taken not to give medicines that are absorbed in the stomach via a nasojejunal tube (Thomson, Naysmith and Lindsay, 2000).

Injections

Registrants must not prepare substances for injection in advance of their immediate use, or administer medication drawn into a syringe or container by another practitioner when not in their presence.

Intravenous medication

Two registrants should check the medication to be administered, one of whom should also be the registrant who then administers the IV medication. Throughout the duration of IV medication therapy, the registered nurse must monitor the patient and their response.

IV injections cannot be administered by unqualified people or student nurses. It is common practice for healthcare organisations to require registered nurses to undertake assessed competencies in the administration of IV medications before they are permitted to administer them independently.

Immediately make a clear and accurate record of all medicine administered, withheld or refused by the patient. Ensure that your signature is clear and legible.

Gloves should be worn when handling certain types of medicines that are irritant or that can be absorbed into the skin, such as cytotoxics, local anaesthetics and antibiotics.

Once a medicinal product has been prescribed and dispensed to an individual the drug is the individual's own property. To use it for someone else is theft.

Contact the prescriber or another authorised prescriber without delay if:

- contra-indications to the prescribed medicine are discovered
- the patient develops a reaction to the medicine
- assessment of the patient indicates that the medicine is no longer suitable.

Where medication is not given, the reason for not doing so must be recorded.

The IV route guarantees rapid delivery of medicine (Fitzsimons, 2001). However this route also carries the highest risk of adverse reactions such as anaphylaxis, the reaction known as 'speedshock' when the medicine is administered too rapidly, extravasation, infiltration, infection and phlebitis (Dougherty, 2002).

The process of administering medicines is:

1 Wash your hands.
2 Give the patient information on the medication and obtain their consent.
3 (In a hospital) check the patient details (name, date of birth and hospital number) on the hospital wrist identification band against the patient details on the drug chart. (In other settings, confirm identity using appropriate methods.)
4 Wash your hands between touching the patient/client and the drug trolley.
5 Check that you have the right medication, for the right route of administration and the right dose against the drug chart.
6 Use the non-touch technique when administering oral medications, pushing or pouring tablets/syrups out of the packaging and into a medicine pot without touching the medication itself.
7 Clean the skin before administering subcutaneous or intramuscular injections.
8 Subcutaneous injections are delivered at a 90 degree angle.

Administering controlled drugs

CDs should be administered in line with relevant legislation and local standard operating procedures. When administering controlled drugs a secondary signatory is required.

The signature of students must be countersigned by a registered nurse when a student has administered medicines (always under supervision).

Storage of medicines

All medicinal products must be stored in accordance with the patient information leaflet, summary of product characteristics document found in medication boxes and in accordance with any instruction on the label.

The area for storage and assembly of medicines should remain below 25 °C, as some drugs decompose above that temperature. Medicines for internal use should be stored in a locked trolley, cupboard or room. CDs must be stored in a locked cabinet, and a dedicated locked medicines refrigerator should be used in hospitals and nursing homes. The refrigerator temperature should be monitored daily.

The registered nurse in charge is responsible for the CD key and should know where it is at all times. Key-holding may be delegated to other suitably trained members of staff but the legal responsibility rests with the registrant in charge.

Medication errors and incident reporting

A medication error is defined as any preventable event that might cause or lead to inappropriate medication use or patient harm while the medication is in the control of a health professional, patient or consumer (NPSA, 2005; DH, 2004). In an ideal world there would be no such thing as errors. However this is completely unrealistic and unachievable. The best we can do is to investigate the causes of errors that are made, and to take actions based on the findings with the objective of minimising future errors.

Causes of medication errors

A number of factors contribute to medication errors:
- inadequate training or knowledge
- lack of drug knowledge and awareness among nurses
- difficulty of measurements or calculations required for administration
- lack of information about the patient
- memory lapse
- fault in identity check
- fault in dose check
- inadequate monitoring
- preparation errors
- shift work (there are high error rates on day shifts)
- lack of standardisation
- environmental factors (lighting, noise, frequent interruptions)
- staff workload and fatigue
- poor communication among healthcare providers
- inadequate documentation and record keeping
- medicine stocking and delivery problems
- increased number or quantity of medications per patient
- dosage form (for instance, injectable drugs are associated with more serious errors)
- lack of effective policies and procedures
- improper drug storage.
- inferior, inadequate or unsuitable equipment.

Types of medication error

Omissions

An omission error (OM) is noted if a patient fails to receive a dose of medication that was ordered by the time the next dose is due. If the patient refuses the medication, it is not usually counted as an omission. Doses withheld according to policy (such as 'nil by mouth') are not counted as errors or OMs.

Wrong time

Any drug given 30 minutes or more before or after it was ordered, up to the time the next dose of the same medication was ordered, counts as a wrong time error. 'As required medications' orders are not included.

Wrong dosage

This applies to any dose either above or below the correct dosage by more than 5 per cent, or any difference from the total number of times ordered by the doctor.

Unordered drug given

This covers the administration to a patient of any medication not ordered for that patient.

The chief medical officer set out a strategy to improve patient safety in the NHS in 'an organisation with a memory' (DH, 2000) in response to a recognition that the NHS was falling short of other industries in its ability to learn from its mistakes. Of particular concern was the recurrence of preventable medication errors.

'Building a safer NHS for patients' encourages reporting and learning through a national reporting scheme for patient safety incidents and near misses. The National Patient Safety Agency (NPSA) was set up to collect and analyse patient safety information submitted by NHS organisations, and aims to ensure that lessons learned are fed back into practice.

NPSA error codes cover:

- patient allergic to treatment
- contra-indication in relation to drug or conditions
- wrong/omitted/past expiry date
- wrong formulation
- wrong frequency
- wrong/transposed/omitted medicine label
- wrong/omitted patient information leaflet
- mismatching between patient and medicine
- omitted medicine/ingredient
- other
- wrong method of preparation/supply
- wrong quantity
- adverse drug reaction when used as intended
- wrong route
- wrong storage
- unknown
- wrong/omitted verbal patient directions
- wrong drug/medicine.

Prevention of medication errors

A number of ways of preventing medication errors are mentioned in this chapter. Nurses (or other persons administering medication) should be familiar with the way that medication is ordered. They should have an adequate knowledge about the specific drug prescribed. If additional information on medication administration is required, this should be obtained from pharmacists.

Transcriptions of orders should be avoided and should be recognised as opportunities for errors.

All discontinued or unused drugs should be returned to the pharmacy department immediately or at patient discharge.

Discharged patients must not be given unlabelled drug products to take home.

If a patient or a relative of a patient objects to or questions a particular drug, the nurse should listen, answer questions and, if appropriate, double-check the medication chart and the product before administering it to ensure that no error is made (for instance: wrong patient, wrong route, dose already administered).

Adverse drug reactions

An adverse drug reaction is any response to a drug that:

- is not an intended response
- is unpleasant or harmful to the person receiving the drug
- occurs at approved dosage levels.

In the event of a drug error, immediate action must be taken to prevent any potential harm to the patient, and the error should be reported as soon as possible to the prescriber, line manager or employer (according to local policies and guidelines). All actions must be documented. If a patient experiences an adverse drug reaction to a medication, immediate action must be taken to remedy the harm caused by the reaction. This must be recorded in the patient's notes and the prescriber must be notified.

Incident reporting

Incident reporting processes will vary according to the place of work. Any drug administration errors must be reported immediately via the local incident reporting system, normally to a relevant member of the team. The doctor should be made aware and the pharmacist may be contacted for advice. Further advice can be found on Toxbase at www.spib.axl.co.uk or from the National Poisons Information Service (NPIS).

Today reporting is often in an electronic format, and is accessed via the local NHS Intranet, but sometimes it involves filling in a paper form. The purpose of incident reporting is not just to ascertain blame, but to identify causes which might show how to prevent a similar incident from happening in the future.

Nurses are in an ideal position to detect and report medication errors because of their direct patient care activities and administration of medications to patients. They therefore play an important role in risk reduction.

The NMC stipulates the importance of creating environments where people can report drug errors without fear of reprimand.

S Scenario continued

Mr Watson has been prescribed paracetamol 1 g to be taken regularly every six hours. It is known that paracetamol can be given at a minimum of four-hour intervals. However a maximum dose of 4 g can be administered in a 24-hour period (a quantity that is the same for IV, oral and rectal routes), so Mr Watson is being prescribed the maximum daily dose. The prescription chart states that the paracetamol is to be given at 06.00, 12.00, 18.00 and 00.00 daily. The prescription has been completed fully, correctly and legibly.

On this particular day the unit is particularly busy. Nurse Anne administers paracetamol to Mr Watson as prescribed but is called away before she has documented that the paracetamol has been administered on the medication chart. She forgets to return and make the entry. The next shift takes over. Nurse Beatrice notices the apparent omission on the drug chart and administers the drug for what she thinks is the first time.

Later that shift Anne phones in to report that she failed to sign the drug chart. Beatrice now realises that Mr Watson has had twice the prescribed dose of IV paracetamol, and that Co-dydramol has also been administered since admission to the ICU.

a Learning activity

Find out what the symptoms would be if Mr Watson had suffered an overdose of paracetamol.

c Professional conversation

Beatrice reports the incident, and asks her senior nurse, Hugh, what are the implications. Hugh tries to assess the situation. 'I know you realise that when Anne didn't sign the drug chart, it meant she didn't meet the legal and professional requirements in relation to the administration of medications. But you didn't do all that you should have done either, Beatrice. When you noticed that nobody had signed off the dose, you should have made enquiries to see what had happened. The rule is that omissions must be reported and clearly documented. So you should have made sure that Anne was contacted to find out the reason for the chart not being signed. You should have held off giving a dose until you knew what had happened, and told the prescriber or the doctor. Of course, if you'd done that, Anne would have told you right away that she had in fact administered the dose, she just hadn't signed the chart. So if there was a complaint against you, there'd be reason to judge that both of you had been negligent, I'm afraid.'

The symptoms of paracetamol overdose

Nausea, vomiting, anorexia, pallor and abdominal pain may present within the first 24 hours. An overdose may cause complete and irreversible necrosis of the liver, which may lead to coma and death.

Pharmacological implications

In the event of an overdose, liver damage is likely to occur if the patient does not receive treatment.

The antidote to a paracetamol overdose is N-acetylcysteine (NAC). If this is given within 12 hours, the patient might make a complete recovery. It has also been shown to have benefits up to 48 hours after overdosing.

There is a risk of poisoning, particularly in elderly patients, in cases of liver disease, in cases of chronic alcoholism, in patients with chronic malnutrition and in patients receiving enzyme inducers. In these cases overdosing may be fatal.

Management of the situation

Emergency measures

With a suspected paracetamol overdose, a blood sample must be taken by a suitably qualified member of the healthcare team for plasma paracetamol assay, as soon as possible after the overdose.

The treatment includes administration of the antidote, N-acetylcysteine (NAC) by the IV or oral route.

Symptomatic treatment

Hepatic tests must be carried out at the beginning of treatment and repeated every 24 hours. In most cases hepatic transaminases return to normal in one to two weeks, with full return of normal liver function. In very severe cases, however, liver transplantation may be necessary.

The paracetamol overdose nomogram

This is a table used to identify whether treatment is required in cases of possible paracetamol overdose. In the scenario other factors were involved which could have affected the patient's response to the administration of paracetamol. The patient is a known alcoholic and therefore is likely to have reduced liver function or liver disease. Antibiotics such as Rifampicin can have an adverse effect on the liver. Add these factors to paracetamol overdose and the risk greatly increases.

Table 14.1 summarises the core issues with paracetamol.

Drug dosage calculations

Students of nursing are required to achieve calculation scores of 100 per cent before they can enter the professional register, as stated within

Table 14.1 Working with paracetamol

Paracetamol (adult)	
Type	Analgesic
Dose	1g
Frequency	Four hourly, four times a day
Used for	Mild to moderate pain Pyrexia
Contra-indications and cautions	Hepatic and renal impairment Other paracetamol products
Side-effects	Very rarely a rash
Advice to patients	Confirm that they cannot take with any other paracetamol product

Part

II

the NMC Essential Skills Clusters which are used alongside the NMC *Standards for Proficiency* (2006).

Drug dosage calculation requires the use of mathematical skills. Some drug administrations can require complex calculations to ensure that the correct volume or quantity of medication is administered. In these situations, it is good practice for a second practitioner (a registered professional) to check the calculation in order to minimise the risk of error. Independent checking must be performed independently, and if the results of the calculations are not the same, the process should be repeated, or if possible a third person should do an independent calculation.

Calculations normally use standard metric units:

- length in metres (m)
- weight (mass) in grams (g)
- volume in litres (l, L)
- temperature in degree Celsius (°C).

Sometimes you might have to convert a quantity from one unit to another. A common example is converting a quantity given in milligrams into grams. Milli means 1000th of the measurement, therefore:

- 1 metre = 1000 millimetres
- 1 gram = 1000 milligrams
- 1 milligram =1000 micrograms
- 1 litre = 1000 millilitres

> **ⓐ Learning activity**
>
> Carry out these simple calculations:
> 1 Convert 0.5 g to mg.
> 2 Convert 500 mcg to mg.
> 3 Convert 50 ml to litres.
> 4 Convert 250 mg to g.
> 5 Convert 0.125 g to mg.

A sample conversion

Let's go step by step through the process to convert 500 mg into grams.

Consider the 500 and the mg as two separate parts. The mg is to be changed to g, and as g are bigger than mg, the number that you end up with will be smaller. To make a number one thousand times smaller, think of the number as a decimal (such as 500.0), then move the decimal point three places to the left. This gives .5000, which would be rewritten as 0.5. So 500 mg can be rewritten as 0.5 g.

To convert the other way, use the same idea in reverse. If the units get smaller, the number gets bigger.

Calculating how to meet a prescription

Prescriptions are usually written giving the total dose a patient is to receive. The nurse must find out the amount of drug in each tablet and then calculate how many tablets to give the patient.

For example, patient is prescribed 20 mg of prednisolone but the tablets are available as 5 mg each. How many tablets are required?

You need to find out how many 5s are in 20, or in other words, 20 divided by 5.

The formula is:

$$\text{no. of tablets} = \frac{\text{what you want}}{\text{what you've got}}$$

The answer is 20 mg (what you want) divided by 5 mg (what you've got) which gives the answer 4, so the patient would be given four tablets.

Drugs in liquid form

When drugs are in liquid form, the prescription is usually given in terms of the concentration of the solution or suspension. For example, morphine sulphate is available as 10 mg/ml. This means that 10 milligrams of morphine sulphate are dissolved in every millilitre of liquid.

If the quantity of drug to be given is known, and the concentration of the drug in solution is known, you can calculate the volume of liquid required using the following formula:

$$\frac{\text{what you want}}{\text{what you have got}} \times \text{what is in it}$$

Dosages for children

There is a risk that errors in dosage calculation might not be detected by the practitioner drawing up the dose if suitable strengths of medications are not manufactured. For example tenfold errors can occur where an ampoule which contains more than ten times the required dose is used to draw up an injection for a neonate (Chappell and Newman, 2004).

Double-checking complex calculations and administration of high-risk drugs such as cytotoxics is thought to be effective for reducing medication errors in hospitals (Miller et al, 2006). In many hospitals the procedure is that two nurses check all drugs for children. However, it is unclear how effective and efficient this is compared with single-nurse administration (O'Shea, 1999). Checking the correct dosage for a particular child often requires multiplying a standardised dose by the child's weight in kilograms. Care needs to be taken if the child is overweight, and in order to calculate the correct dose for the child, the ideal weight for the child's height and age should be used (Cheymol, 2000). The dose may need to be reduced if the child has impaired renal or hepatic function.

Developmental differences in physiology between adults and children correlate more closely with surface area than body weight (Baber and Pritchard, 2003). Therefore when an accurate dose within narrow therapeutic limits is required, for example in cytotoxic chemotherapy, you are recommended to use surface area. Body surface area estimates can be made from nomograms published in the British National Formulatory for Children.

Conclusion

The use of drugs has moved from the hit and miss world of early history into the very precise and well-regulated science that now exists. However it is still very important to consider the key factors of pharmacodynamics and pharmacokinetics. It must be remembered that the liver is a key player in drug metabolism, and must be able to either break down the drug molecule or transform it into an active molecule from a precursor. The metabolites from the breakdown process in the liver must also be removed at an appropriate speed from the body, and this relies on the renal and cardiovascular system being functional. If the liver and or the kidneys are in any way impaired, there is a risk that the patient will move from therapeutic to toxic levels of a drug, even though a standard administration pathway has been used. It is important therefore that these factors are taken into consideration when a patient is assessed so that dose modification can be considered if necessary.

Children and the elderly will need modified dosages based on their capacity to metabolise and remove drugs. In particular children cannot be considered as 'mini adults' when it comes to dose calculation because many facets of their metabolism may still be developing and they will not deal with drugs in the same way as adults. For example the blood brain barrier is still immature, putting the central nervous system at risk.

Safe administration of medicine also depends on good well-organised practice. Drug administration should not be undertaken in a hurry, and each patient should be seen to take their medication before the adminstrator leaves them and completes the documentation. The legal guidelines controlling the use of drugs are there for the protection of both the patient and the administrator. Errors do occur, and there is a set pathway of good practice to follow if they do. It is important to know what these are for the area in which you work. They will give you a clear set of actions to follow.

The use of drugs has always been linked to healthcare practice. Understanding how they work is important, and knowing the desired outcome is vital. If you are to be able to detect changes in a patient's response this may indicate they are having an adverse reaction to a medication. Interventions can then be set in place to minimise the damage caused by such

Part

II

a reaction. Good practitioners know the drugs they are working with, and how they expect a patient to respond to them. If you move into a new clinical area, spend some time finding out about some of the drugs that are regularly used in the treatment of the patients in this field, and their possible side-effects. This will help you be prepared for an unforeseen emergency should it occur.

References

Baber, N. and Pritchard, D. (2003) 'Dose estimation for children', *British Journal of Clinical Pharmacology* **56**(5),489–93.

Bravery, K. (1999) 'Paediatric therapy in practice', pp. 401–45 in Dougherty, L. and Lamb, J. (eds), *Intravenous Therapy in Nursing Practice*, Edinburgh, Churchill Livingstone.

British National Formulary (BNF) (2006) *British National Formulary for Children*, London, BMJ, Royal Pharmaceutical Society of Great Britain, RCPCH,

Campbell, H. and Carrington, M. (1999) 'Peripheral IV cannula dressings: advantages and disadvantages', *British Journal of Nursing* **8**(21), 1420–7.

Chappell, K. and Newman, C. (2004) 'Potential tenfold drug overdoses on a neonatal unit', *Archives of Disease in Childhood Fetal and Neonatal Edition* **89**(6), F483–4.

Cheymol, G. (2000) 'Effects of obesity on pharmacokinetics: implications for drug therapy', *Clinical Pharmacokinetics* **39**(3), 215–31.

Department of Health (DH) (2000) *An Organisation with a Memory*, London, DH.

DH (2004) *Building a Safer NHS for Patients: Improving medication safety*, London, DH.

Dougherty, L. (2002) 'Delivery of intravenous therapy', *Nursing Standard* **16**(16),45–52, 54, 56.

Fitzsimons, R. (2001) 'Intravenous cannulation', *Paediatric Nursing* **13**(3), 21–3.

Grieve, J., Tordoff, J., Reith, D. et al (2005) 'Effect of the pediatric exclusivity provision on children's access to medicines', *British Journal of Clinical Pharmacology* **59**(6), 730–5.

McDonald, C. J. (2006) 'Computerisation can create safety hazards: a bar-coding near miss', *Annals of Internal Medicine* **144**(7), 510–16.

Miller, J., Cross, M., Gerrett, D. et al (2006) 'A prioritisation of the most effective interventions for reducing medication errors in UK hospitals as perceived by senior pharmacists', *European Journal of Hospital Pharmacy Science* **12**(2), 23–8.

National Patient Safety Agency (NPSA) (2003) *Seven Steps to Patient Safety: A guide for NHS staff*, London, NPSA.

NPSA (2005) 'Wristbands for hospital patients improves safety', Safer practice notice, 22 November [online] http://www.npsa.nhs.uk (accessed 27 April 2006).

Nunn, T. and Williams, J. (2005) 'Formulation of medicines for children', *British Journal of Clinical Pharmacology* **59**(6), 674–6.

Nursing and Midwifery Council (NMC) (2005a) *Guidelines for Records and Record Keeping*, London, NMC.

NMC (2005b) *Standards of Proficiency for Nurse and Midwife Prescribers*, London, NMC.

NMC (2007) *Standards for Medicines Management*, London, NMC.

Nursing and Midwifery Practice Development Unit (NMPDU) (2003) 'Nasogastric and gastrostomy tube feeding for children being cared for in the community: best practice statement', Edinburgh, NHS Quality Improvement Scotland.

O'Shea, E. (1999) 'Factors contributing to medication errors: a literature review', *Journal of Clinical Nursing* **8**(5), 496–504,

Rothwell, J. and Hegarty, A. (2007) 'Venous blood sampling', pp. 814–15 in Glasper, E. A., McEwing, G. and Richardson, J. (eds), *Oxford Handbook of Children's and Young People's Nursing*, Oxford, Oxford University Press.

Royal College of Nursing (RCN) (2003) *RCN IV Therapy Forum: Standards for infusion therapy*, Plymouth, Becton Dickinson.

Thomson, F. C., Naysmith, M. R. and Lindsay, A. (2000) 'Managing drug therapy in patients receiving enteral and parenteral nutrition', *Hospital Pharmacist* **7**(6), 155–64.

Legislation

Controlled Drugs (Supervision of Management and Use) Regulations 2006

EU Council Directive 65/65/EEC on the approximation of provisions laid down by law, regulation or administrative action relating to proprietary medicinal products.

Health Act 2006

Medicines Act 1968

Mental Capacity Act 2005

Misuse of Drugs Act (MDA) 1971

Misuse of Drugs Regulations 2001 (MDR)

Misuse of Drugs Regulations Northern Ireland (NI) 2002

Chapter

15

Pain management

Part

II

Eileen Mann

Links to other chapters in _Foundation Studies for Caring_

Links to other chapters in _Foundation Skills for Caring_

Don't forget to visit www.palgrave.com/glasper for additional online resources relating to this chapter.

Introduction

The aim of this chapter is to study the healthcare of patients experiencing pain. Pain is multidimensional, highly complex and individual to the sufferer. To add to pain's complexity it can be experienced in many ways. For example:

- It can be acute, such as the pain associated with infection, trauma or surgery.
- Pain can become chronic, perhaps associated with scarring or adhesions.
- *Neuropathic* pain may develop following nerve damage, which leads to abnormal processing in either peripheral or central nervous systems.
- Pain can be experienced as an acute exacerbation of a chronically painful condition, as may happen with a progressive nonmalignant degenerative disease such as arthritis.
- Pain may be termed *malignant* when it is associated with a life-limiting condition such as cancer.
- Pain can also be present in the absence of obvious pathology, when it is termed *idiopathic*.

Learning outcomes

This chapter will enable you to:

- describe the physiology of pain
- explain the multidimensional nature of pain, exploring the reasons that it is such an individual experience
- identify a selection of methods for assessing pain in a variety of clinical settings
- analyse what makes acute pain different from chronic pain, and why chronic pain may defy effective treatment

- discuss pharmacological and non-pharmacological strategies that can be used to manage pain effectively
- analyse some of the barriers to good pain management
- use appropriate referral channels for pain management outside a practitioner's individual sphere of practice
- use relevant literature and research to inform practice.

Concepts

- The patient
- Nonpharmacological strategies
- Chronic pain
- Information giving
- Acute pain

- Empowerment
- Anatomy and neurophysiology
- Evidence-based practice
- Pain assessment
- Psychosocial influences

- Multidisciplinary teams
- Clinical governance
- Pharmacological strategies
- Interdisciplinary collaboration

Pain is a multidimensional phenomenon. This chapter uses the Johnson family's experiences of pain, in the past and present, to explore many of the factors that can make effective pain control a challenging healthcare issue.

Studying a family's individual experiences of pain provides an opportunity to explore a wide range of scenarios. By understanding the context in which each scenario takes place, we shall be able to define the complexities, analyse the issues and outline the challenges posed.

As a healthcare professional you will encounter patients in pain on a daily basis. It is therefore vital that you feel confident about caring for patients suffering from a vast range of painful conditions. Unfortunately evidence suggests that patients routinely experience

a Learning activity

If you are unsure of the meaning of any words or phrases, refer to a good medical dictionary or a reputable source on the web, such as 'Pain terminology' (International Association for the Study of Pain, 1994).

inadequately controlled pain (Ersek and Poe, 2004; APS, 2003). Despite our rapidly expanding knowledge, poor or absent pain assessment, and inappropriate and ineffectively administered analgesia, continue to be documented in the literature (Pasero and McCaffery, 2004). Even in hospitals where acute pain services have had a positive impact, pain control remains less than optimal (Moss et al, 2005). Of particular concern is the fact that although the control of pain and nursing care are inextricably linked, nurses do not always fulfil the function of good pain managers and are not always familiar with methods of effective pain control (Plaisance, 2007).

Historically pain control has not been accorded a high priority, and the literature is critical of all types of healthcare professional, with their poor knowledge base being cited as a primary cause for concern (Ferrell, McCaffery and Rhiner, 1992; Carr, Brockbank and Barrett, 2003). However, our greatly expanded understanding, particularly of the mechanisms of acute pain, means that effective pain management should now be the norm for the vast majority of patients. As a result, it is acute pain that is explored in greatest depth in this chapter.

S   Scenario: Mary Johnson and her family

The Johnson family is currently having a particularly stressful time. Mary Johnson, who is 42 years old, is in hospital following major bowel surgery. She is anxiously awaiting the results of pathology tests after the removal of a tumour from her ascending colon. Her husband Mark, who is 47, has to take time off work to visit and support his wife, and to look after their three children, Martin (aged 13), Amy (10) and Phillip (5). Mark is also supporting his elderly parents, Clive and Phyllis, who are both in their late 70s and becoming increasingly immobile. Phyllis Johnson suffers from a range of disabling conditions, including rheumatoid arthritis and osteoporosis. Clive Johnson is now experiencing increasing problems associated with his diabetes, and has recently undergone surgery for cancer of the prostate.

Although Mary's postoperative pain is being reasonably well controlled via a thoracic epidural placed in her back, it is taking a large hourly volume of epidural solution to achieve this, and Mary is still not completely pain free at rest. She is tense and finds moving and getting comfortable difficult.

a   Learning activity

Think back to a time you were in pain. Did other factors, such as fear that the pain might signify something serious, or boredom, make a difference to how much pain you felt?

Mary is currently exposed to many stressful factors in her life that could make effective pain control harder to achieve:
- She is anxious about the pathology results as there is a chance that the tumour removed during surgery is malignant.
- Mary is also finding it difficult to relax. She is not sleeping particularly well and worries about how the family is coping without her.
- She is feeling constantly nauseous and finds this very distressing.

Until recently pain was viewed within the medical model: that is, the method was to diagnose the physical condition, prescribe a treatment, and expect it to cure the problem. We now know that pain is a biopsychosocial event, which means that its impact is not just dependent on a physical stimulus. Many other factors can influence how pain is perceived. Before we can explore how pain can be effectively controlled we need to know something of neuroanatomy, physiology and pain psychology as it is currently understood.

a   Learning activity

Share a recent experience of pain. Compare this with the experiences of others.

Part

II

Almost all humans have experienced pain, although there are a very small group of individuals who lack pain-conducting nerve fibres and therefore are unable to feel it (Melzack and Wall, 1996). The rest of us have a 'pain history'. Some people's experience of pain has been transient and short-lived, but others, less fortunate, have experienced a lifetime of unremitting and intractable pain. However, when we try to actually define what pain is, it puzzles and confounds a universally accepted definition. In 1986 the International Association for the Study of Pain (IASP), a group of international leaders in the field, came up with an all-encompassing definition:

> Pain is an unpleasant sensory and emotional experience associated with actual or potential tissue damage.

This definition implies that pain is a multifactorial phenomenon, different for each individual regardless of the cause, and fluctuating according to the time of day, what else is going on around them, and how they are actually feeling. McCaffery (1972) put it very simply, recognising that only those in pain can really know what it is like: 'Pain is whatever the person says it is and exists whenever he says it does.'

The meaning of pain, and why individual experiences of it differ so widely

Even if they are the same age, gender, weight and have experienced similar painful stimuli, individuals vary greatly in their degree of pain tolerance. Some experience intense suffering and distress while others appear almost indifferent. Many factors can influence how much pain we feel, and whether the pain causes suffering or is dismissed as being trivial. Among them are:

- the meaning of the pain: does the person know its cause?
- whether the pain might signify a serious or even life-threatening disease
- whether the person was expecting it and well prepared for it
- the amount of distraction: people feel worse if they are staring at four blank walls all day with little to entertain and distract them, and pain is often worse at night because of the lack of distracting sensory stimulation
- the person's cultural or family background, which might encourage them to openly display 'pain behaviour' such as crying and groaning loudly, or have instilled into them that it is important to maintain a 'stiff upper lip'
- spiritual faith: a strong belief that it is 'God's will' enables some people to endure hours of pain and discomfort with serenity.

Buddhism is a philosophy specifically designed to come to terms with human suffering, and fakirs or 'holy men' will walk on nails, hold a difficult posture for hours, or fast for weeks. These men practise what William James discovered in the early part of the last century: 'that human beings, by changing the inner attitudes of their minds, can change the outer aspects of their lives' (cited in Brand and Yancey, 1993). These and many more factors can contribute to the pain we feel and how we may try to control it using various strategies and coping mechanisms (see also Chapter 3 on child and family health).

⟲ⓐ Learning activity

Try to identify some other factors that might influence the way individuals experience pain. How much of this do you feel is culturally determined?

If you wish to read more on this subject of 'what is pain?', refer to Chapters 1 and 2 in Mann and Carr (2006).

For acute pain, Park, Fulton and Senthuran (2000) provide some easy to understand text. For a slightly more challenging text see Carr and Goudas (1999). For an excellent web resource on many aspects of pain and pain control see Bandolier (2003).

The peripheral nervous system

In order to help Mary manage her pain it is necessary to have an appreciation of the biology of pain. If you are unfamiliar with the anatomy and physiology of the nervous system, it may be useful to access a basic introductory text before working through this chapter.

The peripheral nervous system is made up of nerve endings which have receptors embedded into them. These nerve endings are abundant at the periphery (skin surfaces) and join up like the roots of a tree to form larger branches. The branches then enter the central nervous system (spinal cord and brain) as either spinal nerves entering the spinal cord or cranial nerves that enter directly into the brain. The nerves relay information to the brain, where pain perception takes place and our physical and emotional response is initiated.

The nerve endings associated with transmitting pain are termed *nociceptors*, and can be found extensively on skin, periosteum and joint surfaces, and within arterial walls, subcutaneous tissues, muscle fascia and viscera. There are two types of nerve fibres that specifically transmit painful stimuli. *A* delta fibres transmit fast signals and act as a protective mechanism. The slower *c* fibres respond to the inflammatory chemicals associated with actual tissue injury.

> **(a) Learning activity**
>
> Think about a personal experience of pain. For example, have you ever been burned? What was it like? What did you do to try to lessen the pain?

If you put your hand on a hot plate, you whip it away quickly. The pain is sharp, easy to locate and you respond immediately. This pain comes from *a* delta fibres protecting you by provoking rapid evasive action before further damage occurs. Once there is tissue damage, though, a dull, diffused, throbbing ache develops which is associated with redness, swelling and inflammation of the tissue. The slower *c* fibres have been activated, and send continuous signals which are hard to ignore and almost demand you rest your hand to allow for healing to take place. To lessen the pain, we know that putting your hand under cold running water helps. By doing this, not only are you cooling the area, reducing the blood flow and swelling, you are also stimulating *a* beta fibres (responsible for touch sensations) and this helps to modulate or override the pain that is felt. This mechanism is described on page 264.

The response of damaged tissues

Traumatised tissues release breakdown products, which initiate chemical cascades. Prostaglandin *e* is a potent pain-producing byproduct of one of these cascades. Trauma also affects blood vessels, causing spasm, oedema and the liberation of platelets which break down into a pain-producing neuro-peptide called *substance P*. Many other inflammatory chemicals are also liberated, and these set up a chain reaction of inflammation, swelling, redness and increased sensitivity.

The production of kinins, among the most potent inflammatory chemicals, continues to irritate the nerve endings, amplifying pain. Pain-stimulated nerve endings send messages to the brain of any noxious or potentially tissue-damaging event, such as burning, freezing, crushing, bruising, or the cutting of skin, muscle, fascia and so on.

As well as the *a* delta fibres that transmit pain sensations, there are nerve fibres located on the skin that transmit nonpain sensations. *A* beta fibres transmit feelings of gentle heat, cool, touch and vibration. Stimulation of these nerve fibres can promote well-being, such as the sensation we experience on a warm summer's day with the sun on our bodies, a covered hot-water bottle soothing an aching stomach, the relief of a cool poultice applied to an inflamed area, or even the pleasurable sensation of a massage on aching muscles. Their significance to pain perception was first fully described in gate control theory, which was first outlined in the mid-1960s.

Gate control theory

This groundbreaking theory was the result of the collaborative work of the British professor of neuroscience Patrick Wall and the Canadian professor of psychology Ronald Melzack (Melzack and Wall, 1965). The early 1960s saw a period of intense progress within other fields of medicine, particularly surgery, with the early human organ transplants, but at that time researchers had not really started to unravel the puzzles of pain.

The basis of gate control theory is the interaction of the three different nerve fibres mentioned so far. The pain-transmitting *a* delta and *c* fibres (the nociceptors) and sensations transmitted by *a* beta fibres synapse in a specific area of the spinal cord's grey matter called the *substantia gelatinosa*. Gate control theory proposed that it was in this area that a principal pain-modulating or regulating mechanism took place, acting as a gate. The gate could be either opened by the stimulation of nociceptors, enabling pain signals to reach the brain, or closed by the modulating features of competing nonpainful sensations.

There appears to be a finite capacity for transmitting any sensation along the central nervous system, therefore it was proposed that the sensation of pain can be overwhelmed by bombarding the substantia gelatinosa with nonpainful stimulation. This is achieved because the stimulation transmitted by the *a* beta fibres reaches the brain faster and via fewer synapses, so it takes precedence over painful sensations.

Figure 15.1 shows painful and nonpainful stimulation nerve fibres synapsing within the same areas of the spinal cord. The pain fibres cross over in the cord and have multiple synapses within the central nervous system before reaching the areas of the brain where conscious perception takes place. The nonpain sensation fibres, however, do not cross over, but fast track to the brain's sensory cortex. This helps to explain why practical physical pain-relieving remedies such as rubbing your shin when you have walked into a coffee table can actually be effective. For further information you may wish to view the information on 'the multidimensional nature of pain' on this book's website.

W

Learning activity

For more in-depth text on acute pain neurophysiology, refer to the discussion of acute and postoperative pain in Melzack and Wall (1996).

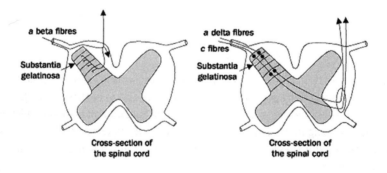

Figure 15.1 Nerve fibres synapsing within the spinal cord

Source: Mann and Carr (2000).

Learning activity

Using the information you have about Mary, consider how psychosocial factors might impact on her perception of pain.

As well as helping to explain why stimulating the skin with a nonpainful and preferably pleasant sensation can help to reduce pain, gate control theory sheds more light on how it is possible for the brain to further regulate how much pain we perceive at any one time. The ability to 'gate' pain sensations found in the substantia gelatinosa seems also to be a feature of other areas of the central nervous system, where similar theoretical gates can also be opened or closed. Apart from sensation at the periphery, chemicals produced within the brain and spinal cord can also activate these additional gates, causing pain perception to be enhanced (as can happen when anxiety accompanies pain) or modulated (for example by the release of endorphins which act like the body's own morphine). This helps to explain pain as a complex biopsychosocial phenomenon which depends on multiple factors, and not just on the intensity of the painful stimuli.

> **a) Learning activity**
>
> From the discussion on the nature of pain and gate control theory, can you suggest any other reasons that Mary's pain is proving difficult to relieve?

Other issues that can usefully be considered are:

- Pain may be resistant to opioids, particularly weak ones, because analgesia containing an opioid has been taken regularly for a long time and tolerance to standard dosing schedules has developed.
- Stress, anger, frustration, fear and anxiety have all been implicated in increasing pain perception.
- What are the strengths and potencies of the pharmacological strategies offered so far?
- Have nonpharmacological therapies been offered and were they effective?
- Is the pain assessment tool adequate and being used in a timely fashion to capture Mary's pain experience and the impact this is having on her potential recovery?

Exploring Mary's recent experience of surgery enables us to track the physiological response of acute pain, as well as explain the impact of some psychosocial influences. Not only did Mary experience extensive tissue damage when her skin and muscle were cut by the surgeon's scalpel, the intermittent visceral pain she experienced prior to her surgery may have resulted in a degree of pain 'wind-up', increasing her sensitivity. *Wind-up* is a term used to describe an increase in the excitability of spinal cord neurones. This excitability means that reduced stimulation can lead to increasing pain when the actual cause of the pain may be resolving normally (Herrero, Laird and Lopez-Garcia, 2000).

> **a) Learning activity**
>
> Talk to a healthcare practitioner who has experienced difficulty helping an individual with their pain control despite the use of strong analgesia. What reasons did they give for this?

> **S) Scenario continued**
>
> Although the bowel does not transmit painful sensations if it is cut or burned, the sensations when it is stretched can be very intense. Prior to her surgery Mary was experiencing intense visceral pain because of a tumour that caused an intermittent blockage of her large bowel. Once the blockage was removed she experienced pain from a range of sources.
>
> One is visceral pain caused by colic as a result of gas build-up in the intestine. Although Mary has a continuous epidural, only a dense nerve block or rendering her semi-comatose would completely remove this intermittent pain. Often referred to as 'wind pain', it is a common complaint following bowel surgery, and can be experienced until function is restored.
>
> Mary is tense and anxious, resulting in the release of stress hormones which contribute to further muscle tension, discomfort and fatigue.
>
> She is also experiencing postoperative pain from the extensive wound site in her abdomen.
>
> A care plan devised with Mary prior to surgery would have highlighted her distress and provided a warning that postoperative pain control might prove challenging. Staff often fail to do this, then have to use large volumes of strong opioids to treat acute pain when a pre-emptive plan might have been more effective. Remember that being in hospital isolates people from their own coping mechanisms and prevents them from using the simple strategies they would use at home.

Nonpharmacological strategies

There is currently a considerable and growing interest in nonpharmacological strategies for pain management. Although for moderate to severe acute pain, nonpharmacological therapies are unlikely to be effective on their own, they can be useful as part of a multimodal approach. Some healthcare professionals can withdraw when a patient's pain is proving to be a challenge, but healthcare professionals with a bedside role and those involved in rehabilitation or function restoration have no such option. Being able to offer comfort strategies can reinforce trust, which is a vital part of developing a therapeutic relationship. Even if these strategies are effective, prescribed medications must be reviewed regularly and any changes deemed necessary acted upon immediately. Effective multimodal analgesia is vital, and there is no substitute after major surgery. Patient advocacy may mean that a healthcare professional needs to question an inadequate prescription. Improving your knowledge will ensure a confident approach in these circumstances.

ⓒ Professional conversation

Marion, a staff nurse caring periodically for Mary, discusses giving information: 'As the staff nurse caring for Mary postoperatively, I was able to reassure Mary that the periodic colicky pain that she was experiencing was a positive sign that gut function was beginning to return to normal. For this "wind pain", early ambulation, peppermint water (Tate, 1997; Pittler and Ernst, 1998) and reassurance that the pain will only be transient are often all that is needed. For Mary, prior knowledge helped reduce some of her fear of any new pain, although she remains very vigilant for any signs of altered sensation.'

Other useful nonpharmacological strategies include:
- simple massage
- ensuring a comfortable position
- listening to music
- watching television
- the distraction of visitors
- knowing prompt attention will follow activation of a call button.

It is helpful to consider the reasons that pain might be relieved by nonpharmacological strategies. Figure 15.2 shows the circular pathways between the sensory cortex, or thinking part of the brain, the midbrain, thalamus and the area of spinal nerve input in the spinal cord.

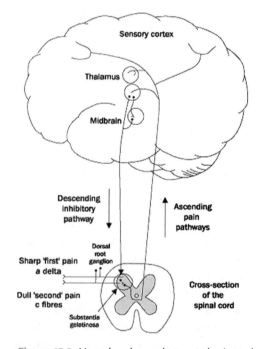

Figure 15.2 Neural pathways between brain and spinal cord showing ascending pain transmission pathways and descending modulation

Source: Mann and Carr (2000).

ⓐ Learning activity

Look at an introductory text on care models and frameworks, and find out how pain management strategies such as information giving can be incorporated into Mary's care plan.

How can distracting attention from the focus of the pain influence the way that it is perceived?

Knowledge of multimodal strategies can provide nurses with a repertoire to enhance analgesia. Useful texts especially on the management of pain after surgery are Gunnar and Helseth (2006), Manias (2003) and Carr and Thomas (1997).

c Professional conversation

Alan, Mary's named nurse, says of pre-operative assessment: 'As Mary's named nurse I tried to ensure that Mary felt as comfortable and relaxed as possible. I believe it is important to find sufficient time to answer queries and address any concerns either as part of routine assessment or separately as the opportunity arises. Listening to patients builds trust and confidence and enables a good rapport to develop. Having pain ignored or disbelieved can render even quite forceful personalities vulnerable and anxious. Mary was certainly eager to have her questions answered, which we tried to do confidently and sensitively. She wanted to know all about her surgery and what was going to happen. Shade (1992) argues that being familiar with the ward routines and what to expect can improve the outcome for patients. Mary was introduced to other patients, and this helped her to feel more relaxed in her strange surroundings. The anaesthetist saw her pre-operatively and explained how epidural analgesia would help to control the pain she would experience. He assured her that with this technique, postoperative pain could usually be well controlled without the ghastly sickness and head spinning that she had experienced in the past.'

S Scenario continued

Mary's pre-operative care was documented in her care plan so that everyone was aware what had been explained, how she was coping, and how well she was orientated to her new surroundings. Mary read, watched television and listened to her iPod before opting for some night sedation which ensured a good night's sleep. An early morning cup of tea, several hours before her surgery, came as a pleasant surprise, but despite all this input it was evident that Mary remained quite anxious.

e Evidence-based practice: nausea and vomiting W

Not all patients need to go without clear fluids for many hours prior to surgery. Studies have showed that for most patients, consuming clear fluids up to two hours before surgery is not only safe, but has also been shown to reduce postoperative nausea (Shevde and Triveldi, 1991; Chapman, 1996).

For further information on postoperative nausea and vomiting please visit the companion website.

S Scenario continued

Postoperative care

Although Mary had previously experienced periods of partial bowel obstruction, on admission to hospital her gut function was relatively normal. Prior to her surgery she received two drugs as pre-medication, a drug to reduce the risk of sickness following surgery (an anti-emetic), and a sedating drug to make her feel sleepy and relaxed. Other patients in the beds around her told her not to worry and were very reassuring. The woman in the bed opposite had experienced an epidural, and told Mary how delighted she had been when on the day of her surgery she had been able to sit out of bed and take a few steps without any significant discomfort.

Epidural analgesia

During Mary's operation, tissue was inevitably cut and damaged, resulting in the chemical inflammatory soup that causes the pain fibres (nociceptors) to transmit pain. However, a general anaesthetic kept Mary asleep so she was not aware of this process.

The epidural catheter sited prior to surgery was used to instil bolus doses of two different drugs into the tissue around Mary's spinal cord where the pain messages would normally enter. One of these drugs was a local anaesthetic, and the other was a powerful opioid analgesic. As a result of these drugs, Mary was able to regain consciousness in the recovery room, initially with no pain at all, and only mild pain when she tried to roll on to her side.

Pain control during Mary's operation

During the operation, the anaesthetist closely monitored Mary's physiological response to pain, carefully recording her heart beat and blood pressure. The epidural space was injected before surgery commenced with a bolus dose of the opioid diamorphine, and local anaesthetic, bupivicaine. Periodically, Mary's epidural was topped up with further doses of bupivicaine. Once the operation was over, a 500 ml bag of normal saline solution containing dilute concentrations of local anaesthetic and the opioid fentanyl was commenced at a rate of 5 ml per hour in the recovery room.

Figure 15.3 shows a cross-section through the spine to illustrate the location of the epidural space and the site of the needle through which a catheter can be threaded to achieve continuous postoperative pain relief.

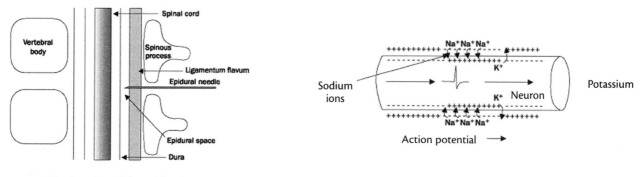

Figure 15.3 The location of the epidural space

Source: Mann and Carr (2000).

Figure 15.4 Local anaesthetic acts on the cell membrane blocking the transfer of sodium ions and potassium which stops the action potential

Source: Mann and Carr (2000).

Figure 15.4 shows how local anaesthetic infiltrated around spinal nerves is able to control pain by blocking the exchange of ions across the nerve membrane, halting the action potential transmitting the signal along the nerve. You may find it helpful to refer to a general anatomy and physiology textbook for a more detailed explanation of these physiological and biochemical processes. For further information on epidurals please visit the companion website.

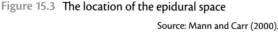

How opioids work

The opioids (such as diamorphine, morphine and fentanyl) prescribed for Mary were able to halt painful transmissions by binding tightly to opioid receptors located on nerve membranes in the central nervous system. Opioids are the principal drugs for potent intra-operative and postoperative pain relief. They have the advantage that they can be chemically reversed with the antagonist drug naloxone should a patient show signs of overdose.

Learning activity

Before you look at Figure 15.3, consider again the terms agonist and antagonist as introduced in Chapter 14.

An *agonist* is a molecule that binds to a specific receptor and triggers a response in the cell. It mimics the action of an endogenous molecule such as a neurotransmitter.

An *antagonist* is a ligand that inhibits the function of an agonist by binding to a specific receptor and thereby 'blocking' the receptor from the agonist.

In your own clinical area, make a list of other pharmacological agents that are regularly used to control pain.

Bandolier (2003) provides some excellent evidence on analgesia.

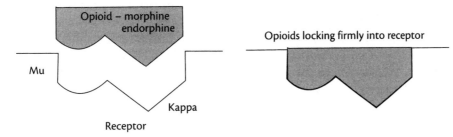

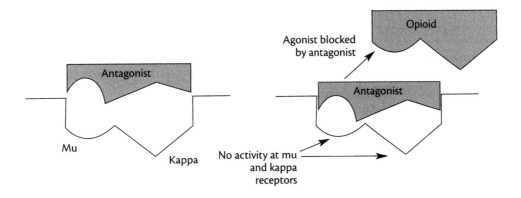

How opioids such as morphine lock onto receptors located on nerve membranes

How the opioid antagonist naloxone can block the action of opioids

Figure 15.5 Opioids locking onto receptors on nerve endings

Source: Mann and Carr (2000).

S Scenario continued

Mary's experience in the immediate postoperative period

In the recovery room Mary awoke virtually pain free. The recovery staff showed her the assessment chart they would be using to monitor her pain and how this would be continued by the ward staff. The family came to see her on the ward later that first evening. Despite Mark's concerns about Mary's diagnosis, the stress of coping with the children, and the demands of his elderly parents, his good humour and the chattering of the children were able to act as a short-term distraction. In truth Mary felt exhausted and was quite pleased when they left. She found the position in which she was most comfortable, and she was able to distract herself a little by watching the television.

Feelings of well-being, the use of distraction, and the use of humour can increase the body's ability to close the pain gates and keep them closed. However, by day two, with Mary waiting to hear the results of her pathology, pain had become more of a problem. The surgeon explained that his initial examination of the tumour suggested it was malignant. However, he was confident that it had been completely removed and Mary's prognosis was good.

Developing a rapport with patients is important if specific needs are to be anticipated and met effectively. Because of the impact that fear and anxiety might have on Mary's experience of pain and her overall recovery, time must be set aside to address these issues.

C Professional conversation

Alan, Mary's named nurse, comments on pain, fear and anxiety: 'I have come to know Mary quite well and although she outwardly appears stoical and in control, I also know that during the past few days she has been consumed with anxiety that the tumour in her bowel may prove malignant and that she could soon die from cancer. Mary wants to see her children grow up and is frightened that they will not manage without her. In her notes I have written that during the ward round, Mary's surgeon explained to her that there was no evidence that the tumour had spread. I have taken some time to explain to Mary that certain bowel tumours treated early enough can usually result in a complete cure. Mary wants to be fully informed with her husband present when discussing various options for treatment, and I have documented this in her notes. I found time to just sit with Mary tonight. She wanted nothing more than to hold someone's hand.'

The amount and type of pain experienced by Mary needed to be assessed throughout the postoperative period in order to ensure her pain control was effective. Mary had been shown the pain assessment chart when she was first admitted as part of her pre-operative preparation. The same chart had been used in the recovery area to give a continuous guide on what drugs and doses were effective or causing unacceptable side-effects.

> **a Learning activity**
>
> Which types of pain assessment tools are available in your own clinical area?

e Evidence-based practice: the assessment of pain

In order for healthcare staff to manage pain effectively, they must have a means of assessing pain and the effects of any treatment that is offered. The best way of assessing acute pain is to use a simple, but validated, pain assessment tool which ideally relies on a patient's verbal response. In Mary's case, staff need to regularly assess the location, intensity and impact on well-being of any pain experienced. The quality or description of pain also helps to signify whether it is resulting from an ineffective epidural or is perhaps the odd spasm caused by trapped wind. A simple verbal or numerical rating system is ideal for assessing the intensity of any pain. In an acute situation it is quick and easy to perform.

For further information on pain assessment refer to Schofield (1995) and Briggs (1995). There is more comprehensive information in 'Pain assessment' in the Clinical Skills section. Although it focuses on more chronic pain assessment, Okifuji et al (2001) might prove useful.

Examples of some of the more commonly used pain assessment tools are:

Visual analogue score

No pain ——————————————————— worst pain

Simple verbal rating

No pain   Mild pain   Moderate pain   Severe pain

Numerical rating
1   2   3   4   5   6   7   8   9   10

Faces chart

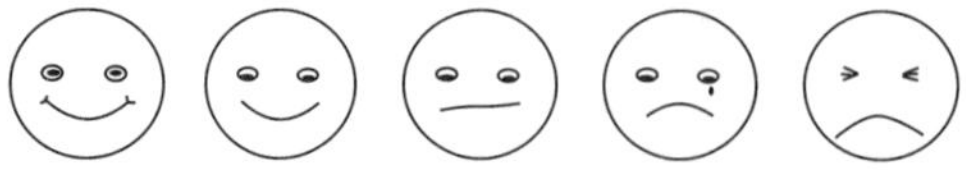

A 'faces chart' may be easier for small children and people with learning disabilities to understand.

> **a Learning activity**
>
> Which of the tools in Figure 15.6 would you select to assess Mary's pain, and why?

Figure 15.6 Pain assessment tools   Source: Mann and Carr (2000).

The use of a simple pain assessment tool combined with questions about Mary's general well-being is all that is needed. An open question asking how she is feeling and then getting her to score her pain intensity is more effective than just asking 'Have you any pain?' A numerical check on a 1 to 10 scale (1 = no pain and 10 = the worst pain ever) will indicate the severity of any discomfort present. If this scoring system is used again after Mary has been asked to move and cough effectively, it will give an indication of whether the epidural is doing its job adequately, or needs adjustment or supplementing with additional analgesia. Remember that some patients may not be able to conceptualise their pain using numbers, so a verbal rating may be more appropriate. This should be ascertained during admission.

Simple verbal numerical rating

Mary's perceived level of pain on movement at 22.00 hrs on the second postoperative day was:

1   2   3   4   5   (6)   7   8   9   10

The vocabulary of pain is also important, and can give a powerful indicator of the cause. Wind trapped in the gut generates a sharp spasm-type pain. Tissue trauma pain tends to be dull and diffused. Nerve damage pain is quite different, and is usually described as a burning, shooting or lancinating pain which has an unfamiliar quality to the patient. These descriptors can act as a powerful diagnostic tool for experienced clinicians.

With more sophisticated methods of pain control, such as epidural analgesia, other assessments have to be made:

- Is the amount of opioid causing sedation?
- Does the patient feel excessively itchy?
- Is the patient nauseous?
- Is the local anaesthetic in the infusion exacerbating any post-operative hypotension?
- Does the patient have normal sensation?
- Is the patient suffering from motor loss?
- Is urine output satisfactory?

> **ⓐ Learning activity**
>
> Why is it that all these factors, not only pain, have to be assessed on a regular basis and any problems encountered acted upon immediately?

Poor analgesia, hazardous or unpleasant side-effects indicate that an immediate review of the current strategy is required. As Mary is reporting her pain severity as 6/10 it should be established whether her epidural is still in the right place, with the infusion rate high enough to provide adequate analgesia without resulting in unwanted side-effects. Could analgesia be improved by giving Mary another drug, such as regular paracetamol or a nonsteroidal anti-inflammatory drug? If other remedies prescribed to control potential side-effects such as nausea, itching or constipation are becoming ineffective, these medications will also need adjustment.

Pain assessment does not just consist of 'Have you any pain?' It needs to ascertain far more than that, and each clinical area will need to devise its own assessment tool, appropriate for the analgesia regimes that are currently used.

> **ⓐ Learning activity**
>
> For further information regarding the management and monitoring of patients with an epidural, refer to a book on the subject, such as Middleton (2006).

Postoperative analgesia

It is often beneficial to combine several pain-relieving drugs that have different modes of action. We have already discussed how Mary's epidural infusion combined a local anaesthetic with an opioid drug. If the epidural fails to provide optimum analgesia, administering additional drugs, such as paracetamol and or one of the non-steroidal anti-inflammatory drugs (NSAIDs) may result in improved analgesia. A protocol should however be in place when NSAIDs are given with an epidural, as there may be a slight increased risk of bleeding when the catheter is removed.

Part II

Should Mary be particularly worried about the removal of drains or of having short procedures carried out that cause pain, entonox may be useful as a way of administering very short-acting pain relief. Entonox is unfortunately often overlooked as a short-term treatment for acute incident pain, although it is extremely safe, and can be used with other drugs as part of a multimodal strategy for brief additional analgesia. It is particularly useful when a patient is waiting for an oral painkiller to work, or is having a painful and unpleasant procedure performed that only takes a few minutes.

Entonox is a 50 per cent mixture of oxygen and nitrous oxide, which has a very rapid onset of action and is excreted almost as rapidly. It comes in a portable cylinder and has been used for many years to help control labour pain in childbirth, by ambulance crews and in Accident and Emergency departments. Entonox is contraindicated for very few people although some may feel a little drowsy, dizzy or sick. (See also page 350 for the use of entonox in childbirth.)

> **(a) Learning activity** **W**
>
> For further information on entonox, see Lawler (1995: 19–21) or Pediani (2003), or visit the companion website.

Analgesic drugs

These are some commonly used analgesic preparations. You can find out their mode of action, normal dose, contra-indications and side-effects by reference to a pharmacology textbook.

There are several ways of classifying analgesics, but usually they are grouped into strong opioids, weak opioids, nonopioids, nonsteroidal anti-inflammatories, local anaesthetics, inhalational analgesia and adjuvants.

Strong opioids include:
- morphine
- diamorphine
- methadone
- oxycodone
- fentanyl
- pethidine (contemporary evidence is questioning the use of this drug).

Weak opioids are:
- codeine and dihydrocodeine (not effective analgesics when given on their own)
- tramadol.

The most common nonopioid analgesic is:
- paracetamol.

Nonsteroidal anti-inflammatory drugs (NSAIDs) include:
- aspirin
- ibuprofen
- diclofenac
- the newer Cox-2 NSAIDs produced to reduce the risk of the gastrointestinal toxicity which can be experienced with traditional NSAIDs.

Local anaesthetics include:
- lignocaine
- bupivicaine.

The main inhalational analgesic is:
- nitrous oxide (when combined with oxygen this produces entonox).

Adjuvants

Occasionally pain can prove difficult to control with analgesic drugs alone. A more in-depth pain assessment can help elicit the reason, and suggest a different drug that is not an analgesic in itself but which could be helpful. These drugs are termed *adjuvant* therapies, and are most often used in chronic pain, or to treat the pain experienced with terminal disease. Examples are:

- buscopan for gut spasm
- an anxiolytic agent such as midazolam or diazepam when anxiety is a major feature
- tricyclic antidepressants and/or anticonvulsants when nerve injury is the primary cause
- an NMDA receptor antogonist such as ketamine for patients who have a very high tolerance of strong opioids.

Evidence is emerging that reinforces the benefits of a multimodal approach to analgesia. The following is an example of an innovative approach using pre-emptive multimodal analgesia for anterior cruciate ligament day case surgery (taken from data presented at the American Society of Regional Anaesthesia and Pain Medicine Annual Spring Meeting 2002 by Reuben et al).

The researchers recruited 1200 patients for the study, to receive either a multimodal pre-emptive analgesia protocol or a standard postoperative protocol. The standard approach included paracetamol, ibuprofen and short-acting opioids before and after surgery prn, which you might quite rightly conclude is already multimodal. However the multimodal approach for the study included paracetamol 1 g 6 hrly and rofecoxib (a Cox 2 NSAID now withdrawn) 50 mg daily for 2 days pre op. Patients were then given a femoral nerve block and intra-articular block of morphine, local anaesthetic and clonidine (not licensed) immediately pre-operatively and paracetamol, rofecoxib, ice and oxycontin (a long-acting opioid) on a regular basic not prn postoperatively. They were also prescribed short-acting opioids prn for breakthrough pain. You might consider this to be unnecessarily multimodal but the results (shown in Table 15.1) make for interesting reading.

Table 15.1 Standard treatment and multimodal treatment

Measured	Standard treatment % of patients	Multimodal treatment % of patients
Same day discharge	58	96
Rehab at six months	68	91
Knee pain at one year	14	4
Developed chronic pain	4	1

Learning activity

For further information on pharmacological strategies, refer to Hawthorn and Redmond (1998: 203). For useful information on acute pain and a compilation of results on the efficacy of various analgesic therapy, visit Bandolier (2003) and the *Oxford League Table of Analgesics in Acute Pain* (Bandolier, 2007). For a general guide on acute pain management see Macintyre and Schug (2007) or Park, Fulton and Senthuran (2000).

Reflect on the way in which Mary's pain has been managed in the scenario and compare it with your own experiences. What lessons can be learned?

Family experiences of pain

How a family responds when a member is in pain helps to shape how children grow up to view pain, either as something to be dreaded and feared, or as a normal part of life, for the most part endurable and not overwhelming. Our upbringing and culture help to formulate this response. We all know of some children who become frightened and distressed by what appears to be trivial pain, but conversely many stoical little souls barely squirm during quite unpleasant and painful procedures.

It is only fairly recently that scientists have confirmed that even premature neonates have the anatomy and function in place to perceive pain, something that for many years was dismissed. As recently as the 1970s surgery was performed on neonates with no or minimal analgesia. Although poor analgesia in infancy or childhood may have a bearing on the intensity of pain perceived later, other factors can be powerful causes of distress, and distress and pain are closely linked. If children pick up the signals from their parents that pain is always to be feared and avoided at all costs, they may not readily develop effective coping strategies when pain inevitably confronts them. This is all part of our central processing of pain. Once the painful stimulation has reached our brains, our brains dictate just how much we will be troubled and distressed as a result.

S Scenario continued

The Johnson family's experiences of pain

Martin's worst memory of pain is of when he was 8 and broke a leg falling out of a tree. The pain was initially severe, but once the leg was splinted and immobile the pain reduced substantially. While in hospital Martin received good multimodal analgesia. He was given a small dose of oral immediate-release morphine syrup with a dose of paracetamol. In order that Martin's leg could be examined he was encouraged to self-administer entonox. When he went home, his mother was given two days supply of paracetamol to be given regularly with the NSAID ibuprofen should paracetamol alone prove insufficient or for any breakthrough pain that might occur. For Martin, this first experience of severe pain was not an unduly negative one; his pain was recognised, believed and acted upon promptly. This has ensured Martin does not view hospitals with fear and anxiety, and he has confidence in the ability of healthcare professionals to manage pain competently and effectively.

Amy's worst experience was following an accident when her fingers were trapped in a car door. The pain was excruciating, sickening and frightening. She had the fragments of one of her fingernails removed in hospital without adequate analgesia, and was then sent home without further advice to her mother regarding pain control. As a result the occasional paracetamol given by her mother was insufficient to control the dull throbbing pain which seemed to be with her for days. For Amy, hospitals are uncaring, frightening places, and she dreads going there again.

Phillip's only real memory of pain is of the occasional earache he has experienced following a cold. It has never been really severe but nonetheless he remembers pain as being 'horrible'. For Phillip a regular dose of paracetamol, lots of cuddles from his mother and a course of antibiotics quickly solved the problem. Getting the infection under control is the key to treating Phillip's pain effectively.

For Mark's father and mother it has been a different story. Their advanced years have brought with them a variety of chronically painful conditions which, for the most part, defy totally effective treatment.

---

a Learning activity

What was your worst childhood experience of pain? Has this left you with any problems such as a fear of needles? You may wish to access further information on the perception of pain. Although most books that explore psychological and sociological approaches to pain tend to reflect chronic pain management, much is to be learned about how we can reduce the risks of chronic pain. Alternatively the information might help us to identify those who are more vulnerable to chronic pain development. A good resource is Main and Spanswick (2000).

S Scenario continued

Mark Johnson's intense pain experience

Mark Johnson has a vivid memory of his first attack of renal colic in his late 30s. Again the pain was very intense, but this time not because of gross tissue damage, but because an area of viscera responded dramatically and painfully to being distended by a trapped kidney stone. Mark's renal colic responded effectively to his general practitioner giving him an intramuscular injection of 100 mg pethidine combined with 50 mg of diclofenac orally.

---

a Learning activity

Have you seen pethidine used in the past? In what way is pethidine different from morphine?

Although pethidine is a short-acting opioid, and therefore of limited use for most pain control, the fact that it is reputed to cause less smooth muscle spasm means it is often given for renal and biliary colic. However, the use of pethidine is now being questioned and it is falling out of favour, especially because its duration of action is often too short and it can lead to cerebral toxicity after repeated doses. A contemporary approach to renal colic, especially in the emergency department of a hospital, would more likely include intravenous rather than intramuscular morphine plus the inclusion of an NSAID (Brown, 2006).

Pain control in the elderly can be far more of a challenge, with comorbidity and polypharmacy adding to the complexity of pain management.

> ## (a) Learning activity
>
> Both morphine and pethidine are controlled drugs. What special arrangements are required for the safe storage and administration of such medication? Does your hospital enable nurses to single check controlled drugs or do the rules require two nurses? If these rules are in place, do you think they hinder rapid and effective pain control?

(S) Scenario continued

Clive Johnson's pain experiences

Clive Johnson's pain experiences have been gained during a lifetime of sport and activity but more recently by illness. In his youth he experienced severe and inadequately controlled pain following injuries sustained during the Korean War. Unfortunately, he also now experiences chronic pain in his feet as a result of nerve damage that has occurred with his late-onset diabetes. Not only does Clive experience neuropathic pain, he has developed a large ulcer above his left ankle. Despite the best efforts of his GP and community health team, no single drug therapy provides long-term, complete pain relief, and dressing the leg ulcer can be particularly unpleasant.

> ## (a) Learning activity
>
> Why is chronic pain so different? Talk to someone who regularly experiences episodes of recurrent periodic pain, such as migraine, or pain that is present on a more or less permanent basis. Find out how they cope with and manage their pain.

As we discussed previously, acute pain is usually related to a specific event or injury which results in immediate pain being experienced. It is accompanied by a response within the autonomic nervous system which will initially leave the sufferer with visible signs such as pallor, sweating, tachycardia and alterations in blood pressure. Acute pain will respond to effective and appropriate analgesia and treatment of the cause of the pain. For instance, pain following the tissue damage of surgery or trauma will usually respond well to psychological preparation, adequate doses of analgesia (Foley, 1993), restorative sleep and effective comfort strategies. Because the pain has resulted from an event, it is self-limiting. Once the event is over or the tissue healing, the pain naturally subsides.

Chronic pain is far more complex and is not just an extension of acute pain. Chronic pain is usually defined as pain that lasts for more than three months, although recent research suggests that its onset can be much quicker than this. It can be associated with a chronic pathological process that ensures pain is ongoing. It can be as a result of changes in the central nervous system that make chronic pain quite different from just a 'long-lasting' acute pain. There may even be a genetic component to the development of chronic pain. Pain may also be present in the absence of any obvious cause, presenting an extremely complex picture with negative psychosocial implications such as not being believed. Patients with chronic pain do not exhibit the autonomic response seen with early acute pain, as their body has adapted; this sometimes leads to inexperienced staff doubting the existence of pain. The experiences of the senior members of the Johnson family enable us now to explore some of these issues in greater depth.

C Professional conversation

Carol, practice nurse, comments on pain and wound management: 'I have been dressing Clive's leg ulcer on and off at the practice for the last three months. He had been having serious problems with hardly any healing taking place, and we became quite worried as Clive has diabetes. During a recent stay in hospital, the tissue viability specialist nurse examined his leg ulcer and dressed it on a few occasions. Clive initially found these dressing changes very painful. The nurse recommended that Clive take combination analgesia of 1000 mg of paracetamol and 20 mg of oral morphine syrup one hour before she arranged to visit him, which helped considerably. She also got him to use entonox while she was dressing the wound. Since Clive has been back with us, he has suffered little pain as the combination analgesia he now takes at home works well, and we have introduced this more widely across the practice.'

a Learning activity

Why is Clive's diabetes a worry to the practice nurses?
For a useful topical review on foot ulceration see Mekkes et al (2003).

S Scenario continued

Clive has had neuropathic pain for many years. Both his feet have lost touch sensation, but he feels unpleasant sensation and pins and needles most of the time. Accepting this as part of his diabetes, he has never really sought further treatment. All the 'painkillers' he has taken in the past have either had no effect whatsoever on his foot pain, or have left him feeling lethargic and constipated.

a Learning activity

What strategies might be useful in controlling Clive's neuropathic pain?

e Evidence-based practice: pain and disability in diabetes

Specialist care may be needed to stabilise chronic conditions such as diabetes with drug adjustments, and this may reduce pain over time. Neuropathic pain which is unlikely to resolve with standard analgesia may also respond to a trial of anticonvulsants such as gabapentin or pregabalin. Other drugs such as a low dose of the tricyclic antidepressant amitriptyline or desipramine may also be beneficial (Backonja and Serra, 2004). When trialling an antidepressant medication, patients need to be assured that these drugs are not being used because staff think the pain is not real and just the result of depression. The drug has a particular action which can be effective in treating painful diabetic neuropathy (McQuay and Moore, 1998). One of the side-effects of both amitriptyline and anticonvulsants is sedation, so when taken at night they may help to establish an improved sleep pattern, enabling patients to cope better with their pain.

A well-evaluated trial of oral morphine or a longer-acting strong opioid such as slow-release oxycodone might be useful when pain is particularly troublesome. Like all of the drugs prescribed for neuropathic pain, opioids will not be effective for everybody, especially prescribed in doses that medical staff are usually comfortable with. However, they may be worth a trial, combined with therapy to control side-effects such as constipation. There are still concerns about addiction even when the evidence does not support this risk (Ferrell et al, 1992). However, effective doses of opioids for chronic pain may lead to intolerable or unmanageable side-effects despite attempts made at controlling these. Furthermore, if pain is a feature of a numb area, there is always less confidence that opioids will be effective (Jadad et al, 1992).

As stated earlier, neuropathic pain often fails to respond to analgesia as the mechanism of pain may be a malfunction in the peripheral or central nervous system and not the nerve terminal stimulation that happens with acute tissue damage, an inflammatory response, or chronic inflammatory conditions such as rheumatoid arthritis. Understanding some of the theories of chronic pain mechanisms enables potentially more effective treatments to be tried.

Not all chronic pain has an identifiable cause or discernible pathology. Gradually we are beginning to understand more about specific chronic pain syndromes. Neuropathic pain is currently attracting considerable research. It is often described as producing a burning feeling with intermittent shock-like sensations. Although not fully understood, it is thought the pain arises from a malfunction or hyperexcitability at the periphery, which can lead to hyperexcitability extending into the spinal cord and brain. It is also theorised that this hyperexcitability can be emphasised by the loss of modulating pathways.

Psychological and sociological factors are also known to contribute to the maintenance of chronic pain. We all seem to equate pain with damage, and the fact that this may not be the case frequently needs reinforcing. Consider that fear of masking damage will often lead to patients not taking analgesia effectively in the early stages of acute pain when it is most effective. This may lead to pain wind-up and the risk of chronic pain. Sufferers of pain may also develop avoidance behaviour and disability, fearing normal mobility may make their condition worse. For musculoskeletal pain especially this fear of pain can be more disabling than pain itself (Crombez et al, 1999), leading to inactivity which may result in a painful disuse syndrome. In addition, the majority of people who develop chronic pain also suffer from depression, anxiety and sleep disturbance, as their pain which fails to be resolved has a negative impact on all aspects of quality of life (Skevington, 1995).

Part

II

S Scenario continued

Phyllis Johnson's pain experiences

Phyllis Johnson's experience enables us to see something of the processes of chronic inflammatory and ongoing musculoskeletal pain. She suffers from rheumatoid arthritis and low back pain following a series of crush injuries to her spine, which has been damaged by osteoporosis. Although Phyllis sees her general practitioner occasionally she doesn't like to be a nuisance and rarely complains, putting her pain down to her age and seeing it as just one of those things you have to live with. She has always assumed there is no specific treatment available for her conditions.

Phyllis's current analgesia is:
- paracetamol as needed
- a Cox 2 inhibitor and codeine have been prescribed for moderate to severe flare-ups of pain.

Traditionally strong opioids have not been prescribed for rheumatoid arthritis pain. However, recent studies are beginning to suggest that good results can be obtained using strong opioids in certain individuals. In light of evidence suggesting the inadequacies of weak opioids, more research is needed on the use of strong opioids, and it is hoped that this will be forthcoming in the future (Walker, 2001).

Phyllis might also benefit from a more extensive range of treatments, as suggested below, for both her rheumatoid arthritis and her osteoporosis. She has recently been referred to a multidisciplinary rheumatology clinic, where the effects of additional prescribed drugs and treatments will be evaluated, adjusted and side-effects monitored.

Treatments for rheumatoid arthritis

The following may be useful.

Corticosteroids

Steroids can improve pain and symptom control but long-term use is associated with osteoporosis, cataracts, poor wound healing, hyperglycemia, hypertension, hyperlipidemia and an increased risk of infection.

Disease-modifying drugs (DMARDS)

These are given to reduce symptoms by slowing down the disease process. There is little evidence that the elderly are at a much greater risk with these drugs, especially methotrexate, provided patients are monitored closely. Routine determination of serum liver enzymes and renal function may reduce individual risk (Hirshberg et al, 2000).

Capsaicin cream

This might help by reducing the influence of substance P, an inflammatory component of rheumatoid arthritis (Konttinen et al, 1994).

Gold injections

These are also thought to affect substance P production (Konttinen et al, 1994).

Tricyclic antidepressants

These drugs can be very problematic in the elderly because of their adverse side-effect profile. They act on descending modulation via the noradrenalin and seratonin inhibition pathway (Konttinen et al, 1994; Shipton, 1999).

- Surgery is an option in rheumatoid arthritis when other treatment has failed and there is joint destruction.

Treatments for osteoporosis

The following may be useful:
- calcium and vitamin D supplements
- bisphosphonates, which prevent bone breakdown and can be very effective in osteoporosis
- calcitonin, which is a natural substance produced by the body that may slow down the loss of bone.

Musculoskeletal pain

S   Scenario continued

Phyllis's osteoporosis means it is vital that she keeps active for as long as possible. With her bones already demineralised and prone to fracture, the less mobility she has, the weaker they become. However, she is now finding it harder to get about and has quite severe damage to her spine. The medications she currently takes for her arthritis pain are of only limited benefit and for the most part, she stoically endures her pain, determined still to find enjoyment in life. She keeps her mind occupied, reading books, watching television, playing cards with her friends and trying to remain cheerful, and these serve her reasonably well as coping strategies. She is well supported by her family, and maintaining her social interactions helps to ensure that she does not become completely overwhelmed by her pain.

As with all chronic pain, nonpharmacological strategies can be vitally important, and both Clive and Phyllis might obtain benefit from:
- heat in the form of warm showers or hot packs to relieve pain and stiffness
- cold packs to reduce swelling and inflammation (although cold is rarely popular with chronic pain sufferers)
- braces and supports
- exercise
- acupuncture and acupressure
- massage
- relaxation
- distraction
- transcutaneous nerve stimulation (TENS).

TENS is traditionally used to help control labour pains, muscular pain and some chronic pains. Although there is currently little strong evidence to support it, some patients do seem to report benefit. Whether this is beyond placebo is yet to be established. If you have a particular interest in TENS you may like to read Carroll and colleagues (2000).

You can see by the scenarios of Clive and Phyllis that their pain is complex. Commonly prescribed pharmacological strategies often prove quite disappointing, and for some chronic pain sufferers improvement in their condition may prove difficult to achieve. Many elderly people view pain as something they have to learn to live with, and suffer in silence. The effect of chronic pain on the family unit is also an important issue that is often overlooked (Snelling, 1994). Considerable numbers of patients are left feeling abandoned, frustrated and helpless by ineffective therapy and the lack of scientific explanation for their pain. This is compounded by the inadequate resources dedicated to the education of clinicians in effective pain management strategies. For chronic pain sufferers pharmacological strategies need to be carefully prescribed, monitored and evaluated, as no two individuals will respond in the same way. However, with appropriate therapy a significant proportion of patients will experience meaningful reductions in their pain and improvements with their quality of life.

> **(a) Learning activity**
>
> What sort of pain assessment tool would be suitable for use with chronic pain sufferers like Phyllis and Clive?

Part **II**

Assessing chronic pain

(See also the section on pain assessment, page 270.)

Many patients with chronic pain never have their pain recognised and fully assessed. Unlike acute pain, where an assessment can be very brief in order to initiate and evaluate treatment, a comprehensive chronic pain assessment can be a lengthy affair. However, assessment of pain location, intensity and impact is vital to establish baseline data prior to the initiation of any sort of treatment strategies. If pain cannot be fully controlled its impact on factors such as quality of life, mobility, sleep, mood and self-efficacy becomes more important. Improving just one or two of these factors can help to reduce the distress associated with pain.

Once assessment has been carried out, assessing the pain on a four-hourly or similar basis as you would for acute pain can be counterproductive. This is particularly the case when an individual has been suffering pain for many years and uses distraction as a coping strategy. Frequent assessment for these people just keeps refocusing their minds on their pain.

> **(e) Evidence-based practice: pain questionnaires**
>
> Most assessment of chronic pain takes the form of questionnaires. One of the best known, which produces a multidimensional scale, is the McGill Pain Questionnaire (MGPQ). This was first devised by Professor Ronald Melzack (1975), and is especially valuable as a research tool or for use by specialist pain clinics. Words that are commonly used to describe pain are grouped together into several categories: sensory, affective and evaluative. Patients are given the questionnaire, which can take up to 20 minutes to complete, and asked to select one word from each subcategory that is most appropriate to describe their pain. For example, one category offers the words dull, sore, hurting, aching and heavy. This particular subcategory describes a sensory aspect of pain. Within each group, the individual words are graded numerically according to increasing intensity: for instance, hurting scores higher than sore. Adding all the numbers gives an overall score or pain-rating index. The chart is combined with a body map to mark the location of pain and can include a visual analogue score for pain intensity.

Pain diaries can be very helpful, but patients need to feel motivated to use them and they can be unsuitable for cognitively impaired patients. The Oxford Pain Chart (McQuay, 1990) is an example of how categorical scales can be incorporated into a pain dairy.

Personality and depression measures are also used in chronic pain management. It is suggested that patients with chronic pain tend to score more highly on hypochondriasis, hysteria and depression scales, although this is controversial (Dolin, Padfield and Pateman, 1996), and most of the time, we have no way of knowing what came first, the pain or the negative psychological fallout.

> **(a) Learning activity**
>
> If you were looking after a patient who complained of uncontrolled chronic pain, whom would you ask for advice?

Interdisciplinary collaboration

Patients may benefit from advice by a specialist pain healthcare professional. Although interdisciplinary advice is ideally based in the community, it is often in hospital that a first contact is made with one or a combination of the following professionals:

- a pain specialist or pain team for assessment, information and a possible trial of therapy
- a specialist who deals with particular chronic conditions that may result in pain such as diabetes or Parkinson's disease
- a palliative care team which may help with analgesia and symptom control for patients with life-limiting conditions
- a dietician for advice on diet: obesity can lead to immobility and this can exacerbate pain, isolate sufferers and reduce social interaction
- an occupational therapist who can help with mobility and independence in the home
- a physiotherapist, who can be an invaluable resource especially when mobility is compromised by musculoskeletal pain and spasm
- a specialist pharmacist who can give advice on analgesia, especially for patients already taking multiple medications which might interact
- a social worker to help families struggling to manage on their own
- voluntary, charitable and self-help organisations which can be particularly helpful in providing specialist support and information.

Effective interprofessional working combines the expertise of several specialities. Good-quality pain management is not just about drugs and therapies. Interprofessional collaboration may often improve the quality of outcome for patients, especially those struggling with chronically painful conditions for which no cure can be found.

> **(a) Learning activity**
>
> How can the effectiveness of any pain management strategies be evaluated?

Using clinical effectiveness and evidence-based research to improve the quality of services to patients

Over the past 20 years the relief of pain has attracted a higher profile than was the case in the 1970s, 1980s and even early 1990s. The evolution of the science of pain, and the development of protocols and guidelines, are beginning to provide us with a 'standard of care' for which healthcare professionals and organisations could well be held accountable. The gradual introduction of a culture of pain assessment using reliable, validated assessment tools provides us with a numerical measure that can be used to evaluate quality initiatives. Regular audit is a way of evaluating the effectiveness of what we are doing at the moment, deciding whether we are satisfied, and if not, devising a standard to aim for in order to improve outcomes in the future. Measuring the quality of care for audit purposes depends on making explicit the quality of practice to be expected. Prior to the development of pain assessment tools, which are still in need of improvement, we lacked a reliable form of measurement, and this probably explained why quality pain-relieving initiatives were slow to take off.

Once an effective system is established to measure the quality of the pain relief, there is a structure in place which can be adapted to measure the effectiveness of interventions. The findings of any evaluation provide evidence of the suitability, or otherwise, of the use of such an intervention. This not only contributes to evidence-based practice but provides evidence for business plans and financial bids for the development of new initiatives.

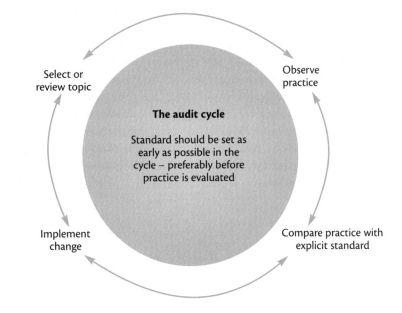

The audit cycle

Standard should be set as early as possible in the cycle – preferably before practice is evaluated

Select or review topic

Observe practice

Implement change

Compare practice with explicit standard

Figure 15.7 The audit cycle

Source: Mann and Carr (2000).

Introducing systematic review and regular evaluation of what you are trying to achieve can help improve the quality of pain relief for patients.

Evidence-based practice is defined as 'the conscientious, explicit, and judicious use of current best evidence in making decisions about the care of individual patients' (Sackett et al, 1996: 2). This would seem fairly straightforward, but applying the principles to good pain management can sometimes prove very frustrating.

> 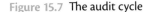 **Learning activity**
>
> Can you think of reasons why healthcare professionals have been slow to realise the value of good pain management and sometimes ineffective in implementing good practice?

Barriers to effective pain relief

There are many barriers to good pain relief, some subtle and others not so subtle.

- Patients can inhibit good analgesia with low expectations about pain relief or feelings that pain is inevitable (Carr, 1997).
- Patients may be reluctant to take analgesia for fear of masking pain and causing damage (Crombez et al, 1999).
- Patients and staff may harbour concerns about perceived untreatable or intolerable side-effects of analgesia.
- There might be unfounded concerns by healthcare professionals, patients and their relatives about addiction and tolerance (Ferrell et al, 1992).
- Access to education in pain management for healthcare professionals has been patchy and haphazard (Sloan, Montgomery and Musick,1998; Griepp, 1992; Bucknall, Marias and Botti, 2001).
- The incorporation of regular pain assessment and evaluation of analgesia into mainstream patient monitoring has been slow. Without good assessment and documentation the needs of the patient cannot be communicated adequately to all those responsible for the patient's care.

> **c** Professional conversation
>
> Theo Greaves, clinical nurse specialist, pain team, comments on organisational barriers to pain management: 'Organisations also create barriers to effective pain management when dated guidelines are incorporated into hospital policy with little if any review (Mann and Redwood, 2000). For example, if two nurses need to check a controlled drug it will often lead to lengthy delays in responding to patients' requests for strong analgesia. The two-nurse check policy was a guideline of the Duthie Report (1988) and not a legal requirement as is often assumed. Questioning what you do and why you do it can often stimulate lively debate and raise previously unidentified issues. Hospitals have traditionally been slow to change, but pressure to review this culture is now widespread. In 1846, the first anaesthetic provided pain-free surgery – 150 years later patients should not have to endure unrelieved pain anywhere in hospital (McQuay and Moore 1998).'

What the future might hold

Nurses have been pivotal in many of the developments to improve pain management. They can continue to exert influence by improving their knowledge and looking to change practice when outcomes fall short of those desired. Pain management is the very essence of caring: incredibly frustrating and stressful when it is poor, but exhilarating for all concerned when it is effective. The development of new therapies could well be on the horizon, but in the meantime an improved knowledge of current pharmacological and nonpharmacological strategies will ensure nursing retains a leading role in pain management.

Extending practice can contribute further to the developments of the last decade. Nurses and other healthcare professionals are already becoming proficient in undertaking pain-relieving procedures such as femoral nerve blocks (Cole, 2005; Layzell, 2007) and providing therapies such as acupuncture (Godfrey, 2006). The introduction of clinical guidelines under which certain drugs may be administered under protocol without a doctor's prescription is already with us (DH, 1989). Nurse prescribing has extended practice way beyond that previously undertaken by nurses (DH, 1999, 2002). The NHS Plan (DH, 2000) cleared the way for nurses to supply medicines under Patient Group Directions and now to prescribe medicines independently. The future holds all sorts of exciting possibilities for the further development of expertise in the field of pain management.

> **a** Learning activity
>
> Look around your clinical area and see whether you can identify any changes that could contribute to improved pain management. How could they be implemented?

Conclusion

This chapter has introduced pain management using a family-based scenario. The scenario incorporated acute postoperative pain, exploring both the physiological and psychological components that help to influence the success or failure of pain management. We touched on the pharmacology of some of the commonly prescribed pain-relieving drugs, and the assessment strategies that need to be in place if therapies are to be evaluated effectively. We looked at how some nonpharmacological strategies can be utilised to help reduce pain, and how coping strategies may increase pain tolerance. We also looked briefly at how interdisciplinary working may enhance patient care, and the barriers that might inhibit a timely or effective response to a patient's plea for pain relief.

Education in pain management has always been one of the major stumbling blocks to establishing good practice. This is now changing, and pain management is becoming more firmly established in both pre-registration and post-registration curricula. Easy access to ongoing education for all healthcare professionals is essential. The development of guidelines based on up-to-date evidence, combined with efforts to improve the way we manage pain, must continue to be a priority for all healthcare practitioners, particularly nurses. The stress that poor analgesia can cause both patients and staff alike should not be underestimated. It is hoped this chapter has helped to introduce this fascinating subject, and the further reading section should provide a guide to sources of more in-depth information.

References

American Pain Society (APS) (2003) 'Principles of analgesic use in the treatment of acute pain and cancer pain', Glenview, Ill., APS.

Backonja, M. and Serra, J. (2004) 'Pharmacologic management part 1: better-studied neuropathic pain diseases', *Pain Medicine* **5**(1), Supplement 1: 28–47.

Bandolier (2003) 'Acute pain' [online] <http://www.jr2.ox.ac.uk/bandolier/Extraforbando/APain.pdf> (accessed 26 February 2009).

Bandolier (2007) *Oxford League Table of Analgesics in Acute Pain* [online] <http://www.jr2.ox.ac.uk/bandolier/booth/painpag/Acutrev/Analgesics/Leagtab.html> (accessed 25 November 2008).

Brand, P. and Yancey, P. (1993) *Pain: The gift nobody wants, a surgeon's journey of discovery*, London, Marshal Pickering/HarperCollins.

Briggs, M. (1995) 'Principles of acute pain assessment', *Nursing Standard*, 9 February (19), 23–7.

Brown, J. (2006) 'Diagnostic and treatment patterns for renal colic in US emergency departments', *International Urology and Nephrology* **38**(1) (February), 87–92.

Bucknall, T., Marias, E. and Botti, M. (2001) *'Acute pain management: implications of the scientific evidence for nursing practice in the postoperative context'*, *International Journal of Nursing Practice* 7, 266–73.

Carr, D. and Goudas, L. (1999) 'Acute pain', *The Lancet* **353**(12), 2051–6.

Carr, E. (1997) 'Overcoming barriers to effective pain control', *Professional Nurse* **12**(6), 412–16.

Carr, E. and Mann, E. M. (2000) *Pain: Creative approaches to effective management*, Basingstoke, Palgrave Macmillan.

Carr, E. and Thomas, V. (1997) 'Anticipating and experiencing post-operative pain: the patients' perspective', *Journal of Clinical Nursing* **6**(3), 191–201.

Carr, E., Brockbank, K. and Barrett, R. (2003) 'Improving pain management through interprofessional education: evaluation of a pilot project', *Learning in Health and Social Care* **2**(1), 6–17.

Carroll, D., Moore, R., McQuay, H., Fairman, F., Tramer, M. and Leijon, G. (2000) 'Transcutaneous electrical nerve stimulation (TENS) for chronic pain', *Cochrane Database of Systematic Reviews*, 4.

Chapman, A. (1996) 'Current theory and practice: a study of preoperative fasting', *Nursing Standard* **10**(18) (20 January), 33–7.

Cole, A. (2005) 'Nurse-administered femoral nerve block after hip fracture', *Nursing Times* **13**(37), 34–6.

Crombez, G., Vlaeyen, J. M. S., Heuts, P. H. T. G. and Lysens, R. (1999) 'Pain-related fear is more disabling than pain itself', *Pain* 80, 329–39.

Department of Health (DH) (1989) *Report of the Advisory Group on Nurse Prescribing*, 1st Crown Report, London, HMSO.

DH (1999) *Review of the Prescribing, Supply and Administration of Medicines*, 2nd Crown Report, London, HMSO.

DH (2000) *The NHS Plan*, London, HMSO.

DH (2002) *Extending Independent Nurse Prescribing within the NHS in England: A guide to implementation*, London, DH.

Dolin, S. L., Padfield, N. L. and Pateman, L. A. (1996) *Pain Clinic Manual*, Oxford, Butterworth Heinemann.

Duthie, Prof. R. (1988) *DH Guidelines for the Safe and Secure Handling of Medicines: A report to the Secretary of State for Social Services*, London, HMSO.

Ersek, M. and Poe, C. (2004) 'Pain', pp. 131–59 in Lewis, S., Heitkemper, M. and Dirksen, S. (eds), *Medical-Surgical Nursing: Assessment and management of clinical problems*, St Louis, Mosby.

Evans, A. (2003) 'Use of entonox in the community for control of procedural pain', *British Journal of Community Nursing* **8**(11) (November), 488–94.

Ferrell, B. R., McCaffery, M. and Rhiner, M. (1992) 'Pain and addiction: an urgent need for change in nurse education', *Journal of Pain and Symptom Management* **7**(2), 117–24.

Ferrell, B., Virani, R., Grant, M., Vallerand, A. and McCaffery, M. (2000) 'Analysis of pain content in nursing textbooks', *Journal of Pain and Symptom Management* **19**(3), 216–28.

Foley, K. M. (1993) 'Pain assessment and cancer pain syndromes', ch. 4.2.2, pp. 148–65 in Doyle, D., Hanks, G. W. C. and MacDonald, N. (eds), *Oxford Textbook of Palliative Medicine*, Oxford, Oxford Medical Publications.

Godfrey, K. (2006) 'Giving pain relief', *Nursing Times* **102**(29), 20–1.

Griepp, M. (1992) 'Under medication for pain: an ethical model', *Advances in Nursing Science* **15**(1), 44–53.

Gunnar, B. and Helseth, S. (2006) 'The gap between saying and doing in postoperative pain management', *Journal of Clinical Nursing* **15**(4), 469–79.

Harmer, M. (2002) *Patient-Controlled Analgesia*, 2nd edn, Oxford, Blackwell Science.

Hawthorn, J. and Redmond, K. (1998) *Pain Causes and Management*, Oxford, Blackwell Science.

Herrero, J., Laird, J. and Lopez-Garcia, J. (2000) 'Wind-up of spinal cord neurones and pain sensation: much ado about something', *Progress in Neurobiology* 61, 169–203.

Hirshberg, B., Mordechi, M., Schlesinger, O. and Rubinow, A. (2000) 'Safety of low dose methotrexate in elderly patients with rheumatoid arthritis', *Postgraduate Medical Journal* 76 (December), 787–98.

IASP (1994) 'IASP Pain Terminology: a sample list of frequently used terms', in Merskey, H. and Bogduk, N. (eds), *Classification of Chronic Pain*, 2nd edn, IASP Task Force on Taxonomy, Seattle, IASP Press [online] <www.iasp-pain.org/AM/Template.cfm?Section=General_Resource_Links&Template=/CM/HTMLDisplay.cfm&ContentID=3058#Anesthesia%20Dolorosa> (accessed 26 February 2009).

International Association for the Study of Pain (IASP) (1986) 'Classification of chronic pain: descriptions of chronic pain syndromes and definitions of pain terms', *Pain*, Supplement 3.

Jadad, A., Carroll, D., Glynn, C., Moore, R. and McQuay, H. (1992) 'Morphine responsiveness of chronic pain: double-blind randomised crossover study with patient controlled analgesia', *The Lancet* **339**(8806) (6 June), 1367–71.

Part

II

Konttinen, Y., Kemppinen, P., Segerberg, M., Hukkanen, M., Rees, R., Santavirta, S., Sorsa, T., Pertovaara, A. and Polak, J. (1994) 'Peripheral and spinal mechanisms of arthritis, with particular reference to treatment of inflammation and pain', *Arthritis and Rheumatism* 7, 965–82.

Lawler, K. (1995) 'Entonox: too useful to be limited to childbirth?' *Professional Care of the Mother and Child* 5(1), 19–21.

Layzell, M. (2007) 'Pain management: setting up a nurse-led femoral nerve block service', *British Journal of Nursing* 16(12) (28 June), 702–5.

Macintyre, P. and Ready, L. (2006) *Acute Pain Management: A practical guide*, 2nd edn, Philadelphia, W. B. Saunders.

Macintyre, P. and Schug, S. (2007) *Acute Pain Management: A practical guide*, 3rd edn, Philadelphia, W. B. Saunders.

Main, C. and Spanswick, C. (2000) *Pain Management: An interdisciplinary approach*, Edinburgh, Churchill Livingston.

Manias, E. (2003) 'Pain and anxiety management in the postoperative gastro-surgical setting', *Journal of Advanced Nursing* 41(6), 585–94.

Mann, E. and Carr, E. (2000) *Pain: Creative approaches to effective management*, Basingstoke, Palgrave Macmillan.

Mann, E. and Carr, E. (2006) *Pain Management* (Essential Clinical Skills for Nurses), Oxford, Blackwell.

Mann E. and Redwood S. (2000) 'Improving pain management: breaking down the invisible barrier', *British Journal of Nursing* 9(19) (26 October–8 November), 2067–72.

McCaffery, M. (1972) *Nursing Management of the Patient with Pain*, Philadelphia, Pa., J. B. Lippincott.

McQuay, H. (1990) 'Assessment of pain, and effectiveness of treatment', in Hopkins, A. and Costain, D. (eds), *Measuring the Outcomes of Medical Care*, London. Royal College of Physicians, Kings Fund Centre for Health Services Development.

McQuay, H. and Moore, A., (1998) *An Evidence-Based Resource for Pain Relief*, Oxford, Oxford University Press.

Mekkes, J., Loots, M., Van Der Wal, A. and Bos, J. (2003) 'Causes, investigation and treatment of leg ulceration', *British Journal of Dermatology* 148(3), 388–401.

Melzack, R. (1975) 'The McGill pain questionnaire: major properties and scoring methods', *Pain*, 1277–99.

Melzack, R. and Wall, P. (1965) 'Pain mechanisms: a new theory', *Science* 150, 971–9.

Melzack, R. and Wall, P. (1996) *The Challenge of Pain*, 2nd edn, Harmondsworth, Penguin.

Middleton, C. (2006) *Epidural Analgesia in Acute Pain Management*, Chichester, John Wiley.

Moss, E., Taverner, T., Norton, P., Lesser, P. and Cole, P. (2005) 'A survey of postoperative pain management in fourteen hospitals in the UK',

Acute Pain 7(1), 13–20.

Okifuji, A., Anderson, K., Cleeland, C., Turk, D. and Melzack, R. (2001) *Handbook for Pain Assessment*, 2nd edn, New York, Guilford.

Park, G., Fulton, B. and Senthuran, S. (2000) *The Management of Acute Pain*, 2nd edn, New York, Oxford University Press.

Pasero, C. and McCaffery, M. (2004) 'Comfort-function goals: a way to establish accountability for pain relief', *American Journal of Nursing* 104(9), 77–81.

Pediani, R. (2003) 'Patient-administered inhalation of nitrous oxide and oxygen gas for procedural pain relief' [online] <http://www.worldwidewounds.com/2003/october/Pediani/Entonox-Pain-Relief.html> (accessed 25 November 2008).

Pittler, M. and Ernst, E. (1998) 'Peppermint oil for irritable bowel syndrome; a critical review and meta-analysis', *American Journal of Gastroenterology* 93(7), 1131–5.

Plaisance L. (2007) 'Nursing students' knowledge and attitudes regarding pain', *Pain Management Nursing* 7(4), 167–75.

Reuben, S., Gutta, S., Tarasenko, V., Steinberg, R. and Sklar, J. (2002) 'Pre-emptive multimodal analgesia for ACL surgery', 27th Annual Spring Meeting and Workshops, 25–28 April, American Society of Regional Anaesthesia and Pain Medicine. Chicago, USA.

Sackett, D., Richardson, W. S., Rosenburg, W. and Haynes, B. (1996) *Evidence-Based Medicine*, London, Churchill Livingstone.

Schofield, P. (1995) 'Using assessment tools to help patients in pain', *Professional Nurse* 10(11) (August), 703–6.

Shade, P. (1992) 'PCA: Can client education improve outcomes?' *Journal of Advanced Nursing* 17, 408–13.

Shevde, K. and Triveldi, N. (1991) 'Effects of clear fluids on gastric volume and ph in health volunteers', *Anaesthesia Analgesia* 72, 528–31.

Shipton, E. (1999) 'Secondary analgesics (Part 1)', pp. 93–107 in Shipton, E. A. (ed.), *Pain: Acute and chronic*, London, Arnold.

Skevington, S. (1995) *Psychology of Pain*, Chichester, John Wiley.

Sloan, P., Montgomery, C. and Musick, D. (1998) 'Medical student knowledge of morphine for the management of cancer pain', *Journal of Pain Symptom Management* 15, 359–64.

Snelling, J. (1994) 'The effect of chronic pain on the family unit', *Journal of Advanced Nursing* 19, 543–51.

Tate, S. (1997) 'Peppermint oil: a treatment for post-operative nausea', *Journal of Advanced Nursing* 26(3), 125–35.

Turk, D. and Melzack, R. (eds) (2001) *Handbook of Pain Assessment*, 2nd edn, New York, Guilford.

Walker, J. (2001) 'Anti-inflammatory effects of s-opioids: relevance to rheumatoid arthritis', *Pain Reviews* 8(3–4) (October), 113–19.

Useful websites

Agency for Healthcare Policy and Research USA: <www.ahcpr.gov/> (accessed 25 November 2008).

British Pain Society: <www.britishpainsociety.org/> (accessed 25 November 2008).

Cochrane Collaboration: <http://www.cochrane.org/index.htm> (accessed 25 November 2008).

Database of systematic reviews of pain relief: <www.jr2.ox.ac.uk/Bandolier> (accessed 25 November 2008).

European Federation of IASP Chapters: <http://www.efic.org/>

(accessed 25 November 2008).

International Association for the Study of Pain: <www.iasp-pain.org> (accessed 25 November 2008).

National Prescribing Centre, *NSAIDS and Gastroprotection* <http://www.npc.co.uk/MeReC_Briefings/2002/briefing_no_20.pdf> (accessed 25 November 2008).

US National Institutes of Health – Pain Research: <http://painconsortium.nih.gov/pain_index.html> (accessed 25 November 2008).

Chapter
16

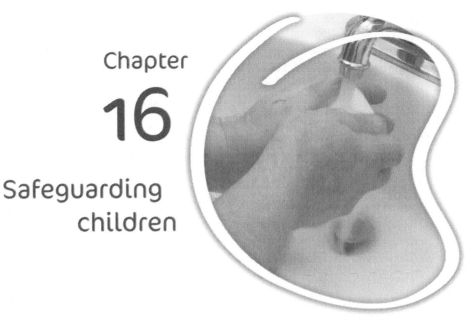

Safeguarding children

Hilary McCluskey and
Melanie Robbins

 Links to other chapters in *Foundation Studies for Caring*

 Links to other chapters in *Foundation Skills for Caring*

W Don't forget to visit www.palgrave.com/glasper for additional
online resources relating to this chapter.

Introduction

All healthcare professionals will come into contact with children at some point in their working lives. This might be because they are working directly with children, or they might be involved with parents, grandparents or neighbours who discuss children with them, or who have children visiting them in hospital. Health professionals working in the community may also see or hear about children in their patients' homes. Sometimes such contacts give rise to professional concerns about the welfare and/or safety of the children.

This chapter provides a basic overview on safeguarding children. It considers what child abuse is in our society and how it can be recognised. It looks at how the law is structured to protect children, and the duties conferred on professionals, with current policy and guidelines on action that needs to be taken.

Please note: this can be a distressing topic, and you might find the material disturbing personally. This is a natural reaction, and if you do find yourself upset by the material, you should access the support of your personal or academic tutor.

Learning outcomes

This chapter will enable you to:

- identify when a child may be in need, or in need of protection
- recognise the need for assessment of the child's needs, and be aware of the tools that are used
- outline categories of abuse and neglect and be able to recognise when there might be concerns
- discuss your role as a student when concerns are identified, including actions that must be taken to promote the child's well-being
- demonstrate good record-keeping principles

- describe the importance of working with children and parents, and of listening to children's understanding of what is happening to them and what they would like to happen
- list five agencies health professionals may work with when safeguarding children
- outline good principles of working together with other agencies
- identify three potential consequences of not taking action.

Concepts

- Childhood
- Children's rights and needs
- Assessment

- Recognition of abuse
- Principles of recording

- Reporting
- Multiprofessional working

> ### ⓐ Learning activity
>
> - What do the terms child, children and childhood mean to you?
> - Are they different? If so how?
> - What do you think these terms might mean for someone of a different culture, religion or social class?

The distressing subject of child abuse is not a new phenomenon. History demonstrates clearly that children's welfare was not always a social priority. Several key aspects have shaped the current position:

- The definition of childhood has changed and developed over the last 200 years.
- Expectations of what a child can do have also altered. In the seventeenth and eighteenth centuries, children were considered able to contribute to the family's economic wealth from approximately the age of 7, for instance by helping on a farm.

- The industrial revolution moved families from a rural to an industrial environment. This moved society from a community focus in the rearing of children, to a more nuclear, 'parenting within the family' approach with minimal state interference (Parton, 1997).
- In the twenty-first century in Britain, we have extended the earliest age at which a child can leave compulsory education from 16 to 18.
- The World Health Organization (WHO) (2003–4) considers that childhood ends at 24 years, when individuals are able more realistically to fend for themselves in all aspects of adult life.
- Social policy has tended to have a see-saw view, reflecting the fears and concerns of the day. In the early child welfare legislation and policy in the early twentieth century, the state wanted to reduce the possibility of juvenile delinquents, and so state intervention was swift and punitive.
- Child abuse came to the public's notice with the Maria Colwell inquiry (DHSS, 1974).
- With each subsequent inquiry, social policy has alternated between a protection/ prevention philosophy and an interventionist perspective, and a more 'softly softly' approach, where the family and parents are to be given support and as much opportunity to change as possible. For instance, the Jasmine Beckford inquiry (Brent, 1985) took the line that the state should intervene as early as possible, and the Cleveland enquiry (Secretary of State for Social Services, 1988) pointed out that there was a 'damned if they intervened and damned if they didn't' position for professionals.
- The focus of current policy aims to combine both approaches, so that prevention and protection work together rather than as either/or alternatives.

(adapted from Parton, 1997; Corby, 2006)

Safeguarding children

> **a Learning activity**
>
> Explore the internet for the term 'safeguarding'. What items does your search engine select, and which client groups are highlighted?

Safeguarding is a term used to refer to a continuum of care for children and young people, which includes:
- promoting healthy emotional, physical, educational and social development of the child, appropriate to the child's age and expected developmental achievement
- ensuring the child is provided with a safe environment, and loving and nurturing care
- protecting children from maltreatment.

Safeguarding is intended to be more encompassing than previous terms such as child protection, as it includes actions to promote the well-being of a child, as well as preventing child abuse and neglect. Actions are based on a belief that although children have certain rights, they are vulnerable as they have not reached an age of maturity and therefore need to be protected in law. Although family structures and lifestyles may vary, it is important that children's needs are met (HMG, 2006).

> Good parenting involves caring for children's basic needs, keeping them safe, showing them warmth and love, and providing the stimulation needed for their development and to help them achieve their potential, within a stable environment where they experience consistent guidance and boundaries.
>
> (HMG, 2006: 31)

Although policies have developed separately in England, Wales, Scotland and Northern Ireland, safeguarding policies in each country are developing rapidly and have been embedded in broader children's policies following similar principles. For the purposes of this chapter, the

English system is used although key differences are highlighted as appropriate. You need to be aware of the national safeguarding children policy guidance governing your place of work, and must also be aware of local guidelines produced by healthcare trusts and local safeguarding children's boards (or their equivalent in Wales, Scotland and Northern Ireland).

Key resources

England	Wales	Scotland	Northern Ireland
HM Government (2006) *Working Together to Safeguard Children: A guide to inter-agency working to safeguard and promote the welfare of children*, London, Department for Education and Skills.	All Wales Area Child Protection Committees (2005) *All Wales Child Protection Procedures*, Cardiff, Wales Child Protection Review Group.	Scottish Executive (2004) *Protecting Children and Young People: Framework for standards*, Edinburgh, Scottish Executive.	Department of Health, Social Services and Public Safety (2003) *Co-operating to Safeguard Children*, Belfast.

All four policies incorporate Articles 3 and 6 of the United Nations Convention on the Rights of the Child (UNCRC, 1989). Article 6 states that every child has an inherent right to life, and that state bodies are obliged to use every possible means to ensure the survival and development of children. There is an obligation for governments to ensure that services are developed and provided to safeguard children from serious harm. Article 3 also states that the best interests of the child must be a primary consideration, and that authorities must provide children with adequate care when parents or others with legal responsibilities fail to discharge their duties.

⚠ Professional alert!

In 2003, the government commissioned a consultation of children and young people in England to determine what they considered to be their key needs to grow and develop safely and to live a fulfilled and productive life. Five outcomes were adopted, and form the basis for all policies and practice to safeguard children, and of the Children Act 2004 (England):

- Be healthy.
- Stay safe.
- Enjoy and achieve through learning.
- Make a positive contribution to society.
- Achieve economic well-being.

(DfES, 2004)

Ⓢ Scenario: Sam and his family

Sam, aged 10 months, lives with both his parents, Jo (aged 17) and Peter (18) on the 14th floor of a high-rise block of local authority flats. The family is living on benefits as neither parent is working. Jo and Peter do not know other young parents in the area, and Jo seldom sees her own parents. She is being treated for postnatal depression which leaves her feeling very tired.

Ⓐ Learning activity

Consider your own experiences of being parented, and the things that you valued most about your parents' care of you. Then think about whether you have any concerns about how Jo and Peter may be able to parent Sam in their current circumstances. How does this relate to the five outcomes outlined in the Professional Alert above?

What a child needs to grow and develop

The obvious first item on a list of requirements for growth and development is nutrition. Children need food, not only for energy but to provide the building blocks of growth and repair. Their nutritional needs differ at each stage of life. Infants feed on milk only (breast or bottle) until they are old enough to be weaned on to solid foods. Infants triple their birth weight in the first year of life, requiring a diet high in fat (Jarvis, 2002). Throughout childhood, energy requirements differ from adults, and there are recognised stages when energy need increases (for example, adolescence). Parents need to recognise the changing nutritional needs of their children, which may not reflect the family's usual dietary patterns.

Children need parents to provide a safe environment for them to grow and develop, taking into consideration the child's age and developmental stage. Each developmental milestone raises different safety issues. For example at around three to four months infants are able to roll (and are in danger of rolling off the bed), while at 12–18 months they take their first steps, introducing risks from stairs, kitchen cupboards, roads and so on.

Exploration allows children to develop imagination, inquisitiveness, and understanding of how to manage risks. Parents need to balance allowing the child the freedom to explore, with assessing risks to the child while at play.

Play and development are fundamental requirements for a child (Smith, Cowie and Blades, 2003). Through play a child is able to rehearse the skills required for adult life:

- Physical skill acquisition: learning to manipulate objects – for example, learning to do and undo buttons – is necessary for a child to learn to dress themselves.
- Social skills: learning to play with others encourages children to learn how to socialise, negotiate conflict and discomfort, and to negotiate difficult emotions. Children also use social play to gain a sense of personal identity, and to learn to empathise with others.
- Play allows the child to tell their story in their own language.

Work by Bowlby (1969, 1973, 1980), and Robertson (1955, 1969, 1970) demonstrated a child's need for a stable, loving bond and secure environment. Bowlby called this *secure attachment*. If children are unable to attach securely to a significant carer, they have more difficulty in forming secure and meaningful relationships in childhood and adulthood, and their reduced responsiveness to the world around them limits their ability to interact, play and learn.

Children who grow up in an environment of low warmth are more likely to have low self-esteem and a poor sense of self-worth. Conversely children who grow up in environments of emotional warmth, demonstrated by lots of praise, statements of love and respect, are more likely to have high levels of self-esteem and be more willing to try new things and explore their environment, unafraid of failure and criticism (DH, 1995).

Poverty significantly affects a child's growth and development in a number of ways (Acheson, 1998; DH, 1999):

- Children's life experiences are likely to be more limited, with fewer family outings to museums, theatre/ cinema, the countryside and so on. There may be fewer educational toys, or the toys might not meet basic safety standards.
- Poverty may limit parents' ability to keep the environment safe, as money for items such as safety gates and childproof locks on kitchen and bathroom cupboards may be beyond the family budget.
- Poverty can influence the quality of the house the family can afford to live in, which may also raise safety issues. Children may be deprived of safe environments in which to play (for example, homes that have no garden or play area, or that open out onto the street, increase the risk of accidents, especially road traffic accidents) (Kendrick, 2002). Children from low socioeconomic backgrounds are at a greater risk of accidents, and this is found across all ages of children and all developed countries (Kendrick and Marsh, 2001).
- Health issues might arise: for example, damp housing may affect the health of the child and family, perhaps aggravating asthma or bronchitis.

Part II

- Low-income families are less likely to be able to afford a balanced nutritious diet, opting for cheaper convenience foods, high in fat and carbohydrates, as these fill the child for longer.
- The effects of poverty can be self-replicating, in that children from poorer backgrounds find it difficult to access education and services, meaning that their children are also born into poverty (Wanless, 2002). The government has made breaking this cycle one of the themes within its policy document *Tackling Health Inequalities: A programme for action* (DH, 2003).

> **a) Learning activity**
>
> In your role as a healthcare professional you will come into contact with children as patients, clients and children of the adults you are working with. What is your role in identifying families who are struggling to meet the five outcomes in *Every Child Matters*?

Children in need

When parents or carers with parental responsibility are unable to meet a child or young person's needs without additional support, the child is known as a 'child in need'. Children who are defined as being 'in need', under section 17 of the Children Act 1989, are those whose vulnerability is such that they are unlikely to reach or maintain a satisfactory level of health or development, or their health and development will be significantly impaired, without the provision of services (section 17(10) of the Children Act 1989), plus those who are disabled (HMG, 2006 section 1.22, p. 36).

Needs might not be met because:

- The child has intrinsic multiple physical, mental or emotional needs or a learning disability.
- The parent is unable to provide for a child's parenting needs because of their own limitations, such as impaired physical, mental, or emotional health, learning difficulties, substance abuse or other forms of abuse within the family (such as domestic violence, or abuse to vulnerable adults) (O'Hagan, 2006; Howe, 2005; DH, 1995; Reder, Duncan and Gray, 1993; Reder and Duncan, 1999; Mullender et al, 2002).

⚠ Professional alert!

Checklists have been devised to identify characteristics of children at risk of abuse, and of families who are more likely to abuse children.

Child	Parent(s)	Social
Pre-term infant	Young	Poor housing
Low birth weight	Lone-parent families	Overcrowding
Difficult feeder	Low educational attainment	Poverty
Required time in special care	Low stress threshold	No social support mechanisms
Wrong gender	Substance dependent	Discriminatory environment – such as racial discrimination
Disability	Mental or physical health needs	
Younger children more likely to be physically abused	Previously abused themselves	
Older children more likely to be sexually abused	Lack of family support	
	Isolated	
	Social exclusion	

Source: adapted from HMG (2006) and McKears et al (2005).

Some children in this position can have their needs met relatively easily by provision of aids in the home, additional living allowances and/or adaptations provided at school. For other families, needs might be more complex and require a range of support services provided by a multi-agency team of professionals, using a family support plan.

Reviews of children who have been seriously injured or have died have repeatedly found an escalation of abuse from mild abuse or neglect to severe abuse, suggesting that early intervention to support parents may help to prevent abuse from occurring and stop children from suffering potential harm (Reder and Duncan, 1999; Reder et al, 1993).

From these reviews a composite of risk indicators was identified (see Professional Alert). It is known that the more risk indicators a family has, the more likely it is that the family will need additional support to prevent abuse or neglect occurring. A family might have a number of these risk indicators, but there is no abuse or neglect; likewise a family might have none of these risk indicators but abuse or neglect has occurred.

Additional attention should be paid:

- where more than one factor is present
- when factors are present over a long period of time (chronicity)
- where the effect of factors on the family is more pronounced (severity).

Some families meet several of the criteria listed here but are still able to provide nurturing and stimulating parenting for their children.

⌐S⌐ Scenario continued

One afternoon Jo presented with Sam at the Accident and Emergency (A&E) department at her local hospital. Sam had a scald to his right hand and fingers and isolated scalds to his chest. Jo reported that she had fallen asleep on the sofa. She stated that when she woke, she saw her coffee cup on the floor and Sam covered in steaming coffee. He was crying. Both Jo and Sam were distressed.

↺a Learning activity

- What information would you need to plan Sam's care?
- What kind of questions might you ask Jo to get more information?
- Consider whether you have any concerns about Sam's current care or his future care.

Assessment

A number of policies aim to enable children and families requiring help to be identified and the support required to be given.

- The *Framework for Assessing Children in Need and their Families* (DfES/DH/HO, 2000) provides for the assessment of three domains (see below). Services should be needs-led and assessment should use a systematic approach, which uses the framework to enable not only the assessment of need, but discrimination between the levels and types of need (Gray, 2002). The prime focus must always be that the child's welfare is protected and promoted.
- *Every Child Matters* (DfES, 2004) details the five targets that underpin work with children and families.
- *Working Together to Safeguard Children: A guide to inter-agency working to safeguard and promote the welfare of children* (HMG, 2006) outlines the roles and responsibilities of each profession and agency to facilitate child and family health. This document also outlines the need for professions and agencies to work together in an integrated way to ensure a seamless service for the child and family.

The three domains under which assessment must be made are:

Infant, child and young person's development

This assesses the infant, child or young person's:

- physical and emotional development, and whether this is age-appropriate
- health and well-being
- ability to identify, which includes their self-esteem
- ability to self-care and develop independence, and whether this is age-appropriate and /or encouraged within any limitations such as disability

- social presentation, including their family and social relationships
- ability for learning, including cognitive reasoning, problem solving, participation, education, employment, progress and achievement of their aspirations.

Parenting capacity of main carers

This assesses the parents':

- ability to provide basic material needs, such as food, clothes and shelter
- ability to respond to the child's changing needs over time
- capacity to meet key psychological needs such as emotional warmth, guidance and provision of consistent boundaries.

Gray (2002) adds that assessment should also consider the role of the father/father figure (rather than assume that a female is the main or only carer). Where one parent does not live with the child, the role that parent will take should also be assessed and agreed. The relationship between the parents and its impact on the child should also be considered.

Family and environmental factors

This assesses the family's:

- Social integration. Poor social integration has been linked with child protection concerns. Families who have access to support, either from the immediate or wider family or from strong neighbourhood sources, are less likely to experience adverse health and educational outcomes.
- Socioeconomic factors including employment, housing and income.
- Coping mechanisms when faced with adversity/stress.
- Relationships with siblings.
- Wider family contacts. The child might have positive contacts with members of the extended family or with adults in their local community, which can help mitigate the effects of adverse influences within the home such as poverty, abuse or violence.
- Family history and functioning. Some families have a long history of dysfunction over several generations, and this increases the risk to the child.

The assessment process should:

- gather and record information systematically, outlining the strengths and challenges within the family
- check the accuracy of the information with the parents and child (if appropriate)
- record any differences in perspective of the information
- identify the vulnerabilities and protective influences available to the child and family
- identify the impact of the current situation on the child
- identify and utilise a 'common language' between agencies and professionals who work with children to ensure the needs of the child are understood and that there is a shared view of what is the child's best interest and a joint commitment to improve the child's outcome.

(adapted from Gray, 2002)

(a) Learning activity

Compare your response to the previous learning activity with the framework of assessment categories outlined.

Do you notice any differences?

Is there information that you might not be able to get just by asking questions?

You might want to search the internet for ideas on possible sources of additional information which could enable a more complete assessment.

Skills of assessment

The skills of assessing children who might be in need, or in need of protection, are no different from the skills of assessment for a physical illness. A lot of information can be gained through observation of the child and family relationships, presentation and behaviour. This allows you to build up a picture of the child's circumstances.

Observation

Watching the child and parents should give you information about:

- The child's presentation. For example, is their clothing appropriate for the time of year? Are their clothes clean? Do they look to be the right height/weight for their age (clothes might be too loose or too tight, perhaps suggesting weight changes)?
- What type of relationship does the child have with the parents? Is there obvious warmth and love demonstrated, or do the parents constantly shout and criticise the child?
- How willing is the child to engage in play with the other children or with adults?

These observations may guide you in your discussions with the parents and in information you may want to explore in more depth. For example, while your observations might suggest the child is underweight, measuring the child's height and weight and plotting these results on a centile chart will give a more accurate picture.

Good listening skills

- Often families use familiar names or phrases to describe shared events or experiences that are unique to them. However calling an abusive event by an innocent name can mean that you do not fully understand what the child is saying. This leaves the child feeling no one is listening to them.
- Using open questions enables the child and family to offer more information, and provides a bigger picture.

Knowledge of expected chronological development

You need to know the expected behaviour and development of children at particular ages, or to know where to access child development expertise, so that an accurate assessment of the child can be made.

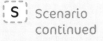

S   Scenario continued

Following assessment in A&E, Sam was admitted to a ward, for assessment of the burns to his fingers.

C   Professional conversation

Twenty-four hours after Sam's admission, on shift handover, staff nurse Imran advised charge nurse Chloe, 'Sam has been restless throughout the night shift. His mother didn't stay the night, although she came in at 11 pm with a teddy for Sam. She left soon after she arrived, without giving Sam a cuddle. She didn't say much to him. We were told she was only on the ward for a couple of hours yesterday. I'm worried about what's going on.'

Chloe asked, 'Has Sam's dad been into the ward at all?'

'No,' Imran said. 'He stood at the door and waited for Jo when she came to give Sam his teddy, but he didn't come in.'

'Have you talked to Jo about your concerns?' Chloe asked.

Imran shook his head. 'There really hasn't been the opportunity as Jo disappeared so quickly. It took us all by surprise – at that time of night we thought she had come to stay for the night.'

Chloe asked, 'Have you discussed your concerns with anyone else?'

Children in need of protection

Children in need of protection might be brought to your attention in any of the following ways:

- A child has previously been recognised as a child in need, and a support package is in place.
- There has been no previous identification of the child as a child in need.
- The child has not previously been identified as a child in need, but they are known to social services and/ or health practitioners.

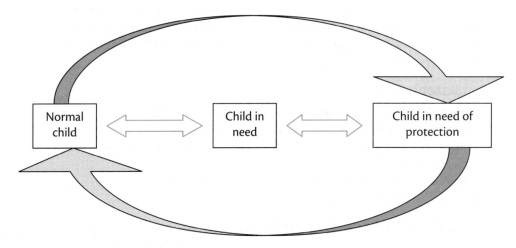

Figure 16.1 Child in need of protection

The WHO regards abuse as:

All forms of physical and/or emotional ill-treatment, social abuse, neglect or negligent treatment or commercial or other exploitation resulting in actual or potential harm to the child's health, survival, development or dignity in the context of a relationship of responsibility, trust, or power.

(WHO, 2003–4)

Initially Sam's situation seemed to be that of a child in need, as Jo and Peter are inexperienced, unsupported parents with some economic difficulties, living in inappropriate accommodation for a young family. However, as the family's situation becomes clearer, there is now some evidence to suggest that Sam is at risk of harm. A systematic approach should be taken to assess Sam's needs (DfES/DH/HO, 2000):

Child development

- Sam has an injury which needs treating. Poor healing might affect future function of his hand and/or cause scarring, therefore Sam needs good nutrition to promote healing and to prevent the possibility of his wound becoming infected.
- Development – there is no indication that Sam is behind with his developmental milestones. However Jo's apparent lack of interaction with Sam might indicate a lack of stimulation and/or poor bonding.

Parenting capacity

- Possible poor bonding – this might be caused by Jo's postnatal depression. Children learn that mothers may not be emotionally available for them, and develop an insecure attachment, which produces uncertainty and anxiety within the child and has the potential to disrupt the child's potential to build relationships (Howe, 2005; Main, 1990).
- Emotional warmth – there is an apparent lack of warmth demonstrated between Jo and Sam.
- Jo is failing to meet Sam's current need for care while he is in the hospital.
- Ensuring safety – Sam's accident demonstrates that Jo did not meet Sam's needs on that occasion, as she did not place the hot coffee safely out of his reach. She lacked vigilance: she should have ensured Sam was somewhere safe before falling asleep.

Environment

- Safety – the accident demonstrates that Sam was not in a safe environment on that occasion.
- Family's social integration – Jo and Peter do not have many support networks which puts them at greater risk of being unable to meet Sam's needs (Garbarino, 1982; Coohey, 1996).
- Employment and income – Jo and Peter are not currently working, which is another stress factor increasing the risk that they may be unable to meet Sam's needs. For example, they might not have been able to afford a playpen to place Sam in when Jo felt sleepy. Research has also demonstrated links between male unemployment and physical abuse of children (Gillham et al, 1998), and Cawson and colleagues (2000) found that children from lower socioeconomic backgrounds were more likely to be physically and emotionally abused and/ or neglected than children from more advantaged homes.

Categories of abuse

Reviewing the outcome of the assessment, a decision needs to be made as to whether this is abuse and if so what kind of abuse it is. There are four categories of abuse under the current legislation (HMG, 2006). When abuse is recognised a set process follows, including the development of a chld protection plan which is to be held on the Integrated Child Protection System (ICS) (the previous system was known as the child protection register) (HMG, 2008).

Physical abuse

> Physical abuse may involve hitting, shaking, throwing, poisoning, burning or scalding, drowning, suffocating, or otherwise causing physical harm to a child. Physical harm may also be caused when a parent or carer fabricates the symptoms of, or deliberately induces, an illness in a child
>
> (HMG, 2006: 38)

Children are sometimes kept away from school until visible signs of physical injury have resolved. Abusers might seek medical aid at different general practitioner (GP) surgeries or A&E departments, and/or move house frequently to prevent previous treatments and suspicions being linked with the presenting injury (Reder et al, 1993; Reder and Duncan, 1999).

Fabricated or induced illness might be suspected, but collecting evidence for proof can be difficult, and poses ethical challenges as children must be protected from harm. Usually medical and nursing practitioners take the key responsibility for obtaining evidence (Munro, 2007). Misreporting of symptoms, falsifying symptoms and induced illness are all used by the parent to attract medical attention. Falsifying symptoms is more common than inducing illness, and there is some indication that the child may become collusive with the parent (Awadallah et al, 2005). Multiple ensuing medical investigations can themselves cause physical harm. Abuse from fabricated illness frequently goes unrecognised for long periods, and children often have poor long-term outcomes: they experience significant emotional and physical harm, sometimes resulting in death (Barber and Davis, 2002).

Signals that could help you recognise a case of fabricated illness are (Barber and Davis, 2002; Munro, 2007; Tamay et al, 2007):

- The child is persistently presented for medical care.
- Symptoms and signs of disease disappear when the child is separated from the perpetrator (that is, the parent).
- Reported symptoms are not explained by any medical condition the child has.
- Results of investigations do not explain signs or symptoms described by the parent or portrayed by the child.
- There is little or limited response to treatment.
- The child's daily activities or schooling are being curtailed unnecessarily.
- The perpetrator may deny the aetiology (that is, the identified causes) of the child's illness.

There has been some controversy around methods used to collect evidence to prove fabricated illness. It is important that ethical principles are followed and that children are not left in a situation where they may be at risk (Munro, 2007).

Emotional abuse

Working Together to Safeguard Children (HMG, 2006: 39) defines emotional abuse as:

> The persistent emotional maltreatment of the child such as to cause severe and persistent adverse effects on the child's emotional development. It may involve conveying to children that they are worthless or unloved, inadequate, or valued only insofar as they meet the needs of another person. It may feature age or developmentally inappropriate expectations being imposed on children. These may include interactions that are beyond the child's developmental capability, as well as overprotection and limitation of exploration and learning, or preventing the child participating in normal social interaction. It may involve seeing or hearing the ill-treatment of another. It may involve causing children frequently to feel frightened or in danger, or the exploitation of corruption of children.

Emotional abuse is hard to prove, and consequently less than 20 per cent of child protection registrations name emotional abuse as the main category of abuse, even though practitioners may directly observe emotional abuse taking place (Howe, 2005). Ongoing observation of the parent treating the child in a way that is hostile, ridiculing, or corrupting is needed to corroborate or confirm suspicions of emotional abuse, and judgements are rarely formed from single incidents. A written chronology of carefully documented events or observations is therefore particularly important. Any child may become a victim of emotional abuse, although those with registered disability or learning difficulties have been found to be up to three times more likely to experience emotional abuse (Sullivan and Knutson, 2000).

Sexual abuse

Working Together to Safeguard Children (HMG, 2006: 39) defines this as:

> Sexual abuse involves forcing or enticing the child or young person to take part in sexual activities, including prostitution, whether or not the child is aware of what is happening. The activities may involve physical contact, including penetrative or non-penetrative acts. They may include non-contact activities, such as involving children in looking at, or in the production of, pornographic material or watching sexual activities, or encouraging children to behave in sexually inappropriate ways.

Most perpetrators of sexual abuse are known to the child, and are likely to be family, friends or acquaintances (Finklehor et al, 1990). Typically, the perpetrator slowly builds up a relationship with the child using coercion and sometimes violence (emotional or physical) to persuade the child to engage in sexual activity. The first touch is likely to appear accidental, or be related to tickling or play, but touch becomes steadily more sexually invasive and more frequent over time, as the child becomes desensitised (Finklehor et al, 1986). This process is known as *grooming*, and children are encouraged to keep the activities secret by either threats or promises. It may be a long time (or post childhood) before a child discloses the abuse (Corby, 2006).

Perpetrators of abuse may abuse large numbers of children over their lifetimes, and some organise social contacts to gain access to children, so that they can abuse them (Munro, 2007). This might be through full-time work with children or helping with children's organisations such as scouts or girl guides, Sunday schools or after-school clubs in a voluntary capacity. Organisations are now becoming more aware of the risks, and most organisations have arrangements in place to try to minimise the risk of employing perpetrators, requiring criminal bureau checks to ensure that potential employees have not previously been prosecuted for offences to children.

Following the Bichard Inquiry Report (HOC, 2004), regulated activity and controlled activity have been identified within the Safeguarding Vulnerable Groups Act 2006. Those carrying out specified activities such as teaching, care, supervision, advice, treatment and transport, and any activity bringing an individual into contact with children or vulnerable adults that is frequent, intense and/or overnight, and those with specified positions of responsibility, such as school governors, will have to be checked via the Criminal Records Bureau and enter the register of the Independent Safeguarding Authority (ISA) which will replace Protection of Children Act (POCA) and Protection of Vulnerable Adults (POVA), List 99. Employers have a duty to check their employees are not barred from working with these vulnerable groups. However while independent workers (such as music teachers) and workers in domestic employment circumstances (such as nannies) will not need to be registered with the ISA, parents will have the right to check the ISA list and if the independent worker/domestic employee is not registered, make a decision whether to proceed to employment, or take their business elsewhere (Singleton, 2007). However Webb-Jenkins (2007) noted that because this is a substantial change to current practice, the government planned a phased introduction, with completion due, at the earliest, by the end of 2008 to enable any problems to be dealt with and any amendments to the Act or alterations to the ISA role to be made as required. As this chapter goes to press, further delays are expected. Meanwhile the current CRB, list 99, POCA and POVA checks for people employed to work with children and vulnerable adults remain.

However, many perpetrators are not discovered, or prosecutions fail to secure convictions, and therefore their records remain unblemished (Corby, 2006), so this is not a foolproof method of preventing abusers from gaining access to children.

Information on sexual abuse is generally obtained through disclosure by the child, although there may also be other emotional and occasionally physical indicators present before disclosure takes place, as identified below. If a child begins to disclose information, practitioners need to be careful not to pose any leading questions as this might lead to evidence being disregarded in court at a later date. Children are very anxious when disclosing any kind of abuse, and may worry about losing control (Corby, 2006). Children who have been sexually abused also feel shame (Finklehor and colleagues, 1986), so it is important that practitioners listen and respond with sensitivity. If the perpetrator is known to the child, the child may be more reluctant to disclose, fearing the potential consequences for family dynamics after the disclosure. The primary concern is always protection of the child, and the child needs to know what is likely to happen and what actions the practitioner is going to take (Corby, 2006; HMG, 2006; DfES/DH/HO, 2003).

⚠ Professional alert!

Children may retract their allegations after disclosure, as they feel vulnerable and worry about losing control. This is a recognised response, and it is important to maintain acceptance of the child while referring on allegations.

The internet and mobile phone technology have enabled abusers to link together to improve access to children. Internet abuse is becoming a rapidly growing problem on an international scale:

- Abusers may 'meet' children through internet chat rooms and conduct their grooming online, arranging a meeting for abuse to take place at a later time when the contact is well established (Durkin, 1997).
- There is a large quantity of online child pornography. Some of the images used are genuine videos or photographs of exploited children, while others are created by technological processes (Quayle and Taylor, 2002). Some men might use these images in place of physical contact with a child (Quayle and Taylor, 2002). However, there is some evidence to suggest that people who access the materials may themselves have their inhibitions desensitised and go on to abuse children directly (Gallagher et al, 2006; Cooper et al, 1999).
- Images may be used to encourage sexual participation in a child, stimulate arousal and show the child how the perpetrator wishes the child to behave (Healy, 1997). Tate (1990) reports that images which feature the child may be used to ensure the child's silence, with threats of showing the images to authority figures or publishing the images against the child's wish.
- Children or young people themselves might be accidentally or deliberately exposed to harmful images (Munro, 2007).
- The internet has enabled paedophiles to form large social networks, allowing communication and collaboration with each other (Quayle and Taylor, 2002; Gallagher et al, 2006).
- Some sites are being used to bully or harass children (Munro, 2007). This is not limited to sexual abuse, and might include scenes of children bullying other children, or children bullying adults (such as teachers), or adults harassing, bullying and controlling children.

Neglect

Neglect is defined in *Working Together to Safeguard Children* (HMG, 2006: 39) as:

> The persistent failure to meet a child's basic physical and/or psychological needs, likely to result in the serious impairment of the child's health or development. Neglect may occur during pregnancy as a result of maternal substance abuse. Once a child is born, neglect may involve a parent or carer failing to provide adequate food or clothing, shelter including exclusion from home or abandonment, failing to protect a child from physical and emotional harm or danger, failure to ensure adequate supervision including the use of inadequate caretakers, or the failure to ensure access to appropriate medical care or treatment. It may also include neglect of, or responsiveness to, a child's basic emotional needs.

Neglect is now the most frequent category of registration for child protection (Stevenson, 1998; Howe, 2005). There is a stronger correlation between neglect and deprivation (Browne and Lynch, 1998) than for other forms of abuse. Often, the child is neglected in more than one area of care, and it is the complex combination of unmet needs that increases the risk to the child. Long-term interventions are frequently needed, and children might enter and leave the Child Protection Register several times during their childhood (Stevenson, 1998).

Stevenson notes that it is rare for families to deliberately neglect a child. Generally, neglect arises from dysfunctional parenting styles, and is often associated with parents who have unrealistic expectations of their children and/or a chaotic lifestyle.

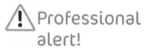

Professional alert!

Some contextual factors significantly increase the risk of a child being neglected:

- social isolation
- larger family size
- single-parent families
- parent(s) with low educational achievement, or learning difficulties
- parent(s) with persistent mental health illness
- substance abuse (including alcohol abuse)
- domestic violence.

Signs of abuse

Common injuries suggestive of physical abuse are:

- Black eyes.
- Grasp marks/fingermarks in clusters to cheeks, upper arms, forearms, legs or chest.

- Petechial haemorrhages across face, neck and chest – associated with slapping and smothering.
- Direct impression outline bruising, delineating an implement such as a belt.
- Bruises of different ages.
- Bruising in uncommon sites, such as the back, inside of legs, buttocks, inside mouth, cheek, ear, abdomen, chest, under arm, genitals or rectal areas.
- Rib fractures (which are usually only present with major trauma such as a road traffic accident), or skull fractures (uncommon in falls of 3 feet or less).
- Previous fractures of different ages. A skeletal survey is usually performed when abuse is suspected and the child is aged less than 2.
- Subdural haematoma (usually caused by shaking) particularly in babies. The signs of this are sudden collapse, fits, or the child is drowsy and or vomiting, followed by an enlarging head.
- Tear to the frenulum.
- Bites (assessment by a specialist dentist is needed as soon as possible after presentation).
- Burns and scalds, in which an object outline might be apparent. Care needs to be taken to distinguish cigarette burns from impetigo, as both can present as small round marks of full skin thickness depth. (Impetigo usually heals quickly when treated but burns take longer to heal and may cause scarring.)

(adapted from Dale, Green and Fellows, 2005)

Health professionals' concerns may be increased if the description of the cause of the injury does not appear to match the physical nature of the injury. For example, a 'black eye' is highly unlikely to be caused by falling to the floor, as the bone around the eye socket protects the eye area from bruising, and the bruising would then be to the nose and possibly forehead, rather than the inner eye orbit. In order to create bruising which includes the whole eye socket, something needs to enter the eye orbit, and this rarely happens accidentally (although occasional unusual injuries do occur).

Possible physical indicators for sexual abuse are:
- female genital circumcision or mutilation (which is unlawful in the UK)
- pain in the genital or anal area
- recurrent pain on passing urine or faeces
- vaginal/penile discharge
- sexually transmitted infections
- bleeding from the genital/anal area (the child may try to hide their underwear to avoid this being noticed)
- pregnancy, with vague references to the father or a refusal to identify the father.

Possible indicators of emotional abuse are:
- children used by violent men to intimidate their wives (continuation of domestic violence), even after separation
- children expected to do inappropriate household tasks for their age
- children who show low self-esteem, anger, withdrawal, apathy, clinging or attention-seeking behaviour, and/or have poor growth and delayed social and language development, with poor concentration at school
- bed wetting, smearing or sleep disturbances.

Possible physical indicators of neglect are:
- failure to thrive, a child who is undernourished and underweight
- red or purple mottled skin on hands and feet in winter
- inappropriate clothing for the weather conditions
- abnormal appetite
- recurrent diarrhoea
- loss of hair, or poor skin condition with possible repeated skin infections
- untreated infections or other medical conditions
- apathy, listlessness.

Part
II

Behavioural signs relating to physical, sexual, emotional or abuse or neglect include:

- Inappropriate sexual behaviour or knowledge for the child's chronological age, or provocative sexual behaviour with adults (which usually signifies sexual abuse).
- Reluctance to participate in physical activities, or to undress for school sports and similar activities (which usually signifies sexual or physical abuse).
- The child sexually abusing other children. (This usually signifies sexual abuse of the child abuser, but may also be related to severe neglect: Masson and Erooga, 1999.)
- Running away from home (this is least common in cases of neglect, but may happen with any form of abuse).
- Self-mutilation and/or suicide attempts (which most frequently relate to sexual or emotional abuse).
- Eating disorders (which are common in sexual abuse in particular, but also found with neglect and emotional abuse).
- Withdrawal, regression, bedwetting, soiling or severe sleep disturbances.
- Poor concentration and/or learning difficulties (which may be present with any form of abuse).
- Loss of self-esteem, which may be present with any form of abuse. When it is accompanied by a reluctance to use mirrors, it most commonly relates to sexual abuse.
- Depression, which can be present with any form of abuse.
- The child might be either unresponsive or over-affectionate with adults, and tends to be nondiscriminating in relationships. This particularly relates to emotional abuse and/or neglect, although it is sometimes present with other forms of abuse.

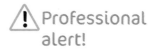

Professional alert!

Some of the behavioural signs listed can occur in children who have not been abused. For example, some children are naturally clingy, or experience sleep disturbance at times. Bed wetting too may be familial rather than a sign of abuse or neglect.

Parental and family behaviour that can be suggestive of abuse occurring includes:

- evidence of hostility towards the child; constant criticism or rejection of the child (emotional abuse)
- siblings who continue hostility towards the child (which suggests emotional abuse or violence in the family)
- a parent/carer who changes their manner with the child when they believe they are out of the hearing of professionals
- failure of a parent to seek medical help when needed, or to take young children for immunisations (suggests neglect)
- a parent's story that does not explain the injury or event, or is inconsistent over time
- parents who avoid professionals having contact with the child or the family (referred to as closure).

Parents may behave in unexpected ways when questioned over their child's condition or over actions they have taken. Sometimes they give responses which appear to indicate abuse even though they are innocent and no abuse has taken place. It is important that the whole picture is considered, taking into account the injury or presentation, what the child says, what the parents say and any other allegations that have been made or any other observations that professionals have made.

Learning activity

Which category of abuse would apply to Sam's situation? Consider your answer before reading on.

There are aspects of three categories – physical abuse, emotional abuse and neglect – in the scenario involving Sam and his family. However, professionals generally specify only one category of abuse or neglect when placing children on the Child Protection Register, although it is recognised that the categories are often interlinked (Corby, 2006; Howe, 2005; O'Hagan, 2006). In Sam's case the category of neglect is the most likely to be specified because his physical injury came as a result of his mother failing to provide adequate supervision.

Professionals must take a holistic approach when working towards meeting the needs of Sam and his family, addressing his physical needs – the aspect he presented with – as well as his emotional and development needs.

Record keeping

Good records provide information that is objective, and informative about events and investigations that have taken place. They include reported contacts and discussions about the concerns, including the time and date of attempted contacts. Poor record keeping has been shown to be a weak link in effective child protection in many case reviews and inquiries (Laming, 2003; Reder and Duncan, 1999; Reder et al, 1993).

Records must:

- be contemporaneous, dated, timed and signed with a printed name underneath the signature
- document who was present and where the incident (or observations) took place
- distinguish between first-hand observation, and observations reported by others
- avoid judgment and supposition
- use precise descriptions, avoiding vague language
- avoid the use of jargon or abbreviations
- note discrepancies between stories
- describe carefully any injuries observed, documenting the size, site and colour of bruising and drawing a body map if appropriate
- include any explanation given for the injuries
- document what was said and by whom, and what actions were then taken
- ideally, record any disclosures or reported allegations of abuse using the actual reported words used by the child or the person alleging abuse, as they may be used in court at a later date for either criminal or care proceedings.

Individual agencies use different structures to support record keeping. For example, nursing records may be based on particular theoretical models. Some records are held by clients (this is usual for community nursing, district nursing and midwifery) or by parents of young children (in the case of health visiting). Usually, information recorded in the client or parent-held records should match any information recorded by practitioners within the clinic base, unless this would compromise the safety of the child or parent (HMG, 2006).

Reporting

You might suspect abuse following a single incident, or concerns might grow over a long period of time. The situation needs to be considered in the context of the family's life, taking into account any disclosure, allegations, signs and symptoms of abuse or neglect, and both the child's story and the parents' story. Systems to record incidents and events or concerns chronologically may help to demonstrate ongoing and chronic failure to provide adequate parenting/care (Stevenson, 2007; Reder and Duncan, 1999).

It is natural for health professionals to feel anxious and uncertain about the judgements they are making (Powell, 2007; Stevenson,1998), and this is even more true of students and inexperienced practitioners. As a student you are in a unique position, in that you are responsible to both the professional organisation(s) with whom you have placements, and

---

a) Learning activity

As one of the health professionals caring for Sam, what would you include in your records to clearly demonstrate what has occurred and why you are concerned?

a) Learning activity

When next out on your placement, find out how the organisation's records are structured, and when health professionals are required to update the information recorded.

a) Learning activity

Writing accurate records will not change Sam's situation, unless other action is taken. What else needs to be done?

your educational organisation, but you are not in a position of employment. Yet you do have responsibilities in respect of safeguarding children (as all professionals do, under the Children Act 2004). Figure 16.2 provides guidelines for students who have any concerns about a child. Once you are a qualified professional you will need to follow the policies laid down by your employer, as these vary between organisations (for example role names may differ from those given here).

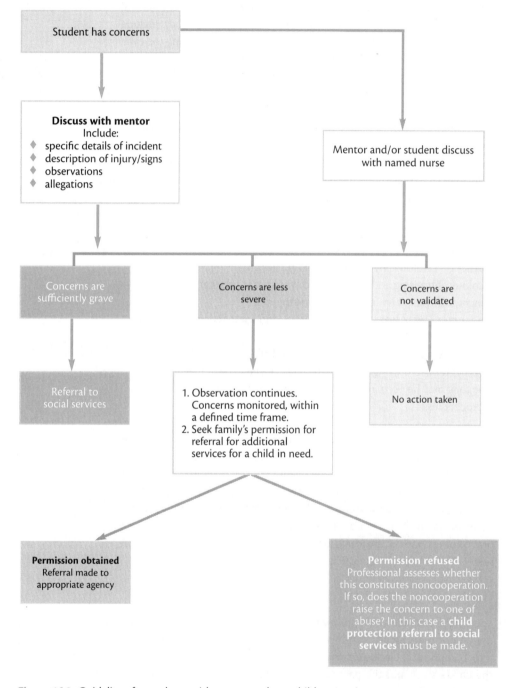

Figure 16.2 Guidelines for students with concerns about child protection

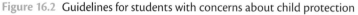

- Your responsibility as a student for your concerns about the child continues until you have discussed your concerns with the mentor and/or other professionals if required, and are aware that the appropriate process has been followed.

- Named and designated nurses, midwives and doctors are appointed by all NHS trusts, primary care trusts and foundation trusts to promote safeguarding children within their areas by offering advice, developing appropriate services for staff support or supervision, and providing training to facilitate staff awareness and understanding of safeguarding issues (HMG, 2006).
- All discussions need to be recorded in the child's records, including any decisions taken or outcomes suggested, detailing who is responsible for carrying out actions.

In England, Wales and Scotland, all health professionals are required by law to refer suspicions of abuse or neglect to social services, or to the police in an emergency situation (Children Act 2004). In Northern Ireland, policy guidance directs professionals to make referrals to social services where there are concerns about a child's welfare.

> **(a) Learning activity**
>
> You have discussed Sam's situation with your mentor, and the named nurse for safeguarding children within your trust, and they validate your concerns. The named nurse suggests that your mentor makes a referral to social services. What information would you include in your referral, and why? Consider your answer before you read on.

Making a referral

Practitioners need to discuss their intention to make a referral with both the child (if they are old enough to have sufficient understanding) and the child's family, unless this would potentially place the child at greater risk of harm. This may be difficult for practitioners who are often anxious about explaining to parents why their parenting is not considered to be good enough. However, it is important that children and parents are able to understand exactly what the issues are. The initial raising of concerns, if executed sensitively, can be an important step in helping the parents to begin to acknowledge and address issues to improve the welfare of their child or children (Stevenson, 2007). It also helps parents to appreciate the significance of parenting issues, and can facilitate their understanding at the beginning of a difficult process (Thoburn, Lewis and Shemmings, 1995).

- Referrals are made by the qualified practitioner responsible for providing care to the child, and not usually by a student healthcare practitioner.
- Referrals are made over the phone to social services, and followed up in writing within 24 hours (follow local procedures).
- There is often a structured approach taken to the written referral, which may use an assessment model, such as the *Framework for Assessing Children in Need and their Families* (DfES/DH/HO, 2000).
- Good record-keeping principles need to be followed when making a referral, such as clearly expressing precise concerns, and differentiating between suspicion of harm and facts, and between observations and allegations (refer back to page 301).
- A copy of the written referral is retained with the child's records. If the records are held by the family, the referring practitioner needs to keep a copy of their referral. Alarmingly, Buckley (2003) identified that the quality of the referral documentation is more important than the nature of the concern when social services determine whether to initiate inquiries.

What happens next?

Social services have a duty to investigate all referrals where there are identified concerns about a child's welfare (section 47, Children Act 1989, England and Wales). Social services may visit the family, talk to the child, and consult with professionals involved with the child and family to gather more information. Once a decision has been reached, social services will inform the referrer of action to be taken.

Strategy meetings may be held, and a case conference convened if it is thought that there is risk of harm to the child. Parents are invited to the case conference, and where children are of sufficient understanding, they are also included in the case conference process. Case conferences provide an opportunity for professionals to share information in a formal meeting, and to evaluate whether or not the child is being harmed or is at risk of being harmed. A decision is then taken on whether the child needs a protection plan. The case conference is followed by a planning meeting which allows professionals and the parents to set out objectives for change, and to develop a support plan to enable the parents to improve the child's well-being. Progress is formally evaluated at subsequent case conferences, and the plan is reviewed and amended when appropriate until sufficient improvement has been made. If the process is unsuccessful, care proceedings may be started to allow the child to be taken into the care of the local authority.

Multi-agency working

A range of agencies may be involved in the child protection process, depending on how many services the child and family have previously been involved with. Good inter-agency working facilitates improved outcomes for the child, but the inquiry reports following child deaths have identified failures in inter-agency working (Reder and Duncan, 1999; Laming, 2003).

Murphy identified a number of key elements that can interfere with inter-agency work (2004: 35):

- Perspective and culture: each professional group has differing perspectives on child protection, which influence their interpretation of data, and the way in which they respond. This may give rise to conflicts between professional groups.
- Role and responsibility: while some responsibilities are shared between organisations, others are different, and the way professionals negotiate overlap and difference sometimes causes tension.
- Stereotyping and prejudice: sometimes our predictions of what type of people take on particular roles or jobs influences our perceptions and interferes with information supplied.
- Professional and organisational priorities: professionals are more likely to give child protection a higher priority if safeguarding children is a fundamental part of their role. For instance, this is more true of social workers and paediatricians than of GPs and school teachers.
- Training: all professionals working with children are advised to have child protection training, but this forms a lower priority for some professional groups than for those who are spending significant amounts of time working with safeguarding children issues.
- Structure and power: different organisations operate in differing ways, and it can be difficult for practitioners to understand the systems operating in another organisation. There are also differences in how much weight is given to one practitioner's opinions and interpretations over another, and although case conferences are designed to try to overcome such power differences, they are not always successful.
- Language: use of language varies between agencies and can obscure rather than aid communication.
- The personal characteristics and anxiety of individual professionals also have an effect.

---

t☆
Practice tip

The who's who of child protection

The main organisations and individuals involved are:

- social services
- the police
- community health, which encompasses health visitors, school nurses, midwives, GPs and practice nurses
- acute health trusts: paediatricians, psychologists, nurses, and allied health professionals such as radiographers, speech therapists, physiotherapists and dieticians
- addiction services
- named and designated nurses for child protection
- education: early years workers, primary and secondary school teachers
- SureStart
- voluntary organisations
- probation services
- youth offending teams
- lawyers
- foster carers.

Recommendations for practice

- Be clear about your role and your responsibility, ensuring that there is a mutual understanding on what you will do, and what others in the multi-agency team will do.
- Respect other practitioners' views, but challenge these if you are in doubt.
- Keep other people informed about any changes, or any actions you have taken.
- Collaborate with other practitioners.
- Communicate effectively, respecting confidentiality where appropriate, without jargon.
- Consider collective judgements that have been made and re-evaluate them at regular intervals.
- Appraise at agreed timely intervals whether the plan for action is effective in improving outcomes for the child.
- Record all interagency communication, contact and assessments.

(adapted from Murphy, 2004)

Domestic abuse

[S] Scenario: Lizzie and her family

Lizzie is a 12-year-old girl who has recently moved to secondary school. Her form teacher is concerned that Lizzie has become more withdrawn over the first term at her new school, and notices that she is increasingly absent from school. She has spoken to Lizzie about this, but Lizzie said there was nothing wrong and became defensive, raising her voice and avoiding eye contact. She then said she needed to get home and rushed away.

At the next parents' evening, the teacher noticed that Lizzie's mother Dawn had four small (1 cm) bruises to the left side of her face and 1 x 1 cm bruise on her right cheek. She was heavily made-up, but there appeared to be some fading bruising to her left eye socket.

[a] Learning activity

Why might the teacher be concerned for Lizzie and for Dawn?

The Department of Health's definition of domestic violence is (DH, 2000: V):

> The term 'domestic violence' describes a continuum of behaviour ranging from verbal abuse, through threats and intimidation, manipulative behaviour, physical and sexual assault, to rape and even homicide. The vast majority of such violence, and the most severe and chronic incidents, are perpetrated by men against women *and their children* [our emphasis].

Signs of domestic violence mirror signs of child abuse, as listed above. Perpetrators use physical violence, intimidation and emotional blackmail, sexual abuse and even neglect to control and abuse their victims. In addition, financial constraints (another form of abuse) may be used to prevent the victim leaving or to increase intimidation and control.

The effects of domestic violence are wide-ranging to both the adult victim and their children. This chapter explores the effects on the welfare of the child, and examines the practitioner's responsibilities. Refer to the next chapter for more detailed exploration of the effects on the adult victim.

Domestic violence is an important issue for children. There is an abundance of literature and studies exploring the effects of domestic violence on women (DH, 2005; Bewley, Friend and Mezey, 1997). Many mothers think they protect their children against the violence, but research indicates that children are aware of what is happening, and even when children are

Part
II

not present at abusive incidents, the abusive environment is damaging to children's emotional health (Mullender, 2000).

- Violent incidents increase in number and severity during pregnancy, posing a threat to the unborn fetus (Bewley et al, 1997).
- Children may not see abuse but they hear the abuse, and imagining what is happening causes psychological distress to the child (Mullender, 2000).
- Children are present in most violent incidents (85–90 per cent), and in more than 50 per cent of incidents, children were also abused (Cleaver, Unell and Aldgate, 1999).
- Older children may get hurt while trying to intervene during an abusive incident (NCH, 1994).
- Children may be drawn into the abuse themselves, either engaging in verbal or physical assaults on their mothers, or trying to conceal assaults from others. An atmosphere of secrecy ensues, increasing vulnerability (Cleaver et al, 1999; McGee, 2000).
- Children are used as a method of keeping the mother silent, as the perpetrator makes threats that the child will be taken away from her or that they will be hurt if the mother does not comply, or if she reports the abuse (Mullender et al, 2002).
- Children may take inappropriate responsibility for parenting younger siblings, particularly if their mother is unable to function as a parent through lowered self-esteem or depression, or through physical disability as a result of the abuse (Mullender et al, 2002).
- Children may be absent from school frequently, either because the abusing parent or the victim keeps them at home to maintain secrecy, or because the child tries to protect the parent who is being abused (Mullender et al, 2002).
- There are strong links between domestic violence and child abuse, so the risk of physical or sexual harm to the child is higher than for households where there is no domestic violence (Farmer and Owen, 1995; Gibbons, Conroy and Bell, 1995; Mullender et al, 2002; Reder and Duncan, 1999).
- Younger children may show developmental delay and/or behavioural difficulties, while older children may display difficulties in concentrating; sleep disturbances; regressive, aggressive, deviant or withdrawn behaviour; anxiety disorders or eating disorders (Mullender et al, 2002).
- Some children may echo the violence by bullying others at school or within the family.

S   Scenario continued

The teacher asked Dawn about the bruising to her face. Dawn said she fell down the stairs and must have bumped her cheek on the way down. The teacher said that the pattern of bruising Dawn had on her face could be caused by fingermarks, and that if Dawn wanted to talk to her at any time about someone harming her, she would be happy to listen and to try to arrange help, if Dawn wanted that. The teacher also said she had become recently concerned about Lizzie's behaviour. As Lizzie had denied that anything had upset her at school, the teacher wondered out loud whether there were difficulties at home. Dawn denied that there were any.

---

a   Learning activity

What ethical dilemmas do you think this situation poses for the teacher, given that Dawn has denied any problems?

What do you think the teacher should do next? Consider your reply before reading on.

The teacher might decide that she has not got enough information to act upon, given that Dawn has denied any abuse. However, we know that the observed injuries are highly suggestive of fingermark bruising, and that the explanation given for the injury is unlikely, as bony prominences such as shoulders and hips are more likely to have been injured through a fall. (Injuries to the face caused by a fall would commonly be on the forehead, and perhaps the nose and/or chin.) Injuries to an eye socket inevitably mean that something has penetrated the socket boundary, so again it is unlikely that this injury could have been caused by falling down the stairs. The teacher also needs to consider that Lizzie is showing disturbed behaviour so she is being affected emotionally, and could be at risk of harm. The teacher might choose to refer the case to social services on this basis, or she could talk to Lizzie again.

If it is known that there is domestic violence, and there are children in the household, a referral must be made to social services. The abused parent might prefer not to take action for themselves, but it is the practitioner's responsibility to ensure that children are protected from harm, and this takes priority over the abused parent's (usually the mother's) wishes. However, referrals need to be made sensitively to avoid placing either the victim or the child at greater risk. Often, social services and health professionals work together to ensure that visits are made at a time when the abuser is not present, and is unaware of social service involvement until a safe plan of action can be determined. A support package may be put in place to help the children and to try to alleviate the effects of the violence at home. If the child is assessed as being in direct danger, this might not be possible. In this instance, the abused parent is encouraged to leave the home and go to a place of safety to protect the child. If they are unable or unwilling to do this, care proceedings might be started (Calder, Harold and Howarth, 2004).

> ⚠ **Professional alert!**
>
> Both the child and the abused adult are likely to feel that they have little control over their lives. It is important the professionals talk to them both and keep them informed on what is happening. Lizzie and Dawn should know that a referral will be made to social services, and possibilities for protective and supportive care should be discussed with them before decisions are reached. The physical danger to the mother and child greatly increases once the abuser becomes aware that other professionals are involved.

Part

II

Bullying

Bullying has become a significant issue. A number of bullied children have attempted and/or have committed suicide. The Department of Health (HMG, 2006) states that professionals must not underestimate the effects bullying can have on children. Bullying has been defined (DH, 2006) as:

> Deliberately hurtful behaviour, usually repeated over a period of time, where it is difficult for those bullied to defend themselves. It can take many forms, but the three main types are physical (e.g. hitting, kicking, theft), verbal (e.g. racist or homophobic remarks, threats, name calling) and emotional (e.g. isolating an individual from the activities and social acceptance of their peer group).

Children usually experience bullying for long periods of time before any action is taken. This can lead to loneliness and school avoidance (Kochenderfer and Ladd, 1996), low self-esteem and increased risk of depression (Hawker and Boulton, 2000). Research also suggests they are at an increased risk of experiencing problems with relationships later in life (Smith et al, 2003). Bullying is not just an issue for secondary school children, but has also been found to occur within the primary age groups. Among the signs are increased reporting by the child of coughs, colds and sore throats, and high levels of behavioural and mental health problems (Wolke et al, 2001).

It has been recognised that good intervention programmes, such as a robust and enforced antibullying programme in schools, can successfully reduce the instances of bullying (HMG 2006; Smith et al, 2003).

> **ⓐ Learning activity**
>
> Reading the key national policy document for your country (refer to the key resources box on page 288) will help you to understand and familiarise yourself with good principles and necessary actions to safeguard children.
>
> Find your local safeguarding children's board website, and explore the contents, to find out what is expected of practitioners in your area.
>
> Who is the designated person (nurse or doctor) responsible for your health practice within your healthcare trust? Try to find their name and contact details on the local safeguarding children's board website.

Conclusion

Supporting children in need and safeguarding children in need of protection are areas of practice that cause anxiety to both new and experienced healthcare professionals. Fears of getting it wrong, or not doing enough, are common issues raised. Evidence from the many inquiries where professionals have failed children demonstrates two key areas. Firstly, all healthcare professionals should be aware of the factors that could indicate that a child is in need, or in need of protection, so that these are not missed or dismissed. Second, health professionals must follow the policies and protocols laid out by government and employers to enable a thorough and accurate assessment, and then fulfil their part when the most appropriate action is agreed, to ensure a positive outcome for the child and family. Health professionals should seek support through support mechanisms such as clinical governance and supervision to ensure they too are supported in what can be an emotionally challenging area of practice.

References

Acheson, D. (1998) *Independent Inquiry into Inequalities in Health*, London, HMSO.

All Wales Area Child Protection Committees (2005) *All Wales Child Protection Procedures*, Cardiff, Wales Child Protection Review Group.

Awadallah, N., Vaughan, A., Franco, K., Munir, F., Sharaby, N. and Goldfarb, J. (2005) 'Munchausen by proxy: a case, chart series, and literature review of older victims', *Child Abuse and Neglect* **29**(8), 931–41.

Barber, M. A. and Davis, P. M. (2002) 'Fits, faints, or fatal fantasy? Fabricated seizures and child abuse', *Archives of Disease in Childhood* 86, 230–3.

Bewley, S., Friend, J. and Mezey, G. (eds) (1997) *Violence Against Women*, London, Royal College of Gynaecologists and Obstetricians.

Brent Borough Council and Brent Health Authority (1985) *Jasmine Beckford: A child in trust. Report of the Panel of Inquiry into the Circumstances Surrounding the Death of Jasmine Beckford*, presented to Brent Borough Council and Brent Health Authority.

Bowlby, J. (1969, 1973, 1980) *Attachment and Loss*, Vols 1, 2 and 3, London, Hogarth Press.

Browne, K. and Lynch, M. (1998) 'The challenge of child neglect', *Child Abuse Review* 7(2), 73–6.

Buckley, H. (2003) **C**hild Protection Work: Beyond the Rhetoric, London, Jessica Kingsley.

Buckley, H., Holt, S. and Whelan,S. (2007) 'Listen to me! Children's experiences of domestic violence', *Child Abuse Review* 16, 296–310.

Calder, M. with Harold, G. T. and Howarth, E. L. (2004) *Children living with Domestic Violence: Towards a framework for assessment and intervention*, Lyme Regis, Dorset, Russell House.

Cawson, P., Wattam, C., Brooker, S. and Kelly, G. (2000) *Child Maltreatment in the United Kingdom: A study of the prevalence of child abuse and neglect*, London, NSPCC.

Cleaver, H., Unell, I. and Aldgate, J. (1999) *Children's Needs – Parenting Capacity: The impact of parental mental illness, problem alcohol and drug use and domestic violence on children's development*, London, HMSO.

Coohey, C. (1996) 'Child maltreatment: testing the social isolation hypothesis', *Child Abuse and Neglect* 20, 241–54.

Cooper, A., Scherer, C. R., Boies, S. C. and Gordon, B. L. (1999) 'Sexuality on the Internet: from sexual exploration to pathological expression', *Professional Psychology: Research and Practice* **30**(2), 154–64.

Corby, B. (2006) *Child Abuse: Towards a knowledge base*, 3rd edn. Maidenhead, Berkshire, Open University Press.

Dale, P., Green, R. and Fellows, R. (2005) *Child Protection Assessment Following Serious Injuries to Infants: Fine judgments*, Chichester, John Wiley.

Department for Children, School and Families (2007) *Raising Expectations: Staying in education and training post 16, from policy to legislation*, London, HMSO.

Department for Education and Skills (DfES) (2004) *Every Child Matters*, London, HMSO.

DfES, Department of Health (DH), Home Office (2000) *A Framework for Assessing Children in Need and their Families*, London, HMSO.

DfES, DH, Home Office (2003) *What to do if You're Worried a Child is Being Abused*, London, HMSO.

DH (1995) *Child Protection: Messages from research*, London, HMSO.

DH (1999) *Working Together to Safeguard Children: A guide to inter-agency working to safeguard and promote the welfare of children*, London, HMSO.

DH (2000) *Domestic Violence: A resource manual for healthcare professionals*, London, HMSO.

DH (2003) *Tackling Health Inequalities: A programme for action*, London, HMSO.

DH (2005) *Responding to Domestic Abuse: A resource manual for health professionals*, London, HMSO.

Department of Health and Social Security (1974) *Report of the Committee of Inquiry into Care and Supervision Provided in Relation to Maria Colwell*, London, HMSO.

Department of Health, Social Services and Public Safety (DHSSPS) (Northern Ireland) (2003) *Co-operating to Safeguard Children*, Belfast, DHSSPS.

Donelly, M. and Robinson, J. (2006) 'Accident prevention', ch. 10 in Peate, I. and Whiting, L. (eds), *Caring for Children and Families.*, Chichester, Wiley.

Durkin, K. (1997) 'Misuse of the internet by paedophiles: implications for law enforcement and probation practice', *Federal Probation* **61**(2), 14–18.

Farmer, E. and Owen, M. (1995) *Child Protection Practice: Private risks and public remedies*, London, HMSO.

Finklehor, D., Araji, S., Baron, L., Browne, A., Peters, S. D. and Wyatt, G. E. (eds) (1986) *A Sourcebook on Child Sexual Abuse*, Thousand Oaks, Calif., Sage.

Finklehor, D., Hotaling, G., Lewis, I. and Smith, C. (1990) 'Sexual abuse in a national survey of adult men and women: prevalence characteristics and risk factors', *Child Abuse and Neglect* 14, 19–28.

Gallagher, B., Fraser, C., Christmann, K. and Hodgson, B. (2006) *International and Internet Child Sexual Abuse and Exploitation*, Research Report, Centre for Applied Childhood Studies, University of Huddersfield and Nuffield Foundation.

Garbarino, J. (1982) *Children and Families in their Social Environment*, New York, Aldine.

Gibbons, J., Conroy, S. and Bell, C. (1995) *Operating the Child Protection System*, London, HMSO.

Gillham, B., Tanner, G., Cheyne, B., Freeman, I., Rooney, M. and Lambic, A., (1998) 'Unemployment rates, single parent density, and indices of child poverty: their relationship to different categories of child abuse and neglect', *Child Abuse and Neglect* 22, 79–90.

Gray J. (2002) 'National policy on the assessment of children in need and their families', in Ward H. and Rose, W. (eds), *Approaches to Needs Assessment in Children's Services*, London, Jessica Kingsley.

Hawker, D. S. J. and Boulton, M. I. (2000) 'Twenty years' research on peer victimisation and psychosocial maladjustment: a meta-analytic review of cross-sectional studies', *Journal of Child Psychiatry and Psychology* 41, 441–55.

Healy, M. A. (1997) *Child Pornography: An international perspective*, Stockholm, World Congress Against Commercial Exploitation of Children.

Her Majesty's Government (HMG) (2006) *Working Together to Safeguard Children*, London, HMSO.

House of Commons (HOC) (2004) *The Bichard Inquiry Report*, London, The Stationery Office.

Howe, D. (2005) *Child Abuse and Neglect: Attachment, development and intervention*, Basingstoke, Palgrave Macmillan.

Jarvis, C. (2002) 'Nutrition', chapter 7 in Polnay, L. (ed.), *Community Paediatrics*, Edinburgh, Churchill Livingstone.

Kendrick, D. (2002) Chapter 22 in Polnay, L. (ed.), *Community Paediatrics*, Edinburgh, Churchill Livingstone.

Kendrick, D. and Marsh P. (2001) 'How useful are sociodemographic characteristics in identifying children at risk of unintentional injury?' *Public Health* 115(2), 103–7 in

Kochenderfer, B. and Ladd, G. (1996) 'Peer victimisation: cause or consequence of school maladjustment?' *Child Development* 67, 1305–17 (also as ch. 7 in Smith, P. K., Cowie H. and Blades M. (2003) *Understanding Children's Development*, 4th edn, Oxford, Blackwell).

Laming, Lord (2003) *The Victoria Climbié Inquiry: Report of an inquiry by Lord Laming*, London, HMSO.

Main, M. (1990) 'Cross-cultural studies of attachment organization: recent studies, changing methodologies, and the concept of conditional strategies', *Human Development* 33, 48–61.

Masson, H. and Erooga, M. (1999) 'Children and young people who sexually abuse others: incidence, characteristics, causation', in Erooga, M. and Masson, H. (eds), *Children and Young People who Sexually Abuse Others: Challenges and responses*, London, Routledge.

McGee, C. (2000) *Childhood Experiences of Domestic Violence*, London, Jessica Kingsley.

McKears, J., Reynolds, M., Forester, S. and Middleton J. (2005) 'Contemporary influences in safeguarding children', in Robotham, A. and Frost, M. (eds), *Health Visiting: Specialist community public health nursing*, 2nd edn, Edinburgh, Elsevier.

Mullender, A. (2000) *Reducing Domestic Violence – what works? Meeting the needs of children*, London, Policing and Reducing Crime Unit.

Mullender, A., Hagues, G., Imam, U., Kelly, L., Malos, E. and Regan, L. (2002) *Children's Perspectives on Domestic Violence*, London, Sage.

Munro, E. (2007) *Child Protection*, London, Sage.

Murphy, M. (2004) *Developing Collaborative Relationships in Interagency Child Protection Work*, Lyme Regis, Dorset, Russell House.

National Children's Homes (NCH) (1994) *The Hidden Victims: Children and domestic violence*, London, NCH.

O'Hagan, K. (2006) *Identifying Emotional and Psychological Abuse: A guide for childcare professionals*, Maidenhead, Berkshire, Open University Press.

Parton, N. (1997) 'Child protection and family support: current debates and future prospects', in Parton, N. (ed.), *Child Protection and Family Support: Tensions, contradictions and possibilities*, London, Routledge.

Powell, C. (2007) *Safeguarding Children and Young People: A guide for nurses and midwives*, Maidenhead, Berkshire. Open University Press.

Quayle, E. and Taylor, M. (2002) 'Paedophiles, pornography and the internet: assessment issues', *British Journal of Social Work* 32, 863–75.

Reder, P. and Duncan, S. (1999) *Lost Innocents: A follow-up study of fatal child abuse*, London, Routledge.

Reder, P., Duncan, S. and Gray, M. (1993) *Beyond Blame: Child abuse tragedies revisited*, London, Routledge.

Robertson, J. (1953) *A Two-Year Old Goes into Hospital*, a scientific film record, Ipswich, Concord Film Council.

Robertson, J. (1955) 'Young children in long term hospitals', *Nursing Times*, 23 September, pp. 63–5.

Robertson, J. (1969) *John, 17 Months, 9 Days in a Residential Nursery*, film, London, Tavistock Institute for Human Relations.

Robertson, J. (1970) *Separation and the Very Young*, London, Free Association.

Robotham, A. (2005) 'Violence – debating the issues', in Robotham, A. and Frost, M. (eds), *Health Visiting: Specialist community public health nursing*, Edinburgh, Elsevier.

Scottish Executive (2004) *Protecting Children and Young People: Framework for standards*, Edinburgh, Scottish Executive.

Secretary of State for Social Services (1988) *Report of the Inquiry into Child Abuse in Cleveland*, Cmnd 412, London, HMSO.

Singleton R. (2007) 'Child protection: the contribution of statutory barring', paper presented at the 'Safeguarding Children? Current debate – Future Prospects' conference, University of Huddersfield, 7 September 2007.

Smith, P. K., Cowie, H. and Blades, M. (2003) 'Play', chapter 7 in *Understanding Children's Development*, 4th edn, Oxford, Blackwell.

Stevenson, O. (1998) *Neglected Children: Issues and dilemmas*, Oxford, Blackwell.

Stevenson, O. (2007) *Neglected Children and their Families*, 2nd edn, Oxford, Blackwell.

Sullivan, P. M. and Knutson, J. F. (2000) 'Maltreatment and disabilities: a population based epidemiological study', *Child Abuse and Neglect* 24(10), 1257–73.

Tamay, Z., Akcay, A., Kilic, G., Peykerli, G., Devecioglu, E., Ones, U. and Guler, N. (2007) 'Corrosive poisoning mimicking cicatricial pemphigoid: Munchausen by proxy', *Child Care, Health and Development* 33(4), 496–9.

Tate, T. (1990) *Child Pornography*, London, Methuen.

Thoburn, J., Lewis, A. and Shemmings, D. (1995) *Paternalism or Partnership? Family involvement in the child protection process*, London, HMSO.

UNCRC (1989) *United Nations Convention on the Rights of the Child*, Geneva, United Nations.

Wanless, D. (2002) *Securing our Future Health: Taking a long term view*, London, HM Treasury.

Webb-Jenkins, C. (2007) 'Safegurding Vulnerable Groups Act 2006: an overview', *Protecting Children* update, February [online] http://

Part

II

www.teachingexpertise.com/articles/the-safeguarding-vulnerable-groups-act-2006-an-overview-1598 (accessed 29 December 2008).

Wolke, D., Woods, S., Bloomfield, L. and Karstadt, L. (2001) 'Bullying involvement in primary school and common health problems', *Archive Disease of Childhood* 85, 197–201.

World Health Organisation (2003/04) *World Report on Violence and Health* [online] www.who.int/entity/violence_injury_ prevention/violence/global_campaign/en/chap3.pdf (accessed 6 December 2008).

Legislation

Children Act 1989
Children Act 2004
Safeguarding Vulnerable Groups Act 2006

Chapter

17

Safeguarding adults

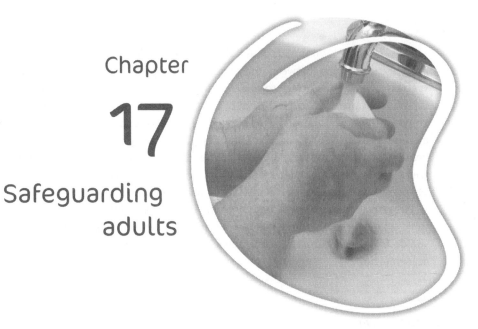

Melanie Robbins, Hilary McCluskey
and Jenny Dedmen

 Links to other chapters in *Foundation Studies for Caring*

 Links to other chapters in *Foundation Skills for Caring*

W   Don't forget to visit www.palgrave.com/glasper for additional
online resources relating to this chapter.

Introduction

This chapter explores domestic abuse, abuse to vulnerable adults and elder abuse, considering links and differences between the concepts. All health professionals, regardless of their speciality (which may relate to adults, children, people with mental health difficulties or those with learning difficulties) need to know about safeguarding both children and adults. You might hear allegations of abuse from neighbours, friends and relatives, or observe abuse in visitors to the people you would normally be working with. There are some similarities between abuse to adults and abuse to children, and to avoid repetition, the chapters are cross-referenced where these similarities occur. It is therefore important that both this chapter and Chapter 16 on 'Safeguarding children' are read in conjunction with one another.

Please note: as with the issues raised in 'Safeguarding children' this can be a distressing topic, and you could find the material disturbing personally. This is a natural reaction, and if you do find yourself upset by the material, you should access the support of your personal or academic tutor.

Learning outcomes

This chapter will enable you to:

- define the terms elder abuse and neglect
- describe the different types of abuse and neglect and develop an awareness of some of the key indicators
- develop an awareness of the stereotypes surrounding older people and how they relate to elder abuse
- explore the concept of vulnerability and what this may mean to you and others
- develop an understanding of the complex issues relating to power relationships and how these affect the older adult
- identify and describe one assessment tool that could provide documentary evidence to indicate potential harm to an older adult
- understand your role as a student in the recognition and reporting of suspected cases of elder abuse.

Concepts

- Social context of definitions with regard to the term 'elderly'
- Vulnerability
- Stereotypes
- Legislation and policy
- Elder abuse including domestic violence
- Safeguarding adults
- Health professional role
- Multi-agency working

Abuse and neglect can occur at any time across the lifecycle, from childhood (refer to Chapter 16) through adulthood and into old age. Some individuals have repeated experiences of abuse across their lifespans, while others' initial experiences of abuse occurs in domestic situations. It might be perpetrated by their partners (boyfriend, girlfriend or spouse), or by siblings, sons or daughters (in which case it is known as *domestic violence* or domestic abuse). There are also those who have successful and fulfilling relationships for most of their lives, but who are at increased risk of abuse as they become more frail and dependent on carers, who might be paid, voluntary or family members (in which case it is known as *abuse to vulnerable adults*). Manthorpe and colleagues (2007) surveyed 2111 people over 65 living in their own homes (in the community), and found that 2.6 per cent reported experiences of abuse or neglect during the last year. Neglect by partners significantly increased over the age of 85, and Manthorpe and colleagues (2007) hypothesised that this was because of the increasing frailty of both partners, leading to an inability to continue to provide support for each other.

Professionals have for many years been attempting to respond to the large numbers of individuals in our society who perpetrate or experience domestic violence (more recently renamed *domestic abuse*), and a significant number of voluntary organisations have emerged to take on specific roles within this complex arena. Public awareness of domestic abuse (violence) has changed rapidly around the turn of the millennium, in response to increased media reporting and campaigns to raise awareness. In response to developing roles, policy guidelines now provide clear recommendations for practice, and some changes have been made to the law to improve protection.

Until recently, abuse to vulnerable adults and elder abuse had received little public attention, with few cases of exploitation, humiliation or abuse being reported by the media. *Hidden Voices* (Action on Elder Abuse, 2004) identifies that 78 per cent of elder abuse occurs over the age of 70 years. Richardson, Kitchen and Livingston (2002) observed that until recently, the focus of attention has been on the characteristics of the abuser rather than protecting the abused. Kalache, coordinator of the World Health Organization (WHO) ageing and life course unit, argues that 'we are today where we were 20 years ago on child abuse and violence against women' (2002). Some have argued that this is because communities in our society are less concerned about older adults, or those with disabilities, than they are about children. The reality might be different, as it could be that the public are too shocked to conceive that individuals are deliberately abusive or neglectful to elderly people (Agnew, 2006). Help the Aged (cited in Agnew, 2006) found that when people were asked to mention social issues that concerned them, elder abuse was not recognised as an issue. The same individuals changed their responses after being shown cards outlining a number of issues including this one: elder abuse was then identified as one of the most important issues.

What is vulnerability?

a) Learning activity

Think about what vulnerability means to you. How does this relate to:

- age?
- a person's ability to care for themselves?
- a person's ability to protect themselves from harm?
- a person's ability to earn money and make financial choices?
- a person's ability to be able to make friends, socialise and/or take part in communal activities?

In carrying out the learning activity you might have decided that children are usually more vulnerable than adults, perhaps because they cannot protect or care for themselves, and because they have no or limited ability to make financial choices. However, using age alone as a way of identifying vulnerability poses problems. When does a person move from being a child into an adult? For the purpose of adult nursing, an adult is defined as somebody who has attained 18 years of age (Brooker and Nichol, 2003) – but unfortunately, a young person who has suffered abuse might continue to be abused after they reach this age. In law, this abuse would no longer be regarded as child abuse, even though the victim and the perpetrator are the same individuals. A person might not feel any more able to protect themselves on the day after their 18th birthday than they did two days earlier.

Perhaps you also consider that ageing makes people more vulnerable to abuse. Generally, 65 years is the most frequently used social construction of old age in our society. This is the age when men and women are expected to retire, and the time at which people may expect to draw a pension, or receive a local bus pass for free or subsidised fares. However, some hospitals do not admit people to their care of the elderly wards unless they are over 75, and the level of benefits changes at 75, as people are able to claim an enhanced heating allowance during the winter, personal taxation rules change, and benefits relating to disability also differ. Alternatively, some organisations offering financial benefits (such as reduced prices for car or house insurance, or national bus tickets) use the age of 50 as their criterion. If being old makes people in the United Kingdom more vulnerable, which of these ages, if any, should be used as an indicator of when the risk increases?

a) Learning activity

- Identify a time in your life when you have felt vulnerable, frightened or unprotected.
- Reflect on what made you feel vulnerable at this time, identifying all the factors that contributed to your feelings.
- Did you take any unnecessary risks, or had you put yourself in some danger by ignoring previous advice given to you?

- Did you feel in any danger during the event?
- Were the circumstances outside your control, or did you feel as though they were?

Note down words to capture your answers, and use your response to try to work out a definition of what vulnerability is, from your perspective.

All adults feel vulnerable in particular situations, new events, new roles, or when taking on different responsibilities. Think about when you began your student role, moving away from home; this may have been a time when you felt vulnerable and unsure about yourself. However as individuals regain control, they adjust to the new situation and alter their thought processes to accommodate the changes in everyday life.

A definition of vulnerability

Going back to the Activities you may have decided that a person's function is important, and that people need to be able to make choices and decisions for themselves. Some people are automatically seen as vulnerable under such an interpretation. People who require the care and protection of others, and who are not fully independent, as a result of physical or cognitive impairment (that is, learning difficulties), or certain mental health difficulties (including people who abuse substances) are vulnerable as both children and adults. Ageing may lead to a decline in cognitive and physical ability, reducing a person's ability to make decisions or look after themselves, therefore increasing vulnerability.

The Department of Health defines a vulnerable adult as:

> A person who is or may be in need of community care by reason of mental or other disability, age or illness, and who is or may be unable to protect him or herself against significant harm or exploitation.
>
> (DH, 2000b: 8, 9)

Safeguarding Adults (ADSS, 2005) recognised that there is ambiguity in this definition. The definition emphasises adults who require community care services – that is, those adults who need health or social care support to maintain or achieve their independence, including unpaid carers, as well as individuals with learning disability or physical, sensory or mental impairments. In addition, the term 'vulnerable adults' may present difficulties as it could suggest that the vulnerability causes or explains the abuse. No one can be responsible for another's violence, and the cause of abuse always lies with the perpetrator, whatever the circumstances are.

The House of Commons Health Select Committee's inquiry into elder abuse (2004) called for an expansion of this definition of vulnerability, to include older adults experiencing abuse, but who do not need community care services, and who live in their own homes and are able to take care of themselves (paragraph 14). However, the government responded stating that its definition is wide, and includes individuals who receive either health or social care services; people who fall outside this definition and who are able to take care of themselves are covered by guidelines for domestic violence or other forms of harm (DH, 2004).

It is therefore important to stress the following points:

- Some independent adults experience harm from a person who is related to them or who lives with them or maintains a close relationship – this is domestic abuse or domestic violence.
- Some dependent adults (requiring community care) experience harm or neglect from a carer, or from a person who is related to them or who lives with them or maintains a close relationship – this is abuse/ neglect to vulnerable adults (and may include abuse of carers).
- Older people might experience abuse or neglect as above, which may be classed as either domestic violence or abuse/neglect to vulnerable adults, depending on whether or not the older person requires community care – this is frequently termed *elder abuse*.

The law and adult protection

a Learning activity

- Which pieces of legislation are you aware of that relate to individual safety?
- What types of actions by one person on another would you consider to be unlawful?

In England, Wales and Northern Ireland, adult protection is governed by community care legislation and related social service guidance, with application of criminal justice legislation for types of abuse which come under criminal offences:

> Substantially no new social services legislation was passed concerning adult protection, equivalent for example to child protection provisions contained in The Children Act 1989. Indeed, central government has failed to adopt proposals made by the Law Commission (1995) that local authorities should be given such protective powers in respect of adults.
>
> (Mandelstam, 2005: 402)

Responding to adult abuse or to the need for adults to be protected is therefore complex, and there are often a series of criteria to be met before certain laws can be applied, so some individuals are not protected by the law. For example, the court can apply inherent jurisdiction to intervene when people lack the capacity to make decisions for themselves, to protect them from self-neglect or neglect or abuse by others.

In England and Wales:

- The National Assistance Act 1948 allows people (with or without full mental capacity) to be removed from the home if they are not able to care for themselves or are not receiving adequate care, provided that the move is necessary to prevent injury.
- The Mental Health Acts allow detention under certain circumstances for assessment or treatment, if people have a mental disorder, and to procure the protection of the individual or of others. They also allow the appointment of guardians where appropriate and available.
- The Environmental Protection Act 1990, the Public Health Act 1936 and the Public Health Act 1961 can be used when it is necessary to abate issues that present a nuisance to the public or that cause potential health risks to others, such as excessive accumulation of verminous debris and filth.
- The Family Law Act 1996 provides for regulation on occupation of homes, and allows perpetrators of abuse to be removed from the home or to have restricted occupation rights. It can also cause termination of matrimonial home rights where abuse has been found. The court has to consider the respective needs of both parties and of children, whose welfare is paramount.
- Criminal offences include application of the Sexual Offences Act 2003, the Protection from Harassment Act 1997, the Domestic Violence, Crime and Victims Act 2004, the Theft Act 1968 (in cases of financial abuse) and also include offences of assault and battery, and manslaughter. Notably, there is no criminal offence of neglect to adults.

Scotland has a specific statute to protect adults, the Adult Support and Protection (Scotland) Act 2001, and the application of this legislation will develop over time.

> **a** Learning activity
>
> Look at your list from the earlier reflection. Does your list reflect the legislation above or are there any differences that surprise you?

Domestic abuse

Domestic abuse from the child's perspective was explored in Chapter 16. When someone mentions domestic abuse, the usual image (stereotype) is not a child or older person or even a man, but a young woman, usually from a lower socioeconomic group. Yet domestic violence can happen to anyone, from any culture, social class, age or gender, and forms 25 per cent of all violent crime (ADSS, 2005).

One useful definition is:

> Domestic violence is the 'continuum of behaviour ranging from verbal abuse, through threats and intimidation, manipulative behaviour, physical and sexual assault, to rape and even homicide. The vast majority of such violence and the most severe and chronic incidents, are perpetrated by men against women and their children.
>
> (DH, 2000a: V)

A later definition describes it as:

> Any incident of threatening behaviour, violence or abuse (psychological, physical, sexual, financial or emotional) between adults who are or have been intimate partners or family members, regardless of gender or sexuality.
>
> (ADSS, 2005: 10)

In 2005 the government stated that the term 'domestic abuse' should be used rather than 'domestic violence', as this terminology more easily incorporates the variety of abusive situations people find themselves in, whereas the term 'domestic violence' tends to lead people to consider the physical effects only. This section uses the term 'domestic abuse', but when referenced literature has used the term domestic violence (for instance in relation to crime statistics) that terminology is echoed here. Statistics rely on reported cases of domestic abuse, and as it is known that abuse is under-reported, they are an underestimation of actual cases.

> **S** Scenario: Valerie's case
>
> Valerie, aged 50, arrives at the local Accident and Emergency (A&E) department early on Sunday morning, with her friend Jane. She says she tripped in her slippers and fell down the stairs, late the previous night. Her arm has been hurting her since and so she thought she needed to 'get it checked'. She keeps apologising for taking up everyone's time, stating that she is just 'a silly middle-aged woman who doesn't look where she is going'. After examination the doctor suspects a broken shoulder and sends Valerie for an x-ray. The doctor notes that Valerie has been in A&E before with minor injuries, and every time she has claimed she has fallen, tripped or walked into objects.

> **a** Learning activity
>
> What do you think should be recorded about Valerie's injury and presentation?
>
> Referring to the material on reporting/record writing in Chapter 16, try to prepare a draft record of this event.

Although it is acknowledged that there are cases of domestic abuse being perpetrated on men by women or by same-sex partners (about 8 per cent of male murder victims are murdered by their female partners, according to Home Office *Criminal Statistics 2000/01*), 81 per cent of reported domestic violence is perpetrated by men against women (BMRB, 2004/05). The prevalence rates for domestic abuse are the same across all economic levels and ethnic backgrounds (Walby and Allen, 2004). Statistics suggest that one in four women will experience domestic abuse (Council of Europe, 2002) and that two to three women a week, in the United Kingdom, are murdered by a man they know (usually a partner or ex-partner). These deaths account for 42 per cent of women murder victims (Home Office, 2000/01). These figures have remained more or less constant, with almost 40 per cent of the female murder victims in 2003/04 being killed by their current or ex-partner (and about 5 per cent of male murder victims being killed by their partners in the same year) (Povey, 2005). Therefore this section concentrates on the needs of women experiencing domestic abuse.

⚠ Professional alert!

Healthcare professionals need to be cautious when interpreting statistics. For example, the figures of men killed by female partners and women killed by male partners are not directly comparable as there are many more male homicides in any one year than female homicides.

Health professionals need to be alert to the possibility of violence perpetrated by women on either male partners or relatives, or their female partners or relatives, and to the possibility of male to male violence between partners. There is also incidence of violence by adolescent children against their parents (Cottrell, 2001).

⌷S⌷ Scenario continued

Valerie returns from x-ray. The film confirms the doctor's provisional diagnosis: she has fractured her clavicle (shoulder). The radiographer's written comment says that she noticed some bruises on Valerie's upper body (chest and abdomen), which were a variety of colours, indicating that they were of differing ages. The doctor asks Valerie about the bruises and how she got them. Valerie starts to get flustered and tries to avoid answering the questions.

At times she appears confused about how the bruising occurred. The bruising was a result of the fall, she keeps insisting, and all her fault.

Valerie's friend Jane beckons the nurse to one side and says she is very concerned about Valerie, and the number of bruises and falls she has been having lately. Jane adds that if she hadn't called to collect Valerie for church that morning, Valerie would not have come in to A&E.

⌒a⌒ Learning activity

What is the health professional's responsibility here? If you were in this position, what would you do with Jane's statement? Is there any additional information you would want to collect, and where would you obtain it from? Consider your answer before reading on.

There are several elements that need to be assessed in Valerie's case.
- Her physical injury – her fractured clavicle will need treatment.
- Her bruising – the bruises should be documented, and mapped against a body chart, with size and colour noted. The bruising could be photographed.
- Valerie's confusion. An assessment needs to be made on whether this is caused by a medical issue or by psychological or emotional distress. It may also be an attempt to divert staff attention from the physical injuries, as by appearing confused, Valerie can avoid giving a coherent story or explanation.
- Jane's concern about Valerie and the number of falls she is having. Note that Jane has not raised concerns about Valerie being 'confused'.

Just as in safeguarding children in need of protection (see the section on record keeping/ documentation, page 301 in Chapter 16, for more detail), a key responsibility here is to document your observations and assessment accurately. Wherever possible, you should note the explanations Valerie provides and Jane's concerns using the exact phrases used by Valerie and Jane. The same principles of record keeping used in child protection situations apply in this situation.

It is not unusual for victims of domestic abuse to try to keep the abuse hidden. There are a number of possible reasons, including:

- embarrassment
- fear of not being believed
- feeling ashamed
- not knowing where to go or whom to ask for help
- fear that if they seek help it might make the situation worse
- anxiety about living on their own if the relationship breaks down or their partner is sent to jail
- fear about finances, both the amount of money they would have if the relationship broke down, and managing it themselves (if they did not do so within the relationship)
- the abuser having control of the family finances
- still loving the abuser
- in some cases, having experienced abuse for so long that they feel that their situation is 'normal'.

(adapted from DH, 2000a; ADSS, 2005)

⌐S⌐ Scenario continued

Valerie's husband Robert arrives at the A&E department. He appears to be very concerned that Valerie has been taken to hospital. He says he was not at home the previous night when she fell, and since he left home early that morning, he had not realised till then that Valerie was hurt. He also confirms Jane's statement that Valerie has been falling a lot lately, but adds she has always been clumsy, right from the beginning of their marriage.

Robert sits next to Valerie and talks continuously to her. The nurse tries to engage Valerie in conversation while she is taking some physical observations (temperature, pulse, blood pressure), but Robert keeps answering for her. Valerie avoids eye contact with the nurse or Robert, and appears to defer to him, even checking with him when she needs to use the toilet.

⌐a⌐ Learning activity

- How would Robert's behaviour make you feel?
- What strategies could you use to enable Valerie to answer for herself?

Domestic abuse, abuse to vulnerable adults and elder abuse include the same types of abuse outlined in Chapter 16 (please refer back to that chapter): that is, physical, sexual, emotional abuse and neglect, with the additional categories of psychological and financial abuse.

Table 17.1 outlines the different types of abuse and how these may manifest in a client/patient. As you can see, the signs and symptoms are wide and variable, but this does not remove your responsibility to look and listen to the client/patient's story to identify any of them so that appropriate action can be taken.

Many of the signs listed in Table 17.1 are generic to most types of abuse. In addition, the following factors should be considered and may arouse suspicion for the healthcare professional:

- The story or explanation given does not explain the injuries or the circumstances.
- The story changes over time, or it is retold in exactly the same way as though it has been rote-learned.

Table 17.1 **Signs and symptoms of abuse**

Abuse	Signs and symptoms
Physical abuse comprises:	
Hitting, slapping, smacking, punching, kicking	Bruising, which may be in shape of fist/hand or foot, or show fingermarks – often 1–1.5 cm apart, three or four bruises of about 1 cm diameter. May be multiple bruising of different colours/ages. Fractures – differing ages, no treatment sought; spiral fractures; repeated fractures; head injuries. Injuries to covered parts of body, or in sites where accidental injuries are uncommon, such as ear pinna, eye sockets, abdomen, inner thighs. Explanation does not match injury, or story is incoherent or changes over time.
Biting	Break in skin or bruising showing teeth marks which can often be clearly detected initially – may be in areas hidden by clothing.
Burning	Could be scalds, splashed burn marks – or may show shape of hot object pressed against skin. First, second or third-degree burns.
Pushing, throwing objects near someone, restraining	May or may not be signs of bruising; the victim may display fear when the perpetrator approaches.
Tying up, throwing objects at the person, using objects as weapons, strangling	May be bruising showing cord or object outlines.
Suffocation	Usually no signs, but there may be petechiae (small red pinprick threads on skin or whites of eyes) in extreme circumstances around the eyes and/or upper chest.
Stabbing/shooting	It can be difficult to detect stabbing if a long fine implement is pushed into the abdomen. Otherwise, bleeding, and wounds indicative of the weapon used.
Starving	Failure to thrive, signs of malnutrition such as thin hair, increased hair loss, poor skin condition, frequent fractures.
Genital mutilation	Injury to genitals – particularly common with female circumcision.
"Honour violence" – 'retribution' in some cultures where a woman's behaviour is deemed unacceptable	Dependent on type of violence.
Making the survivor work excessively	Signs of physical exhaustion.
Waking the survivor at night	Tiredness, irritability, irrational behaviour.
	General signs: may include poor health, poor nutrition, depression, eating disorders, suicide attempts, chronic pain, attempts to cover up the injury with clothing or make-up, fear, miscarriage. Incontinence (in the elderly).
Sexual abuse comprises:	
Forced sexual acts (no consent), such as rape, buggery, unwanted touching/oral sex, bondage, forced masturbation	There may be injury to genitals/breasts or other tissue suggesting physical force, or physical manipulation/injury; but often there are few signs. Presence of semen or blood in the genital area. Sexually transmitted diseases. Psychological distress including shame, humiliation and fear.

Part

II

Abuse	Signs and symptoms
Forcing the victim to participate in group sex, or have sex unwillingly in front of others, or forcing them to have sex with others while being watched	As above.
Forced prostitution	As above.
Ignoring religious prohibitions about sex	Encourages feelings of shame, humiliation and fear.
Refusal to practise safe sex	Pregnancy, sexually transmitted disease.
Sexual insults	Humiliation, shame and sometimes fear.
Preventing breastfeeding	May interfere with bonding. The woman has little control.
Forced pornographic involvement (may be shown images or filmed to make images)	Shame, humiliation, fear, may include public degradation.
Portraying sexual images on the internet/forcing use of sexual images on the internet/sexual bullying through internet chat sites	Any of these could occur in same-sex relationships as well as heterosexual relationships.
	General signs: Any sexual abuse may lead to self-harming, eating disorders, or even suicide attempts. There may be fear or reluctance at being asked to undress, or fear of male healthcare staff, or a reaction to being touched. Sometimes individuals may present in chaotic or inappropriate dress, with or without accompanying poor hygiene, to try to divert attention away from themselves by making themselves appear unattractive. There may also be a fear of using mirrors. Sleeping disorders are common. Lowered self-esteem, recurrent depression or unexplained physical pain (somatic). Pregnancy, termination of pregnancy, or miscarriage. Note that violence escalates during pregnancy (Mezey and Bewley, 2000). Midwives are now required to ask all women whether they are experiencing domestic abuse. Incontinence (particularly in the elderly).
Psychological and emotional abuse comprises:	
Intimidation, insulting, shouting, swearing, frightening, blaming, humiliation, denying the abuse, threatening to harm children or to take them away and/or report so-named 'inadequate' parenting to social services, enforcing a distorted perspective – no one will believe the victim, buying gifts to say sorry and create a feeling that it will be all right, or over a time a feeling of being unsure who to trust (fostering distrust of the person's judgements). Isolating a woman from friends and family, moving frequently, preventing a woman from learning English or from going to places alone where she may be able to ask for help, eroding independence. Keeping the person locked in a room, or removing mobility aids so they are unable to get around. Undermining confidence, making racist remarks.	**General signs for both psychological and emotional abuse:** Women usually experience lowered self-esteem. They may be depressed and appear withdrawn, or may present anger and hostility. Unexplained physical pain (somatic). Sleeping disorders, self-neglect. Eating disorders, particularly bulimia. Attempts at self-harming or suicide attempts. Lack of confidence, inability to make decisions, unsure of their own judgement. Attempts to justify the relationship or cover up the perpetrator's rudeness if it is displayed in public. Difficulties in socialising, fear. Incontinence (in the elderly).
Financial	
Not letting a woman work, undermining efforts to find work or study, refusing to give money, asking for an explanation of how every penny is spent, making her beg for money, gambling, not paying bills, using her money/valuables illegally, removing pension books or bank books.	Changes in demeanour or in possessions or in dress, obvious changes/restriction in spending power. Inability to afford food, which in extreme circumstances may lead to malnutrition. Inability to afford medication.

Abuse	Signs and symptoms
Neglect	
Deprivation of food, comfort, clothing, heat or medication	May be associated with emotional/psychological abuse (as well as other forms of abuse), or may be unintentional. For example, a daughter who is working full time and also acts as carer to a confused parent may fail to notice or not respond to the increasing needs of her parent, to the point of neglect. At this point, they may not be able to shop or feed themselves and may start to lose weight, or they may sit in wet clothes for portions of the day while the daughter is at work if they become incontinent, for example. Loss or excessive gain of weight. Unkempt appearance. Loss of false teeth, spectacles, hearing aids or mobility aids. Medical conditions which go unresolved for a long time because person has no access to health care, or written prescriptions are not 'exchanged' for medication. Failing to attend pre-arranged medical appointments, X-rays and so on. In the elderly or vulnerable, meals and drinks being placed out of reach of the person and then removed untouched. Lack of stimulation, not providing access to books, television and the like.

- There has been significant delay between the time of injury and seeking medical help.
- One partner appears to talk over the other partner, or appears to talk for the other partner – indicating undue exertion of control. The perpetrator will not leave their partner alone.
- One partner appears to be looking to the other partner all the time for permission to respond to questioning.
- Nonverbal signals do not match the verbal story. For instance, the victim might look away and not make eye contact while talking, or lean away from you when answering questions.
- The abused person may minimise the violence or take the blame on themselves.
- Fear, indicated again by nonverbal signals and body posture, or by moving suddenly when touched.
- The woman appears evasive, ashamed, embarrassed or apologetic (Campbell and Soeken, 1999).
- Frequent attendance at A&E.
- A functionally impaired patient who arrives without their main carer.
- The perpetrator might overtly threaten staff trying to treat the abused person.
- Alcohol/drug abuse (women experiencing violence are 15 times more likely than others to abuse alcohol and nine times more likely to abuse drugs: Stark and Filcraft, 1996).
- Suicide/parasuicide (women experiencing violence are five times more likely than others to attempt suicide: Stark and Flitcraft, 1996).

Looking at Valerie again, we can see that she clearly has some of the presentation aspects that should make us question her situation more closely:

- She has had frequent attendances at A&E.
- Her explanation of events is not consistent with her injuries (in fact her account is very confused).
- She blames herself.
- Robert will not let her answer for herself.
- She appears ashamed and/or embarrassed about her injuries.

Part II

a Learning activity

Which aspects of domestic abuse would you consider could be happening to Valerie?

You might hear people stating forcefully, 'Well, she chooses to stay,' or 'Why doesn't she leave him?' Look again at the types of abuse and the abusive acts, especially the physiological and emotional categories. It is difficult for women who feel everything is their fault, have low self-esteem, no money and nowhere to go, and who maybe fearful their partner will be able to find them if they leave and that things will be worse afterwards as a result, to find the courage and skills to plan to leave. The time immediately before and after a woman leaves an abusive home is the most dangerous in terms of the risk of a serious assault or murder (DH, 2005). Women often seek help from health services first, but do not always receive a supportive response (Du Plat-Jones, 2006).

James-Hanman (1998) found that many health professionals are reluctant to ask a woman whether she has experienced domestic abuse, even when they suspect abuse. Their fear of confrontation was explained as:

- Fear that they will not be able to respond appropriately to the situation and that it will exceed their ability to control.
- Lack of knowledge about the options available, or about local agencies that might be able to provide support.
- Concerns that questioning will cause offence.
- Fear of interfering, as some regarded this as a private matter between partners.
- Anxiety about the effects on a family, and particularly fear that they might be responsible for causing the break-up of a family.

Table 17.2 summarises some of the factors affecting disclosure of abuse by both men and women.

Table 17.2 Factors affecting male and female disclosure

Factors affecting female disclosure	**Factors affecting male disclosure**
Fear – the perpetrator may have threatened further violence if she asks for help.	Disempowerment – those in authority are reluctant to believe that a man is being abused by a female partner, and might mistrust what he is saying.
Shame: belief that the violence is her fault, or that it is normal among couples.	Shame: men feel ashamed because they cannot protect themselves from their partners.
Low self-esteem and powerlessness – repeated emotional and physical violence reduces a woman's belief in her ability to make decisions, and she comes to believe she does not deserve a life free from violence.	Police are more likely to believe a woman who accuses the man of being the aggressor, and men are then blamed and sometimes charged incorrectly.
A belief that the partner will change or that he intends to change. Episodes of violence are interspersed with episodes of calm which may be signalled by gifts and loving gestures from the perpetrator, and leave the woman feeling confused.	Men do not want to admit to themselves or others that they are being abused.
Women may be unaware of services or help available to them, and find it hard to access this information.	Men have not been encouraged to disclose abuse and do not know who to turn to.
Women see the role of the health visitor as being concerned with children rather than other problems.	There is limited public (media) information on female abuse of men, and little has been done to encourage men to disclose abuse.
Adapted from Ingram (2001) cited in Du Plat-Jones (2006), and Robotham (2005).	Adapted from Cook (1997) cited in Du Plat-Jones, (2006).

Sufferers from domestic abuse want (DH, 2005):

- to be safe
- to be believed, taken seriously and respected
- interventions to be at the right time and proactive – you should ask the victim what is happening

- to have information provided
- to have independent advocates (from the voluntary sector, for example)
- to liaise with the different agencies and to keep the overview of the case
- a single person or agency as contact/provide help and support to prevent having to repeat their story
- to be given clearly explained options based on their circumstances, so they can make choices
- to have contact with other sufferers
- to be kept informed of developments – such as when an abuser is released from a police station or turns up at the child's school
- to be given support to cope with the effects of abuse on their children
- to have their views listened to, respected and incorporated into services that are offered to them.

Safeguarding vulnerable adults

Safeguarding adults is the current terminology that aims to identify an adult who is in need for support or intervention because they are 'at risk'. Just as in child protection and domestic violence, our terminology has changed and developed as our knowledge of the issue increases, so our growing knowledge of adults who suffer abuse has led us to the current term 'safeguarding vulnerable adults'.

⭐ Practice tip

Questions to ask if domestic abuse is suspected:

- Is everything all right at home?
- Are you being cared for properly?
- Is your partner (or carer, daughter, son etc.) taking care of you?
- Can you tell me who hurt you?
- Can you tell me how you got those injuries?
- Can you show me how this happened?
- Have you ever been in a relationship where you were hit or where someone hurt you in any way?
- Does your partner (carer, son or daughter etc.) lose their temper with you, and if they do, can you describe what happens?
- Has your partner (carer, son or daughter, etc.) ever broken things that you care about, threatened to hurt you or those you love (such as your children), or forced you to have sex or manipulated you to have sex when you didn't really want it, or in a way you didn't want?

Source: DH (2000a).

[S] Scenario: Tom and his family

Tom Smith is a 75-year-old man who lives with his wife. Tom and Judith have been married for many years and looked forward to a happy retirement. Tom was a university professor and Judith was a primary teacher at the local school. They have one married daughter and three grandchildren who live a great distance away, and family conflict limits the amount of contact they have. Tom's health started to decline in his mid-60s, when he developed Parkinson's disease followed by a series of small strokes, just after he retired at the age of 65. This has left him with limited mobility and language problems. Judith has cared for him without any help, and the couple have financed alterations to their home to enable Tom to remain at home.

This caring process has not always been easy for Judith as Tom is a strong-willed man, who has found it difficult to adjust to being dependent upon his wife.

Tom has a lack of awareness about his abilities and consequently has had numerous falls. He has sustained some injuries, mainly lacerations to his head which have required overnight hospital stays and suturing of the wounds. Tom gets very frustrated at not being able to express himself, showing annoyance both at himself and at Judith who finds it difficult to understand him at times.

a) Learning activity

- Who do you consider to be 'vulnerable 'in the Smith family, and why?
- Do any of your reasons reflect the definitions of vulnerability outlined earlier in this chapter?

Consider your reply before reading on.

In the scenario Tom and Judith are vulnerable, Tom because of his illness and poor health, and Judith because as the sole carer, she has extra demands placed on her. This may challenge her physically and emotionally as she provides practical care to Tom, manages his frustration and adjusts to her new 'role' within the family – no longer wife, but nurse to Tom's injuries and carer for his physical needs. However, this couple would need to access community support in order to achieve vulnerability as defined by the government in *No Secrets* (DH, 2000b). It is likely that Tom is accessing medical services and so he would be classed as vulnerable, but Judith would not be unless she is having ongoing medical treatment, as there are no other care services being provided.

The importance of carers' contributions to meeting the needs of people within illness and/or disability has been recognised in many research studies, who identify that this group of people provide a significant contribution, saving the NHS and social services vast amounts of money (Carers UK and University of Leeds, 2007). Service users and carers (and those speaking for them) have long complained that their needs are ignored, to the detriment of their health (Wilson, 2004). The Carers (Equal Opportunities) Act 2004 means that carers are entitled to have their needs assessed, and for their needs and interests to be considered when assessing the services available to the service user and carers. The Carers and Disabled Children Act 2000 enables local councils to offer services that will support the carer in the caring role, while maintaining the carer's health and well-being, although it does not place an obligation on councils to make provision.

S) Scenario continued

Tom arrives early at his rehabilitation session with the occupational therapist (OT), and Judith leaves quickly without her usual chat with the staff at the centre. During the session the OT notes a number of bruises on Tom's arm, and that he has lost some mobility in his functioning arm. When the OT tries to touch the arm, Tom yells out and pulls away. The OT asks Tom what is the matter. Tom tries to communicate but he is incoherent and is very difficult to understand.

a) Learning activity

- What would be your concerns here?
- What would you need to do next?

c) Professional conversation

Alison, the OT caring for Tom, comments, 'I noticed Tom was not moving his functional arm as easily as in previous therapy sessions. When I touched his arm to encourage him to use it, he yelled out in pain, and that was when I noticed the bruises. Tom was trying to tell me what had happened but his distress increased his speech problems and made it more difficult for me to understand what he was saying.

'I spoke clearly and slowly to Tom to reassure him that I had seen he was in pain. I asked him closed questions so that he only had to concentrate on 'yes' or 'no' responses, and I gave him time to respond before asking the next question. I was then able to get an understanding of what Tom was trying to tell me. He had been falling and his wife had to help him up, which was how he hurt his arm. I suggested to Tom that we needed to check his arm was not broken, as he had hurt it following a fall, and that this would mean getting it x-rayed at the local hospital. Tom agreed, but said he did not want to stay in hospital but to go home afterwards. I reassured Tom that I would pass on his request, but that he should take the advice of the doctor.

'I felt that giving Tom enough time to express his needs helped him to regain control of the situation, and together we planned the next step.'

Elder abuse

a) Learning activity

Consider the relevant terms you may have read or heard about, other than the term 'elder abuse'.

Think about the following terms and decide what they have to offer in relation to defining elder abuse. Please note: these terms that have been previously established in the field of elder abuse and neglect are listed in chronological order (first column, then second column) (Biggs, Phillipson and Kingston, 1995).

- Granny battering
- Elder abuse
- Elder mistreatment
- The battered elder syndrome
- Elder mistreatment

- Granny bashing
- Old age abuse
- Inadequate care of the elderly
- Granny abuse
- Elder mis-care

The term 'elder abuse' is problematic, as it forces a demarcation line in terms of age. When does a person become elderly? (Think back to the section on what is an adult, and on how old age is established.) Other terminology can also be misleading; for example 'granny battering' implies that is it only females that are affected, and the abuse is of a physical nature leading to physical harm. However both sexes are subjected to abuse, and just as in child abuse and domestic abuse, this takes many forms, not just physical violence. Definitions of elder abuse therefore create some problems and have changed over time. They include:

> A single or repeated act or lack of appropriate action, occurring within any relationship where there is an expectation of trust, which causes harm or distress to an older person.
>
> (Action on Elder Abuse, 2007)

> Abuse may consist of a single or repeated acts. It may be physical, verbal or psychological, it may be an act of neglect or omission to act, or it may occur when a vulnerable person is persuaded to enter into a financial or sexual transaction to which he or she has not consented, or cannot consent. Abuse can occur in any relationship and may result in significant harm to, or exploitation of, the person subjected to it.
>
> (DH, 2000b: 9)

In trying to encapsulate the complexity of abuse and the range of victims, the ADSS (2005) document reframes the term elderly abuse to cover safeguarding vulnerable adults. Mowlan and colleagues (2007) highlight the difficulties in defining elderly abuse because of the very varying sets of circumstances that older adults experience, which reflect the different types of relationships between the perpetrator and the abused.

- For some victims, elder abuse is an extension of the domestic abuse they have suffered throughout the relationship with that perpetrator.
- For others the abuse started when they became frail, and unable to care for themselves completely because of physical or mental health issues.
- Some abuse begins when it is the perpetrator who becomes frail because of physical or mental health issues.

- The abuse might be perpetrated by other family members,
- The abuse might be perpetrated by someone the older adult trusts such as the next-door neighbour or a friend,
- The perpetrator might be a stranger (the issue of con men and 'cold callers' are frequently the topic of television programmes such as the BBC's *Rogue Traders*)
- The issue is further complicated by the definition of vulnerability (see previous section).

Robotham recognises that elder abuse can be difficult to detect or be hidden.

> Elderly people do not live public lives and there is far less likelihood of contact with external agencies [*compared with children*]. In addition, there are few developmental parameters against which one can measure adult progress and thus there are problems in discerning the difference between frailty caused by age and/or illness and the effects of abuse.
>
> (Robotham, 2005: 255–6; material in brackets added)

Multi-agency working

All abuse requires a multi-agency response to ensure that victims of abuse do not fall between services (DH, 2005). Since 2004, primary care trusts have had a statutory duty to work with other local agencies to reduce crime (with crime and disorder reduction partnerships, under the Crime and Disorder Act 1998).

Safeguarding Adults: A national framework of standards for good practice and outcomes in adult protection work (ADSS, 2005) tries to encapsulate all of these areas and provide a framework for good practice, recognising the need for integrated and multiprofessional working to deliver services that will enable vulnerable adults to be identified and receive appropriate help and support. There are 11 standards addressing the need for setting clear local interagency policies to ensure effective delivery.

Standard 3 states:

> The 'Safeguarding Adults' policy includes a clear statement of every person's right to live a life free from abuse and neglect, and this message is actively promoted to the public by the Local Strategic Partnership, the 'Safeguarding Adults' partnership, and its member organisations.
>
> (ADSS, 2005: 3)

Staff should follow a simple plan:

- Be alert to potential vulnerable adults and unsafe situations.
- Address immediate protection concerns.
- Refer concerns to the multiple agencies that need to be involved.
- Decide which *Safeguarding Adults* procedure will be the most appropriate to address the concern. This is similar to assessing whether there is a child in need situation or a safeguarding child in need of protection situation.
- Implement the local safeguarding assessment strategy from which multi-agency involvement and contribution to the assessment will be identified.
- Assist in developing a multi-agency safeguarding plan, and in its implementation.
- Review the plan.
- Record and monitor the process and outcome.

The different types and indicators of elder abuse and abuse to vulnerable adults

Review the section on types of abuse on pages 319–21. Abuse of vulnerable adults and of elderly people mirrors domestic abuse, including physical, sexual, emotional, psychological and financial abuse. Mowlan and colleagues (2007) note that elderly people who viewed issues of relationships, social support and religious beliefs, with positive feelings of social 'connectedness' tended to have more protection from long-term harm than those who had fewer social connections or positive feelings about their social network.

S Scenario continued

Tom is taken to the local A&E department accompanied by one of the workers at the centre. At A&E it is noted that although his arm is not broken, there is extensive bruising. It is noted that Tom also has older bruising on his chest. Judith arrives and is very flustered and distracted. She breaks down and confides to the worker that she can't cope any longer. She struggles to pick Tom up when he falls, and has permanent backache from helping Tom with his daily needs. Tom gets up at least three times in the night and she feels as if she hasn't slept for months. She admits Tom's frustrated outbursts are difficult to manage and that she has responded aggressively on a number of times, hence the bruising on Tom's body.

a Learning activity

What do you feel are the key issues about Tom and Judith's situation? Consider your answer before reading on.

In order to assess the situation the following questions need to be asked (DH, 2000a):

- Who is the vulnerable person?
- What is the nature and extent of the abuse?
- How long has the abuse been going on?
- What is the impact of the abuse on the individual?
- Will the abuse be repeated and/or progress to more serious abuse?

a Learning activity

What are the answers to these questions for Tom and Judith?

In the scenario, Tom and Judith are vulnerable, Tom because of his illness, reduced independence and reliability on Judith, and Judith as sole carer for Tom. The abuse consists of physical and psychological abuse. Tom's criticism of Judith and frustration affect both him and Judith, and Judith's tiredness and frustration at Tom have led to her hitting him. The abuse might have been occurring for a number of years, but has progressed slowly as Tom's dependence on Judith has increased. Both appear distressed by the situation they find themselves in, but without support the abuse is likely to continue.

Just as in children in need/safeguarding children in need of protection, the assessment of Tom and Judith highlights that the couple need help with the day-to-day management of Tom's disabilities so that Judith can regain her strength. Tom and Judith would qualify for community care/respite care, and with these needs provided for, the abusive incidents are likely to cease.

Your responsibility as a student and professional

The same principles outlined in Chapter 16 apply here. Please re-read those sections (pages 301–303). There are some additional points for you to consider when dealing with vulnerable adults, which are outlined in Table 17.3.

a Learning activity

- Find out your local policy on safeguarding vulnerable adults.
- Who is your adult protection coordinator, responsible for safeguarding vulnerable adults?
- Read the Department of Health *No Secrets* document (DH, 2000b).

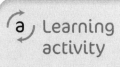

Part

II

Table 17.3 Reporting concerns about vulnerable adults

	Vulnerable adults	**Adults experiencing domestic violence**
Responsibility of students	Work with professionals to meet the person's health need. Report concerns to your mentor. Do not question the person – this must be done by a trained/experienced member of staff. If a person discloses abuse, let them know you believe them but say you need to get someone better able to help. DO NOT QUESTION anyone about suspected abuse in front of anyone else. Document any concerns/injuries/comments the person makes about the cause of the injury.	Report concerns to the designated person.
Responsibility of trained professionals	Ensure the person's health needs are met. Tell the individual you believe them. Use clear questions when asking the individual whether they have been abused, stating clearly why you suspect this: for example, that bruising does not reflect their story. Create opportunities to speak to the individual alone if someone else is with them. Ask what the individual wants to happen. Encourage the individual to make phone calls to relevant agencies if that is what they want. Follow local policy to assess the person in terms of level of vulnerability – if this is a case where the individual would be classified as a vulnerable adult because of unmet community care needs or an individual experiencing abuse. Safeguard the vulnerable adult by: 1 Community care: assessment of need and appropriate services put in place. Where the assessment suggests the individual is vulnerable and abuse is occurring: 2 Remove them from the home situation into residential care, or 3 Remove the carer (especially if the carer is a paid carer or the individual is in an institutional setting) until a full investigation has been conducted, or 4 Ensure that alternative care arrangements are made in the home. Remember to collect evidence for any criminal proceedings. Involve the police where this is local policy, the individual wishes to take legal action or a criminal offence has been committed. Do not guarantee confidentiality as the record may need to be disclosed to protect the vulnerable adult.	While it is the individual's choice not to follow through with a complaint or to leave the situation, where there are children in the house, confidentiality to the individual cannot be maintained and safeguarding the child procedures must be followed. Ensure a plan to leave the abusive environment safely is agreed and in place before the individual leaves.

Conclusion

Abuse occurs where one person abuses a position of power over another person. This chapter has explored the effect of abuse within adult domestic relationships, and of other vulnerable adults including the elderly. Our society has become increasingly responsive towards domestic abuse, but is only recently beginning to recognise that abuse occurs to the elderly and to vulnerable adults. There are no specific protection laws to safeguard most adults including the elderly, and there is only limited protection for some vulnerable adults.

Your role as a health professional is clear. As with safeguarding children, you must be aware of the signs and situations when an elderly person presenting to you could be in an abusive situation. You need to act on your concerns by following policy and protocol to ensure a full assessment of the situation is undertaken and an appropriate action plan agreed. As a health professional, you need to ensure that you are supported through support mechanisms such as clinical governance and supervision, as this can be an emotionally challenging area of practice.

References

Action on Elder Abuse (2004) *Hidden Voices* [online] www.elderabuse.org.uk (accessed 10 December 2007).

Action on Elder Abuse (2005)*Adult Protection Data Monitoring* [online] www.elderabuse.org.uk (accessed 10 December 2007).

Action on Elder Abuse (2007) 'Definition of elder abuse' [online] www.elderabuse.org.uk(accessed 10 December 2007).

Agnew, T., (2006) 'Beating abuse', *Nursing Older People* **18**(1), 10–12.

Association of Directors of Social Services (ADSS) (2005) *Safeguarding Adults: A national framework of standards for good practice and outcomes in adult protection work*, London, ADSS [online] http://www.adss.org.uk/publications/guidance/safeguarding.pdf (accessed 4 December 2008).

Biggs, S., Phillipson, C. and Kingston, P. (1995) *Elder Abuse in Perspective*, Philadelphia, Open University Press.

British Market Research Bureau (BMRB) (2007) British Crime Survey, 2003–2004 [online] http://www.esds.ac.uk/Government/bcs/ (accessed 1 December 2007).

Brooker, C. and Nichol, M. (2003) *Nursing Adults: The practice of caring*, Edinburgh, Mosby.

Campbell, J. C. and Soeken, K. L. (1999) 'Forced sex and intimate partner violence', *Violence Against Women* **5**(9), 1017–35.

Carers UK and University of Leeds (2007) *Valuing Carers: Calculating the value of unpaid care*, London, HMSO [online] http://www.carersuk.org/Newsandcampaigns/Valuingcarers/Fullreport/ValuingcarersFINAL.pdf (accessed 10 December 2007).

Cottrell, B. (2001) *Parent Abuse: The abuse of parents by their teenage children*, Canada, National Clearing House on Family Violence,

Council of Europe (2002) Recommendation of the Committee of Ministers to Member States on the protection of women against violence, adopted 30 April 2002 and explanatory memorandum, Strasbourg, Council of Europe.

Home Office (2000/1) *Criminal Statistics 2000/01*, London, HMSO.

Department of Health (DH) (2000a) *Domestic Violence: A resource manual for healthcare professionals*, London, The Stationery Office.

DH (2000b) *No Secrets: Guidance on developing and implementing multi-agency policies and procedures to protect vulnerable adults from abuse*, London, The Stationery Office.

DH (2004) *The Government's Response to the Recommendations and Conclusions of the Health Select Committee's Inquiry into Elder Abuse*, London, HMSO.

DH (2005) *Responding to Domestic Abuse: A resource manual for healthcare professionals*, London, The Stationery Office.

Du Plat Jones, J. (2006) 'Domestic violence: the role of health professionals', *Nursing Standard* 21 (13 December), 44–8.

Hanmer J. (1994) Policy Development and Implementation Seminars, Patterns of Agency Contact with Women, Research Paper No. 12, Leeds Metropolitan University.

House of Commons Health Select Committee (2004) *Elder Abuse*, London, HMSO.

James-Hanman, D. (1998) 'Domestic violence: breaking the silence', *Community Practitioner* **71**(12), 401–7.

Kalache, A. (2002) *Ageing and Life*, course unit, Geneva, World Health Organization.

Law Commission (1995) *Mental Incapacity Law*, Law Com. No. 231, London, HMSO.

Mandelstam, M. (2005) *Community Care Practice and the Law*, 3rd edn, Jessica Kingsley, London.

Manthorpe, J., Biggs, S., McCreadie, C., Tinker, A., Hills, A., O'Keefe, M., Doyle, R., Constantine, R., Scholes, S. and Erens, B. (2007) 'The UK national study of abuse and neglect among older people', *Nursing Older People* **19**(8), 24–6.

Mezey, G. and Bewley. S. (2000) *An Exploration of the Prevalence and Effects of Domestic Violence in Pregnancy*, London. ESRC.

Mowlan, A., Tennant, R., Dixon, J. and McCreadie, C. (2007) *UK Study of Abuse and Neglect of Older People: Qualitative findings*, prepared for Comic Relief and the Department of Health, Kings College, University of London.

Povey, D. (ed.) (2005) 'Crime in England and Wales 2003/04, Supplementary volume: homicide and gun crime', Home Office Statistical Bulletin no. 02/05.

Richardson, B., Kitchen, G. and Livingston, G. (2002) 'The effect of education on knowledge and management of elder abuse: a randomized control trial', *Age and Ageing* **31**(5), 335–41.

Robotham, A. (2005) 'Violence: debating the issues', pp. 239-–62 in Robotham, A. and Frost, M. (eds), *Health Visiting: Specialist community public health nursing*, 2nd edn, Edinburgh, Churchill Livingston.

Stark, E. and Flitcraft, A. (1996) *Women at Risk: Domestic violence and women's health*, London, Sage.

Walby, S., and Allen, J. (2004) *Domestic Violence, Sexual Assault and Stalking: Findings from the British Crime Survey 2001*, London, Home Office.

Wilson, V. (2004) 'Supporting family carers in the community setting', *Nursing Standard* **18**(29) (31 March), 47–53.

World Health Organization (WHO)/ International Network for the Prevention of Elder Abuse (INPEA) (2002) *Missing Voices: Views of older persons on elder abuse*, Geneva, WHO.

Part

III

Insights into care with client groups

Chapters

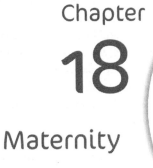

Chapter

18

Maternity

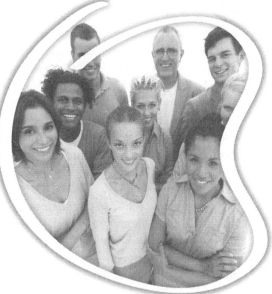

Brenda Rees and Colin Rees

Links to other chapters in *Foundation Studies for Caring*

Links to other chapters in *Foundation Skills for Caring*

W Don't forget to visit www.palgrave.com/glasper for additional online resources relating to this chapter.

Part

III

Introduction

Women receiving maternity care are usually healthy, and are not seeking a 'cure' for a medical condition. This makes pregnancy and birth different from other situations involving health professionals. For the majority of women, pregnancy and birth are normal physiological processes. However, for others health risks do exist. Some women may have an existing medical condition, or a complication develops during pregnancy that requires special attention.

Each pregnancy and birth is affected by a number of variables. These include cultural, historical and practical influences, the woman's health, previous obstetric history, and the way the pregnancy and birth progresses. This is what makes maternity care a varied and richly rewarding area of work.

Although normal pregnancy and childbirth is the responsibility of midwives (NMC, 2008), nurses and other healthcare professionals also encounter pregnant women and their families in a number of community and hospital settings. It is therefore important to have an insight into a woman's journey through pregnancy and childbirth, and the way health services respond to her needs. The aim of this chapter is to provide an insight into maternal care as provided by a midwife, and the policies, values and philosophy on which that care is based.

Learning outcomes

The chapter will enable you to:

- understand some of the common terminology surrounding maternal health
- identify some of the principles of midwifery care
- identify some of the health policies that shape maternal care
- outline some of the major physical, and psychosocial changes experienced by women (and their partners) in this period
- demonstrate a broad knowledge of the growth of the fetus in pregnancy

- identify the contact points between women and midwives during pregnancy
- access sources of literature on issues related to a healthy pregnancy and birth
- explain the purpose of antenatal screening procedures
- outline the varied role of the midwife
- describe the birth process
- identify some of the events that take place following the birth.

Concepts

- Pregnancy
- Midwifery care
- Transitions to parenthood
- Normal pregnancy
- The developing fetus
- Education for a healthy pregnancy and labour
- Women-centred care

- Fatherhood
- Choice
- Empowerment
- Maternity services
- Obstetric services
- Antenatal care
- Screening and monitoring in pregnancy

- Birth plan
- Stages of labour
- Intrapartum care
- Partogram
- APGAR scores
- Postpartum care
- Breastfeeding
- Postnatal care

Background to maternity services in the United Kingdom

National Health Service (NHS) policies control the provision of maternity services in the United Kingdom. Over the last 40 years, substantial changes in these policies have led to a transformation in where most births take place. In 1957, 36 per cent of all births took place in the home, and a further 13 per cent in nursing homes under the care of a midwife or general practitioner (GP). Within 20 years, the number of hospital births had increased to 66 per cent, and those at home had declined to 12 per cent (DH, 2007). By 2005, the figure for home births in England had dropped to 2.5 per cent (Hansard 2007). In other words, most babies are now born in a hospital setting.

Other notable health changes include an increase in the number of medically controlled and influenced labours. During the early 1980s a high proportion of labours were routinely induced, using powerful drugs such as oxytocin. At the time, the NHS supported this increasingly medicalised approach to birth. The Peel Report (SMMAC, 1970) recommended that 100 per cent of births should be in hospital. This was seen as a way of improving maternal and baby outcomes. The same view was put forward nearly 15 years later, when the *Maternity Care in Action* report (DH, 1984) stated that every woman should be encouraged to have her baby in a maternity unit. Clearly, policy makers saw birth as a high-risk medical condition, and one needing hospitalisation and the control of an obstetrician, with support from midwives. This led to a rapid decline in, and finally closure of, maternity homes and the discontinuation of GP-assisted deliveries in the United Kingdom. For many women, pregnancy and childbirth continues to be a medicalised event, involving a complex range of professional support, and the use of technical equipment (DH, 2007).

Almost in contradiction to this, the 20 years to 2009 have seen a drive by some consumer and professional groups towards less invasive births, and a challenge to the idea that all births are high-risk and require medical supervision. To support this, there is clear evidence that some of the technical developments, such as continuous electronic fetal monitoring (EFM), have had little effect on improving birth outcomes (Thacker, Stroup and Chang, 2001). The government accepted these arguments and policy has changed in line with the evidence. Legislation now promotes a greater involvement of the midwife in the entire birth event, and a central role for women in having choice, continuity and control in their care. This was the central theme of *Changing Childbirth* (DH 1993), and is reiterated in the *National Service Framework for Children, Young People and Maternity Services* (DH, 2004) and the National Institute for Health and Clinical Excellence (NICE) guidelines for intrapartum care (NICE, 2007a).

Despite the criticism of the unnecessary use of technical intervention, there has been a rise in the number of caesarian section births, not only in the United Kingdom but also worldwide. While the World Health Organization (WHO) recommended that caesarian sections should form no more than 15 per cent of all deliveries, in 2002–03 the rate was around 22 per cent for England. This suggests caesarian sections were becoming a 'normal' mode of delivery. In response, consumer groups and midwifery bodies, including the International Confederation of Midwives (ICM) and the Royal College of Midwives (RCM), campaigned for a greater focus on normal birth, and a reduction in unnecessary clinical interventions (Lavender and Kingdon, 2006).

This has resulted in policy support for midwifery-led birth centres, and, for those who require it, the centralising of consultant-led units. Policy is now based on the principle that 'all women will need a midwife, but some need a doctor too' (DH, 2007).

In the United Kingdom, the *National Service Framework (NSF) for Children, Young People and Maternity Services* (DH, 2004) sets the agenda for maternity care. The guiding principles are set out in Standard 11 (see the evidence-based practice box below). This chapter illustrates the NSF standard through a case study.

(e) Evidence-based practice

NSF Standard 11

Ensure that pregnant women receive high-quality care throughout their pregnancy, have a normal childbirth wherever possible, are involved in decisions about what is best for them and their babies, and have choices about how and where they give birth.

Source: DH (2004).

a Learning activity

Talk to friends and relatives who have had babies in different decades, going back as far as you can. Consider who was involved at the birth, where it took place, and how it unfolded. Compare descriptions of the births over time, and take note of any similarities or differences.

S Scenario: Introducing Kerry

Kerry is 19 years old and has just discovered she is pregnant. She works part time in a supermarket and for two nights a week in a local pub. She lives with Dave, her boyfriend of two years. He is a 26-year-old van driver who is divorced. She has a reasonable relationship with her parents, although it has recently been a little strained.

She has a body mass index (BMI) of 31, which is on the border of making the pregnancy high risk, as she is overweight. A BMI of over 29 in nonpregnant women is considered obese (WHO classification of normal and abnormal body weight using BMI). A BMI of over 35 at the start of pregnancy is considered a high-risk factor (NICE, 2007a). Kerry has always enjoyed drinking and going out to bars and clubs with her friends. She started smoking when she was 14 and smokes about 15 cigarettes a day: more, if it is a long drinking evening. Now she lives with Dave, they tend to eat takeaways or convenience meals. During the day, she snacks on crisps and chocolates.

Kerry's medical history is good. Her major health problems are her weight, and her drinking and smoking. This is her first pregnancy, although she has been having unprotected sex with Dave for some time.

Kerry confirmed her suspicions that she was pregnant by buying a pregnancy testing kit from her local chemist. Pregnancy tests identify the presence of beta-human chorionic gonadotrophin (ß-hCG) in the urine (or blood) (Medforth et al, 2006). Her first reaction was one of disbelief, although on reflection it came as no real surprise to her. When she moved in with Dave, she was using the contraceptive pill, although not consistently. When nothing happened when she forgot to take it, she began to have unprotected sex with Dave, believing that for some reason, perhaps because of her size, she just could not become pregnant. They had not been planning to have a baby; it was something that just happened.

Dave was initially a little stunned at the news, but soon became thrilled at the idea of becoming a father. He had no children from his previous marriage. Kerry also shared the news with her parents, who, after a short silence over the phone, also became very excited about becoming grandparents. Kerry was unsure at first what she thought herself, as she felt it would make a big difference to her life, but was unclear in what way.

As this is her first pregnancy, the impact that pregnancy and baby will have on her current life is something of an unknown. Kerry decides to use their home computer, which Dave usually uses as part of his work, to search for information about pregnancy on the web.

a Learning activity

Using a web search engine such as Google, put in the search words "I'm pregnant" to see what information might be available to women who learn they are pregnant. Make a list of things from your search that she and Dave may have to consider in terms of Kerry's health, and their new role as parents.

The transition to motherhood is a complete physical and psychosocial process. Each aspect will have different consequences, and the aspects cannot be taken in isolation from each other. Early physical signs of pregnancy include:

- missed periods
- nausea and vomiting especially first thing in the morning
- abdominal pains
- a 'metallic' taste in the mouth

- changes to the breasts including tenderness, increase in size, 'heaviness', sensation of tingling
- feeling tired
- increased frequency of micturition
- constipation
- increased vaginal discharge
- heightened sense of smell in relation to food
- changes in the taste of certain food
- may go off foods
- possibly a craving for unusual foods or unusual combinations of food (pica).

Although the list contains mainly physical factors, many of these also have consequences for other aspects of life. Pregnancy in one way or another becomes a major part of life for those concerned, as it touches so many aspects. Some physical signs, such as morning sickness, may be seen as distressing, but it must be stressed that not all of the symptoms of pregnancy are wholly negative. The very physical shape of the pregnant body can evoke positive reactions in others towards the pregnant woman.

Early in pregnancy the physical developments taking place inside the body are small, but important. Changes take place in the uterus, where a fertilised egg develops into a viable fetus. Around six to ten days following conception, the fetus triggers changes in the level of hormones, such as oestrogen and progesterone, in the body. These protect the fetus by ensuring that menstruation does not take place. They also prepare the body for breastfeeding (Coggins, 2005).

Later signs of pregnancy include movements of the fetus, felt at first as 'fluttering', at around 18–20 weeks for first-time mothers, and 16–18 weeks for those with previous pregnancies (Fraser and Cooper, 2003; Medforth et al, 2006).

> ### a) Learning activity
>
> Kerry thought that her size might have had something to do with her ability to conceive. Using a search engine, establish if there is a relationship between BMI and the ability to conceive. Then search to see what effect a high BMI might have on pregnancy and labour.
>
> You might find it useful to read Irvine and Shaw (2006).

The developing fetus

During pregnancy, the midwife is responsible for both the woman's health and that of the baby. Midwives are experts on the normal development of the fetus, as well as lifestyle and health factors that can affect the woman's health, and in turn that of the baby.

We can divide pregnancy into three major time periods, or trimesters (see Table 18.1). Each stage has implications for the development of the baby, the woman, and contact with health services. It is important to note that screening procedures are not compulsory, and in accordance with NICE guidelines (2003), are first discussed with the woman, who then makes an informed decision on whether to accept or decline them. Similarly, the extent to which women experience the symptoms listed varies.

> ### S) Scenario continued
>
> At seven weeks pregnant, Kerry already feels different, as her role is now changing to that of a pregnant woman. The pregnancy also has social consequences for others. For instance, Kerry's parents now have the additional role of prospective grandparents, and Dave's role is changing to that of prospective father. For each role, there are a set of implications in the form of expectations and obligations on how individuals should play that role.
>
> For Dave and Kerry, this can be summed up in the word 'responsibility', not only for the developing fetus (already being thought of as 'our baby'), but also responsible for the baby's health in the womb. Kerry is now the main carer for this developing baby, although she is unsure of everything that she can do to protect the physical safety of her unborn child.

Table 18.1 Developments during the three trimesters of pregnancy

Trimester	Baby's development	Women's experiences	Contact with health services
First (weeks 0–13)	Starts as an 'embryo' and at 10 weeks is called a fetus (young one). The first four weeks show fastest rate of growth. Visible on ultrasound from six weeks. Begins sucking and swallowing surrounding fluid. Kidneys begin to function and from week ten small amounts of urine are passed back into the amniotic fluid in which it is floating. At 12 weeks following conception the fetus is fully formed. The fetal heart can be heard using sonic aid from around nine weeks and on ultrasound scan.	Symptoms of early pregnancy: missed periods, morning sickness, tiredness, breast size changes, and some mood swings. Adjustments to lifestyle to protect pregnancy (changes to smoking, drugs, alcohol, caffeine levels).	Contact with midwife around 10–12 weeks at booking visit. Screening tests for Down's syndrome (11–14 weeks). Blood tests for Hb, blood group, HIV, syphilis, sickle cell and thalassaemia. Dating ultra-sound scan, enables accurate expected date of delivery. Free dental treatment available throughout pregnancy and for a year after the birth.
Second (weeks 14–26)	Rapid skeletal development. Fetal heart can be heard on auscultation. Most organs capable of functioning. Responds to sound from 20–24 weeks. At about 22 weeks covered in very fine soft hair called 'lanugo'. Later covered in white, greasy 'vernix'. Both disappear before birth. Around week 26, eyes open for first time.	Reduction in morning sickness. Breasts continue to increase in size. May develop backache and constipation. Baby's movements felt.	Screening tests including alfa-feto protein (AFP) 16–18 weeks. Amniocentesis (not routine) (week 16). Routine check on BP and urine at all antenatal visits. Early pregnancy 'classes' may be available. If in employment, employer must be notified of pregnancy in writing, GP or midwife will supply maternity certificate (MAT B1) from about week 20.
Third (weeks 27–40)	Clear sleep and wake times result in movements being more obvious at some points of the day. Towards the end of the pregnancy settles into a head down position, and moves further down pelvis. There should be gradual fetal weight gain over this entire period. Movement will continue where there is sufficient amniotic fluid circulating to facilitate this despite space restrictions.	Steady but not excessive weight gain and some postural oedema in lower limbs. Hormonal changes cause the joints in the pelvis to loosen in preparation for the birth. This can be experienced as joint pain and present as backache or a pain in the symphysis pubis making mobility increasingly difficult. Increased tiredness, forgetfulness and heartburn. Difficulty sleeping. Braxton Hicks contractions at around week 28 (these are mild contractions that help the uterus prepare for labour and occur for short periods of time). If working, paid maternity leave organised. May feel uncomfortable with size because of the pressure of the baby's weight on nerves in the legs and pelvis. May also increase frequency of micturition.	More blood tests for haemoglobin level. Offered preparation for parenthood education sessions around 8–10 weeks before due date. Frequency of antenatal visits varies depending on any problems found or suspected. Focus on fetal growth and maternal well-being, especially any changes from baseline BP reading. More visits may be offered if it is a first pregnancy. After week 36, the midwife checks the position of baby to ensure the head-down position is maintained. Delivery between weeks 37 and 42. If not delivered by week 41 may be offered a sweep of the membranes to encourage labour. Induction may be suggested if this is not successful.

Sources: based on Fraser and Cooper (2003), Bounty (2006) and DH (2006).

Many women gain information about pregnancy from a variety of sources such as family and friends, as well as health professionals. From your earlier search of the web, you will have seen there are a number of websites providing factual information on physical changes, and some of the things that will happen in the coming weeks and months before the birth. Some of this information is from commercial sites that try to sell prospective parents a range of products, while others are 'official' health sites. There is also a range of leaflets and booklets women receive once in contact with their midwife, produced by a variety of sources such as Bounty booklets (Bounty, 2006), MIDIRS informed choice leaflets (http://www.midirs.com), and the Department of Health's *The Pregnancy Book* (DH, 2006).

W

> ### (a) Learning activity
>
> Visit a newsagent and look for magazines aimed at mothers and parents. Scan the index pages to gain an idea of the topics they cover. Look particularly at readers' questions and letters pages for the issues raised by readers.

The role of the midwife

> ### (a) Learning activity
>
> What would you list as the main aspects of the midwife's role?

Midwives are often associated merely with the birth of a baby. This is a limited view of their work, as their role is far more extensive (NMC, 2008). The International Confederation of Midwives (ICM) provides a comprehensive definition of the role (see below). The professional responsibilities of midwives are slightly different from those of nurses. Although some roles in nursing have changed and are still evolving, with nurses now taking responsibility in some areas of care, for example in prescribing and in specialist roles, the role of the midwife has had a recognised degree of autonomy in the United Kingdom for over 100 years. This is set out in the terms of a statutory document that enables midwives to operate as practitioners in their own right, and so act independently of medical cover (NMC, 2008).

> ### (e) Evidence-based practice
>
> **Definition of the role of the midwife**
>
> A midwife is a person who, having been regularly admitted to a midwifery educational programme, duly recognised in the country in which it is located, has successfully completed the prescribed course of studies in midwifery and has acquired the requisite qualifications to be registered and/or legally licensed to practise midwifery.
>
> The midwife is recognised as a responsible and accountable professional who works in partnership with women to give the necessary support, care and advice during pregnancy, labour and the postpartum period, to conduct births on the midwife's own responsibility and to provide care for the newborn and the infant. This care includes preventative measures, the promotion of normal birth, the detection of complications in mother and child, the accessing of medical care or other appropriate assistance and the carrying out of emergency measures.
>
> The midwife has an important task in health counselling and education, not only for the woman, but also within the family and the community. This work should involve antenatal education and preparation for parenthood and may extend to women's health, sexual or reproductive health and childcare.
>
> A midwife may practise in any setting including the home, community, hospitals, clinics or health units.
>
> (Adopted by the International Confederation of Midwives Council meeting, 19 July 2005, Brisbane, Australia)

Part

III

The midwife's role is that of lead professional for women with low-risk pregnancies: that is, those with no complication in pregnancy or childbirth. Where women do have complications in pregnancy and childbirth, midwives work in partnership with the obstetrician. In these cases, the obstetrician is the lead professional. The line between the risk categories is decided by criteria defining what constitutes a high-risk pregnancy, such as those listed in Table 18.2.

Table 18.2 High-risk pregnancy criteria

Factors that mainly affect maternal well-being:	Factors that are more likely to affect fetal outcomes:	
→ Hypertension → Renal disease → Respiratory disease → Cardiac disease → Haemoglobinopathy → Psychiatric conditions → Infections (e.g. varicella) → Drug misuse → Extremes of age → Obesity (BMI>35) → Maternal diabetes	→ Poor obstetric history (for instance, miscarriage or preterm labour) → Pre-term labour maturity (including rupture of membranes and labour) → Rhesus disease → Maternal diabetes → Monozygotic multiple pregnancy → Fetal abnormality → Assisted conception	→ Some of the common complications developing during pregnancy that are linked to serious fetal compromise: → Pre-eclampsia → Placenta praevia → Fetal growth restriction

Source: based on DH (1999).

The concept of risk in pregnancy and birth is particularly important, as it will influence the type of care provided, and who is involved in managing that care. Where the risk of complications arising in pregnancy is considered to be low, the midwife's role is to promote the normality of pregnancy and labour. The beliefs underpinning this are clear from reading the extract of the Royal College of Midwives' position paper on normal childbirth (RCM, 2004) in the evidence-based practice box below.

e Evidence-based practice

Royal College of Midwives Position statement on normal childbirth

- The Royal College of Midwives defines normal childbirth as one where a woman commences, continues and completes labour physiologically at term (between 37–42 weeks). The College believes that a policy of maximising normal birth in the context of maternal choice is safe. Further, that it offers short and long-term health and social benefits to mothers, children, families, and communities. Such a policy is more likely to succeed if childbirth is placed within a social and family context.
- The majority of women with uncomplicated pregnancies are fit and healthy and have the potential to give birth normally with healthy newborns as the expected outcome. This is best met within a social model of care.

- Midwives are expert professionals skilled in supporting and maximising normal birth and their skills need to be promoted and valued. The role of the midwife is integral to models of care, which promote normality. Maternity services can enhance midwifery skills and autonomous practice by providing the appropriate practice settings.
- The RCM recommends that maternity service providers review their policies, guidelines, practices and models of care to ensure that they are based on a philosophy committed to maximising normal birth and to ensure that a range of options are available to women.
- The RCM recommends that midwives value, support and develop their own skills and knowledge and those of their colleagues, in the area of normal childbirth.

Source: RCM (2004).

In pregnancy, the first meeting between a women and her midwife takes the form of a 'booking' visit. This is based on the time prior to the NHS, when a women had to book or make a reservation for a bed in a maternity home or for the services of a midwife. This meeting can be in the home or on health premises, and is a detailed exploration of the woman's physical, emotional and social background. Initial health assessments between those using health services and a health professional are important as they enable the professional to obtain or identify:

- clear details on health indicators that might point to unmet needs
- the basis to plan further care
- the individual's understanding of the situation
- any current or future risk factors
- the need for information or education
- the level of support needed to manage the situation
- the need to involve other health professionals or services.

> **a) Learning activity**
>
> Make a list of the possible topics Kerry might need to discuss with the midwife at her booking visit.

This booking session provides the midwife and the pregnant woman with information to help them both consider some options to increase the chances of a healthy pregnancy, and consider the kind of birth the woman would like, and that will be suitable for her needs.

> **S Scenario continued**
>
> Kerry's contact with her midwife followed a phone call to the GP receptionist, who referred her to the midwife. The midwife then contacted Kerry and arranged to see her at home. The following week, Kerry met the midwife, who introduced herself as Sally. Kerry was pleased that the two of them got on immediately. Sally was in her late 20s. She was enthusiastic and seemed genuinely to want the best for Kerry. This is Kerry's 'booking visit' where she starts her relationship with the midwife. It provides Kerry with the opportunity to raise questions about her pregnancy and the birth.

The kind of things that are at the top of a woman's list to discuss are confirmation of the due date of delivery, and the options surrounding where she can give birth. The due date can quickly be calculated by the midwife from the last menstrual cycle date. A dating scan is also offered, as it gives a precise dating of the pregnancy, and most women accept this offer.

The booking visit follows the principles of the NICE guidelines for England on antenatal care (2003), which state:

> Pregnant women should be offered evidence-based information and support to enable them to make informed decisions regarding their care.

The topics discussed at the booking visit will include:

- routine care during the antenatal period
- family medical history
- personal medical history
- social history
- previous obstetric history
- screening options
- options for place of birth
- maintaining a healthy approach to life
- eating habits including certain foods to avoid
- levels of alcohol consumption
- smoking habits
- possible domestic abuse
- rest and exercise
- employment issues (notifying employers of pregnancy and entitlements for paid maternity leave)
- maintaining a healthy sex life
- taking medication
- mental health
- planning for the future and looking after the baby
- choice in feeding the baby.

It is important to achieve a complete health profile at this point, and this includes mental health symptoms or problems. The NICE Guidelines for England on *Antenatal and Postnatal Mental Health* (NICE, 2007b) suggest that the first booking session is an ideal time to ensure that there are no outstanding mental health problems that may need to be considered during the pregnancy. If a woman is already taking medication for a mental health problem, there is the risk that it could cross the placenta and affect the health of the baby.

Other questions that midwives must ask concern the possibility of domestic violence or abuse. This can be triggered for the first time in pregnancy. Where there is already a history of abuse in a relationship, there can be an increase in its extent and frequency in pregnancy (Medforth et al, 2006). The discovery of potential or actual abuse will have repercussions for the safety of the woman, and also involve the baby being put on the 'at-risk' register. This will affect safety procedures surrounding the pregnancy and birth, and may involve an action plan being set up. This will require the midwife to liaise with the police and social services. Ultimately, this may lead to the baby being taken into care following the birth.

This illustrates the sensitive issues surrounding the booking visit, some of which might continue throughout the pregnancy and birth. The midwife will also include the father of the baby where present, so that care will be provided for the couple. Clearly, some discussions may need to take place in private where appropriate. The relationship established by the midwife will affect the nature and quality of the care provided during this period. This has implications for both the clinical and social skills of the midwife.

The midwife will carefully record the details discussed at the booking visit in the woman's hand-held notes, providing accurate documentation (NMC, 2008). Producing clear documentation is a priority skill for health professionals and a legal responsibility. If there are any problems or queries following the care received, the record will be part of the evidence demonstrating what happened.

⌷S⌷ Scenario continued

There was one health problem on Kerry's mind that was causing her some concern. Ever since she was young she has had a problem with injections, and 'needles' generally. These cause an immediate physical reaction, often a faint, followed by vomiting and feelings of nausea for around 12 hours. She has been told that she is 'needle phobic'. The question she has is, 'How would this affect my pregnancy and the birth?'

↻a Learning activity

Search for information on 'needle phobia', and consider where in her pregnancy and labour Kerry is likely to encounter a problem. If possible, find out how this could be dealt with. Think about it from Kerry's point of view, and how this might impact on how she experiences the coming events. What kind of support do you think she might look for from the health professionals around her?

The journal article by Searing and colleagues (2006) might be a useful source of information.

Antenatal clinical attendances

The purpose of antenatal care is to monitor the health of both the mother and the baby to ensure everything progresses smoothly. Care is usually provided at a clinic, which can be in a GP surgery or at a hospital, but it can also be provided in the woman's home where this is appropriate. There is a common timetable for appointments throughout the pregnancy with a midwife, GP or consultant obstetrician. Visits to the antenatal clinic provide an opportunity for the woman to be offered a number of screening tests, at various times during the pregnancy. These include blood tests (see Table 18.3), tests to determine conditions such as diabetes, tests for small or large for gestational age babies, (sometimes called 'small/large for dates'), and Down's syndrome.

(a) Learning activity

What implications of screening might need to be explained to women before they make a decision on whether to accept it?

Routine checks during pregnancy, such as those in Table 18.3, are influenced in England by the NICE guidelines on *Routine Care for the Healthy Pregnant Woman* (2003). These suggest that for women having their first baby with uncomplicated pregnancies, a schedule of ten appointments for antenatal clinic should be adequate. Those with uncomplicated previous pregnancies might require only seven.

The guidelines also outline the screening tests that should be offered to women, and at what points in the pregnancy. It is stressed that women should receive an explanation of the purpose of any screening test when it is offered, and they should have the opportunity to discuss any issues and ask questions about the implications of such tests.

Clinic visits usually include routine urine analysis, blood pressure monitoring to screen for hypertension, and a check for any oedema after week 36. The position of the baby in the womb is also examined to determine whether it is head down. One of the reasons for monitoring is to exclude the development of pre-eclampsia, a multisystem disorder unique to pregnancy. Its severity depends on the woman's blood pressure (BP) and proteinurea. A BP of 140/90mmHg and a proteinurea dipstick reading of 1+, or 3g in 24 hours are defining characteristics (Medforth et al, 2006).

Table 18.3 Tests in early pregnancy

Before 16 weeks of gestation:
Blood tests for:
→ Blood group, rhesus status and red cell antibodies
→ Haemoglobin to screen for anaemia
→ Hepatitis B virus
→ Sickle cell and thalassaemia
→ HIV
→ Rubella susceptibility
→ Syphilis serology
Urine test to screen for asymptomatic bacteriuria Ultrasound scan to determine gestational age Down's syndrome screening:
→ Nuchal translucency at 11–14 weeks
→ Serum screening at 14–20 weeks
Between 18 and 20 weeks of gestation:
Ultrasound scan for detection of structural anomalies

Source: NICE (2003).

Antenatal education

One of the topics discussed at the booking visit is attending a 'Preparation for Parenting' group. These are called different names in different places, and are generically called antenatal classes. According to the NICE guidelines in England on antenatal care (NICE, 2003), all women should be offered the opportunity to attend antenatal classes. They are an ideal opportunity to consider health and social options, and help make informed decisions about parenthood issues. The type, format and content of groups can vary enormously. Recent guides on how to conduct antenatal education show that much has changed in relation to the content and structure of such sessions (Schott and Priest, 2002; Nolan, 2005).

Part

III

[S] Scenario continued

Kerry has not had a great deal of contact with babies and feels a little out of her depth. At the same time she feels that a 'group' session might turn out to be a little like school, which was not a favourite time in her life. When she discusses this with the midwife, Sally reassures her that the groups are relaxed, and very useful. Sally gives her details of National Childbirth Trust (NCT) classes held locally in the house of the organiser. There is a fee to be paid for these. However, as Sally said she would be involved in the next NHS ones to be held in the local health centre, Kerry chose to go to them. In both situations she was told that Dave would be an important member of the sessions, although Kerry could attend on her own if that was what they preferred.

Antenatal education is part of the maternity services' public health role, and supports people in making informed health decisions. It also covers the wider issues of parenting, and not just the birth. In some areas there may be early sessions in pregnancy available.

Antenatal classes have a number of advantages. The most important is having a greater understanding of the options surrounding the pregnancy and birth. They also provide the opportunity to meet both staff who are can answer a wide range of questions, and other women who are likely to give birth around the same time. Some maternity services offer follow-up postnatal groups to encourage women in the same neighbourhood to make contact with each other and reduce possible effects of isolation in the early weeks after the birth. Although research suggests that there is little difference in the clinical outcomes of the birth, the information gained and the opportunity to know and practise methods of relaxing in labour are evaluated as helpful. The inclusion of fathers is an important aspect of the sessions, and is recognition that fathers have information needs too, and need to feel ready for the birth (Wöckel et al, 2007).

> **ⓐ Learning activity**
>
> What skills do you feel a midwife will need in order to conduct such group sessions?

> **ⓒ Professional conversation**
>
> Brenda, a senior midwife, says, 'My mother inspired me in my ambition to become a midwife. I used to listen to her talk about my eldest brother's birth, and how brilliant the midwife had been. She had got my mother to walk around, and encouraged her to have a bath when she was in pain. My mother talked so fondly about that midwife and the positive experience of that first birth that I wanted to be a midwife, just like my mother's first midwife, and help women have a positive birth experience.
>
> 'I first trained as a nurse and then became a midwife. Once I qualified, I developed an understanding of the art and science of midwifery. For me, the key words are partnership with women, giving them information so that they can make informed choices, and empowering them to make decisions. I try to help them believe in themselves, and understand that for most of the time birth is a normal physiological process. I believe women have to be prepared for this journey, and some years ago I was able to introduce antenatal yoga classes into my work, preparing women for that positive experience.
>
> 'My goal is always to develop a trusting relationship with the woman and her family. Gaining their confidence in you is a big part of their gaining confidence in themselves to birth normally. If they feel you are supporting them, they will trust you, and keep relaxed in labour. This can help keep things normal and reduce the risk of complications occurring. Thanks to my mother, I have been able to help so many women have a positive birth experience.'

Becoming a father

> **Ⓢ Scenario continued**
>
> Dave has a problem. Initially he was delighted to learn he was to become a father, but now he is beginning to feel uncertain about his role, particularly his part in the labour. He is also anxious about seeing Kerry in pain. He feels he might not able to do much about helping her cope with it. His worst fear is that he will feel a total outsider at the birth, almost an intruder at the event. He wants to be there for Kerry, but he also feels he needs to be there in his own right for the birth of his first child.

> **ⓐ Learning activity**
>
> What might be Dave's role at the birth and how can staff ensure he feels an integral part of the events?

Health services tend to concentrate on the person requiring help and support. In maternity care, the focus has traditionally been on the woman. In some cases, of course, the father is not in a continuing relationship with the mother, or is not able to be present. However, where he is part of the situation, he can be unsure of his role, and feel he is not really included in the event. There can also be a feeling of 'awkwardness' at being there in what traditionally has been defined as 'women's business'. The events surrounding the birth involve a degree of intimacy not always shared even with partners. Up to the late twentieth century, men were not allowed to be with their partner at the birth. However, towards the end of the last century, things were made a lot more civilised and the father, or birth partner, was seen as a vital part of childbirth. This was because it was shown that birth outcomes were better, and the course of the birth was smoother where the woman was relaxed and had the support of someone close.

> **ⓐ Learning activity**
>
> Look at some of the books and leaflets aimed at preparing mothers, and examine the information aimed at fathers. Look particularly at how much space is given to the topic, and whether there is a clear role outlined for the father. How helpful do you feel the information you find might be to fathers?

Feeding the baby

The most natural way to feed a baby is by breastfeeding, which has many advantages, especially for the baby (Hale, 2007). However, the United Kingdom does not have a strong breastfeeding culture. This is evident because it has one of the lowest breastfeeding rates in the world, especially amongst disadvantaged families (Dyson et al, 2006). Many factors might be involved in this: for example, a woman's views on the role of breasts, the way breasts are portrayed in the media, the attitude of those around a woman, family members and friends, the degree of privacy available when feeding, and of course the experience of seeing other women breastfeed. However, there is evidence to suggest that GPs and midwives are influential in shaping the decision on feeding (Dyson et al, 2006), and this is why the promotion by health professionals of breastfeeding as the healthiest choice for infant feeding is so important.

This last point is supported by Chapple (2006), who identifies the promotion of breastfeeding as part of the public health role of the midwife. She points out that there are two challenges facing health professionals, and these are to increase:

- the number of women who start breastfeeding (initiation)
- the length of time that women breastfeed (continuation).

The midwife's role is to encourage women to breastfeed through giving clear information on its advantages. They are also charged to help the mother provide a successful first feed following a birth, which is Step 4 in the Baby Friendly Initiative 10 Steps (UNICEF, 1998), and to provide advice and support with feeding both immediately after the birth, and once home in the community.

In addition to the midwife, there are a number of voluntary groups, including the National Childbirth Trust and La Leche League, which provide breastfeeding support for women. Despite this combined effort, figures for women starting and maintaining breastfeeding continue to be low. There are clear differences in the level of breastfeeding by social class, with the higher classes having a higher rate of breastfeeding. As this is a cheaper feeding option, the reluctance to breastfeed is not related to income. Teenage and young mothers are a particularly vulnerable group, as they are only half as likely as older mothers to initiate any breastfeeding (Dyson et al, 2006). The complexity of the factors involved in this problem suggests that multifaceted changes are essential if the situation is to improve (Renfrew et al, 2006).

> **ⓐ Learning activity**
>
> Over the next week or so, note how many adverts, news items and features you spot on breastfeeding compared with other ways of feeding a baby, then examine some of the parenting magazines for how they approach the issue of feeding.

Part

III

Nonphysical aspects of pregnancy

During the antenatal period, health professionals must avoid simply concentrating on the physical aspects of pregnancy. For prospective parents, there are not only a large number of physical changes to accommodate, but also a number of psychological and social concerns. These include (Coggins, 2005):

- issues surrounding whether the pregnancy was planned or is wanted
- changing body image
- frequent feelings of being unwell
- relationship issues with partner and/or parents
- fears of miscarriage
- anxiety regarding the transition to parenthood
- anxiety regarding screening and fetal well-being
- career/employment issues
- housing/environmental issues
- financial issues
- altered lifestyle issues (including reducing or stopping smoking, alcohol and drug use)
- religious/cultural issues concerning the baby.

This list clearly illustrates the wide-ranging changes during this period, many of which have substantial consequences. An important issue then, is how well as a society we can prepare people for these changes, and indeed whether it is even possible to do this.

> **(a) Learning activity**
>
> What might be the consequences if health professionals only conceptualise pregnancy as a biological event?

> **[S] Scenario continued**
>
> Throughout her pregnancy, the midwife helped Kerry to address some of her risk factors and challenges. Kerry decided to quit smoking and got Dave to stop with her, to give her support. Sally referred her to the smoking cessation specialist and was able to support Kerry throughout the pregnancy with the quit smoking programme designed for her.
>
> An important part of Kerry's care was dietary advice on a healthy approach to eating. It is inadvisable for women to go on a weight-reducing diet in pregnancy, as this may affect the baby's health. Normal weight gain is one of the most positive signs of a healthy pregnancy. Sally advised Kerry to try to cut out chocolates and crisps, and consider the amount of fat in the food she eats. She should also try to ensure that her diet included the recommended five-a-day portions of fruit and vegetables.
>
> When it came to the alcohol, Kerry found she had gone off the taste of her favourite drink, so it was a relief to find there was a range of non-alcohol alternatives.
>
> Sally also encouraged Kerry to discuss how needles were to be used with those involved, in an attempt to reduce the needle phobia. Kerry always explained to them that her needle phobia could lead to a sudden faint or vomiting. Care was taken that she was sitting or lying down when needles were used, and she did not have to walk anywhere until she was fully in control. She also carried a small bottle of water with her, so she could sip it if she felt faint when bloods were taken. The progress of her labour was also discussed, so she understood that Syntometrine would be used for active management of the third stage of labour, which is the delivery of the placenta and membranes.

Preparing for the birth

During pregnancy, women are encouraged to write a personal birth plan detailing the main features they would ideally like included in the birth. This may include (Medforth et al, 2006):

- preferred place of birth
- birth companion
- positions for labour and birth they would prefer to adopt
- pain relief alternatives

- management of the third stage of labour (delivery of the afterbirth)
- suturing of any tears
- prophylactic administration of vitamin K for the prevention of haemorrhagic disease of the newborn
- cultural or religious customs to be observed.

One important aspect is the place of birth. According to NICE (2007a), in England all women should be offered a choice of planning to birth at home, in a midwife-led unit (or 'birth centre': Kirkham, 2003) or in an obstetric unit. Full information should be given on each option so that an informed decision can be made.

As was shown in Table 18.2, a number of risk factors can influence the choice of the place of birth. Other considerations can relate to culture and tradition. For instance, despite evidence to show that a home birth can be a safe option for women at low risk of complications (DH, 2003), the number of home births is still a very small proportion of the total.

> **(a) Learning activity**
>
> Why do you think home births are not currently part of the UK culture, and yet for some countries, a home birth is seen as the preferred option?

Midwifery-led units

These are now available in many areas. They differ from an obstetric unit in a number of important ways, as well as in the absence of doctors. There is a clear philosophy influencing the midwife's relationship with women, and how the birth is managed. Although there are several models of care applied in different units (Kirkham, 2003), one of their main aims is to maintain normality in childbirth and reduce unnecessary clinical intervention. Fundamental to this is the belief that the birth environment is key to facilitating a normal birth. There is a more relaxed atmosphere in such units, where women are encouraged to mobilise, adopt different positions, use the bath/pool, and continue to have light snacks to maintain their stamina. The whole environment and atmosphere is more like that of a home than a clinical setting. For example, some women and their partners choose to have music of their choice playing to create a more familiar, relaxed atmosphere.

> **S Scenario continued**
>
> Kerry wants her birth to have as few medical interventions as possible, and so wants to go to the local midwifery-led unit. This is a short distance away on a hospital site. If the course of the birth changes, she knows that she will have to be transferred in labour in an ambulance to the obstetric unit five miles away.

Hospital-based obstetric unit

The short history of maternity services at the start of this chapter outlined the way births moved from home to hospital, where they came under the control of obstetricians. Although some of the reasons for this have been successfully challenged, the greatest proportion of births are still in hospital. For some women, a high level of monitoring and assistance during the birth is essential. All women who fall into the 'high-risk' category should give birth in such a unit, as well as those women who choose this option. For the remainder, clear judgements need to be made on the appropriate path for each woman, and the extent to which they require the support and specialist expertise of the obstetrician. In such units, midwives still play a fundamental part of the birth experience and work in partnership with the obstetrician, as appropriate.

Part

III

The birth

Two days after the baby's due date, Kerry experiences some of the symptoms of early labour she had been prepared for as part of the birth preparation group. She contacts the midwives' office, and the midwife asks her about the signs of labour she is experiencing, how she is coping and whether the baby is active. The midwife is confident it is safe for Kerry to stay home for the time being, and tells her to carry on as normal, to eat, drink fluids, try to get some rest, and to have baths to help her with any pains. Above all it is important to keep relaxed and to allow labour to establish. Going into the unit too soon could delay this process.

Dave stays with her, and when the contractions are more painful and regular they check again with the midwives' office and are told to make their way to the midwifery-led unit. Kate, one of the midwives, meets them. She will be responsible for managing Kerry's care during labour. Kate takes them both to one of the small number of birthing rooms in the unit.

The birth of a baby is a life-changing event. This is recognised by RCM (2005), which states that for women, labour is not 'just normal' but actually 'extraordinary', and will have implications for all aspects of life, as we saw earlier. Few single events in our life have such a range of consequences as this one occasion. For this reason Lavender and Kingdon (2006: 335) stress:

> It is so important that midwives do not lose sight of the immensely special, unique and life-changing event each and every birth is.

The midwife will influence the experience of a particular birth, and the quality of care received to an important extent. Women can recall exactly what was said and done to them during a birth for a long time to come.

Intrapartum care

Kate makes some notes when they arrive, and asks whether Kerry has a birth plan. Kerry produces one, and she reads it. She then examines Kerry and takes a history of how and when the labour started. She asks questions to determine when the contractions started, how long they are lasting, whether Kerry has experienced a 'show', and whether her waters have broken. Kate checks her blood pressure, pulse and temperature, and tests Kerry's urine. Kate then performs an abdominal examination to establish the lie and position of the baby, and determine how much of the head can be palpated abdominally. An important part of the check is listening to the fetal heart, using either a pinnard, a trumpet-shaped hollow instrument, or a Sonicaid, as Kerry's pregnancy is low-risk. This information is recorded as part of the birth notes. Kate explains to Kerry that as the contractions are coming on a regular basis and she has had a show, labour is possibly now established. They can then decide the best way to manage the labour.

One and a half hours after arriving at the unit, Kerry's contractions are coming every three minutes. Although she is coping with her contractions well, she is becoming distressed. Kate obtains consent to perform a vaginal examination (VE), which confirms that Kerry is in established labour. Her cervix is fully effaced: that is, instead of being tubular and thick, it has become flat and thin, and has dilated (opened up) to 7 centimetres.

Kate shares the information with Kerry and Dave, and encourages Kerry to spend some time in the birthing pool to help her cope with the contractions (NICE, 2007a) and keep relaxed. As the contractions become more regular, Kerry finds it difficult to stay in the enclosed space of the pool, so she decides to come out of the water. She is encouraged to walk around the room a little or squat. With each contraction, Kerry begins to get the urge to push, and her waters rupture. The liquor is clear, which indicates that all is normal. Throughout the labour Kate listens to the fetal heart, which is seen to maintain good beat-to-beat variability and to be within the normal limits (usually between 120 and 160 bpm).

The stages of labour

Labour can be defined in purely physiological terms as the process by which the fetus, placenta and membranes are expelled through the birth canal (Medforth et al, 2006). It is divided into the three stages shown in Table 18.4.

Table 18.4 The three stages of labour

First stage	Second stage	Third stage
The transition from pregnancy to labour begins gradually (McCormick, 2003). Although it is difficult to identify the exact point at which the first stage of labour starts, established labour is confirmed by the onset of regular painful uterine contractions, and there is progressive cervical dilatation from 4 centimetres (NICE, 2007a).	The second stage of labour is defined as being from the full dilation of the cervix, and is complete following the birth of the baby. Onset of the active second stage is confirmed when: → the baby is visible → expulsive contractions with a finding of full dilation of the cervix or other signs of full dilation of the cervix → active maternal effort following confirmation of full dilation of the cervix in the absence of expulsive contractions (NICE, 2007a). Birth is expected to take place within three hours of the start of the active second stage in most women (NICE, 2007a).	The third stage follows the birth of the baby, and involves the uterus contracting and reducing in size. The placenta is expelled in this phase. This is either as part of the normal physiological process (physiological third stage), or following the administration of an oxytoxic injection given after the birth (active management of the third stage) (Chapman, 2003).

Throughout labour, the midwife constantly assesses progress and does everything possible to ensure that the labour and birth remain normal. There are a number of ways of optimising this, including (Lavender and Kingdon, 2006: 336):

- creating a positive atmosphere and environment
- presence, comfort and encouragement
- assessment of labour
- assessment of the heath of the fetus
- mobility and encouraging suitable positions for labour and birth
- helping women to cope with the pain of labour.

We could add to this, helping the birth partners find a role and contribute to the birth experience. From the initial point of contact between the labouring woman and the midwifery services, the midwife must ensure that everything is accurately recorded in the notes.

One feature of record keeping at birth is the completion of the 'partogram'. This is a graphical representation of the physical elements in a woman's labour (Chapman, 2003). Its advantage is that at a glance it captures the main points of the progress of the labour and the maternal and fetal monitoring throughout the birth process. As with other forms of recording, it is a legal document, and should include (Medforth et al, 2006):

- time of birth, gender and weight of the baby
- any abnormalities identified at birth
- Apgar score (see below)
- any resuscitation or intervention or drugs given to the baby
- length of each stage of labour
- any blood loss
- repair to the perineum, or status of perineum
- any meconium or urine passed during or post birth
- feeding intentions and summary of feeding/skin to skin contact.

> **a Learning activity**
>
> What implications do all these activities have for the type and extent of skills required of the midwife?

Part III

Scenario continued: Kerry's labour

Throughout the labour, Kerry is encouraged to drink plenty of fluids to keep hydrated. The labour continues to progress well once she is out of the pool. Her contractions become stronger and closer together, coming about every two minutes. Now out of the pool, she feels she requires something to help her cope with the contractions. She is finding it difficult to keep focused on her breathing. Kate suggests she tried to breathe entonox with each contraction. Entonox is an inhalation analgesia consisting of nitrous oxide and oxygen, which Kerry has control of herself, breathing it with each contraction. With its help, Kerry relaxes, and becomes more focused on her breathing with each contraction.

It is now four hours since Kate first examined Kerry, and as the contractions are now becoming expulsive, she performs a further VE. This reveals that the cervix is fully dilated. This happens at 10 cm, and indicates that Kerry is in the second stage of labour. The VE also reveals the baby's head is below the ischial spines and in the normal anterior position. Kate tells Kerry that when she feels the urge to push, she should use this with each contraction. Kerry naturally adopts a squatting position with each contraction.

After she has pushed for just over an hour, Kerry's baby boy is born, and breathes spontaneously once he is in air. His skin colour changes from an initial dusky blue/purple to a normal skin shade, to indicate he is oxygenating his lungs. Kate makes an assessment of his condition at birth, known as the Apgar score, which is 9 at one minute, and 10 at five minutes – top scores! She places the baby on Kerry's stomach and helps her put him to the breast and feed him.

The midwives then give the parents time to get to know their son before they proceed to weigh him and to check that he is in a good condition after the birth and that there are no congenital malformations. Kerry and Dave have already decided to call him Sam.

The midwife assesses and records the baby's condition at one minute and five minutes after the delivery, using the Apgar score to record the result of the assessment. This is carried out to identify the need for any immediate action, such as resuscitation. The Apgar method of assessment was developed in 1953 and consists of observations on five indicators that make up the acronym (Fraser and Cooper, 2003; Medforth et al, 2006):

- **A**ppearance (colour)
- **P**ulse (heart rate)
- **G**rimace (response to stimuli)
- **A**ctive (muscle tone)
- **R**espirations.

Each indicator is given a score of 0, 1 or 2, where 0 means an indicator is absent or indicative of a serious situation (such as a blue or pale-coloured baby, or limp muscle tone), 1 indicates a slow or minimal situation, and 2 indicates a good or positive situation (heart rate of over 100 bpm). A combined Apgar score of between 1 and 3 means the baby needs immediate resuscitation, between 4 and 7 indicates mild or moderate asphyxia, and scores from 8 to 10 indicate that the baby is in good physical condition.

The baby is handed to the mother following the birth and skin-to-skin contact is encouraged. This has a large number of physiological as well as psychological benefits, and from a social point of view reinforces the arrival of the baby. The physical contact is also positive for the baby, as babies who have had a traumatic birth appear a lot calmer following this contact. All babies breastfeed better if this contact has taken place. They also exhibit less distressed behaviour and cry less than babies who do not have early skin-to-skin contact. Additionally, it provides a good method of guarding against hypothermia in the newborn, and is an effective measure against hypoglycaemia (Medforth et al, 2006). It is also Step 4 of the Ten Steps of the Baby Friendly Initiative (UNICEF, 1998). The establishment of emotional attachment through skin-to-skin contact has also been seen as an advantage for the father (Chapman, 2003).

The final stage of the labour is the delivery of the placenta and membranes, usually following an injection of Syntometrine 1 ml, which is know as active management of the third stage of labour. The mother is encouraged to breastfeed the baby immediately.

A critical examination of the newborn takes place when the baby is weighed to ensure that no abnormalities can be detected. It is at this stage, if the woman has consented, the baby is injected with vitamin K to prevent haemorrhagic disease of the newborn. Once the initial care of the mother and baby has been achieved, the midwife can then complete the documentation of the birth.

S · Scenario continued

Kerry's birth is a positive experience and no complications occur. Following the birth Kerry is given help and support with breastfeeding. The midwife carries out an examination of the baby, including the usual check for any birth abnormalities and defects. Sam is in excellent condition and nothing unusual is detected. Kerry is also checked to ensure that her blood pressure is normal, that her uterus had contracted, that the blood loss following birth is normal, and she is able to pass urine. Kerry is fortunate that her perineum is intact and sutures were not required. Although she is relieved at this, Kerry's needle phobia had become less of a problem, because she has confidence in the midwives, such as Kate, who managed her care. In addition, as part of her birth plan, an anaesthetic cream has always been used prior to any procedure that might have brought on an attack.

Before going home, Kerry enjoys a refreshing shower and has something light to eat. Four hours after the birth, Kerry and Sam are discharged home accompanied by Dave.

The postnatal period

The postnatal period can be defined as the period after the end of labour. Once home, regular contact with a midwife lasts not less than ten days after the birth, and for such longer periods as the midwife considers necessary (NMC, 2008).

Key priorities for the midwife

- Carry out full examination of the baby within 72 hours of birth.
- Monitor any health indicators showing deviations for mother and baby.
- Give support with feeding.
- Give parents help in adapting to parenting roles.
- Carry out neonatal screening between seven and ten days, including tests for Phenylketonuria (PKU) and hypothyroidism.
- Health education, including contraceptive advice (NICE, 2006).

The PKU screening test involves taking a blood sample from the baby's heel. This is to detect a deficiency of phenylalanine, a metabolic disorder. If not treated within the first few weeks following birth, the condition will result in brain damage. As with all tests the procedure has to first be clearly explained, and consent must be freely given.

S · Scenario continued

Once Kerry is home, she relaxes and really enjoys looking after Sam, with the support of Dave. The breastfeeding goes well, and she is able to arrange with the midwife when she will visit her to check her breastfeeding technique. Kerry feels emotionally a little down on day three after the birth, but realises that this is normal and the result of hormonal changes. She is advised and supported with her postnatal exercises, and at day ten is discharged to the care of the health visitor, as all is normal with both Kerry and Sam.

Most health needs are met by a team approach including the midwife, health visitor and GP, amongst others. At the appropriate time, the midwife hands over the care to the health visitor, and this is done in a formal capacity. There must be documentary evidence for the handover of care from the midwife to health visitor.

Part III

Conclusion

Kerry has provided an example of a reasonably uncomplicated pregnancy and labour. If there had been more serious challenges to her health, such as developing pre-eclamsia, early rupture of membranes, failing to progress in labour or going into premature labour, then she would have had her care transferred to an obstetrician, and given birth under very different circumstances. This might have included more assisted delivery methods, such as the use of a Ventouse, where suction is applied with each contraction to help deliver the head, or the use of forceps to help the head out, or even a caesarian section. As a result the Apgar score might have been different. If there had been any problems with the baby, such as breathing difficulties, there might have been a transfer to a neonatal intensive care unit (NICU).

(a) Learning activity

Summarise in bullet form what you feel are the important principles of maternity care illustrated through Kerry's experience of maternity care.

Now you have followed Kerry through her pregnancy and birth experience, return to the learning outcomes at the beginning of the chapter to ensure that you feel you have achieved them, and visit the linked website for this chapter where you will find further information and the opportunity to test your knowledge.

References

Bounty (2006) *Your Pregnancy*, 2nd edn, Diss, Bounty (UK) Ltd.

Chapple, J. (2006) 'A public health view of the maternity services', in Page, L. A. and McCandlish, R. (eds), *The New Midwifery: Science and sensitivity in practice*, 2nd edn, Edinburgh, Churchill Livingstone. Elsevier.

Chapman, V. (ed.) (2003) *The Midwife's Labour and Birth Handbook*, Oxford, Blackwell Science.

Coggins, J. (2005) 'Early pregnancy care', in Wickham, S. (ed.), *Midwifery: Best practice, Volume 3*, Edinburgh, Books for Midwives.

Department of Health (DH) (1984) *Maternity Care in Action Report*, London, DH.

DH (1993) *Changing Childbirth: Report of the Expert Maternity Group*, London, HMSO.

DH (1999) *Delivering the Future: Report of the High Risk Pregnancy Group*, London, DH.

DH (2003) *Choice in Maternity Services, Ninth report of session 2002–03, Vol. 2*, London, DH.

DH (2004) *National Service Framework for Children, Young People and Maternity Services*, London, DH.

DH (2006) *The Pregnancy Book*, London, DH.

DH (2007) *Managing It Better: For mother and baby*, London, DH.

Dyson, L., Renfrew, M., McFadden, A., McCormick, F., Herbert, G. and Thomas, J. (2006) *Promotion of Breastfeeding Initiation and Duration: Evidence into practice briefing*, London, NICE.

Fraser, D. M. and Cooper, M. A. (2003) *Myles Textbook for Midwives*, 14th edn, Edinburgh, Churchill Livingstone.

Hale, R. (2007) 'Infant nutrition and the benefits of breastfeeding', *British Journal of Midwifery* 15(6), 368–71.

Hansard (2007) *Home Births: Written answers, 2 March* [online] http://theyworkforyou.com (accessed 2 April 2007).

Irvine, L., and Shaw, R. (2006) 'The impact of obesity on obstetric outcomes', *Current Obstetrics and Gynaecology* **16**(4), 242–6.

Kirkham, M. (2003) *Birth Centres: A social model for maternity care*, Edinburgh, Books for Midwives.

Lavender, T. and Kingdon, C. (2006) 'Keeping birth normal', in Page, L. A. and McCandlish, R. (eds), *The New Midwifery: Science and sensitivity in practice*, 2nd edn, Edinburgh, Churchill Livingstone.

McCormick, C. (2003) 'The first stage of labour: physiology and early care', in Fraser, D. and Cooper, M. (eds), *Myles Textbook for Midwives*, 14th edn, Edinburgh, Churchill Livingstone.

Medforth, J., Battersby, S., Evans, M., March, B. and Walker, A. (eds) (2006) *Oxford Handbook of Midwifery*, Oxford, Oxford University Press.

National Institute of Clinical Excellence (NICE) (2003) *Antenatal Care: Routine care for the healthy pregnant woman*, Clinical Guideline 6, London, NICE.

NICE (2006) *Routine Postnatal Care of Women and their Babies*, London, NICE.

NICE (2007a) *Intrapartum Care: Care of healthy women and their babies during childbirth*, Clinical Guideline 55, London, NICE.

NICE (2007b) *Antenatal and Postnatal Mental Health: Clinical management and service guidance*, Clinical Guideline 45, London, NICE.

Nursing and Midwifery Council (NMC) (2008) *Midwives Rules and Standards*, London, NMC.

Nolan, M. (2005) *Birth and Parenting Skills: New directions in antenatal education*. London. Elsevier Science.

Royal College of Midwives (RCM) (2004) *Position Statement Number 4: Normal childbirth* [online] http://www.rcm.org.uk/info/docs/PS4-Normal-Childbirth.doc (accessed 21 March 2007).

RCM (2005) *Midwifery Practice Guideline No.1: Evidence-based guidelines for midwifery-led care in labour*, London, RCM.

Renfrew, M., Herbert. G., Wallace, L., Spiby, H. and McFadden, A. (2006) 'Developing practice in breastfeeding', *Maternal and Child*

Nutrition **2**(4), 245–61.

Searing, K., Baukus, M., Stark, M. A., Morin, K. H. and Rudell, B. (2006) 'Needle phobia in pregnancy', *Journal of Obstetric, Gynecologic and Neonatal Nursing* **35**(5), 592–8.

Schott, J. and Priest, J. (2002) *Leading Antenatal Classes: A practical guide*. Hale, Books for Midwives.

Standing Maternity and Midwifery Advisory Committee (SMMAC) (1970) *Domiciliary Midwifery and Maternity Bed Needs* (Peel Report), London, The Stationery Office.

Thacker, S., Stroup, D. and Chang, M. (2001) 'Continuous electronic heart rate monitoring for fetal assessment during labour', *Cochrane Database of Systematic Reviews* Issue 2.

UNICEF (1998) *Implementing the Ten Steps to Successful Breastfeeding: A guide for UK Maternity service providers working towards baby friendly accreditation*, London, UNICEF UK BFI.

Wöckel, A., Shäfer, E., Beggel, A. and Abou-Dakn, M. (2007) 'Getting ready for birth: impending fatherhood', *British Journal of Midwifery* **15**(6), 344–8.

Further reading

Henderson, C. and Macdonald S. (eds) (2004) *Mayes' Midwifery: A Textbook for Midwives* (13th edn.), Edinburgh, Ballière Tindall.

Medforth, J., Battersby, S., Evans, M., March, B., Walker, A. (2006) (eds) *Oxford Handbook of Midwifery*, Oxford, Oxford University Press.

Peate, I and Hamilton, C (2008) *Becoming a Midwife in the 21st Century*, Chichester, John Wiley.

Walsh, D (2007) *Evidence-based Care for Normal Labour and Birth*, Abingdon, Routledge.

Useful website

MIDIRS www.midirs.org

Part

III

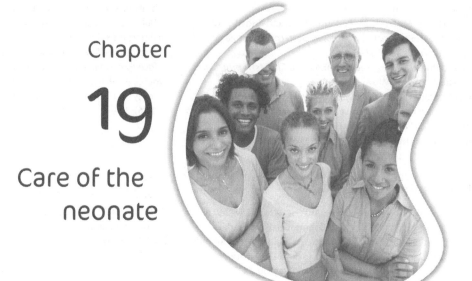

Chapter

19

Care of the
neonate

Marion Aylott

W Don't forget to visit www.palgrave.com/glasper for additional online resources relating to this chapter.

Introduction

'Neonate' is the term for the first 28 days of life, and that is the core subject of this chapter, with particular reference to preterm infants who require medical care in this period.

Infants born preterm – that is, before 37 weeks gestation, especially those born very early before 30 weeks gestation – often face a host of medical, health, developmental and social challenges, and so do their families. Those requiring time in the neonatal unit (NU) have problems ranging in seriousness from minor to life-threatening. Because the range is so varied, some infants may stay only hours and others for months until they are ready to go home.

Infants born preterm face a greater risk of serious health problems for a number of reasons relating to lower birth weights and underdeveloped organs (Mangieterra, Materro and Dunkelberg, 2006). The NU is a highly specialised and complex clinical area that requires a multidisciplinary team approach to the provision of care, including a neonatologist, neonatal medical and nursing staff, pharmacists, physiotherapists, occupational and speech therapists and dieticians.

Preterm birth is the leading cause of developmental disability in children. However, the majority of infants who leave the intensive care unit (ICU) grow up to be healthy adults (Marlow et al, 2005). But no incubator, no matter how high tech, will ever replace the womb.

The broad goals of nursing care in this period are to provide physiologically based care to the preterm newborn, to support parents in their transition to parenthood under stressful and emotive, often unexpected circumstances, and to teach them how to care for their preterm infant.

This chapter gives you an introduction to the world of neonatal nursing through a scenario in relation to the newborn period (first 24 hours of life) to help you locate fundamental issues in neonatal nursing. It explores the main philosophies and essential elements in the care of the mildly preterm, low-birthweight neonate.

Learning outcomes

This chapter will enable you to:

- identify the type of information found in the pregnancy history, labour and delivery history that is likely to be clinically significant in the care of preterm infants, including the Apgar score
- identify normal values for the vital signs and signs and symptoms of respiratory distress
- describe important features of the prevention and early recognition of common problems met by the preterm infant; hypothermia, hypoglycaemia and hypoxia.

Concepts

- Neonate
- Low birthweight
- Preterm
- Newborn
- Family-centred care
- Transition
- Thermoregulation
- Hypoglycaemia

The preterm neonate

Not every pregnancy makes it to the due date. In fact about 12 per cent of all babies born in the United Kingdom are 'premature' or 'preterm' (sometimes caregivers will refer to a preterm infant as a 'prem': Hass, 2007). A 'term pregnancy' is defined as 37 to 42 weeks. Infants born within this time frame are generally regarded as 'being ready to be born'. The term 'preterm' refers to infants born before 37 weeks of the pregnancy. Most infants are fully developed and ready for birth within one or two weeks of their estimated due date, so a full-term pregnancy is defined as anything between 38 and 42 weeks of pregnancy (WHO, 2004).

The infant's 'gestation' refers their 'age' in relation to how many weeks pregnant the mother is. For example an infant born at 32 weeks in the pregnancy is referred to as an infant of '32 weeks of gestation'.

The term 'newborn' denotes the first 24 hours, and 'neonate' the first 28 days of life after birth (see Figure 19.1). This period bears clinical significance as it is a time of transition for both the infant and the family. The neonate, whose human needs have been met entirely by the mother up until birth, now has to survive and adapt to extra-uterine life. This period poses a physiological challenge for the baby born at term, but for the infant born preterm and/or of low birthweight (LBW) (less than 2500 g) this time is extremely hazardous (Madar, 2005).

(a) Learning activity

How do we classify prematurity? The World Health Organization (WHO) (2004) classifies preterm infants into three categories. Go to this reference and look up the definitions for:
- mildly preterm
- moderately preterm
- extremely preterm.

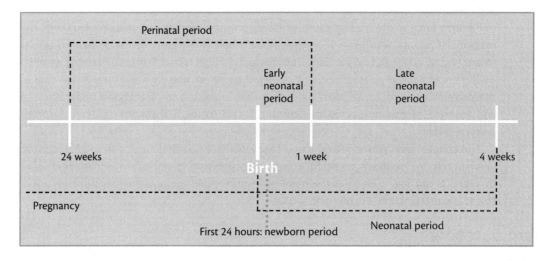

Figure 19.1 Defining the neonatal period

Each extra week an infant can grow in utero (that is, in the mother's womb) will usually translate to a considerable increase in their chances for good health and survival. For ease of reference, pregnancy is also divided into trimesters:
- The first trimester is 0–12 weeks.
- The second trimester is 13–27 weeks.
- The third trimester is 28–40 weeks.

t☆ Practice tip

Caregivers and many parents often refer to their premature infants as '29-weekers' or '34-weekers', referring to the gestational age at which they were born.

What is low birthweight?

When an infant is born preterm, their weight can affect their chances of survival. Generally the heavier the infant for their gestational age, the better off they tend to be. In the case of twins or triplets (and higher-multiple births), often the smallest of the set experiences more difficulties than their larger sibling(s) (although this is not always the case). Infants less than:
- 2,500 g (or 5 lb 9 oz) are regarded as having a low birthweight (LBW)
- 1,500 g (or 3 lb 5 oz) are regarded as having a very low birthweight (VLBW).
- 1,000 g (or 2 lb 4 oz) are regarded as extremely low birthweight (ELBW).

What causes prematurity and low birth weight?

Preterm birth may occur for a combination of reasons, not all of them clear (ONS, 2007). Although about 30 per cent of preterm births are unexplained and spontaneous (Hass, 2007), there are many factors thought to account for them, and for the recent increase in the proportion of them, including:

- increased number of multiple births
- increased number of infants conceived with assisted reproductive technology
- uterine infection
- maternal high blood pressure
- previous preterm delivery
- increasing maternal age.

Even so, half of preterm births are from unclear causes (NICE, 2003). Many questions about preterm birth remain unanswered, and it is unlikely that we will ever find a single answer to the question how we can prevent preterm birth.

A few lifestyle factors are thought to possibly increase the woman's risk of having her infant before 37 weeks (Wen et al, 2004). Be aware that these factors do not 'cause' preterm birth, they only 'increase the risk' of an infant being born prematurely. They include:

- chronic maternal illness
- maternal smoking
- drug and alcohol misuse.

The health of the mother has an important influence on fetal growth. Any chronic maternal illness such as hypertension can impair the growth of the fetus by affecting the function of the placenta. Maternal smoking and alcohol abuse are also known to impair the growth of the fetus (Hussain and Preece, 2006). Antenatal health promotion activities, including expectant mother awareness of preterm labour symptoms, and smoking cessation programmes, may help to reduce the rate of preterm and LBW births (Moore, 2002).

Sometimes a preterm infant is born because the labour is induced or a caesarean section is performed to end the pregnancy early. This is called an 'elective preterm birth', and can happen if the mother and/or the infant are unwell, leading to a decision by the obstetrician to deliver the infant(s), even though they are preterm. Careful consideration goes into weighing up the health of the mother and/or infant(s) as well as the infant's estimated gestation and weight. It usually boils down to the belief, on balance, that the infant(s) are better off 'out than in'. Elective preterm births account for approximately 25 to 40 per cent of preterm births (Mangieterra et al, 2006).

> **a) Learning activity**
>
> Make notes on your current understanding of the problems associated with prematurity before reading on.

Part III

Prematurity and low birthweight: the size of the problem

Currently approximately 12 per cent, that is 80,000 of all babies born in the United Kingdom, or put more simply one in eight infants, require some level of special care, and 2.5 per cent (17,000) of all babies born need some level of neonatal intensive care (BLISS, 2007a).

> **a) Learning activity**
>
> The world of neonatal care has a language all of its own. Nurses in this field, and other health professionals who may come into contact with the newborn from time to time, need an understanding of the normal parameters of pregnancy, labour and delivery and the normal newborn. This provides a framework for the problems that are identified in the high-risk neonatal. Study Table 19.1 to begin to familiarise yourself with some of the terms used.

Table 19.1 Glossary of terms

Term	Definition
Corrected age (CA)	Calculated from the expected date of delivery. For example, a baby born at 33 weeks gestation who is now nine weeks of age has a corrected age of two weeks.
Extremely preterm	Infant born between 24 and 28 weeks gestation.
Gestational age (GA)	Calculated from the first day of the last normal menstrual period to the date of birth, and normally expressed in completed weeks.
Gravida	The number of times a woman has been pregnant (including the current pregnancy), regardless of duration or outcome.
Low birthweight (LBW)	An infant who weighs less than 2500 grams (5 lb 5 oz) at birth.
Very low birthweight (VLBW)	An infant who weighs less than 1500 grams (3 lb) at birth.
Extremely low birthweight (ELBW)	An infant who weighs less than 1000 grams (2 lb 2 oz) at birth.
Extremely very low birthweight (EVLBW)	An infant who weighs less than 500 grams at birth.
Neonate	The first 28 days of life after birth.
Newborn	The first 24 hours of life after birth.
Mildly preterm	An infant born between 32 to 37 weeks gestation.
Moderately preterm	An infant born between 28 to 32 weeks gestation.
Para	The number of pregnancies a woman has completed past 20 weeks, regardless of whether the infant(s) is/are born alive or dead.
Perinatal	The perinatal period commences at 22 completed weeks (154 days) of gestation and ends seven completed days after birth.
Preterm	An infant born before 37 completed weeks gestation.
Term	An infant born after 37 and before 42 completed weeks gestation.
Trimester	A division of pregnancy into three equal parts of 13 weeks each.

Short and long-term problems

Preterm and LBW infants may face serious health problems in the short term, such as:
- breathing difficulties, known as respiratory distress syndrome (RDS)
- intraventricular haemorrhage
- infection.

Possible long-term problems include:
- neurodevelopmental disability
- impaired lung function
- impaired sight and hearing
- malnutrition
- congestive heart failure.

(a) Learning activity   W

Go to the website for BLISS, the premature baby charity (http://www.bliss.org.uk).
BLISS offers support to parents whose babies are born preterm or sick. This website also provides general information and statistics on preterm birth.

The UK survival rate of LBW and preterm infants is 85 per cent (Rees and Inder, 2005). Thus, preterm delivery is a major cause of neonatal death and causes nearly 50 per cent of long-term neurologic morbidity (Wen et al, 2004) (see Table 19.2). Neonatal nurses are in a unique position to promote the welfare of the infant born preterm and/or with LBW in both the short and long term (BLISS, 2007a, 2007b).

Table 19.2 Survival and disability rates

Gestational age	% survival	% major disability	% mild disability
23	11	40	40
24	26	30	20
25	44	32	35
26	60	25	30
28	80	15	25
30	90	10	20
> 31	95	2	4

Source: Office for National Statistics website: www.statistics.gov.uk. Crown Copyright material is reproduced with the permission of the Controller Office of Public Sector Information, OPSI.

W

S Scenario: Introducing Jane

Jane Jones has had two miscarriages in the first trimester. She has one son, aged 5 (born at 35 weeks). She is now pregnant again, and at 31 weeks.

a Learning activity

Reread the glossary on p. 358.
- What is Jane's gravida?
- What is her para?

t☆ Practice tip

A preterm infant has two ages. The first is their 'actual age'. This is also known as the 'chronological age', and is the measure that parents use, as it starts from their birth date. The second is their 'corrected age'. An infant's corrected age is the age they would be had they been born at term (estimated from the 40th week). The corrected age means that if the infant was born two months preterm and is now 12 months old (their actual age), their corrected age is 10 months. Medical professionals often use the corrected age of a premature infant to assess their milestones for growth and development.

Part

III

The philosophy of neonatal care

Preterm infants, irrespective of their degree of prematurity, are like children and adults regarded as having their own rights, although they are acknowledged to be vulnerable individuals (for instance, in the Human Rights Act). There is an increasing body of evidence which demonstrates that the needs and development of preterm infants can be better addressed not just by focusing on their medical needs, but also by respecting the infant as an individual who can communicate and has social and emotional needs (BLISS, 2007b).

An NU, particularly one providing neonatal intensive care, can be a very traumatic and intimidating place for parents who are already bewildered and under great stress from having a preterm or sick neonate, who might stay there for anything between four and 140 days (BAPM, 2007). Stress and distress at this time has been shown to have significant consequences for the mother, child and family in both the short and long term (Price et al, 2007). The emerging care delivery model for neonatal care is family-focused, developmentally supportive care, a philosophy which attempts to incorporate human caring and relationship building into a high-tech environment.

a Learning activity

Go to the March of Dimes prematurity website (http://marchofdimes.com/prematurity/prematurity.asp). This provides easy-to-follow information on the facts surrounding prematurity and some of the research that is being carried out into premature births.

Jane is 41 years old. She is gravida⁴, para¹ and has presented with premature prolonged rupture of membranes (PPROM) at 31 weeks gestation. She is given antibiotics and Betamethasone, a corticosteroid, and admitted for bed rest.

A threatened preterm birth

As we have seen, preterm birth can be the end result of multiple pathways. In some women, labour begins early for reasons that are clear, such as multiple gestation pregnancy, abnormalities of the mother's cervix or uterus or infection, or for no apparent reason (Moore, 2002). In about 30 per cent of preterm births, women experience ruptured membranes prior to the onset of labour and prior to 37 weeks gestation. Women with PPROM are given antibiotics to prevent infection in both the mother and fetus, and to prolong the pregnancy and reduce the chance of labour starting soon after the waters break, thereby lengthening gestation (Roberts and Dalziel, 2006). Corticosteroid injections, for example Betamethasone, are recommended for women from 24 to 32 weeks gestation. They help to mature the fetus's lungs and reduce the infant's risk of having breathing difficulties and brain haemorrhages (RCOG, 2004).

S   Scenario continued

Jane and her partner Peter are seen by the neonatologist (a consultant specialist in neonatal medicine) and neonatal nurse. The neonatologist speaks frankly with them, giving them information regarding the likely survival and long-term morbidity at this gestation. The neonatal nurse facilitates a visit to the NU.

Open and honest communication

When a neonatologist suggests that delivering a couple's infant preterm is recommended, one of the most common concerns for parents, is 'Will my baby be all right and will they survive?' The health and survival prospects for a baby born preterm depend on many factors. These can include:

- the infant's gestation and birthweight
- whether there are twins or more
- the mother's health and actual/potential complications
- the infant's health and actual/potential complications
- where the infant(s) is/are born.

The outcomes for preterm infants have improved dramatically in recent decades because of improvements in modern technology and the advancements in treatments now available. However, there remain health risks associated with being born too early, and the 'older' in gestation the infant, the better off they tend to be. Predicting how (or whether) preterm infants will recover can be difficult even for an experienced neonatologist. They will usually advise parents to take each hour and each day, one at a time. The most critical times for the survival of preterm infant(s) are typically the first week after birth and the days or hours before the birth.

Women, their partners and family can experience many diverse emotions around episodes of threatened preterm labour, preterm labour and birth of a preterm infant (Amankwaa, Pickler and Boonmee, 2007; O'Shea and Timmins, 2002). Most parents find it hard even to come to terms with what is happening at the time, and are likely to be overwhelmed with the reality of having a baby who is less than perfect and who is in a life-threatening situation. Feelings of denial, helplessness, fear, hostility, guilt and blame may emerge and interfere with their ability to communicate with each other or with health care personnel (Boyd, 2004). It is important to remember that these intense parental reactions are normal (Heermann, Wilson and Wilhelm, 2005). Open and honest communication is especially important at this time (Spencer and Edwards, 2001).

> **a) Learning activity**
>
> To learn more about parental experience of preterm birth, see *Born too Soon* (Channel 4, online).

> **t☆ Practice tip**
>
> From the moment a perinatal problem is recognised and a preterm or sick neonate is anticipated to the point of its resolution, there is a continuum of care.

> **S Scenario continued**
>
> Three weeks later (at 34 weeks gestation), Jane develops a fever of 38 °C and starts contracting. The fetus is a breech presentation and a caesarian section is performed. At delivery, Molly has a lusty cry and her Apgar scores are 6 and 7 at one minute and five minutes respectively, as a result of her poor respiratory effort, cyanosis, decreased tone and decreased response to stimulation. Her heart rate is 140 bpm.

What is an Apgar score?

Upon birth, infants are assessed and stabilised by a team of neonatal specialists including a neonatologist, neonatal nurses and others. Infants are given an Apgar score to reflect how they adjust at various intervals to immediate changes outside the womb. The Apgar score is a method of assessing an infant's clinical condition after delivery (see Table 19.3, and also page 350). It is based on five vital signs:

- heart rate
- respiratory effort
- presence or absence of central and peripheral cyanosis
- muscle tone
- response to stimulation.

Each vital sign is given a score of 0, 1 or 2. A score of 2 is normal, a score of 1 is mildly abnormal and a score of 0 is severely abnormal. The individual vital sign scores are then totalled to give an Apgar score out of 10. The best possible score is 10 and the worst 0. Normally the Apgar score is from 7 to 10. Infants with a score between 4 and 6 have moderate depression of their vital signs, while infants with a score of 1 to 3 have severely depressed vital signs and are at great risk of dying unless they are actively resuscitated. The Apgar score should be performed on all infants at one minute after birth to record the infant's clinical condition and to assess whether the infant requires resuscitation. If the one-minute Apgar score is below 7, then the Apgar score should be repeated at five minutes to document the success or failure of resuscitation efforts (Resuscitation Council UK, 2005).

Table 19.3 Apgar score

Score	0	1	2
Heart rate	No	< 100 bpm	> 100 bpm
Respiratory effort	No	Hypoventilation	Good
Presence of cyanosis	Central	Peripheral	No
Muscle tone	Toneless	Decreased tone	Flexion
Response to stimulation	No	Some movement	Good crying

Part

III

An overview of common problems

The preterm infant is physiologically different from those born at term and has a tendency to have difficulty with transition compared with the term infant because:

- they are more vulnerable to cold stress
- they are at risk for hypoglycaemia
- they have immature lungs.

Preterm infants have significant problems related to thermoregulation. The preterm infant has a greater surface area to mass ratio, and loses heat quickly. Production of heat greatly increases oxygen consumption (Wyllie, 2006). This is known as 'cold stress'. The risk of cold stress is reduced by ensuring a warm, draught-free environment. This is usually provided by an incubator. The incubator reduces radiation and convective heat losses as well as providing exogenous heat. Prewarming the incubator and thus materials that come into contact with the preterm infant reduces conductive heat loss. Lastly, keeping the infant dry or from lying in wet nappies reduces evaporative heat losses (Aylott, 2006a, 2006b).

> **t** ☆
>
> ### Practice tip
>
> Exposure to cold can increase oxygen consumption by 100 per cent (Wyllie, 2006). Therefore, keep the baby warm.

The preterm infant is at risk of hypoglycaemia after birth because they have limited glycogen and fat stores. Moreover, high metabolic requirements mean higher calorie requirements, so the preterm infant requires an immediate supply of calories. If the infant is sufficiently stable, a nasogastric tube is passed and the infant is commenced on a small volume of enteral milk feeds. The remainder of the infant's requirements are supplied by intravenous dextrose. If however, the infant is very sick and unlikely to be starting enteral milk feeds in the first few days, total parenteral nutrition (TPN) is administered.

A deficiency of surfactant in the preterm infant's lungs interferes with normal exchange of oxygen and carbon dioxide. Surfactant deficient lungs are inelastic or 'stiff', and therefore require more pressure to inflate them (Dunn and Reilly, 2003). This substantially increases the work of breathing for the preterm infant with little if any glucose, fat and protein reserve. The resulting condition of respiratory distress is referred to as respiratory distress syndrome (RDS), and is discussed in more detail later in this chapter.

> **S** **Scenario: Molly's progress**
>
> Molly, born at 34 weeks gestation, is transported to the neonatal unit in a transport incubator with 30 per cent ambient oxygen. On admission she weighs 2.23 kg. She is placed in a prewarmed incubator with humidified ambient oxygen. Her head circumference is 30 cm and her length is 41 cm.

Examining LBW

There are standards or averages in weight for unborn infants according to their age in weeks. LBW means an infant with a birth weight of less than 2500 g (5 lb 8 oz). Their low birth weight can be proportionally appropriate for gestational age, or large or small for gestational age.

> **a** **Learning activity**
>
> Birth weight = gestation duration + intrauterine growth
>
> Through plotting of weight, head circumference and length versus gestational age, each infant is classified as small, appropriate or large for gestational age. Using the chart in Figure 19.3, plot Molly's birth weight, length and head circumference against her gestational age. Determine whether she is:
>
> - large for gestational age (LGA)
> - appropriate for gestational age (AGA)
> - small for gestational age (SGA).
>
> These parameters are influenced by genetic factors and intrauterine conditions.

SGA (see the Learning activity below) occurs when the fetus is at or below the tenth weight percentile for their age (in weeks). Seventy per cent of infants who are SGA are small simply because of constitutional factors such as female sex or maternal ethnicity, parity or body mass index. The remaining 30 per cent are small as a result of intra-uterine growth deficit (IUGD) (Fang, 2005). IUGD is defined as failure of normal fetal growth. Thus, how much an infant weighs at birth depends not only on how many weeks old it is, but also on the rate at which it has grown. The neonate with IUGD has been affected by a pathologic restriction in its ability to grow and is consequently at a higher risk of mortality than those who are AGA (Marlow, 2004). The causes for IUGD include:

- maternal factors such as high blood pressure
- fetal factors such as multiple pregnancy
- placental factors such as placental haemorrhage.

Complications of preterm birth are amplified by the effect of suboptimal fetal growth (Fang, 2005). SGA neonates have experienced chronic stress in utero and possess diminished reserves to withstand the stresses of labour, delivery and transition to ex-utero life. They are therefore at risk for significant hypoglycaemia after birth because they have limited glycogen and fat stores. Their lack of fat deposits results in difficulties with thermoregulation. A high metabolic rate means higher calorie requirements and high oxygen demand, and therefore places an extra demand on the respiratory system. This triad of challenges is described as the neonatal energy triangle (see Figure 19.2) (Aylott, 2006a, 2006b).

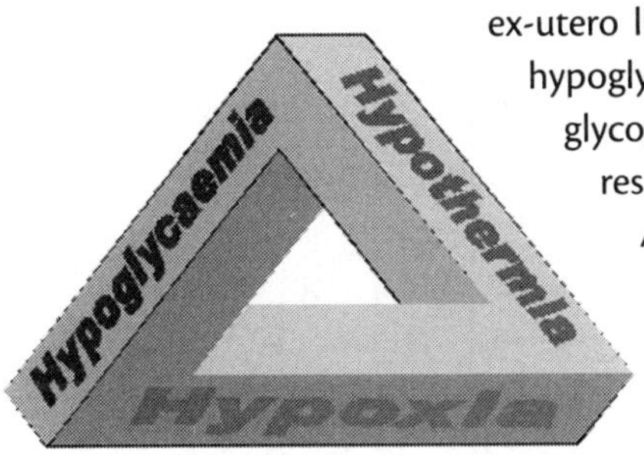

Figure 19.2 The neonatal energy triangle

t☆

Practice tip

An accurate assessment of age is important for two reasons:
- Age and growth patterns appropriate to that age aid in identifying neonatal risks.
- It helps in developing management plans.

(a) Learning activity

More neonatal terms have been introduced. In your vocabulary notebook, enter these terms and provide definitions for them:

- Apgar score
- Average for gestational age (AGA)
- Hypoglycaemia
- Hypoxia
- Intra-uterine growth deficit (IUGD)
- Premature rupture of membranes (PROM)
- Prolonged premature rupture of membranes (PPROM)
- Respiratory distress syndrome (RDS)
- Small for gestational age (SGA)
- Thermoregulation

Part

III

(S) Scenario continued

On admission Molly's observations were:

Temperature	36.2 °C	
Heart rate	140	Pulses are equal, 2+ in strength
Respiratory rate	50	Fair aeration over both lung fields with clear breath sounds
Blood pressure	45/30	(mean of 38)
Capillary refill time	2	
Oxygen saturation	96 per cent	

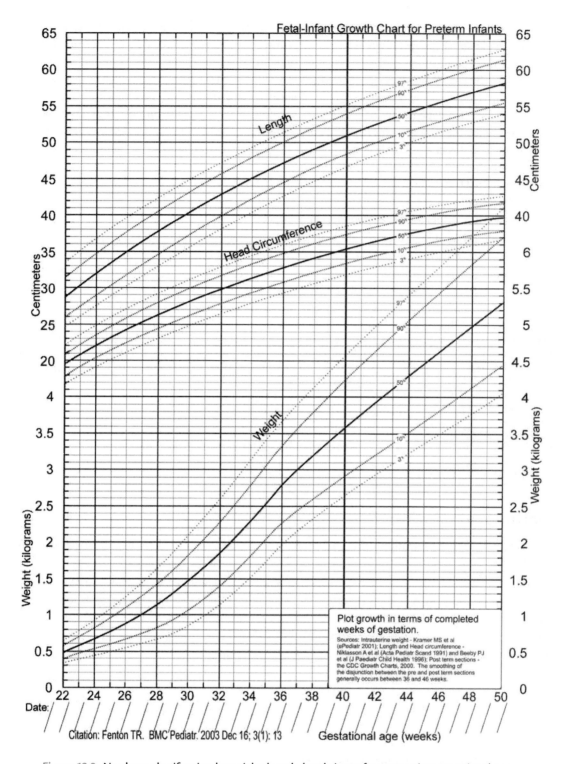

Figure 19.3 Newborn classification by weight, length, head circumference against gestational age
Source: Fenton (2003).

Common clinical problems

Like newborn infants born at term (over 37 weeks gestation), preterm infants need to make adjustments to life after birth. This means maintaining their body temperature, breathing and adjusting to feeding through suckling. However, they miss out on the final five weeks of gestation, which are an important time for the maturation of the physiologic processes that ready the fetus for life outside the womb (Neill and Knowles, 2004). During this remaining time of gestation, the fetus lays down subcutaneous tissue and brown fat, deposits glycogen stores in the liver, absorbs antibodies from across the placenta, and as the intra-uterine environment becomes less spacious, fetal muscle tone is increased (Pados, 2007). As the brain and lungs are the last organs to mature, most preterm infants under 34 weeks gestation experience problems that relate to central nervous system and lung immaturity (Blackburn, 2004). Therefore, these final weeks are important for neurological maturation, which results in improved sleep–wake state regulation and coordination of suck, swallow and breathing patterns. In summary, the increased risk of developing clinical problems described as the 'three Hs' – hypoglycaemia, hypothermia and hypoxia – for preterm infants like Molly is primarily because of organ system immaturity (Aylott, 2006a). To a certain extent, these problems are to be expected, and a good neonatal nurse will anticipate and prevent them in order to maintain stability. Let's look at the neonatal energy triangle in depth now.

t☆
Practice tip

The final five weeks of gestation are an important time for the maturation of the physiological processes that ready the fetus for life outside the womb. Although the major organ systems are functionally mature and allow for almost certain survival, the importance of the final weeks of gestation should not be underestimated.

The neonatal energy triangle: hypoxia

The most common health concern for the preterm infant is their ability to breathe on their own. Preterm birth at less than 34 weeks gestation is a risk factor for a common newborn respiratory problem known as respiratory distress syndrome (RDS), which significantly increases the need for intensive care (Clark, 2005). Preterm infants develop RDS primarily because their lungs are immature and have insufficient time to develop enough surfactant (deMello, 2004). Surfactant is a protein fluid that is produced by the lining of the infant's lungs. Having adequate surfactant reduces the surface tension of their lungs, contributing to the elasticity of their lung tissue. This is needed for the lungs to completely inflate at birth. A lack of surfactant makes it more difficult for the infant to inflate and maintain lung expansion when breathing. In addition, the connective tissue of the infant's lungs is also immature, making them 'stiff'.

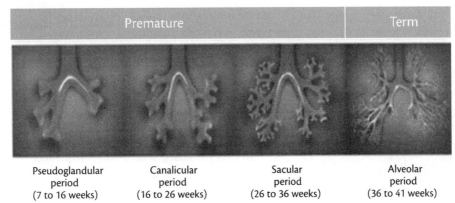

Figure 19.4
Fetal lung development

| Pseudoglandular period (7 to 16 weeks) | Canalicular period (16 to 26 weeks) | Sacular period (26 to 36 weeks) | Alveolar period (36 to 41 weeks) |

The lungs of a preterm infant have significantly decreased volume and surface area, together with increased air space wall thickness, inhibiting gas exchange (Hislop, 2005). The preterm lung has decreased airway diameters contributing to increased airway resistance. This means that high artificial ventilation pressures are often needed to open up the alveoli on inspiration and prevent collapse on expiration. Furthermore, when this immature lung is exposed to the mechanical stress of artificial ventilation, subsequent airway and alveolar development are significantly altered (Hjalmarson and Sandberg, 2002). Consequently, a fibrous membrane like scar tissue known as hyaline membrane forms. These hyaline membranes appear like 'ground glass' on chest x-rays, and are typical of RDS (see Figure 19.5).

Part
III

Mothers who it is thought might give birth to preterm infants less than 34 weeks, like Jane, are given Betamethasone injections 24 to 48 hours before the birth. These stimulate the production of surfactant and therefore 'mature' the infant's lungs for breathing (Clark, 2005).

In summary, RDS is characterised by problems associated with immaturity of the lungs: first, immature alveoli and second, a deficiency of surfactant lining the air spaces of the lung. This disease process can be further exacerbated by the fact that the preterm neonate is at risk of hypothermia and hypoglycaemia which 'switch off' surfactant production.

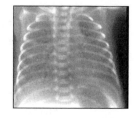

Figure 19.5 A neonatal chest x-ray which shows the typical 'ground glass' appearance of RDS

t☆
Practice tip

Hypoglycaemia and hypothermia can exacerbate hypoxia, and vice versa.

Respiratory assessment

Many neonatal nurses begin with examination of the heart and lungs when the infant is quiet at the beginning of the assessment. The respiratory system is evaluated by counting respirations over a full minute because breathing in neonates is irregular. The normal respiratory rate for newborns is between 40 and 60 breaths per minute (Pados, 2007). The normal respiratory rate decreases as gestational age increases. Neonatal respiratory rates are higher than those of older infants and children because of the mechanical properties of their chest walls and airways.

Respiratory distress causes the following signs and symptoms:

- Tachypnoea: rapid shallow breathing greater than 60 breaths/minute.
- Recession with each inspiratory breath:
  - intercostal recession: sharp in-drawing of skin between the ribs
  - subcostal recession: sharp in-drawing of skin below the rib margin
  - sternal: sharp in-drawing of skin beneath the sternum
  - substernal: sharp in-drawing of skin below the bottom of the sternum
  - supra-clavicular: sharp in-drawing of skin above the clavicles
- Nasal flare: flaring of the nostrils during inspiration.
- Cyanosis: bluish coloured mucous membranes around the nose and mouth.
- Grunting: a moaning sound, 'ugh', when the baby exhales.
- Apnoea: cessation of breathing for a period of 15 to 20 seconds.

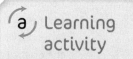
ⓐ Learning activity

Neonates have a compliant chest wall. What kind of recession can you identify in Figure 19.6?

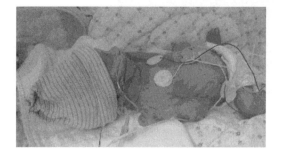

Figure 19.6 A neonate

ⓐ Learning activity   W

To learn how to evaluate a baby's work (effort) of breathing, accurately and reliably, please see the chapter information on the website that accompanies this book.

Nasal flaring during inspiration represents the infant's attempt to achieve airway dilation and reduce airway resistance, thus achieving a higher tidal volume. Although an obligatory nasal breather, the infant may also have an open mouth to decrease resistance to airflow (Kumar and Bhatnagar, 2005).

Grunting is a noise heard at the end of expiration, and is the infant's natural method of preventing alveolar collapse. This reduces their work of breathing with subsequent inspiration (Merenstein and Gardner, 2006). The infant accomplishes this by occluding their airway with premature glottic closure and actively exhaling against the closed glottis. The grunt sound is made when the infant opens the glottis, inhales, quickly exhales, and again closes the glottis against expiration (Panitch, 2005).

An important respiratory pattern of note for the newborn is periodic breathing. During periodic breathing, a baby has multiple episodes of respiratory pauses or apnoea (less than 6 seconds) interspersed with normal respiration. This is normal and can occur in preterm and term infants up to three months of age (Sly and Collins, 2005). However, a long period of apnoea that exceeds 20 seconds in duration is always abnormal. Such prolonged episodes of apnoea are frequently accompanied by cyanosis, bradycardia, pallor or hypotonia. Apnoea is a common finding in preterm infants, and if prolonged, can lead to hypoxemia and bradycardia. The exact cause is unknown but it is thought to be caused by an immature central nervous system, specifically the medulla in infants born at less than 34 weeks gestation (Sly and Collins, 2005). Because of this risk, preterm infants under 34 weeks gestation have continuous cardiorespiratory monitoring until there are no recorded apnoeic episodes for five to seven days. During this period, the neonatal nurse documents the frequency and severity of any apnoeic episodes, and the type and amount of stimulation required to interrupt the event (Martin, Abu-Shaweesh and Baird, 2004).

In the event of an apnoeic episode the nurse first provides gentle skin stimulation in the areas where nerve endings are most responsive (see Figures 19.7 and 19.8). If skin stimulation is not effective (that is, the infant does not start breathing), the nurse provides bag-valve-mask ventilation until the episode is passed (Stokowski, 2005). Therefore, the neonatal nurse must ensure that bag-valve and mask set-ups with oxygen are readily available at the infant's cotside. Infants born at less than 32 weeks gestation and those having frequent apnoeic episodes are prescribed daily caffeine citrate (Fraser et al, 2005).

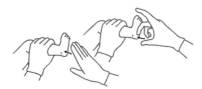

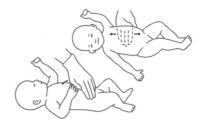

Figure 19.7 Providing skin stimulation to the feet

Figure 19.8 Providing skin stimulation along the spine and abdomen

Pulse oximetry is a simple noninvasive method of measuring peripheral oxygenation. However, accurate interpretation of pulse oximetry must utilise the relationship between SpO_2 saturation and oxygen tension (PaO_2) as described by the oxyhaemoglobin dissociation curve (see Figure 19.9). Care must be taken when interpreting high levels of oxygen saturation. Since blood is almost completely saturated at a PaO_2 of 11-13kPa it becomes very difficult to

Part

III

estimate oxygen tensions above 8kPa since the dissociation curve begins to reach a plateau (DiFiore, 2004). Baseline oxygen saturation levels of 97–99 per cent can be expected in healthy preterm infants nursed in room air. However oxygen saturations in this same range in infants receiving supplemental oxygen are problematic. Oxygen saturations at this level may be too high and may lead to retinopathy of prematurity, blindness that affects preterm infants, which is thought to be caused by damage to the retina as a result of hyperoxia (too high levels of oxygen) (Mack, 2006). Therefore, upper alarm limits of 95 per cent are set in practice when an infant is receiving supplemental oxygen therapy (Bohnsorst, Peter and Poets, 2002).

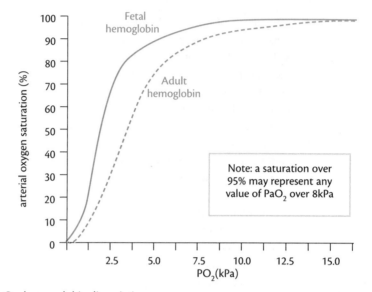

Figure 19.9   Oxyhaemoglobin dissociation curve

To assess the impact of increased work of breathing on the cardiovascular system, the neonatal nurse continually monitors the infant's heart rate. A normal heart rate is usually between 100 and 160 beats/minute. The normal resting heart rate is higher in young gestational age infants (McChance and Huether, 2006). The resting heart rate also decreases with increasing chronological age. *Tachycardia* in the newborn is defined as a heart rate greater than 160 beats/minute, and *bradycardia* as a heart rate less than 100 beats/minute (DiFiore, 2004). Be aware that tachycardia in the newborn can be caused by crying, pain, hypovolaemia (decreased circulating volume), hyperthermia and drugs. Bradycardia in the newborn can be caused by hypoxia, hypothermia or vagal stimulation, for example caused by passing a nasogastric tube.

Correct measurement of blood pressure in infants is essential because blood pressure is an important indicator of cardiovascular status (Stebor, 2005). The normal values for blood pressure (BP) depend on the infant's gestation (Dannevig et al, 2005). Usually a term newborn's systolic BP is around 70 mmHg, with a diastolic BP of around 50 mmHg. It is still impossible to define exactly what a normal preterm BP should be. It is generally recommended that the infant's gestational age is the desired minimum mean blood pressure (Weindling and Bentham, 2005).

Babies who are mildly preterm (33 to 36 weeks) can develop RDS within the first 24 hours after birth, but will often be able to cope with just receiving supplemental oxygen for a few days (Fraser et al, 2005). Infants with more severe forms of RDS may need to be treated with more aggressive therapy. Continuous positive airway pressure (CPAP) is usually indicated if the inspired oxygen concentration exceeds 50 per cent (Barclay, 2005).

t☆
Practice tip

The condition of a sick neonate can take a turn for the worse in a matter of minutes. Being able to constantly monitor and immediately react to detrimental changes can help to avoid organ damage and failure.

However, if the neonate develops increased respiratory distress despite these medical interventions, doctors may administer surfactant replacement directly into the lungs and instigate mechanical ventilation (McGuire, Fowley and McEwan, 2005).

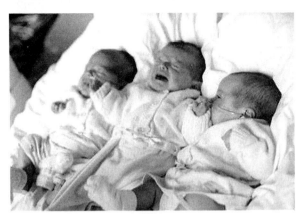

Figure 19.10 Newborn triplets

The neonatal energy triangle: hypothermia

Keeping infants warm is an essential part of neonatal nursing care. The range of normal body temperature in the newborn does not differ from that of the child or the adult. However, the newborn loses much more heat to the environment than the child or adult, because heat loss is determined by their:

- large surface area to total body mass ratio
- minimal subcutaneous tissue
- skin permeability to water.

For infants younger in gestational age, the problem becomes even more significant, as you can see in Figure 19.11. A 28-week gestation infant has a surface area in relation to mass which is almost double that of the term infant and six times that of the adult. Thus newborn babies, especially those born preterm, lose heat easily and are extremely dependent on the environment to help them to maintain body temperature.

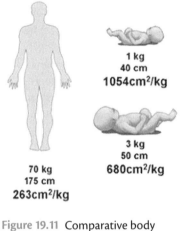

1 kg
40 cm
1054cm²/kg

3 kg
50 cm
680cm²/kg

70 kg
175 cm
263cm²/kg

Figure 19.11 Comparative body surface area to body mass ratio

Preterm infants are not able to regulate their body temperatures as well as term infants because of their immature hypothalamic regulatory centre (Ellis, 2005). Birth also occurs before the deposition of subcutaneous fat and sufficient glycogen stores in the last trimester of pregnancy, so the infant lacks sources of energy for maintenance of homeostasis (Lyon, 2004). Additionally, the preterm infant is less able than term infants to maintain a less flexed posture, which helps to reduce surface area, and this places them at increased risk for hypothermia (Laptook and Jackson, 2006). Normally, a full-term infant exposed to cold stress is able to increase metabolism to maintain a neutral body temperature without significant physiological consequences. However, the preterm infant exposed to cold stress must rely on immature mechanisms and inadequate stores of glucose, which is required for increasing metabolism for heat. Hypothermia stimulates brown fat metabolism, a process that requires glucose, resulting in rapid depletion of glucose and thus hypoglycaemia when limited glucose stores are exhausted (Aylott, 2006b). At the same time, increasing metabolic rate leads to increased oxygen consumption and therefore increased respiratory rate. Ultimately, in an effort to maintain a neutral thermal body temperature the preterm infant is likely to become hypoglycaemic and develop respiratory distress; remember the neonatal energy triangle (Aylott, 2006a, 2006b).

Part
III

Temperature assessment

The normal body core temperature of newborns is between 36.6 °C and 37.2 °C. Hyperthermia is defined as a core temperature of more than 37.5 °C, and hypothermia is a core temperature of less than 36.5 °C (McCall et al, 2006). In order to maintain homeostasis, the neonatal nurse aims to care for the infant in a neutral thermal environment (NTE). An NTE is the environmental temperature at which the infant's metabolic demand and therefore oxygen consumption is minimal (McCall et al, 2006).

Temperature measurement is an essential part of monitoring a preterm infant's health status, as abnormal temperature is strongly associated with increased morbidity and mortality (Bailey and Rose, 2000). Temperature measurement in preterm infants needs to be accurate, non-invasive, safe and speedy, with an emphasis on minimal disturbance, and the thermometer should be simple to use and clean. It is recommended that a central and a peripheral temperature are monitored simultaneously, and the difference charted. This is because the intermittent measurement of a central (axilla) temperature will only detect cold stress at a late stage. When cold, an infant attempts to reduce heat loss by constricting blood capillaries in the skin, thus keeping blood in the central circulation. When peripheral vasoconstriction can no longer compensate, the central temperature falls. Therefore, the peripheral body temperature falls long before the central body temperature. Measuring both a central and a peripheral temperature and continuously monitoring the difference between these two readings enables cold stress to be detected at a much earlier stage. The difference between central and peripheral temperature in homeostasis should be less than 2 °C. This is often referred to in practice as the 'toe–core differential'. Figure 19.12 demonstrates how the toe–core differential is first increased before the core temperature begins to fall. As the toe–core differential increases, cold stress is already beginning and intervention is needed immediately before the infant uses vital glucose stores and has increased oxygen consumption (Waldron and MacKinnon, 2007).

The peripheral temperature probe is usually placed on the sole of the foot, and is protected from convective heat loss by a pad or sock (see Figure 19.13). This is especially important when the infant is being nursed under an overhead radiant heater or phototherapy.

Learning activity

Babies lose heat to the environment by four mechanisms:

- conduction
- convection
- evaporation
- radiation.

Define each mechanism and give two examples of how each can occur in practice.

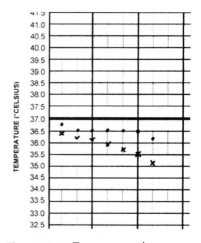

Figure 19.12   Temperature chart

Practice tip

Be aware that peripheral temperature probe accuracy can be directly affected by its positioning, most commonly when the infant's feet get wet from their nappy.

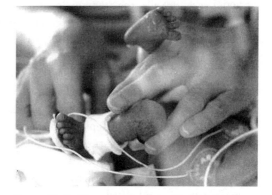

Figure 19.13   Covering a peripheral temperature probe with a protective shield

For a long time until recently, rectal temperature measurement was accepted as the gold standard for accurate core temperature measurement. However, there is a large body of knowledge that identifies the risks associated with rectal temperature taking, such as rectal perforation and vagal stimulation (Smith, 2004). The proven site of preference and greatest accuracy for core temperature measurement is the axilla or the abdomen, remembering that these sites under-read core temperature by up to 0.5 °C (Smith, 2004). Normal axillary or abdominal temperature falls between 36.5 and 37 °C. Again an abdominal temperature probe placed over the liver can be affected by a radiant heater and phototherapy, and therefore should be covered usually with a reflective shield. A manual axilla temperature is also taken, usually four-hourly, as a quality check of probe accuracy.

Incubators and radiant warmers are the universally accepted method of maintaining a NTE for term and preterm infants (Flanady and Gray, 2005).

t☆

Practice tip

Possible causes of cold stress include open incubator doors and handling of the infant. A small preterm infant can take up to two hours to recover from a period of handling.

ⓐ Learning activity

The baby's temperature is maintained using two common methods. In relation to the principles of heat loss – evaporation, conduction, convection and radiation – and practical considerations, consider the advantages and disadvantages of a radiant warmer compared with an incubator.

The neonatal energy triangle: hypoglycaemia

Hypoglycaemia is the most common metabolic problem occurring in preterm SGA infants (Hawdon, Nugent and Angel, 2000). In the fetus, serum glucose levels are about 70 per cent of those in the mother, and almost all of this comes from facilitated diffusion across the placenta (Noerr, 2001). Stores of glucose in the liver accumulate slowly through gestation, with a marked increase during the last trimester (Beardsall et al, 2003). A term infant is estimated to have only enough hepatic glycogen stores to support metabolic demands for about 24 hours without an exogenous energy source (Hewitt et al, 2005). However, the preterm infant is at great risk for hypoglycaemia because of limited glycogen stores and relatively immature glucose homeostastic mechanisms. If glycogen stores are insufficient, and the infant's intake is not sufficiently adequate to maintain blood glucose, the infant will develop hypoglycaemia. Neonatal nurses must be aware of the increased risk of hypoglycaemia in these babies (Williams, 2005). Left untreated, hypoglycaemia leads to reduced central nervous system blood glucose levels which may result in seizures and long-term neurological impairments (Blackburn, 2004). Also, remember the neonatal energy triangle: any alteration in metabolic processes, including hypothermia or hypoxia, will increase glucose needs and accelerate this process (Aylott, 2006a, 2006b).

Part

III

t☆

Practice tip

In preterm infants and those born SGA, adequate fetal glycogen storage has been interrupted or impaired, placing these infants at risk for hypoglycaemia in the first 36 to 48 hours of life.

ⓐ Learning activity

Refer to Chapter 6, 'Fundamental aspects of nursing assessment and monitoring' in Glasper, Aylott and Prudhoe (2007) to learn the correct technique for blood glucose testing and obtaining a sample by neonatal heel lance.

The preterm infant should be monitored closely for signs and symptoms of hypoglycaemia and should be supported appropriately. Signs and symptoms of hypoglycaemia might be subtle and nonspecific such as:

- apnoea
- jitteriness
- exaggerated Moro (startle reflex)
- irritability
- poor sucking or feeding
- cyanosis
- hypotonia
- lethargy
- hypothermia.

Similar signs occur with a variety of other important neonatal conditions such as hypoxia and infection. Additionally, hypoglycaemic preterm infants may be entirely asymptomatic. Therefore, it is important that clinical judgements and interventions are based on individual assessments of blood glucose at regular intervals in at least the first 36 hours of life (Noerr, 2001). Generally, glucose levels are maintained above 2.6mmol/L in (Hawdon et al, 2000).

> **[S] Scenario continued**
>
> To prevent hypoglycaemia and hypovolaemia, Molly is immediately commenced an intravenous infusion of 10 per cent dextrose (60ml/kg/24 hours) on admission. Once her respiratory distress settles, she will be commenced on nasogastric tube feeds of expressed breast milk. Early enteral feeding also helps to prevent hypoglycaemia.

Coordinated sucking, swallowing and breathing (see Figure 19.14) begins to emerge at 34-36 weeks postconceptual age, but may not become well coordinated until 37 weeks (Mizuna and Ueda, 2003). Therefore, feeding must often be done by gastric tube until the infant has developed coordination of the suck, swallow and breathe reflex. This coordination is gained by repeated supervised exposure of the infant to breast or bottle feedings (Pinelli and Symington, 2007). There is growing evidence to support the view that non-nutritive sucking at the breast or on a pacifier (a dummy) helps to promote functional sucking skills (Harding et al, 2006).

Gastric emptying in the preterm infant is delayed compared with the term infant. Immaturity of the small intestinal motor function prolongs gut transit time and is volume limiting (McCain, 2003), and for this reason enteral feeds are started at 1ml/kg/hour bolus feed, This is progressively given in increasing volumes (for example increased by 1ml/kg eight-hourly) and the hourly intravenous fluid rate reduced accordingly as the increased volume of feed is tolerated.

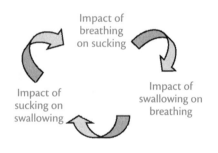

Figure 19.14   The suck, swallow, breathe triad

Conclusion

This chapter has given you the opportunity to begin to explore the common clinical challenges faced by the preterm and LBW infant. Every major organ system is anatomically and functionally immature in the term newborn but is especially so in the preterm infant. Successful newborn transition to extra-uterine life for the preterm infant persists beyond the first few days of life. Comprehensive care of preterm infants therefore requires an understanding of immature anatomy and physiology and the corresponding needs of the preterm infant.

Preterm and LBW neonates, especially those that are classified as SGA, do not possess the reserves to withstand the stresses of transition to extra-uterine life. They are therefore at risk for significant hypoglycaemia after birth because they have limited glycogen and fat stores. Their lack of fat deposits results in difficulties with thermoregulation. Their high metabolic rate means higher calorie requirements and high oxygen demand, and therefore places an extra demand on the respiratory system. This triad of challenges is described as the neonatal energy triangle. These problems can be anticipated, and a good neonatal nurse will apply clinical risk management strategies for the early identification and management of hypoxia, hypoglycaemia and hypothermia in order to maintain stability.

References

Amankwaa, L. C., Pickler, R. H. and Boonmee, J. (2007) 'Maternal responsiveness in mothers of preterm infants', *Newborn and Infant Nursing Reviews* **7**(1), 25–30.

Aylott, M. (2006a) 'The neonatal energy triangle part 1: metabolic adaptation', *Paediatric Nursing* **18**(6), **38–42**.

Aylott, M. (2006b) 'The neonatal energy triangle part 2: thermoregulatory and respiratory adaptation', *Paediatric Nursing* **18**(6), **38–42.**

Bailey, J. and Rose, P. (2000) 'Temperature measurement in the preterm infant: a literature review', *Journal of Neonatal Nursing* **6**(1), 28–32.

Barclay, L. (2005) 'Early use of surfactant, NCPAP improves infant respiratory distress syndrome', *Medscape Medical News* [online] http://medscape.com/viewarticle/480012?src=mp (accessed 9 February 2009).

Beardsall, K., Yuen, K., Williams, R., and Dunger, D. (2003) 'Applied physiology of glucose control', *Current Paediatrics* 13, 543–8.

Blackburn, S. T. (2004) *Maternal, Fetal and Neonatal Physiology: A clinical perspective*, 2nd edn, St Louis, Miss., Mosby.

BLISS (2007a) *Facts and Figures* [online] http://www.bliss.org.uk/page.asp?section=135&sectionTitle=Facts+and+figures (accessed 9 February 2009).

BLISS (2007b) *BLISS Baby Charter* [online] www.bliss.org.uk/core/core_picker/download.asp?id=64 (accessed 9 February 2009).

Bohnsorst, B., Peter, C. S. and Poets, C. F. (2002) 'Detection of hyperoxaemia in neonates: data from three new pulse oximeters', *Archives of Disease in Childhood: Fetal and Neonatal Edition* 87, 217–19.

Boyd, S. (2004) 'Within these walls: moderating parental stress in the NICU', *Journal of Neonatal Nursing* **10**(3), 80–4.

British Association of Perinatal Medicine (BAPM) (2007) *Standards for Hospitals Providing Neonatal Intensive and High Dependency Care and Categories of Babies Requiring Neonatal Care*, London, BAPM.

Chamley, C. A., Carson, P., Randall, D. and Sandwell, M. (2005) *Developmental Anatomy and Physiology of Children: A practical approach*, Edinburgh, Elsevier and Churchill Livingstone.

Channel 4 (nd) *Born too Soon* [online] http://www.channel4.com/health/microsites/B/borntoosoon/why.html (accessed 9 February 2009).

Clark, R. H. (2005) 'The epidemiology of respiratory failure in neonates born at an estimated gestational age of 34 weeks or more', *Journal of Perinatology* 25, 251–7.

Dannevig, I., Dale, H. C., Liestol, K. and Lindemann, R. (2005) 'Blood pressure in the neonate: three non-invasive oscillometric pressure monitors compared with invasively measured blood pressure', *Acta Paediatrica* **94**(2), 191–6.

DeMello, D. E. (2004) 'Pulmonary pathophysiology', *Seminars in Neonatology* 9, 311–29.

DiFiore, J. M. (2004) 'Neonatal cardiorespiratory monitoring techniques', *Seminars in Neonatology* 9, 195–203.

Dunn, M. S. and Reilly, M. C. (2003). 'Approaches to the initial respiratory management of preterm neonates', *Paediatric Respiratory Reviews* 4, 2–8.

Ellis, J. (2005) 'Neonatal hypothermia', *Journal of Neonatal Nursing* 11, 76–82.

Fang, S. (2005) 'Management of preterm infants with intrauterine growth restriction', *Early Human Development* **81**(11), 889–900.

Fenton, T. R. (2003) 'BMC', *Pediatrics* **3**(1), 13.

Flanady, V. J. and Gray, B. H. (2005) 'Chest physiotherapy for preventing morbidity in babies being extubated from mechanical ventilation', Cochrane Library (banco de dados), 4th edn.

Fraser, J., Walls, M. and McGuire, W. (2005) 'ABC of preterm birth: respiratory complications of preterm birth' *Student British Medical Journal* 13, 278–80.

Glasper, A., Aylott, M. and Prudhoe, G. (2007) *Fundamental Aspects of Children's and Young People's Nursing Procedures* London, Quay Books.

Hajunal, B. L., Braun-Fahrlander, C., von Siebenthal, K., Bucher, H. U. and Largo, R. H. (2004) 'Improved outcome for very low birth weight multiple births', *Pediatric Neurology* **32**(2), 87–93.

Harding, J. E., Miles, F. K., Becroft, D. M., Allen, B. C. and Knight, D. B. (2006) 'Chest physiotherapy may be associated with brain damage in extremely premature infants', *Journal of Pediatrics* **132**(3), 440–4.

Hass, D. M. (2007) 'Preterm birth', *British Medical Journal Clinical Evidence* [online] http://www.clinicalevidence.com/ceweb/conditions/pac/1404/1404_background.jsp (accessed accessed 9 February 2009).

Hawdon, J. M., Nugent, M. and Angel, P. (2000) 'Controversies regarding definition of neonatal hypoglycaemia', *Journal of Neonatal Nursing* **6**(5), 169–71.

Hawdon, J. M. (2005) 'Blood glucose levels in infancy – clinical significance and accurate measurement', *Infant* **1**(1), 24–7.

Heermann, J. A., Wilson, M. E. and Wilhelm, P. A. (2005) 'Mothers in the NICU: iutsider to partner', *Pediatric Nursing* **31**(3), 176–81, 200.

Hewitt, V., Watts, R., Roberton, J. and Haddow, G. (2005) 'Nursing and midwifery management of hypoglycaemia in healthy term neonates', *International Journal of Evidence Based Healthcare* 3, 169–205.

Hislop, A. (2005) 'Developmental biology of the pulmonary circulation', *Paediatric Respiratory Reviews* 6, 35–43.

Hjalmarson, O. and Sandberg, K. (2002) 'Abnormal lung function in healthy preterm infants', *American Journal of Respiratory and Critical Care Medicine* 165, 83–7.

Hussain, K. and Preece, M. (2006) 'Applied physiology: understanding growth', *Current Paediatrics* 16, 430–3.

Kumar, A. and Bhatnagar, V. (2005) 'Respiratory distress in the neonate', *Indian Journal of Pediatrics* 72, 425–8.

Laptook, A. and Jackson, G. (2006) 'Cold stress and hypoglycaemia in the late preterm ("near-term") infant: impact on nursery admission', *Seminars in Perinatology* 30, 24–7.

Lissauer, T. and Fanaroff, A. (2006) *Neonatology at a Glance*, Oxford, Blackwell.

Lyon, A. (2004) 'Applied physiology: temperature control in the newborn infant', *Current Paediatrics* 14, 137–44.

Mack, E. (2006) 'Oxygen administration in the neonate', *Newborn and Infant Nursing Reviews* **6**(2), 63–7.

Madar, J. (2005) 'Clinical risk management in newborn and neonatal

Part

III

resuscitation', *Seminars in Fetal and Neonatal Medicine* 10, 45–61.

Mangieterra, V., Mattero, M. and Dunkelberg, E. (2006) 'Why and how to invest in neonatal health', *Seminars in Fetal and Neonatal Medicine* 11, 37–47.

Marlow, N. (2004) 'Outcome following extremely preterm birth', *Current Paediatrics* 14, 275–83.

Marlow, N. (2007) 'UK neonatal networks – how far have we gone?' *Paediatrics and Child Health* **17**(2), 1–4.

Marlow, N., Wolke, D., Bracewell, M. and Samara, M. (2005) 'EPICure Study Group: neurologic and developmental disability at six years of age after extremely preterm birth', *New England Journal of Medicine* 352, 9–19.

Martin, R. J., Abu-Shaweesh, J. M. and Baird, T. M. (2004) 'Apnoea of prematurity', *Paediatric Respiratory Reviews* 5 (Suppl A), S337–82.

McCain, G. C. (2003) 'An evidence-based guideline for introducing oral feeding to healthy preterm infants', *Neonatal Network* 22(5), 45–50.

McCall, E. M., Alderdice, F. A., Halliday, H. L., Jenkins, J. G,. and Vohra, S. (2006) 'Interventions to prevent hypothermia at birth in preterm and/or low birthweight babies', *Cochrane Review* 3.

McChance, K. L. and Huether, S. E. (2006) *Pathophysiology: The biologic basis for disease in adults and children*, 5th edn, St Louis, Miss., Elsevier Mosby.

McGrath, J. and Bodea Braescu, A. V. (2004) 'State of the science: feeding readiness in the preterm infant', *Journal of Perinatal and Neonatal Nursing* 18: 353–68.

McGrath, J. M. (2007) '"He's just a little small": helping families to understand the implications of caring for a late preterm infant', *Newborn and Infant Nursing Reviews* **7**(2), 120–1.

McGuire, W. and Fowlie, P. W. (2005) *ABC of Preterm Birth*, Oxford, BMJ Publishing.

McGuire, W., Fowlie, P. W. and McEwan, P. (2005) 'ABC of preterm birth: care in the early newborn period', *Student British Medical Journal* 13, 320–2.

Merenstein, G. B., and Gardner, S. L. (2006) *Handbook of Neonatal Intensive Care*, 6th edn, London, Elsevier.

Mizuna, K. and Ueda, A. (2003) 'The maturation and coordination of sucking, swallowing and respiration in preterm infants', *Journal of Pediatrics* **142**(1), 36–40.

Moore, M. L. (2002) 'Preterm birth: a continuing challenge', *Journal of Perinatal Education* **11**(4), 37–40.

National Institute for Clinical Excellence (NICE) (2003) *Antenatal Care: Routine care for the healthy pregnant woman*, Clinical Guideline 6, London, NICE.

Neill, S. and Knowles, H. (2004) *The Biology of Child Health: A reader in development and assessment*, Basingstoke, Palgrave Macmillan.

Noerr, B. (2001) 'State of the science: neonatal hypoglycaemia'. *Advances in Neonatal Care* **1**(1), 4–21.

Office of National Statistics (ONS) (2007) *Maternity Statistics*, May 2006/7. London, ONS.

O'Shea, J. and Timmins, F. (2002) 'An overview of parents' experiences of neonatal intensive care: do we care for both parents?' *Journal of Neonatal Nursing* **8**(6), 178–83.

Pados, B. F. (2007) 'Safe transition to home: preparing the near-term infant for discharge', *Newborn and Infant Nursing Reviews* 7(2),106–13.

Panitch, H. B. (2005) *Pediatric Pulmonology: The requisites in pediatrics*, Philadelphia, Penn., Elsevier Mosby.

Pinelli, J. and Symington, A. (2007) 'Non-nutritive sucking for promoting physiologic stability and nutrition in preterm infants', *Cochrane Library* 4, 54.

Price, S., Lake, M., Breen, G., Carson, G., Quinn, C. and O'Connor, T. (2007) 'The spiritual experience of high-risk pregnancy', *JOGNN Clinical Research* **36**(1), 63–70.

Rees, S. and Inder, T. (2005) 'Fetal and neonatal origins of altered brain development', *Early Human Development* 81, 753–61.

Resuscitation Council (UK) (2005) Resuscitation Guidelines: Newborn life support, London, Resuscitation Council, [online] http://www.resus.org.uk/pages/nls.pdf (accessed 9 February 2009).

Roberts, D. and Dalziel, S. (2006) 'Antenatal corticosteroids for accelerating fetal lung maturation for women at risk of preterm birth', *Cochrane Database of Systematic Reviews* 2.

Royal College of Obstetricians and Gynaecologists (RCOG) (2004) 'Antenatal corticosteroids to prevent respiratory distress syndrome', London, RCOG.

Sly, P. D. and Collins, R. A. (2005) 'Physiological basis of respiratory signs and symptoms', *Paediatric Respiratory Reviews* 7, 84–8.

Smith L. S. (2004) 'Temperature monitoring in newborns: a comparison of thermometry and measurement sites', *Journal of Neonatal Nursing* **10**(5), 157–65.

Spencer, C. and Edwards, S. (2001) 'Neonatal intensive care unit environment: a review from the parents' perspective'. *Journal of Neonatal Nursing* **7**(4), 127–31.

Stebor, A. D. (2005) 'Basic principles of noninvasive blood pressure measurement in infants: cultivating clinical expertise', *Advances in Neonatal Care* **5**(5), 252–61.

Stokowski, L. A. (2005) 'A primer on apnea of prematurity', *Advances in Neonatal Care* **5**(3), 155–70.

Thureen, P. J. and Hay, W. W. (2001) 'Early aggressive nutrition in preterm infants', *Seminars in Neonatology* 6, 403–15.

Tin, W., Walker, S. and Lacamp, C. (2003) 'Oxygen monitoring in preterm babies: too high, too low?' *Paediatric Respiratory Reviews* 4, 9–14.

Tucker, J. and McGuire, W. (2005) 'ABC of preterm birth: Epidemiology of preterm birth', *Student British Medical Journal* 13, 133–76.

Waldron, S. and MacKinnon, R. (2007) 'Neonatal thermoregulation', *Infant* **3**(3), 101–4.

Wang, M. L., Dorer, D. J. and Fleming, M. P. (2004) 'Clinical outcomes of near-term infants', *Pediatrics* 339, 313–20.

Ward Platt, M. and Deshpande, S. (2005) 'Metabolic adaptation at birth', *Seminars in Fetal and Neonatal Medicine* 10, 341–50.

Weindling, A. M. and Bentham, J. (2005) 'Blood pressure in the neonate', *Paediatrica* **94**(2), 138–40.

Wen, S. W., Smith, G., Yang, Q. and Walker, M. (2004) 'Epidemiology of preterm birth and neonatal outcome', *Seminars in Neonatology* **9**(6), 429–35.

Williams, A. F. (2005) 'Neonatal hypoglycaemia: clinical and legal aspects', *Seminars in Fetal and Neonatal Medicine* 10, 363–8.

World Health Organization (WHO) (2004) *Unsafe Abortion: Global and regional estimates of the incidence of unsafe abortion and associated mortality in 2000*, 4th edn, Geneva, WHO.

Wyllie, J. (2006) 'Applied physiology of newborn resuscitation', *Current Paediatrics* 16, 379–85.

Chapter

20

Care of the child and young person

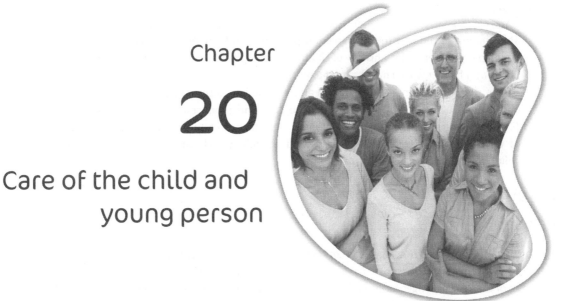

Alan Glasper, Janet Kelsey and Gill McEwing

Links to other chapters in *Foundation Studies for Caring*

Links to other chapters in *Foundation Skills for Caring*

W Don't forget to visit www.palgrave.com/glasper for additional online resources relating to this chapter.

Part

III

Introduction

This chapter introduces the fundamental principles underpinning the care of children and young people. It provides a history of children's nursing and considers ways in which children's needs may be met within healthcare today.

The aim of the chapter is to give you an introduction to the world of child health nursing and explore a number of prevailing philosophies and practices. When you go on to read Chapter 21 you will find a scenario relating to an asthmatic child. The health/illness paradigms of childcare are therefore fully investigated to help you locate contemporary issues in childhood nursing.

Learning outcomes

This chapter will enable you to:

- consider the origins of children's nursing in the context of the changing concepts of childhood
- examine some of the key challenges facing child health nurses in the twenty-first century
- appreciate some of the recent innovations in the care of sick children
- use relevant literature and research to inform the practice of nursing
- describe the importance of play

- discuss different approaches to the management of care for the sick child
- recognise the role of the family in a child's life and well-being, and propose strategies to work collaboratively with the child and family
- appreciate the importance of immunisation in children
- recognise the essential requirements of nutrition in the infant and child
- discuss the effect of hospitalisation on children.

Concepts

- Childhood
- Play
- Hospitalisation

- Children's rights
- Children's nursing and the nurse's role

- Immunisation
- Family-centred care
- Nutrition

History of children's nursing

The history of children's nursing begins with Captain Thomas Coram, who after working in shipping, mainly in the America, became a successful merchant in London in 1832 (Nichols and Wray, 1935). Coram was embarrassed at the way in which abandoned children were treated in society, and in response worked with the influential people of his time for a Royal Charter to establish a Foundling Hospital in modern-day Bloomsbury in London in 1841 (Glasper and Mitchell, 2006). In accommodating abandoned infants and children in the Foundling Hospital, Coram wanted to stop the practice of parents abandoning their infants and children to die on the streets of London. The primary aim of the Foundling Hospital, which was not a hospital for sick children, was to provide care and education until the child was old enough to work. Sadly the Foundling Hospital had high mortality rates mainly because of the appalling state of ignorance about the spread of disease. Of the 15,000 children admitted to the Foundling Hospital during the years 1856–60, only 4400 lived to adulthood.

In the absence of in-patient facilities for sick children, charitable dispensaries similar to modern outpatient departments were established, and one of the first was developed in 1869 in Red Lion Square London by Dr George Armstrong, now regarded as the father of ambulatory care. The main aim of dispensaries was to reduce mortality rates among poor children by providing advice and administering medicines. Children were not allowed to be treated as in-patients in most hospitals because they were feared to be harbingers of disease. In reality many children succumbed to the normal infectious diseases of childhood exacerbated by poor nutrition. George Armstrong himself was not a supporter of in-patient care for children in hospital. He is credited with saying, 'If you take a sick child away from the parents, you break its heart immediately' (Miles, 1986).

Although dispensaries offered a modicum of care, the desperate state of housing for the poor ensured that their success in reducing the mortality rates of sick children was at best modest. There was a gradual realisation that specialist in-patient care for sick children was needed.

The establishment of children's hospitals

The National Children's Hospital in Dublin was founded as a hospital for sick children in 1821 by Dr Henry Marsh (later Sir Henry Marsh), Dr Philip Crampton (later Sir Philip Crampton), and Dr Charles Johnson, as the first teaching children's hospital in the British Isles. Dr Charles West, a young paediatrician working in one of the London dispensaries, had seen what could be achieved for in-patient sick children during a visit to Dublin. He was appalled that an international city the size of London should not have the facilities to treat children with acute illnesses. West's friend was the author Charles Dickens, and at the time of the opening of the Hospital for Sick Children in Great Ormond Street in 1852, nursing was still at the Sairey Gamp stage of development, graphically portrayed in Dickens' novel *Martin Chuzzlewit*. This character was a domiciliary working-class nurse who was a drunkard and stole from her patients, totally at odds with today's image of nursing. After much fundraising, a lot of it attributed to Dickens himself, the Hospital for Sick Children, Great Ormond Street in London opened in 1852 with ten beds. Today, like many children's hospitals and units across the United Kingdom, it exists to serve the sick children of society. Its mission statement, 'The child first and always', is indicative of this commitment to caring for sick children.

The growth of children's hospitals

- National Children's Hospital Dublin (1821)
- Hospital for Sick Children, Great Ormond Street, London (1852)
- Royal Manchester Children's Hospital (1855)
- Royal Hospital for Sick Children, Edinburgh (1860)
- Birmingham Children's Hospital (1862)

- Evelina Children's Hospital (1869)
- Children's Hospital Temple Street (1893)
- Sunderland Children's Hospital (1910)
- Alder Hey (1914)
- Booth Hall (1915)

An important function of hospitals such as the National Children's Hospital, Dublin and the Hospital for Sick Children, Great Ormond Street was the training and education of nurses with the special skills required to nurse ill children. The legacy of Florence Nightingale, who came to notice in 1854 during the Crimean war when she led a team of adult nurses to care for sick and injured British soldiers, ensured that the emerging nursing profession was built on cleanliness and discipline. However, fears of infection and the growing professionalism of nursing began to erode the lay care role of parents and carers, and within 20 years of the establishment of the children's hospitals, parental visiting was limited to an hour per week.

Although West and Nightingale corresponded on the optimum way to care for sick children, she was an opponent of his initiative, believing that children should not be in hospital wards. She did acknowledge in her famous *Notes on Nursing* that 'Children: they are affected by the same things (as adults) but much more quickly and seriously' (1859: 72).

The subsequent Nightingale-designed schools of nursing concentrated on adult care, and the battle by children's nurses for a professional recordable qualification was protracted and hard. Nightingale actually opposed registration, and registration for children's nurses was effectively delayed until after her death. Ethel Bedford Fenwick, the founder of the British Nurses' Association, led the fight for nursing registration, and although she had trained as a children's nursing probationer at Nottingham children's hospital she was not supportive of a nursing register that included children's nurses.

After a number of acrimonious amendments to the clauses of the Nurses Bill, Dr Christopher Addison, the Minister for Health, introduced his own Bill for the State Registration of Nurses in which children's nursing became part of a supplementary register. The Act was passed in December 1919. Importantly, two nurses out of the 16 appointed to the General Nursing Council were to be experienced children's nurses.

The struggle to protect the direct-entry Registered Sick Children's Nurse (RSCN) qualification continued, with general nurses insisting that children's nursing was a specialist area best suited to a post-registration qualification. A Royal College of Nursing (RCN) commissioned report chaired by Lord Horder (RCN, 1943, cited in Glasper and Charles-Edwards, 2002a) recommended that children's nursing become a post-registration qualification. The impending threat of Horder's report galvanised the senior sick children's nurses towards a protectionist lobby. The central thrust of their argument was that 'paediatric nursing is not a speciality but general care at a special age period'. This mantra has stood the test of time and helped stave off the recommendations of Horder. It did not however save the direct-entry RSCN qualification. This was because there was inequity towards nurses holding a single RSCN qualification, who tended to have poor promotion prospects. Getting beyond staff nurse was almost impossible without a State Registered Nurse (SRN) qualification. Hence many went on to do additional training.

In 1964 the direct-entry RSCN course was abolished at the Hospital for Sick Children, Great Ormond Street and was gradually phased out all over England. The direct entry route was abolished in Northern Ireland in 1978 (Wales never had a three-year programme) with only Scotland retaining the single RSCN until the advent of Project 2000. Sick children's nursing only survived through the introduction of integrated courses combining general nursing with children's nursing. This three-year, eight-month course was very popular but there were only a very limited number of places available in a small number of children's hospitals. To gain more children's nurses, hospitals in England introduced the 13-month post-registration route to RSCN. After more than a quarter of a century, the pre-registration child branch was reintroduced in 1989 with the advent of Project 2000.

Concepts of modern children's nursing

The environment of care

The importance of the therapeutic environment in the reduction of psychological trauma associated with hospital admission for children has long been recognised. This reflects a long sequence of government white papers and Department of Health publications commencing with *The Welfare of Children in Hospital* (Ministry of Health, 1959) developed under the chairmanship of Sir Harry Platt, and now encompassing such policies as the *National Service Framework for Children, Young People and Maternity Services* (DH, 2004b).

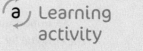

Learning activity

Go to http:www.dh.gov.uk/en/Healthcare/NationalServiceFrameworks/Children/DH_4089111 and **read the summary document.**

Hospitals remain frightening places for children, who because of their relative emotional immaturity may find the whole experience psychologically damaging. During a hospital admission children may experience hostile sights and sounds, especially in areas such as the emergency department.

Learning activity

In your learning group consider why environments such as the emergency department might be particularly upsetting for a child.

Do hospitals harm children?

Glasper and Haggarty (2006) have indicated that there is much evidence to indicate that hospitals can have a detrimental effect on sick children. Such effects in the young child are known as *maternal deprivation*.

Maternal deprivation occurs when the sick child is separated for long periods of time from their primary care giver, who is usually the mother. Robertson (1970) has articulated the stages of separation anxiety that occur during maternal deprivation.

Protest

This stage can last from a few hours to a few days. The child has a strong conscious need of their mother, and the loud crying exhibited is based on the expectation built on previous experience that their mother will respond to their cries. During this stage of the maternal deprivation sequence the child will cry noisily and look eagerly towards any sound that might come from their mother.

Despair

This stage succeeds protest, and can best be compared to clinical depression. It is a sign of increasing hopelessness and despondency. The child becomes less active and vocal, and in the past this was interpreted by the nursing staff as a sign that the child was settling into the ward.

Denial/detachment

In this, the final stage of maternal deprivation, the child represses their longing for their mother and begins to lose their attachment. They appear, at least superficially, to have settled into the hospital routine and will respond positively, if shallowly, to kind adults who take an interest in them. Importantly they react badly to brief reappearances of their mother, for example during the weekly visiting periods, giving rise to the fallacy that parents actually made matters worse. There is no wonder that generations of children's nurses dreaded 'Sunday afternoon visiting'.

Burr (2001) stresses that the environment of care should be based on the child's needs and not on those of the adults who care for them. Many children's nurses throughout the United Kingdom now wear a more relaxed uniform, such as brightly coloured polo shirts, in an attempt to appear more approachable to families, and similarly doctors have abandoned their white coats. Some hospitals such as the Hospital for Sick Children, Toronto and the Children's Hospital of Eastern Ontario have employed experts in child environmental design to create settings in which children can be cared for without detriment to the carers, and that mitigate the potential harmful effects of hospitalisation. Creating such child-friendly hospitals requires strategic thinking in which signage to aid family navigation from one department to another is given high priority. Carlyle (cited in Glasper, 2002) emphasises the need to involve all potential users of a child health facility, including children and their families, in determining a design that provides solutions that support caring.

Part
III

[S] Scenario: introducing Leanne

Leanne is 11 months old. She is admitted to hospital for a planned minor operation.

(a) Learning activity

How would you expect Leanne to respond to this experience? What can be done to alleviate any distress she shows?

Children's rights

Moving beyond the rhetoric of the many documents published that recommend change in the way children are cared for in health environments has been perennially difficult. Although the publication of Platt's *The Welfare of Children in Hospital* (Ministry of Health,

1959) was a high-water mark in the postwar chapter of child care, it was many years before it was fully implemented. It can be argued that the successful implementation of many of the findings of this and other subsequent reports owes much to the activities of the National Association for the Welfare of Children in Hospital (NAWCH). Founded in 1961 as a pressure group predicated upon the widespread implementation of the Platt Report, this charitable consumer organisation evolved into Action for Sick Children (ASC) in recognition that sick children are not only cared for in hospital. Perhaps the most important vehicle for enshrining children's rights into healthcare settings over the first decade of the twenty-first century has been the enthusiastic incorporation of children's charters, bills of rights and other such explicit acknowledgements of their enfranchisement into the day-to-day world of child healthcare (DH, 1996). The ratification by the United Kingdom of the United Nations Convention on the Rights of the Child in 1992 (UN, 1992) can be seen as the precursor to many of these developments.

Many children's units and hospitals have subsequently developed their own explicit charters for children, which now form an integral component of clinical governance.

Preparing children for admission to hospital and stressful procedures

Throughout the first decade of the twenty-first century, children's nurses have come to recognise the benefits of preparing children and their families for stressful healthcare life events wherever they occur. The role of parents throughout these components of a child's healthcare career should not be underestimated. Although families come in all shapes and sizes, all would appear to benefit from some type of preparation for stressful life events such as a hospital admission.

> **a** **Learning activity**
>
> Have you or a member of your family been in hospital as a patient? How did it feel when you were in hospital? Do you think there are any differences between children and adults in this respect?

> **e** **Evidence-based practice**
>
> **Features of hospital that can worry children**
> Visintainer and Wolfer (1975) placed the features of hospital that can worry children into five categories:
> - physical harm or bodily injuries in the form of discomfort, pain, mutilation, or death
> - separation from parents and the absence of trusted adults, especially for preschool children
> - the strange, the unknown and possibility of surprise
> - uncertainty about limits and expected 'acceptable' behaviour
> - relative loss of control, autonomy and competence.

Cross (1990) looked at the short-term effects of hospitalisation after the child has been discharged. Of children aged between 2 and 7 years, 54 per cent experienced some difficulties, including nervousness about separation, more demanding behaviour, sleeping difficulties, and difficulty with mother–child relationships. However, McClowry and McLeod (1990) found no changes in the behaviour in children between the ages of 8 and 12 years.

There might be many reasons for this difference:
- Older children might be more resilient to the stress of hospitalisation.
- Older children might be disguising their real feelings.
- The measuring tool used in the research might not have been broad enough to encompass this age group.

Changes in a child's routine such as admission to hospital exposes them to stress, and it should be remembered that certain categories of children, such as those with special needs, might not be able to articulate their needs, likes and dislikes, fears and discomforts adequately (Tippett, 2001).

Other factors can increase child and family anxiety. An emergency admission means that the child has had no preparation for it, thus potentially increasing anxiety. It is important to remember that 'routine tests and observations' can be very stressful for the child and family, and time should be spent at this stage preparing the children for what is going to happen.

Preschool children are less able to cope positively with hospitalisation than school-age children, so preparation cannot be left to schoolroom activities. Although the school classroom is an excellent environment for teaching the skills necessary to cope with hospitalisation, other methods have to be adopted for younger children. This is highly pertinent when it is known that by the age of 5 years, 25 per cent of children will have had a stay in hospital, with a third of these caused by accidents. Glasper and Haggarty (2006) have argued that preparation through play or rehearsal of activities associated with distressing healthcare interventions can mitigate their effects, acting as stress innoculators.

> **ⓐ Learning activity**
>
> Much has been written about different methods of preparation. Read the useful text 'How to prepare', in Taylor and colleagues (1999).

Not all parents feel able to help their children in this context, and it must be recognised that they too may need preparation. In these ways children's nurses have adapted to work through the medium of the parent(s) as proxy deliverers of care in full recognition that most children are dependent on their parents' emotional support for help in coping with anxiety. If those whose role is one of protection become frightened themselves, this fear can be transmitted to the child. Such emotional contagion can be reduced by preparing the whole family for the event, since it is believed now that a well-prepared parent(s) results in a better prepared child. A variety of strategies have been developed by children's nurses to help families cope with the emotional traumas of hospital admission and other related healthcare interventions.

Many children's units send out written material in the mail to parents and their children, some time prior to the admission. Preadmission programmes purport to provide families with opportunities to experience first hand in a nonthreatening manner the complexities of the healthcare environment. These programmes use therapeutic play as one mechanism for the child and parent(s) to explore a number of healthcare situations (or healthcare apparatus).

The therapeutic value of play confers a crucial sense of normality for children who find themselves in abnormal environments such as hospitals, and helps the child to adapt and thus cope. Therapeutic play is of great value not only to assist in the preparation of the child and family for the admission to hospital, but also to reduce stress throughout the hospital stay. Play can be used to aid communication, prepare for procedures, and create a more relaxed environment for the child. It was first introduced into paediatric wards in 1963.

Part III

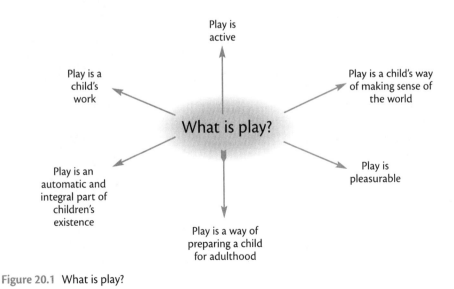

Figure 20.1 What is play?

Play is an activity that is for pleasure rather than for a serious or practical purpose. It is an essential tool by which children learn about the world around them, and forms an important part in growth and development. It can also provide the child with a sense of control (Chambers, 2006). Sometimes adults think they have forgotten how to play. If you relax and let the children take the lead you will find it easier, nevertheless, you should be aware that your own expectations and inhibitions might get in the way. Of course, children play for many reasons, some of which are described as to:

- have fun
- communicate
- make sense of and master the environment
- socialise
- solve problems
- get distraction from anxiety-provoking situations
- practise adult behaviours and skills
- aid development: this includes social, moral, physical, cognitive and emotional development.

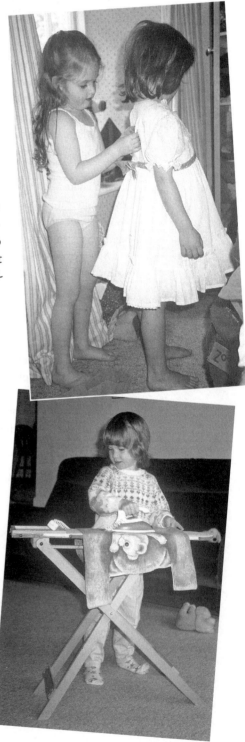

a) Learning activity

Before reading on consider, what particular function play can have for Leanne whilst she is in hospital.

Play can also be an important child-centred communication tool. Sometimes it is seen as a type of language between the child and the carer. By giving up adult-focused language we can gain a child's-eye perspective of their experiences (Webster, 2000). Play specialists in areas caring for children work in partnership with parents and other staff, educating them to develop their own play vocabulary. However, they are not the only people who play with children in hospital. Play is a useful strategy because:

- It is an excellent form of communication.
- It is something that the child normally does in their everyday life, therefore it is familiar.
- It is usually safe and nonthreatening.
- Anyone can be involved.

As part of their emotional development children can learn through play to cope with anxiety-producing situations, such as hospitalisation. This is known as *therapeutic play*. Therapeutic play is used to help children to cope or develop their coping skills when they are faced with often overwhelming stress , and has been defined as a pleasurable activity that contributes to the general well-being, especially the mental well-being, of the player (Chambers, 2001). Its purpose is therefore to help achieve emotional and physical well-being (Chambers, 2008). Therapeutic play is different from child-led play in that it is structured by adults and it has extrinsic goals.

We can use therapeutic play to:

- assess the child's knowledge of a medical condition and treatment
- identify and rectify misunderstandings
- address issues which cause anxiety or concern
- help the child understand what will be expected and what to expect

- provide information.

All of these are achieved by sharing information with the child in a developmentally appropriate manner. Therapeutic play employs a variety of techniques to achieve this (Chambers, 2008):

- Projective play, which is described as helping children, can communicate by scaling down their experiences to a manageable size.
- Role-play can help identify any hidden misunderstandings, fears or feelings the child may have. It allows the child to try on adult roles, and one of its aims is to help them as they seek to gain a sense of control.
- Messy play is a great kick against the system and an outlet for the expression of emotion.
- Distraction techniques are acknowledged to help limit anxiety and stress. Their aim is to help the children develop coping strategies in a developmentally appropriate way.

Some examples of distraction techniques are:

- blowing bubbles
- counting
- hangman (hang the person you are angry with!)
- puppets
- imagining
- breathing
- relaxation tapes
- shouting.

Visualisation techniques are also used with some children. However, they should only be undertaken by health professionals familiar with the procedure, as particular skills are needed.

Learning activity

Have you ever used any of these techniques? Did you recognise what you were doing? Try to write a short reflective account of your feelings at the time. Can you think of any other ways you could maintain Leanne's link with home?

Table 20.1 Play materials for different ages

Play material	Uses	Benefits	Age
Dolls	Role play, discussion, good for checking knowledge	Easy for the child to identify. Allows concrete thinking and uses visual and aural memory.	2–10 years
Books	Information and good for parents to read to child	Can use again at their own pace.	2 years onwards
Photo Diary	Discussion and detailed explanation	Can make their own. Can involve and show to others.	6–7 years onward
Video	Discussion and detailed explanation	Good for those reluctant to play. Can use at their own pace.	6–7 years
Leaflets	Information-specific to procedure	Can use again.	2 years onwards

The use of special dolls can allow children and their parents to make sense of their own internal anatomy and external body appearance. Although anatomical dolls require skilful and careful use, it is accepted nevertheless that when discussing with children certain procedures involving parts of their anatomy, especially if they cannot normally see, touch or hear the body part, it is necessary to use things that they can see, touch, hear and relate to concretely. Similarly toys that encourage interactive medico-nursing play are freely available at low cost. Although new media formats are constantly evolving in an attempt to clarify information for children and their families, the use of books remains a cheap and popular medium through which children can be prepared for an eventual healthcare intervention.

Children in hospital can meet many new people as a result of their admission, and every effort should be made to reduce this added stress.

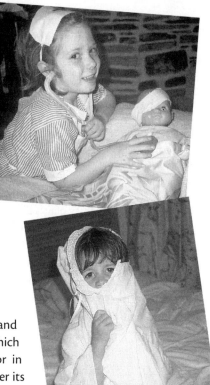

Management of care

Family-centred care is the hallmark of the children's nurse (Callery and Smith, 1991). Although it was implicit in the 1959 Platt Report, which recommended sweeping changes in the way children were cared for in hospital, family-centred care was almost nonexistent for many years after its publication. The work of NAWCH (now renamed ASC) in the early years of the movement concentrated on the removal of the barriers to family-centred care, such as restricted visiting arrangements and a lack of basic facilities for parents to stay with their sick children. With the publication of subsequent reports came fresh evidence that basic recommendations to foster family-centred care were being implemented only slowly.

The transition of first allowing parents unrestricted visiting to hospital wards, followed by the provision of parental accommodation which was more than a simple chair at the bedside, paved the way for a philosophy of care in which the child and family were perceived as an indivisible unit. Meadows' (1969) classic description of UK resident parents as captive mothers is one reiterated by Darbyshire (1994), who reaffirms the wishes of parents for greater involvement in the direct care of their children in hospital. To bolster the concept of family-centred care, the development of a partnership model of nursing care (Casey, 1993), through which the care of children, either well or sick, is carried out by their families with varying degrees of help from suitably qualified members of the healthcare team whenever necessary, helped turn government rhetoric into a practical reality.

Family-centred care

The Department of Health (2004b) suggests that children's wards practise within a philosophy of family-centred care. The main concepts of family-centred care are:

- The unit of care is the family, not just the child.
- The individuals that make up the 'family' are decided by each individual family.
- The nursing care and the environment should support and enable the family to care for their child.

The involvement of parents and other family members in the care of the child benefits the child both physically and emotionally (Casey, 2007; Glasper and Ireland, 2000). This is also beneficial to the family as it maintains the family unit, and enables them to continue in their parenting role and to develop the knowledge and skills required to care for their sick child (DH, 2004b).

However, there has been some evidence to suggest that parents attempting to care for their sick child in hospital can find it distressing because of the unfamiliar environment and conflict of interests between family members. Therefore it is important that the nurse works towards what is in the best interests of the child and the family, and that the family decide the level of involvement that is right for them.

Children's wards frequently use a model of care based on Casey's partnership model of care' (1988); family-centred care is fundamental to this model. The philosophy behind Casey's partnership model is that the best people to care for the child are the family. To do this the family may require varying degrees of support and assistance from the healthcare team. The model also acknowledges that the family can consist of any of its members, and anyone else who is emotionally close to the child. You can read more about this, and family-centred care is general in Chapter 6.

> ### (a) Learning activity
>
> It is now generally accepted that a parent or another family member should be resident in hospital with a sick child, and that they will assist in the care of the child. Discuss the possible advantages and disadvantages of this with the following individuals:
> * parents
> * children
> * nurses
> * doctors.

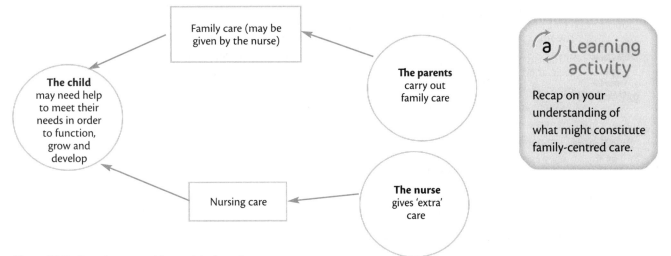

> ### (a) Learning activity
>
> Recap on your understanding of what might constitute family-centred care.

Figure 20.2 Casey's partnership model of nursing
Source: Casey (1988).

> ### (c) Professional conversation
>
> Wendy, a paediatric ward sister, discusses the issues that characterise family-centred care:
> 'Having been a ward sister for a number of years I really appreciate the recognition of this concept. Of course, many of us feel that we have always recognised that parents or other primary carers satisfy the child's important basic care needs in the normal situation until the child has developed the ability to do this themselves. It's important that we appreciate that parents can usually learn to care for the child's enhanced needs brought about by a change in health status, but that they may need help, support and guidance to learn these skills.
>
> 'We also have to accept that if parents are to care for their child's needs they may require supportive care themselves. The real challenge for some is the recognition that the nurse's role in this form of care may move from that of care deliverer to that of care facilitator. Most important is the acceptance that the child is an integral part of the family unit, and to improve the child's health involves addressing that family unit as a whole.'

Part
III

The parent requires the knowledge and skills necessary to care for the child. Dealing with a child in a hospital setting is very different from caring for the child at home, and the parent may need help and support to learn new care skills, and implement them confidently.

> ### (a) Learning activity
>
> What strategies could you use to support parents when they are on the children's ward? Take a look at the facilities that are available in the hospital where you work.

Don't forget that parents will also have needs that you should consider. Assisting parents to feel as relaxed and supported as possible will help to prevent stress transferring to the child, and so limiting recovery. Parents will have physical needs, including access to:

- Somewhere to rest and sleep.
- Somewhere to wash and change clothes.
- Somewhere to find food and drink.
- Means of communicating with those at home.

The role of the nurse is also crucial in terms of meeting parents' emotional needs. Parents will need reassurance that they are behaving appropriately, and that their actions are facilitating their child's recovery. It is by working closely with parents through a family-centred care approach that health care professionals can ensure these needs are met.

There are many reasons why family care may be delivered by a nurse. We discussed these in Chapter 6, but to recap:

- The parent might be stressed and tired, and the priority is that they are able to rest so that they can soon continue to care for the child.
- The child's situation might require adaptation of the parent's normal care practices. For example, if the child has a plaster cast on a leg, helping the child to bathe or go to the toilet will become more complicated. The parent might need to have this adapted procedure demonstrated, and the opportunity to practise it while being supported by the nurse.
- The parent might have competing responsibilities. The need to go to work or to care for other children at home can mean that a parent cannot stay in hospital to participate in the child's care. The nurse will then have to explore other methods of ensuring that the parent's participation continues as far as conditions allow.
- On rare occasions, the parent's actions are not in the child's best interests.

Family-centred care is not static, and the healthcare team acknowledge this, continually review the situation, and amend care accordingly. The key to family-centred care is communication, between all parties involved (parent, child and professional).

As we know from Chapter 6, Action for Sick Children (ASC) (2000) has summarised the important principles of child healthcare from their perspective in the *Millennium Charter*. These ideas might be seen as the prerequisites for, and the underpinning of, family-centred child healthcare.

The Millennium Charter (see also p. 103)

- All children shall have equal access to the best clinical care within a network of services that collaborate with each other.
- Health services for children and young people should be provided in a child-centred environment separately from adults so that they are made to feel welcome, safe and secure at all times.
- Parents should be empowered to participate in decisions regarding the treatment and care of their children through a process of clear communication and adequate support.

- Children should be informed and involved to an extent appropriate to their development and understanding.
- Children should be cared for at home with the support and practical assistance of community children's nursing services, unless the care that they require can only be provided in hospital.
- All staff caring for children shall be specifically trained to understand and respond to their clinical, emotional, developmental and cultural needs.

- Every hospital admitting children should provide accommodation for parents, free of charge.
- Parents should be encouraged and supported to participate in the care of their child when they are sick.
- Every child in hospital should have full opportunity for play, recreation and education.
- Adolescents should be recognised as having different needs from those of younger children and adults. Health services should therefore be readily available to meet their particular needs.

Learning activity

Now you have considered the themes introduced in this chapter, can you suggest the principles that should be observed to ensure that Leanne receives family-centred nursing care?

Children's nurses as health promoters and information givers

It is important that children's nurses are able to provide information to parents, not only about their child's illness but also current recommendations and guidelines to enable healthy growth and development. Parents frequently request information about immunisation and nutrition.

Immunisation

During the assessment of any child you should always ask about the child's immunisation status. Immunisation of children is the single most cost-effective form of prevention and a positive health benefit for children. It saves the lives of more than 3 million people worldwide each year, and it saves millions more from suffering illness and lifelong disability (World Health Organization (WHO) estimates). The WHO states:

> Before the introduction of routine childhood vaccination, infectious diseases were the leading cause of child death, and epidemics were frequent. Even today these diseases cause suffering and death, with measles, Haemophilus influenzae type b (Hib), pertussis and neonatal tetanus being the great killers. Every year, 10.6 million children die before the age of five years; 1.4 million of these are due to diseases that could have been prevented by vaccines. Taking into account both children and adults, vaccine-preventable diseases kill 3 million people around the world every year (WHO estimates). Even though the WHO European Region has the lowest incidence of such diseases, vaccine-preventable diseases continue to cause an estimated 32,000 unnecessary deaths in young children across the Region every year (WHO estimate).
>
> In the WHO European Region all of the member states have agreed to try to eliminate measles, rubella and congenital rubella syndrome by 2010.

(WHO, 2007)

Part
III

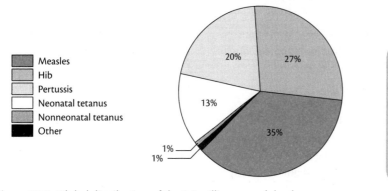

Legend:
- ■ Measles
- ▨ Hib
- ▨ Pertussis
- ☐ Neonatal tetanus
- ▨ Nonneonatal tetanus
- ■ Other

27% | 20% | 13% | 35% | 1% | 1%

Figure 20.3 Global distribution of the 1.4 million annual deaths in children under 5 years from vaccine-preventable diseases

a Learning activity

Find out about the incidence of the major vaccine-preventable diseases in your area.

Protecting children against infectious disease is dependent on the development of safe and effective vaccines. Once a licence has been granted and the vaccine is in general use, surveillance continues to detect less common reactions or problems associated with the vaccine. All vaccines can give rise to side-effects, although it is rare that these are severe. However, the complication rate for each disease is greater than that of the vaccine. But no vaccine is 100 per cent effective, although the reasons for this are not fully understood. A proportion of primary vaccine failures might be caused by impotent vaccine arising from poor vaccine handling.

- More than 95 per cent of the people who receive a single dose of measles, mumps and rubella (MMR) vaccine will develop immunity to all three viruses. A second gives immunity to almost all of those who did not respond to the first dose (CDCP, ndb).
- If sufficient individuals in a population are immunised, those who cannot receive vaccine because of medical contraindications and those who did not respond to the vaccine will be protected from disease by herd immunity.
- The level of vaccine coverage required varies for different diseases, and is partly dependent on the infectivity of the causative organism.
- Anaphylactic reactions to vaccines are extremely rare, but have the potential to be fatal. Between 1997 and 2003, 118 million doses of vaccines were dispensed, and during this period 130 cases of anaphylaxis were reported to the Medicines and Healthcare products Regulatory Agency (MHRA) . No deaths were reported (Bohlke et al, 2003).

Immunisation should be postponed for any child who is suffering an acute illness. However, minor infections without fever or systemic upset are not reasons to postpone immunisation. Any vaccine is contraindicated when an individual has had a severe local or general reaction to a preceding dose. Some individuals cannot be given live vaccines because they are unable to make a normal immune response and could suffer disseminated infection. Similarly, inactivated vaccines, while not being dangerous, can be ineffective (DH, 2006).

S Scenario continued

Leanne is due to receive her 12-month vaccinations.

a Learning activity

What vaccinations would you expect Leanne to receive? What advice would you expect to be given to the mother regarding whether this vaccination should go ahead? Consider your response before reading on.

Those who should not receive vaccinations, or for whom there are special requirements, include (DH, 2006):

- Children undergoing treatment for malignant disease with chemotherapy or generalised radiotherapy, or within six months of terminating treatment.
- Children who have received an organ transplant and are currently on immunosuppressive treatment.
- Children who have received a bone marrow transplant should have their immunity to diphtheria, tetanus, polio, measles, mumps, rubella and Hib checked six months after transplantation and be immunised accordingly.
- Children on high-dose corticosteroids: 2mg/kg/day for at least a week or 1mg/kg/day for one month. Live vaccines should be deferred for at least three months following cessation of treatment. Children on lower-dose steroids for prolonged periods need to be assessed individually.
- Live vaccines should not be given within three months of immunoglobulin.
- Live vaccines should either be administered simultaneously at different sites or a three-week interval should be allowed.

A multidisciplinary team approach to immunisation provision has been found to be particularly beneficial. This includes opportunistic immunisation of children in contact with health professionals for other reasons and domiciliary services. These additional approaches can be useful in increasing the uptake of vaccinations.

Table 20.2 Routine childhood immunisation programme

Each vaccination is given as a single injection into the muscle of the thigh or upper arm.

When to immunise	Diseases protected against	Vaccine given
Two months old	Diphtheria, tetanus, pertussis (whooping cough), polio and + *Haemophilus influenzae* type b. (Hib) Pneumococcal infection.	DTaP/IPV/Hib Pneumococcal conjugate vaccine (PCV)
Three months old	Diphtheria, tetanus, pertussis, polio and *Haemophilus influenzae* type b. (Hib) Meningitis C.	DTaP/IPV/Hib+ MenC
Four months old	Diphtheria, tetanus, pertussis, polio and *Haemophilus influenzae* type b. (Hib) Meningitis C. Pneumococcal infection.	DTaP/IPV/Hib + MenC + PCV
Around 12 months	*Haemophilus influenzae* type b. (Hib) Meningitis C.	Hib/MenC
Around 13 months	Measles, mumps and rubella. Pneumococcal infection.	MMR + PCV
3 years four months to 5 years old	Diphtheria, tetanus, pertussis and polio. Measles, mumps and rubella.	DTaP/IPV or dTaP/IPV + MMR
13 to 18 years old	Tetanus, diphtheria and polio.	Td/IPV

Part

III

S Scenario

Leanne's mother has looked up information on the MMR vaccine on the internet, and is confused. She wants to know, are there are any risks that she should consider? What advice would you give her?

Table 20.3 Non-routine immunisations

When to immunise	Diseases protected against	Vaccine given
At birth (to babies who are more likely to come into contact with tuberculosis than the general population)	Tuberculosis	BCG
At birth (to babies whose mothers are hepatitis B positive)	Hepatitis B	Hep B

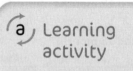

Learning activity

Find out the percentage immunisation uptake for different vaccinations of children in your area. Would you consider asking about a child's siblings' immunisation status? When do you think this topic should be approached?

Nutrition

During the first year of life growth is rapid and it is essential that the nutritional needs of the infant be met. The infant requires:

- Protein, which is used in infants almost entirely for growth, unlike in adults where it can be used as an energy source or converted to fat. An adequate intake of protein with a balance of amino acids is essential.
- Carbohydrate as the main energy source.
- Fat, which is stored by babies to act as an emergency energy food and used for insulating them from the cold. Fatty acids are also essential to ensure normal growth. Fat reduction should not be considered for children under the age of 2 years.
- Minerals: although the infant's iron store will last for approximately the first six months it is essential to provide an iron source when mixed feeding is introduced.
- Calcium is needed for the development of the bones and teeth.
- Other trace elements such as copper and zinc must be provided to enable normal development.
- A full range of vitamins is required for normal development.

Exclusive breastfeeding for the first four months of life has been associated with significant reduction in the risk of asthma by the age of 6 years. Public health interventions to promote and increase the duration of breastfeeding may help to reduce the prevalence and severity of childhood asthma (Oddy et al, 1999). Weaning is defined by the Department of Health (1994) as the 'process of expanding the diet to include food and drinks other than breast milk or infant formula'. Thus weaning allows the infant to meet their growing nutritional requirements. The WHO recently changed its recommendation that 'infants should be exclusively breast-fed for the first four to six months of life' to 'exclusive breast-feeding for six months, with introduction of complementary foods and continued breast-feeding thereafter'. In the United Kingdom the Department of Health (2004) recommends that six months (26 weeks) is the age for the introduction of solid food for all infants, whether formula fed or breast fed. Some parents may wish to wean earlier, and four months should be regarded as the earliest age at which solids could be introduced (DH, 1994). Not weaning before four months of age does mean waiting until the infant is at least four calendar months old, which is 18 weeks, not 16 weeks.

Learning activity

To find out more about weaning, read BDA (nd).

The aims of weaning are to:

- introduce a wide range of tastes and textures
- teach the infant to take food from a spoon
- teach the infant to take fluids from a cup
- provide a more energy dense diet
- provide iron.

Initially weaning should commence by giving one or two teaspoons of food that is a smooth, thick-cream consistency. Half of the breast or formula feed should be given first, and no salt or sugar should be added. New flavours are gradually introduced.

The next stage is to introduce food that has soft lumps or is mashed, and by about nine months, minced or finely chopped food can be introduced, ensuring the infant gets lots of different textures so that they can learn to chew. By 12 months of age children should be getting a good mixed diet, with about three meals and two to three healthy snacks in between.

> **ⓐ Learning activity**
>
> Leanne's family are vegetarians. How can her mother ensure that Leanne receives all the nutrients required for healthy growth and development?

Problems that may be associated with weaning include:

- failure to thrive
- risk of choking
- rejection of solids
- faddy children
- constipation
- diarrhoea
- obesity
- dental caries.

There are many excellent booklets available from your local health promotion resource centre about the dietary needs of babies and children. You should use these to guide your learning about how to wean infants on to solid food. Another excellent source of information about nutrition is the European Food Information Council at www.eufic.org/fr/home/fhome.htm.

> **ⓐ Learning activity**
>
> Plan a weaning menu for a eight-month-old for one day. Compare your menu with a colleague's.

Conclusion

Children today are regarded as having their own rights, but are acknowledged as vulnerable individuals. This is recognised in contemporary society through robust legislation to protect them. Despite this, the developing child is always at risk in an increasingly dangerous environment, and healthcare settings may present particular risks.

Children's nursing is practised within a philosophy of child-focused and family-centred care in which, whenever possible, the child, parents and carers are equal partners. This partnership enhances self-esteem, enables children to reach their full potential and encourages the development of autonomy in care and decision making. Although this branch of the nursing profession has a long history which predates that of modern adult nursing, the future of the children's nurse at the pre-registration level remains unclear (Ellis et al, 2008).

Changes in the care of sick children have been spurred by the realisation of the harmful effects of admitting children to hospital and a greater identification of their developmental needs, including those of psychosocial care.

Children differ from adults intellectually, emotionally and physically. Childhood is a period of rapid growth and development, and children of varying ages from birth to adolescence have very different needs (Bee, 2000). Children are particularly vulnerable to the effects of illness and hospitalisation, and therefore require specialised and individualised care (Taylor et al, 1999; Glasper and Haggarty, 2006).

Part

III

References

Action for Sick Children (ASC) (2000) *Millennium Charter for Children's Health Services*, London, ASC.

Bee, H. (2000) *The Developing Child*, 9th edn, London, Allyn & Bacon.

Bohlke, K., David, R. L., Marcy, S. H. et al. (2003) 'Risk of anaphylaxis after vaccination of children and adolescents', *Paediatrics* 112, 815–20.

British Dietetic Association (BDA) (nd) *Position Statement on Breastfeeding and Weaning on to Solid Foods*, BDA Paediatric Group [online] www.bda.uk.com/resources/PositionStatementWeaning.pdf (accessed 23 December 2008).

Burr, S. (2001) 'Passing on the passion: influences and change in children's services', *Paediatric Nursing* 13(10), 19–22.

Callery, P. and Smith, L. (1991) 'A study of role negotiation between nurses and parents of hospitalised children', *Journal of Advanced Nursing* 16, 772–81.

Casey, A. (1988) 'A partnership with child and family', *Senior Nurse* 8(4), 8–9.

Casey, A. (1993) 'Development and use of the partnership model of nursing care', in Glasper, E. . and Tucker, A. (eds), *Advances in Child Health Nursing*, London, Scutari Press.

Casey, A. (2007) 'Partnership model of nursing', in Glasper, E., McEwing, G. and Richardson, J. (eds), *Oxford Handbook of Children's and Young People's Nursing*, Oxford, Oxford University Press.

Centres for Disease Control and Prevention (CDCP) (nd a) Information on vaccination [online] http://www.cdc.gov/vaccines/ (accessed 2007).

CDCP (nd b) 'Measles – Q&A about disease &and vaccine' [online] www.cdc.gov/nip/diseases/measles/faqs.htm (accessed 23 August 2007).

Chambers, M. (2001) 'Towards a definition of therapeutic play: a concept analysis', unpublished MSc paper, London, RCN Institute.

Chambers, M. (2006) 'The importance of play', in Glasper, E. A., McEwing, G. and Richardson, J. (eds), *Oxford Handbook of Children's and Young People's Nursing*, Oxford, Oxford University Press.

Chambers, M. (2008) 'Therapeutic play in hospital', in Kelsey, J. A. and McEwing, G. (eds), *Clinical Skills in Child Health Practice*, Edinburgh, Churchill Livingstone.

Committee of the Central Health Services (1959) *The Welfare of Children in Hospital*, London, HMSO.

Cross, C. (1990) 'Home and hospital', *Nursery World* 90(3228), 22–3.

Darbyshire, P. (1994) *Living with a Sick Child in Hospital: The experiences of parents and nurses*, London, Chapman & Hall.

Department of Health (DH) (1994) *Weaning and the Weaning Diet*, Report on Health and Social Subjects 45, London, HMSO.

DH (1996) *The Patients' Charter: Services for children and young people*, London, HMSO.

DH (2004a) *Infant Feeding Recommendation*, London, DH.

DH (2004b) *National Service Framework for Children Young People and Maternity Services: Core standards*, London, The Stationery Office.

DH (2006) *Immunisation against Infectious Disease* (The Green Book), London, DH.

Ellis, J., Glasper, E. A., Horsely, A., McEwing, G. and Richardson, J. (2008) 'NMC Review of pre-registration nursing education: views of the children's and young people's nursing academic community', *Journal of Children's and Young People's Nursing* 2(2), 56–60.

Glasper, E. A. (1995) 'The value of children's nursing in the third millennium', *British Journal of Nursing* 4(1), 27–30.

Glasper, E. A. (2002) 'Contemporary issues in the care of sick children', *British Journal of Nursing*, 11(4), 248 –56.

Glasper, E. A. and Charles-Edwards, I. (2002a) 'The child first and always: the registered children's nurse over 150 years, part 1', *Paediatric Nursing* 14(4), 38–42.

Glasper, E. A., and Charles-Edwards, I. (2002b) 'The child first and always: the registered children's nurse over 150 years, part 2', *Paediatric Nursing* 14(5), 38–43.

Glasper, E. A. and Haggarty, R. E. A. (2006) 'The psychological preparation of children for hospitalization', in Glasper, E. A. and Richardson, J. (eds), A *Textbook of Children's and Young People's Nursing*, London, Elsevier.

Glasper, E. A. and Ireland, L. (2000) *Evidence-Based Child Healthcare: Challenges for practice*, Basingstoke, Macmillan.

Glasper, E. A. and Mitchell, R. (2006) 'Historical perspectives of children's nursing', in Glasper, E. A. and Richardson, J. (eds), A *Textbook of Children's and Young People's Nursing*, London, Elsevier.

McClowry, S. G. and McLeod, S. M. (1990) 'The psychological responses of school age children to hospitalization', *Children's Healthcare* 19(3), 155–60.

Meadows, R. (1969) 'The captive mother', *Archives of Disease in Childhood* 44(235), 362–7.

Miles, I. (1986) 'The emergence of sick children's nursing, part 1: sick children's nursing before the turn of the century', *Nurse Education Today* 6, 82–7.

Ministry of Health (1959) *The Welfare of Children in Hospital* (the Platt Report), London, Ministry of Health.

Nightingale, F. (1859/1970) *Notes on Nursing: What it is and what it is not*, London, Duckworth.

Nichols, R. H. and Wray, F. A. (1935) *The History of the Foundling Hospital*, London, Oxford University Press.

Oddy, W. H., Holt, P. G., Sly, P. D., Read, A. W., Landau, L. I., Stanley, F. J., Kendall, G. E. and Burton, P. R. (1999) 'Association between breast-feeding and asthma in six-year-old children: findings of a prospective birth cohort study', *British Medical Journal* 319, 815–19.

Robertson, J. (1970) *Young Children in Hospital*, London, Tavistock.

Swallow, V. M. and Jacoby, A. (2001) 'Mothers' evolving relationships with doctors and nurses during the chronic childhood illness trajectory', *Journal of Advanced Nursing* 36(6), 755–64.

Taylor, J. Muller, D., Wattley, L. and Harris, P. (1999) *Nursing Children: Psychology, research and practice*, 3rd edn, Cheltenham, Stanley Thornes.

Tippett, A. (2001) 'All about me: documentation for children with special needs', *Paediatric Nursing* 13(10), 34–5.

United Nations (1992) Convention on the Rights of the Child, Geneva, United Nations.

Visintainer, M. A. and Wolfer, J. A. (1975) 'Psychological preparation for surgical pediatric patients: the effect on children's and parent's stress responses and adjustment', *Paediatrics* 56, 187–202.

Webster, A. (2000) 'The facilitating role of the play specialist', *Paediatric Nursing* 12(7), 24–7.

World Health Organization (WHO) (1985) *Targets for Health for All*, Copenhagen, WHO.

WHO (2007) EURO/03/07 [online] http://www.euro.who.int/vaccine/20080415_5 (accessed 23 December 2008).

Websites

European Food Information Council: www.eufic.org/fr/home/fhome.htm.

Chapter

21

Care of the acutely ill child

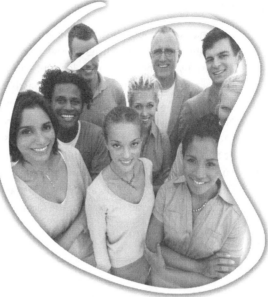

Gill McEwing and Janet Kelsey

W Don't forget to visit www.palgrave.com/glasper for additional online resources relating to this chapter.

Introduction

Asthma is a serious health problem which affects adults and children of all ages and throughout all the countries of the world. When asthma is uncontrolled it creates severe limitations on the individual's life and can be fatal. Early diagnosis of asthma and effective management can reduce the burden of asthma and improve the person's quality of life. When a child has a chronic illness and experiences acute exacerbations, it is stressful for the child and their family. This chapter follows the care of a child presenting to their GP with an acute exacerbation of asthma, through their admission to hospital, to the management of their care at and after discharge. It uses this scenario to investigate the care required for a child during an emergency admission to hospital, the assessment procedures, and management of the child's condition. The skills and care necessary to meet the child's needs are presented, as are guidelines to provide support for the family.

Learning outcomes

This chapter will enable you to:

- use relevant literature and research to inform the practice of nursing
- recognise and meet the potential care needs of a child with acute asthma
- demonstrate knowledge of physiological measurements in children

- identify the signs of respiratory distress
- discuss the importance of nursing assessment
- understand the methods for administering the medications required for a child with asthma
- discuss the ongoing care of a child with asthma.

Concepts

- Childhood asthma
- Acute children's nursing and the nurse's role

- Assessment of children
- Chronic illness in childhood
- Family-centred care

[S] Scenario: Introducing Tom Brown

Tom is 8 years old. He has a sister Emily, aged 5, and a three-month-old baby brother, Samuel. Tom was admitted to hospital at the age of 3 with an attack of wheezing. By the age of 5 he had been diagnosed as a severe asthmatic.

Asthma

Asthma is a chronic inflammatory condition of the airways, the cause of which is still not completely understood (Kieckfeler and Ratcliffe, 2004). It can be described as 'airway obstruction that is reversible, airway inflammation, and increased airway responsiveness to a variety of stimuli'.

(a) Learning activity

Make notes on your current understanding of asthma before reading on. Remember to write down words to check out or cues to pick up on, for example 'What stimuli?'

The asthmatic response includes:

Bronchospasm

This is a narrowing of the bronchial walls as a result of the contraction of the smooth muscle. It is more severe in the smaller bronchi and bronchioles where there is no cartilage in the walls.

Inflammation

This causes the airways to become hyper-responsive and narrow easily in reaction to a wide range of stimuli. There is further narrowing of the airways by the invasion of the mucosa, submucosa and muscle tissue by inflammatory cells.

Inflammatory cells

These cells are mainly eosinophils, but also contain neutrophils, macrophages and mast cells. They contain chemical mediators, including histamine, prostaglandins and leukotrienes, which cause vasodilation and increased capillary permeability. This leads to mucous production and oedema.

The lumen of the airways is therefore narrowed by contraction of the smooth muscle, mucosal oedema and the hyper-secretion of mucus (Hockenberry et al, 2003).

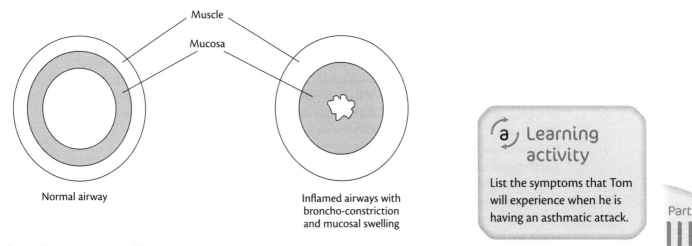

Muscle

Mucosa

Normal airway

Inflamed airways with broncho-constriction and mucosal swelling

Figure 21.1 Normal and inflamed airways

> **ⓐ Learning activity**
>
> List the symptoms that Tom will experience when he is having an asthmatic attack.

Part

III

There are two phases of the asthmatic response (Kieckfeler and Ratcliffe, 2004). The first phase occurs within minutes of the exposure to the stimuli, reaches a peak in about 30 minutes and subsides after approximately two hours. It includes bronchospasm, oedema and mucous secretion. The second phase occurs about 4–12 hours after the exposure. It reaches a peak after about 4–8 hours, but can last for more than 24 hours. There is an inflammatory reaction, which can lead to damage to the lung tissue. The airways are hypersensitive to allergic stimulation, which can result in further inflammation and bronchoconstriction.

Asthma is the commonest medical condition of childhood (Newacheck and Halfon, 2000). It affects as many as one in 11 children in the UK (Asthma UK, 2004), and is a major cause of morbidity in children. The incidence and severity of the disease increased dramatically over the latter part of the twentieth century (Kaur et al, 1998), with statistics demonstrating a small decline in recent years (ONS, 2004). The increase was thought to be caused by environmental factors (Caldwell. 1998), and evidence of underdiagnosis and treatment was thought to be a contributing factor (Kaur et al, 1998). Changes in the prevalence of asthma in children are difficult to determine owing to changes in diagnostic

> **ⓐ Learning activity**
>
> Why do you think Tom was diagnosed as an asthmatic?

a) Learning activity

Identify environmental factors that might increase the incidence of asthma.

practice (Magnus and Jaakkola, 1997), but however defined, asthma and wheezing in children has increased dramatically over the past few decades.

There are approximately 1500 deaths (adults and children) as a result of asthma each year in Britain, of which 80 per cent are thought to be preventable (BTS SIGN, 2008). When asthma is not properly controlled, it results in disturbed sleep, absence from school and inability to participate in leisure activities. Severe childhood asthma can cause disfigurement, with chest wall deformities (Cross, 1999). Asthma is a chronic disorder that can affect a child's quality of life by restricting their existence physically, emotionally and socially (Rydstrom et al, 2005).

a) Learning activity   W

Find out how many children have been diagnosed with asthma in the United Kingdom. Go to http://www.asthma.org.uk for information and key statistics. The Globe Initiative for Asthma (GINA) aims to reduce asthma prevalence, morbidity and mortality. Useful reports and guidelines can be accessed at www.ginasthma.org.

Asthma in children aged under 5

Diagnosis of asthma under the age of 5 years is difficult because wheezing and coughs are common in this age group even when the child does not have asthma. Wheezing is often related to viral illnesses, particularly respiratory syncytial virus in children under 2 (GINA, 2007). Transient wheezing has been linked to parental smoking and prematurity, and often disappears after the age of 3 years. A diagnosis of asthma is strongly suggested if the child suffers from:

- frequent episodes of wheezing, more than once a month
- activity-induced coughs or wheezes
- nocturnal cough when free of viral infections
- no seasonal variation in wheeze
- symptoms persisting after the age of 3 years.

Other possible causes of wheezing must be taken into consideration, such as cystic fibrosis, chronic rhino-sinusitis and gastroeosophageal reflux.

a) Learning activity

For additional information about children presenting with asthma under 5 years and a full list of alternative causes of symptoms, look up GINA (2007) and BTS SIGN (2008).

The course of the disease

The age of onset varies, but the first symptoms usually show before the child is 4 years old. Boys are affected more than girls before the teenage years, then the trend reverses (Hockenberry et al, 2003). A better prognosis is associated with an earlier onset, except when the age of onset is less than 2 years (BTS SIGN, 2008).

Symptoms begin to decline in the teenage years. In some individuals they disappear, but others may suffer relapses in later life (Strachan, 1999). Asthma is more likely to resolve in boys than girls (BTS SIGN, 2008).

Key points

- Two main factors are involved in the development of asthma, atopy and allergy. *Atopy* is when an individual readily develops antibodies of the IgE class against common materials present in the environment. Genetic and environmental factors affect IgE levels. Evidence suggests that growing up in a 'clean' environment may predispose to asthma, and that early life exposure to inhaled and ingested products of microorganisms may be critical in reducing the risk (Frew and Holgate, 2005). Repeated upper respiratory tract viral infections in early life appear to stimulate the immune system and reduce the risk of asthma up to school age (Sabina et al, 2001).

- There is no test available to distinguish between acute bronchial infection and asthma.
- If a child is suffering from a persistent recurrent cough or wheeze that responds to treatment with bronchodilator therapy, this indicates that the cause might be asthma (Caldwell, 1998; BTS SIGN, 2008).
- The child might suddenly develop a cough, which can follow a viral infection. It can be dry or productive, sometimes paroxysmal, and is frequently worse at night.
- The sputum is often thick and gelatinous. This is mainly caused by plasma leakage and the damaged epithelium (Hockenberry et al, 2003).
- Wheezing is caused by air being forced through the narrowed airways, but if the child's chest is silent this may be the result of exhaustion and not a sign of lack of severity of the attack.
- The course of asthma varies from child to child. Most children have discrete episodes of the disease with symptom-free periods in between; however, some children appear to suffer constantly from the symptoms (Hockenberry et al, 2003).
- The degree of symptoms can vary from mild to severe.
- The severity may change depending on the time of year. If the child is sensitive to pollens, then spring and summer could be the time when they experience most episodes of the disease. However, if the child reacts to cold air, the winter months could cause the most concern.

> **a) Learning activity**
>
> Find out more about atopy, and what other allergic conditions are associated with asthma in this syndrome.

Treatment of asthma focuses on supportive care to ensure that the child receives adequate oxygen and does not tire excessively. Therapy centres on the use of medication to reverse the physiological changes of asthma in order to ease breathing and return the situation to normal.

> **S) Scenario continued**
>
> Tom was very happy at his previous school, but the family have now moved house and Tom is due to start his new school tomorrow. Tom is anxious about starting at his new school, and was upset when he went to bed. Several hours later his mother realises that Tom is having some difficulty with his breathing. Tom uses his inhaler to try to improve his breathing.

Children with asthma appear to have more difficulty with coping with psychological stress than other children. Experiences such as moving house, birth of a sibling and changing school can be stressful for all children. However when they are combined with a hospital admission, it may create more stress than the child can cope with (Meadow and Newell, 2002).

There are some predisposing factors related to a child developing a hypersensitivity to specific stimuli or triggers. The general predisposing factors include:

- strong genetic factor (Frew and Holgate, 2005)
- family atopy (Frew and Holgate, 2005)
- maternal smoking
- not breastfed for the first four months of life (Oddy et al, 1999).

Indoor triggers are:

- Allergy to house-dust mite and fungal spores. The allergen is the faeces of the mite. The mite feeds on dead skin cells which can collect on pillows and mattresses (Frew and Holgate, 2005). Modern houses with double-glazing tend to lack ventilation, and moisture levels allow moulds to grow (Zuriek et al 2002). The fungal spores from Aspergillus Fumigatus are a causative factor in asthma (Frew and Holgate, 2005).

- Allergy to animal dander (Caldwell, 1998).
- Tobacco smoke (Simon, Everitt and Kendrick, 2005).

Outdoor triggers are:

- Allergy to pollen. The most troublesome time for pollen from flowers and grasses seems to be May and June. It is difficult to stay indoors for these months, but it is recommended that the child avoids being outside in the early evening when the pollen count is at its highest.
- Cold air.
- Air pollutants.
- Industrial chemicals.
- Ozone levels (Camargos, Castro and Feldman, 1999).

Other triggers are:

- Viral infections. This is the most common trigger in children (Cates and Fitzgerald, 2001).
- Exercise. A study carried out by de Bisschop and colleagues (1999) showed that children suffering from exercise-induced asthma could significantly reduce post-exercise bronchoconstriction by carrying out a short warm-up programme prior to exercise.
- Food allergies. These include food colourings (tartrazine), nuts, eggs, and drinks containing ice or carbon dioxide (Simpson, Glutting and Yousef, 2007). Food allergies should be investigated thoroughly before the specific foodstuff is eliminated from the diet.
- Stress, emotion and laughing. It is hard to evaluate the effect psychological factors have on childhood asthma, but excitement and anxiety can precipitate or aggravate attacks (Meadow and Newell , 2002).
- Paracetamol. Weekly or daily use of paracetamol has been linked with increasing the severity of asthma in some individuals. The advice is to reduce intake of the drug (Shaheen et al, 2000).

> **(a) Learning activity**
>
> Consider which of these triggers might have caused Tom's asthma attack, giving your rationale.

> **(S) Scenario continued**
>
> Tom and his parents were careful to ensure that he took his normal medications during the recent move.

All medications should be delivered by inhalation whenever possible. This ensures that the drug acts directly on the bronchioles and therefore has an immediate effect. and a lower dose of the drug is required (Rudolf and Levene, 1999).

> **(a) Learning activity**
>
> Find out what medications are used to treat asthma.

There are two main groups of drugs, 'relievers' and 'preventers'. Relievers include beta 2-agonists such as salbutamol and terbutaline, and in some cases ipratropium bromide is used. The preventers are prophylactic drugs such as sodium cromoglycate and steroids (Rudolf and Levene, 1999).

> **(S) Scenario continued**
>
> Tom's condition worsens. His breathing becomes more rapid and his mother can hear an audible wheeze. The general practitioner (GP) is asked to visit.

Table 21.1 Drugs used to control asthma

Drug group	Effect	Examples	Method
Beta2 agonists	Dilates the smooth muscle of the bronchioles. Reduces muscle spasm and leads to an increase in the size of the lumen of the airways. Increases movement of the cilia. Decreases chemical mediators.	SalbuDeepakol Epinephrine Albuterol Metaproterenol Terbutaline Salmeterol long-acting	Inhalation (can be given intravenously and orally)
Anti-cholinergic bronchodilator	Blocks the vagal stimulus to the bronchi, reduces muscle constriction and mucus production (BTS, 1997).	Ipratropium bromide	Inhalation
Methylxanthines	Weak bronchodilator. Increases movement of mucus in the airways. Increases the contraction of the diaphragm and respiratory muscles. Inhibits the release of mediators from the inflammatory cells.	Aminophylline Theophylline	Inhalation (intravenously as life-saving measure)
Corticosteroids	Suppresses the inflammatory process, reduces mucus secretion and mucosal. Reduces hyper-responsiveness of the airways (Hunter, 1995).		Inhalation (prophylactically)
Corticosteroids	Reduces the inflammatory response. Encourages damaged epithelium to heal.		Orally or intravenously. Used in acute attacks.
Other drugs	Stabilisation of mast cells.	Sodium cromoglycate Cromolyn sodium Nedocromil sodium	Inhalation However, this needs to be taken more frequently and is not so effective in some children (Caldwell, 1998).

Learning activity

Tom is very breathless. What signs and symptoms will he present to the GP?

Asthma is one of the respiratory illnesses of childhood that commonly presents as a lower airway obstruction causing respiratory distress. The signs and symptoms of respiratory distress caused by asthma can be differentiated from those of other causes. The clinical features of severe asthma can be identified as:

- breathlessness
- being unable to talk in sentences
- chest recession
- peak flow reduced to less than 50 per cent of expected
- wheezing may or may not be a prominent feature.

Learning activity

What treatment would you expect the GP to administer? Check for the most up-to-date advice regarding the management of acute asthma at http://www.sign.ac.uk/pdf/sign101.pdf. Consider your response before reading on.

If an acute attack fails to respond to the child's usual treatment, urgent treatment is required. Frequent doses of Beta2 agonists are safe in the treatment of an acute asthmatic attack. Two to four puffs repeated every 20 to 30 minutes according to response may control a mild attack, increased to 10 puffs in a severe attack. If the child's condition is not improving after 10 puffs, the child should be transferred to hospital. More Beta2 agonists can be given while awaiting the ambulance. During the transfer the child should be given nebulised Beta2 agonists using compressed oxygen (BTS SIGN, 2008).

S Scenario continued

The GP finds that Tom is not responding to the treatment. He has received 10 puffs of Beta2 agonists using his metered dose inhaler (MDI) and spacer. There is evidence that nebulised Beta2 agonists are more likely to cause tachycardia and hypoxia than if the patient is given the Beta2 agonists via MDI and spacer (BTS SIGN, 2008). The GP decides to admit him to hospital, and while waiting for the ambulance to continue administration of the Beta2 agonists via MDI and spacer.

The hospital's policy is to admit acute medical admissions directly to the children's ward. The GP reminds Tom's parents to take all Tom's medications with them. Tom's mother accompanies him to hospital with his three-month-old brother.

---

a Learning activity

Find out from your local hospital whether emergency medical admissions are admitted directly to the children's ward, or go to Accident and Emergency (A&E) first and then to the ward following assessment and emergency care. What do you think are the advantages and disadvantages of each approach to admission, for the child and their family?

S Scenario continued

On arrival at the ward the hospital doctor assesses Tom. The assessment includes a brief history and examination. The aim is to identify whether Tom is at risk of developing a severe exacerbation of his asthma. Tom is very anxious, as he has not attended this hospital before.

a Learning activity

Identify what questions the doctor needs to ask in order to ascertain the history and severity of Tom's condition. You might be able to arrange to listen in on the doctor's assessment of such a child.

Asthma can be categorised by degree (Cross, 1999):

- **mild asthma**: children who do not have continuous symptoms and only experience occasional short attacks
- **moderate asthma**: children who may have continuous mild symptoms and more frequent exacerbations which can last for several days or weeks
- **severe asthma**: children who have continuous symptoms and frequent, severe attacks.

Adverse features in the patient's history could include:

- previous episodes of respiratory failure or hypoxic-related seizures as a result of asthma
- deterioration despite the use of oral steroids or frequent inhalation of bronchodilators at home
- recent hospitalisations or emergency-room visits for asthma
- dependence on multiple medication, particularly oral steroids
- noncompliance or psychosocial problems.

S Scenario continued

Once Tom is settled on the ward, the nurse allocated to him carries out a full nursing assessment.

a Learning activity

What can the nurse learn from looking at and listening to Tom? What would you expect Tom's vital signs to be? Consider your responses before reading on.

Normal respiratory rates are given in Table 21.2, normal heart rates in Table 21.3 and systolic blood pressure (BP) by age in Table 21.4.

Respiratory rates should be measured over a full minute. It should be remembered that young children breathe diaphragmatically, and therefore are observed by watching abdominal movement rather than the movement of the chest.

An accurate pulse should be measured for a full minute. When measuring the heart rate of children less than 2 years of age, a stethoscope should be placed over the apex of the heart and the beats counted for a full minute.

The size of the child's limb must be taken into consideration when taking blood pressure (BP). The cuff bladder length should cover 90–100 per cent of the circumference of the arm (Morgenstern and Butani, 2004), and the bladder width to length ratio must be at least 1:2. The most common cause of error in BP measurement for both manual and automated methods is the selection of an incorrect cuff size (Beevers, Lip and O'Brien, 2001: 22–48). The use of a too small cuff leads to erroneously high BP readings, whereas overly large cuffs do not seem to generate significant errors (Morgenstern and Butani, 2004).

The National Institute of Clinical Excellence (NICE) (2007) states that 'normal body temperature varies within and between individuals' and that measurement of body temperature can vary with the site of measurement and type of thermometer used. It acknowledges that it is difficult to define fever based on a fixed body temperature, and defines fever within the guideline as 'an elevation of body temperature above the normal daily variation'. Anderson, Peterson and Wailoo (1990) described this variation as ranging between 36 °C at night and 37.8 °C during active periods in the day for infants. NICE recognises that in scientific studies the criterion for fever is typically a fixed body temperature such as 38 °C or higher.

It is important to remember that a good assessment is much more than just the recording of numbers; the best information is gained from well-developed observational and listening skills. The assessment of the respiratory system involves the assessment of the rate of breathing, type of respirations, any noise on breathing, cough, chest movement, colour of the child, ability to feed and talk, the oxygen saturation level, nasal flaring and position of the child. A large amount of the assessment of breathing can and should be done from a distance, without even touching the child (Syers, 2008).

Physical signs such as wheeze and respiratory rate are poor indicators of the severity of an asthma attack. Contraction of the sternomastoids, chest retraction, pulse rate, peak expiratory flow rate and arterial oxygen saturation are better guides. Cyanosis is a late sign, and an indication of a life-threatening attack (Advanced Life Support Group, 2000).

Table 21.2 Normal respiratory rates

Age (years)	Breaths/min
0<1	30–40
2–5	20–30
5–12	15–20
>12	12–16

Table 21.3 Normal heart rates

Age (years)	Breaths/min
0<1	110–160
2–5	95–140
5–12	80–120
>12	60–100

Table 21.4 Systolic blood pressure (BP) by age

Age (years)	Systolic BP
0<1	70–90
2–5	80–100
5–12	90–110
>12	100–120

Expected systolic BP = 80 + (age in years x 2)

a Learning activity

What are the different methods of assessing the vital signs of temperature, heart rate, respiratory rate and blood pressure? Why are certain methods more appropriate for different groups of children? Go to NICE (2007).

Part

III

> ⌐S⌐ Scenario continued
>
> At this time Tom has not responded well to the initial treatment of beta2 agonists. He is
> unable to drink and is finding it increasingly difficult to carry out a conversation.

Assessment

Before the nurse can plan the client's care, the client's problems must be defined and
identified. Consequently, the assessment phase of planning care begins with the collection
of data about the health status of the client, and ends with a statement of their problems.
The assessment process involves the nurse collecting data. This data can be gathered from
a number of sources. *Primary data* is from the client, and *secondary data* is from other
sources. It also involves the data being validated; for example, Tom might say that his only
health problem is his asthma, yet when you talk to him with his parents, they state he has had
recurrent ear infections. The data gathered also needs to be recorded in an organised fashion.

There are two different types of data collected, subjective and objective. *Subjective* data
includes thoughts, feelings, beliefs and sensations that the client is experiencing. *Objective*
data is that gathered by the use of observation and examination.

It is important to remember that the admission process might be the first time that a child
patient and their family meet the nursing staff. First impressions can lay the foundation for
the future relationship. For this reason, care should be taken to use the opportunity to get to
know the child. Questions should be asked in language understandable to those being asked.
The nurse should be sensitive to the needs of the child and their
family, and time should be given for them to both answer and
ask questions.

There are many different tools available to aid a nursing
assessment. Often they are based on the nursing model that is
used to underpin practice.

Go to the chapter website and look at an example of
nursing documentation for the assessment of a child (which is
reproduced by kind permission of the Royal Cornwall Hospital
Trust).

In the learning activity you might include in your list of
priority issues, for example:

- Safety: it is important to ensure that Tom is supported,
  monitored and receives appropriate treatment to improve
  the situation but also to prevent deterioration.
- Information: Tom and his mother need to know both what
  is happening and why the steps being taken to support Tom
  are important. It is equally important that the nurse is able to
  establish the priorities and concerns of Tom and his mother.
- Comfort: it will be helpful to Tom and his mother if they are
  treated in a gentle and respectful manner. If the nurse is calm
  and efficient in her approach to Tom and his mother's care
  needs, this should also communicate a reassuring message.

> ⌐a⌐ **Learning activity**
>
> Consider what other sources might
> be used to gather information about
> Tom. In your current placement find
> out how information is gathered on
> assessment, recorded and organised.
> Detail the objective data that you
> would need to carry out Tom's
> assessment adequately.

> ⌐a⌐ **Learning activity**
>
> Can you identify the nursing needs
> of Tom and his family utilising the
> information you have been given?
>
> Make a list of the initial priority
> issues for this family. Do this activity
> before reading on.

One of the problems that is often identified from the assessment
is that the child is very anxious about coming into hospital.
What causes this anxiety? Much of the research examining the effects of hospitalisation on
children has focused on why children react differently to hospital experiences. A variety of
strategies have been developed by children's nurses to help families cope with the emotional
traumas of hospital admission and other related healthcare interventions. Changes to a child's

routine such as hospital admission can expose them to stress, and it should be remembered that certain categories of children, for example those with special needs or those for whom English is not the first language, might not be able to articulate their needs adequately (Glasper, 2002).

It is important to realise that although the lung is obviously the primary target of respiratory distress, when respiratory failure follows there may be impairment of other vital organs as a result of decreased arterial blood gases, acidosis and hypercarbia.

The general clinical signs of respiratory distress in children can be described within the systems they affect: see Table 21.5.

> **S**   Scenario continued
>
> Tom's condition does not improve, and the nurses need to monitor the level of his respiratory distress.

Table 21.5 Clinical signs of respiratory distress

Respiratory		Cardiac	General	Cerebral
→ Tachypnoea → Altered depth and pattern of breathing → Intercostal, subcostal and suprasternal inspiratory retractions → Nasal flaring → Cyanosis → Decreased or absent breath sounds → Expiratory grunting	→ Wheeze and or prolonged expiration → Dyspnoea → Cough → Head bobbing → Stridor → Seesaw respirations → Decreased chest expansion → Decreased breath sounds	→ Tachycardia or bradycardia → Hypertension or hypotension → Duskiness → Cyanosis → Cardiac arrest	→ Poor skeletal muscle tone → Fatigue → Abdominal pain → Increased sweating → Altered consciousness level	→ Restlessness → Irritability → Headache → Confusion → Diminished response to parents or pain → Coma

It can be seen from this discussion that carefully looking at and listening to a child is invaluable in assessing their respiratory status. In addition the measurement of capillary refill, oxygen saturation and peak expiratory flow rate are helpful in making a nursing assessment.

Other systems may also be affected by altered respiratory status. Following the ABC criteria for assessment in conjunction with neurological observations provides a framework for rapid and effective nursing assessment of the child with respiratory problems.

> **a**   Learning activity
>
> For all the systems, check your understanding of the terminology by, for example, checking definitions in a dictionary. Also write key points to explain why breathing difficulties may lead to all these signs and symptoms.

Part

III

Capillary refill

Syers (2008) describes capillary refill as:

> The time taken for the capillary bed to refill with blood after being exposed to pressure to empty the bed. Cutaneous pressure is applied to a digit or centre of the sternum for five seconds. The pressure is then released and the number of seconds that it takes for the capillaries to refill and the skin colour to return to normal is counted. This should be less than two seconds. A slower time indicates poor perfusion, which can be a sign of shock. However a low ambient temperature can reduce the specificity of this test. Additionally if the child has a fever that is in the rising stage, the peripheral circulation may well be shut down and the refill time will be delayed. In this instance it is advisable to use the centre of the sternum. This test should be undertaken alongside other assessment tools and the results interpreted accordingly i.e. a prolonged CRT and raised HR could indicate a fever, anxiety, hypoxia or hypovolaemia.

Oxygen saturation

The administration of oxygen may be prescribed to maintain oxygen levels during an asthmatic attack. In a severe asthmatic attack, oxygen should be administered using a tight-fitting face mask or nasal cannula (BTS SIGN, 2008). The most suitable one will be chosen depending on the child's age and condition. Oxygen should be humidified whenever possible.

How much oxygen is in the blood depends on:

- the haemoglobin concentration in the blood (Hb g/dl)
- the oxygen saturation of the haemoglobin (Sao2)
- the partial pressure of oxygen: that is, how much is dissolved in the plasma (Pao2).

Carbon dioxide is transported to the lungs dissolved in the plasma, or as bicarbonate, or carbamino compounds. Carbon dioxide is acidic, therefore if the level of carbon dioxide in the plasma rises, the child becomes acidotic.

Analysis of the blood pH and the arterial blood gases provides information of the child's gas exchange and acid-base status. The normal partial pressure of oxygen (Pao2) in the arterial blood is 11–14kPa (Kilo Pascals). It is lower in neonates: Pao2 = 8-10kPa. Normal partial pressure of carbon dioxide (Paco2) in the arterial blood is 4.0–5.5kPa (Rudolf and Levene, 1999).

Disturbances in acid-base balance can be caused by respiratory disorders. If respiration is inadequate, the child's blood pH will fall and result in acidosis. Assessment of arterial blood gas values can assist in deciding the best course of treatment (Frew and Holgate, 2005).

In asthma the monitoring of arterial blood gases may be necessary. If the child shows signs of severe respiratory distress, it will help determine whether the child is in respiratory failure and needs respiratory support. Controlled ventilation using endotracheal intubation may be necessary for a short period of time, usually 8 to 12 hours. Transcutaneous measurement of oxygen saturation is used for continuous oxygen assessment (Frew and Holgate, 2005).

Pulse oximetry measures the arterial blood saturation by calculating the percentage of haemoglobin that is saturated with oxygen. Because haemoglobin is photosensitive and has the capacity to absorb different amounts of light, changes in oxygen levels can be detected rapidly. A light-emitting sensor and a photodetector are placed in an opposing position around a digit, hand, foot or earlobe. The diode emits red and infrared lights, which pass through the skin to the photodetector. Oxyhaemoglobin absorbs more infrared light than deoxyhaemoglobin. This is detected by the microprocessor, which displays the percentage of oxyhaemoglobin (Bloxham, 2006). To enable the sensor to 'pick up' a reading, the patient needs to have an adequate pulsatile blood flow to the periphery. The site chosen for the sensor should be warm, with good capillary perfusion, and comfortable for the child.

Carrying out pulse oximetry on a site that is already being used for BP monitoring or as access for an arterial catheter will produce inaccurate recordings. Using a sensor that is too tight will restrict perfusion, leading to an inaccurate result, and movement of the sensor or child will lead to motion artefact (Bloxham, 2006). The probe site should be checked every hour and changed every two hours to prevent pressure necrosis or burns from incompatible sensors and oximeters (Bloxham, 2006).

Children like Tom should have their oxygen saturation recorded on arrival on the ward. Saturations of less than 90 per cent are indicative of a severe attack.

> **a) Learning activity**
>
> Find out normal values for oxygen saturation. If possible measure your own.

Fluid management

A child such as Tom is at risk of dehydration, and the assessment should identify this. It is important to ensure the child has a sufficient fluid intake. Oral fluids may be difficult when the child has severe breathing problems. Therefore fluids are administered intravenously to meet normal fluid requirements and to replace additional losses caused by hyperventilation. The amount and type of fluid administered is prescribed according to the individual child's size and hydration needs. Measurements of blood gases, pH and serum electrolytes will be used to determine the extent of the child's dehydration, acidosis and electrolyte imbalance. The insertion of an intravenous cannula is a stressful experience for both the child and the parent, therefore age-appropriate preparation for the procedure needs to be given (Lane, 2006a). The cannula should be inserted into a site that takes into consideration the child's age and level of activity, and it should be secured to ensure it remains stable, but in a way that leaves the insertion point visible (Lane, 2006b).

An infusion pump is normally used to reduce the risk of circulatory overload. The nurse should, on a regular basis, monitor the rate of the infusion and the infusion site for signs of phlebitis and extravasation. There are many risks associated with the administration of intravenous fluids. Comprehensive protocols should be available in the ward area, and these should be complied with to improve safety (Bloxham and Kelsey, 2008).

> **a Learning activity**
>
> Find out the recommended intravenous fluid requirements for a child of Tom's age.

> **S Scenario continued**
>
> After Tom's initial poor response to his treatment, he responds well to nebulised Beta2 agonists two-hourly, driven by oxygen. He also commences oral prednisolone.
>
> During the next 24 hours Tom's condition continues to improve. He is wheezing less, his respirations are between 18 and 22 breaths per minute, his pulse is 90 beats per minute at rest, and his oxygen saturation is above 90
>
> per cent. He is able to recommence oral fluids and his intravenous infusion is discontinued. The next day, he is discharged home and his GP is informed of his progress. Tom is a moderate to severe asthmatic; therefore he will be advised to follow the national guidelines for chronic asthma management.

Principles of asthma management

The management of asthma is focused on controlling the underlying inflammatory response using prophylactic therapy, and breakthrough symptoms being treated with bronchodilators. It is essential that the child and family are aware that asthma cannot be cured. The aim is to control the symptoms so that the child can lead a full and active life (Kieckfeler and Ratcliffe, 2004).

National and international guidelines for the management of asthma in children advise a step approach to drug management (BTS SIGN, 2008). Using this protocol, children are assessed and assigned to a level of treatment related to the severity of their asthma. The treatment is subsequently adjusted to meet the child's changing needs, and control is maintained with the lowest possible dosages of drugs. There is a step approach to the treatment of asthma which has been adopted nationally by British Thoracic Society/Scottish Intercollegiate Guidelines Network (2008), available at http://www.sign.ac.uk/pdf/sign101.pdf.

The step approach for children aged from 5 to 12 years is outlined below, but as evidence increases this programme of therapy might be updated, so it is important that you check the website to confirm the most up-to-date plan for treatment. There are step approaches for children under 12 years and for adults (children over 12 are considered adults).

Step 1: Inhaled beta2 agonists to relieve symptoms, administered no more than three times a week.

Step 2: Low dose 200–400 mcg/day inhaled steroids initially twice daily. A once-daily dose can be considered if good control is achieved.

Step 3: Consider add-on therapy of long-acting beta2 agonists. If there is some benefit from long-acting beta2 agonists but control is inadequate, increase the dosage of inhaled steroids to 400mcg/day and continue with long-acting beta2 agonists. If there is no benefit from the long-acting beta2 agonists, stop the dosage, and increase the dosage of inhaled steroids to 400mcg/day. If there is still poor control, consider leukotriene receptor antagonist or theophylline.

Step 4: Increase to 800mcg/day inhaled steroids.

Step 5: Continuous or frequent use of oral steroids at as low a dose as possible plus 800mcg/day inhaled steroids. Refer to a respiratory physician.

Good inhaler technique is essential for effective treatment, and it is important that the most suitable device is chosen for each individual child. It may be necessary to try out a variety of devices before the child is able to find the correct device (Caldwell, 1998). The choice of inhaler is affected by the age of the child, prescribed treatment, the child's lifestyle and the child's preference. Over 90 per cent of asthmatics take all the medications they require by inhalation. However, inhaled drugs are not effective during severe asthmatic attacks because the airways are completely obstructed by inflammation and mucus (Jordan and White, 2001). Bronchodilators are most effective when delivered as inhaled aerosols. This route of delivery also decreases the amount of the drug entering the systemic circulation, and therefore reduces side-effects (Jordan and White, 2001).

a Learning activity   W

The British Thoracic Society (BTS, 2008) has published guidelines on asthma management which are also available on its website at http://www.brit-thoracic.org.uk. Having read these guidelines, satisfy yourself that you understand the forms of therapy used to treat asthma, their modes of administration and actions.

The Medline Plus site (www.nlm.nih.gov/medlineplus/asthma.html) has comprehensive information, and you can read the latest news and articles on treatments.

NICE (2000) has published a useful review of the use of inhaler systems/devices for   W
children. This can be accessed on the website at http://www.nice.org.uk. This is also a good example of how the effectiveness of a healthcare intervention is evaluated.

a Learning activity

Which type of inhaler do you think would suit Tom best?

Inhaler technique

Inhaler devices require different levels of skill and coordination to administer effectively. The method of administration for inhaled drugs varies with the child's age and ability. Nebulisers are the method of choice for infants and young children. When inhalers are prescribed, the child and family need to be taught how to use the device. This involves giving careful instructions, demonstration and then assessing their ability to administer the drug correctly (Caldwell, 1998), as poor technique is one of the main reasons for lack of control of symptoms. In many cases only a very small percentage of the medication reaches the lungs and the rest is swallowed.

This percentage can be radically improved by the use of spacer devices (Holliday and Kierulff, 2008). Spacer devices are the best method of delivery for inhaled drugs in young children as they provide a holding chamber from which the child can repeatedly breathe, increasing the opportunity for the child to inhale the drug (Jordan and White, 2001). It is important to note that when steroids are inhaled, the child should be encouraged to rinse out their mouth or clean their teeth after administration to remove any medication left in the mouth (Holliday and Kierulff, 2008). Inhaler technique is clearly demonstrated on the website http://www.asthma.org.uk/health_professionals/interactive_inhaler_demo/index.html.

Using a spacer with a face mask

For children under the age of 3 years, prescribed metered dose inhalers are best used in conjunction with a spacer and a facemask:

1 Ensure the holes in the face mask are occluded.
2 Attach the inverted spacer plus inhaler to the face mask.
3 Place the facemask over the infant's nose and mouth.
4 Inverting the spacer ensures that the one-way valve falls open.
5 Activate the inhaler.
6 The infant inhales during normal tidal breathing, at least six breaths.
7 Wait 30 seconds to repeat the sequence if a second dose is required.

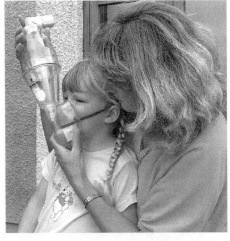

Figure 21.2 Using an inhaler

Spacer devices

Children over 3 years can usually use spacer devices directly via the mouthpiece. To aid administration the child should stand up to enable full diaphragmatic excursion and look upwards to reduce pharyngeal angle, and therefore minimise depositing the medication in the mouth. Encouraging the child to bite on the mouthpiece avoids their closing their teeth behind it. Another problem can be that the child occludes the mouthpiece with their tongue.

To use a spacer device:

1 Remove the inhaler cap, shake the canister and insert it into the device.
2 The child should stand up and look upwards. Place the mouthpiece in the child's mouth. Encourage the child to bite on the mouthpiece, Advise the child to try to keep their tongue down (Holliday and Kierulff, 2008).
3 Encourage the child to breathe in and out gently (tidal breathing). This will open and close the valve and a clicking noise will be heard.
4 Keeping the device in the same position, depress the canister once to release a dose of the drug.
5 The child should continue to tidal breathe for five breaths.
6 Remove the device from the child's mouth.
7 Wait 30 seconds to repeat the sequence if a second dose is required.

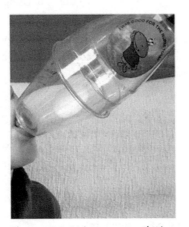

Figure 21.3 Using a spacer device

By the age of 5 years children can usually generate enough inspiratory flow to activate dry powder devices and have the skills of coordination to use metered dose inhalers.

To use a metered dose inhaler:

1 Shake the canister before use. The child should stand up and look upwards.
2 Have the child exhale to functional reserve capacity.
3 Activate the inhaler at the start of the inspiration.
4 Have the child take a slow, deep breath.
5 Have the child hold the breath for 5 to 10 seconds.
6 Have the child take one puff at a time, and break for 30 seconds between puffs (Holliday and Kierulff, 2008).

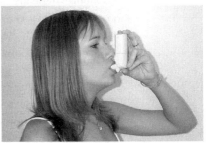

Figure 21.4 Using a metered dose inhaler

To use a turbohaler:

1 Unscrew and lift off the outer white cover.
2 Hold the turbohaler upright.
3 Twist the grip forwards and backwards as far as you can until you hear the click.
4 The child should stand up and look upwards, then breathe out.
5 Put the mouthpiece between the lips and have the child breathe in deeply.
6 Remove the inhaler from the mouth and have the child hold the breath for 10 seconds.
7 Replace the white cover on the turbohaler.

To use an accuhaler:

1 Hold the outer casing of the accuhaler with one hand while pushing the thumb grip away until a click is heard.
2 Hold the mouthpiece towards you.
3 Slide the lever away until it clicks.
4 The child should stand up and look upwards. Hold the inhaler level.
5 Have the child breathe out gently away from the device.
6 Have the child put the mouthpiece in their mouth and breathe in steadily and deeply.
7 Remove the device from the mouth and have the child hold their breath for 10 seconds.
8 Close by sliding the thumb grip back until it clicks.

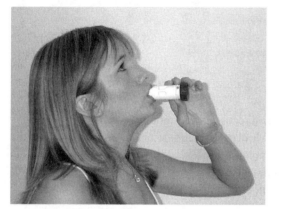

Figure 21.5 Using a turbohaler

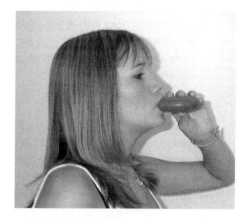

Figure 21.6 Using an accuhaler

W The Asthma and Allergy Foundation of America's website (www.aafa.org) has interesting videos, featuring health professionals discussing core issues such as treatment in children of 5 to 12 years of age, and in adolescents.

S Scenario continued

The step plan is explained to Tom and his parents. Tom's mother is worried about the adverse effects of steroids.

a Learning activity

How could you reassure Tom and his parents regarding this issue? Look up a recognised pharmacology book to find out the side-effects that Tom might experience.

Some of the side-effects of steroids

The most common side-effects of inhaled corticosteroids are oropharyngeal thrush and dysphonia. These are not common and are caused by the drug coming in contact with the oropharynx. They can be reduced by rinsing the mouth after inhalation or using a large-volume spacer with the metered dose inhaler (Holliday and Kierulff, 2008).

A study by McCowan and colleagues (1998) showed that high doses of inhaled steroids may adversely affect growth rates. However, the reduction in stature may be caused by a combination of influences which would also include the severity of the asthma and the degree of control (Kieckfeler and Ratcliffe, 2004).

Although use of prophylactic steroids has been demonstrated to be safe and effective in the treatment of childhood asthma (Sharek and Bergman, 2000), some parents may feel a little reluctant to give these medicines to their children.

Long-term management of asthma

Many asthmatic children remain undiagnosed, and those that are diagnosed are often inadequately treated (Cross, 1999; Caldwell, 1998). The greater willingness of doctors to diagnose asthma in children is probably the single most important factor in improving treatment. There is no permanent cure for asthma, but appropriate drug regimes abolish symptoms for most asthmatics (Cross, 1999).

The British Thoracic Society (2008) has produced principles for the management of asthma. These include family and child participation in care, avoiding identified triggers, and using the lowest effective dosages of drugs. They state that the most important aspect of management is that the child and the family understand asthma, the forms of treatment available, and what to do when changes in condition occur. There is a need to educate the child and parents so they understand the difference between preventive and relief treatment, are able to administer inhaled drugs effectively and use a peak flow meter, and are able to monitor symptoms and use a drug usage diary. The primary care team are closely involved in managing the child's asthma, and can develop a personalised action plan together with the child and parents which helps improve the management of the condition. Personal action plans can be requested from www.asthma.org.uk. Many randomised controlled trials and a Cochrane review suggest that action plans appear to be one of the most effective interventions available in the routine management of asthma (Wolf et al, 2003).

W

Peak flow measurement

Many children are unable to perceive their degree of airway obstruction, so to assist in the monitoring of their condition a peak expiratory flow meter is used. This is a relatively cheap way of making an objective measurement of the rate at which the child can empty their lungs in litres per minute. Peak flow meters can be used to monitor the child's asthma at home and to check on diurnal variation or fall, which makes it possible to anticipate an impending asthma attack and the need for treatment (BTS SIGN, 2008; GINA, 2007). As the airways become more inflamed, more air becomes trapped within them, making it difficult to blow out. This results in a reduced peak flow reading. The BTS recommends that, where appropriate, every patient with asthma should have their own peak flow meter and should be encouraged to use it to monitor their asthma and the efficacy of inhaled or nebulised medication. In September 2004, a new standard European Union (EU) peak flow meter was introduced. The readings obtained on an EU scale meter have been shown to be more accurate than those from other meters because changes in airflow will result in peak expiratory flow (PEF) readings changing uniformly for the whole range of the meter.

Children can usually learn to use these devices from about 4 years of age. Peak expiratory flow rates (PEFR) vary with age, sex, height and race. A variation of up to 8 per cent of normal values is considered acceptable. PEFR is a good marker of severity of asthma in children who use these meters regularly; however, in children who have not used the meters previously the results should be interpreted with caution. PEFR should be compared with either the best previous PEFR when well or the predicted PEFR for height.

Table 21.6 Peak flow normal values

Reproduced with permission of Clement Clarke International www.clementclarke.com

Paediatric Normal Values

Peak expiratory flow rate
For use with EU/EN 13826
scale PEF meters only

Height (m)	Height (ft)	Predicted EU PEFR (L/min)
0.85	2'9"	87
0.90	2'11"	95
0.95	3'1"	104
1.00	3'3"	115
1.05	3'5"	127
1.10	3'7"	141
1.15	3'9"	157
1.20	3'11"	174
1.25	4'1"	192
1.30	4'3"	212
1.35	4'5"	233
1.40	4'7"	254
1.45	4'9"	276
1.50	4'11"	299
1.55	5'1"	323
1.60	5'3"	346
1.65	5'5"	370
1.70	5'7"	393

Part

III

The predicted PEFR can be calculated for the height from the formula:

Expected PEFR = (5 × height in centimetres) − 400

Peak flows should be recorded before and 10 minutes after each dose of nebulised salbutamol. The peak flow meter is therefore an important aid in assisting in the management of asthma, but the child's clinical condition must always be taken into account (Caldwell, 1998; BTS SIGN, 2008; GINA, 2007).

To use a peak flow meter:
1 Stand.
2 Take a full breath in.
3 Place the mouth tightly around the mouthpiece.
4 Huff out hard and fast.
5 Repeat three times.
6 Record the highest reading.

> **ⓐ Learning activity**
>
> Try to obtain a peak flow meter and record your own peak flow recordings for a period of time. Do your recordings vary? If so, can you identify why?

> **Ⓢ Scenario continued**
>
> This part of the scenario focuses on the issues that need to be considered in family-centred care of Tom.
>
> In the acute phase Mrs Brown might be helped and supported to deliver care that satisfies Tom's basic needs. She can help Tom to drink small amounts of fluids, she can help him to wash, and she can help to reassure and comfort him. As Mrs Brown's understanding of the tasks of management improve she can begin to take responsibility for monitoring Tom's condition using observation and peak flow measurement, and ensure that his medication is administered effectively. In the longer term she can work to ensure the normality of their everyday experience by, for example, minimising the effect of trigger factors that provoke Tom's asthma. Over time, Tom and his family will learn to be flexible and to adapt these care practices to integrate them into family life. This will give them confidence to make the changes necessary to meet new situations.

> **ⓐ Learning activity**
>
> How would you ensure that Tom's family can meet these needs?

Ongoing care

Before a child like Tom is discharged there are several aspects that can be addressed to help reduce future exacerbation of his asthma.

Reducing exposure to triggers

* When specific triggers are known, it is recommended that exposure is avoided wherever possible (Harrop, 2003).

The eradication of house-dust mites

* The bedroom should be well ventilated; there should be no signs of dampness or mould. The bedding should be laundered frequently to at least 60 °C.
* The mattress, duvet and pillows can be covered with material that is not porous to house-dust mites.
* Ideally, the floor should not be carpeted. If necessary, a minimal-pile carpet of synthetic fibre should be used.
* The room should be vacuumed regularly with a cleaner that retains dust particles below 5 microns. In some cases desensitisation to specific triggers is possible.

Immunotherapy

Allergen-specific immunotherapy involves injecting an extract of the allergen under the skin. Research shows that there can be a significant reduction in asthma symptoms and medication following immunotherapy (Abramson, Puy and Weiner, 1999). However the therapy is not practical for some children as they find the injections unpleasant, and children often have multiple sensitivities.

It is important to take a positive approach when caring for children with asthma. This, combined with effective prevention, can enable the child to lead a normal life. Parents need to support their children and encourage them to express their feelings about having asthma, and develop strategies to cope with these feelings (Caldwell, 1998).

One way of ensuring effective high-quality care for the child with asthma is the multidisciplinary team approach. The team includes the child, parents, specialist nurse, GP, hospital staff, school teachers and pharmacists (Cross, 1999).

The importance of teachers understanding the needs of the child with asthma

Children spend 40 per cent of their waking life at school. It is therefore important that teachers understand the disease and can support the child with their treatment.

Teachers appear to restrict asthmatic children more than is necessary, especially regarding their involvement in sporting activities. Kieckfeler and Ratcliffe (2004) also found teachers lacked confidence in how to manage an acute asthmatic attack. Therefore it is important to educate teachers to form part of the care team.

a) Learning activity

Reflect on your knowledge of caring for a child with asthma. Before you completed this chapter, would you have been confident dealing with a child having an asthma attack? How much training do you think teachers receive about caring for children in school with asthma? Try to find out from one of your local schools about training offered to teachers (it might be a good idea to speak to the school nurse for this information).

In caring for the asthma of a child like Tom and ensuring their well-being, both the child and their mother (or other carer) will have to master several tasks.

Do the learning activity on the right. Did your list include:

a) Learning activity

From the knowledge you have built up about childhood asthma, list what you think are the important knowledge and skills that Tom and his mother will need to manage this situation.

- Monitoring Tom's condition to detect early any signs of deterioration so that action can be taken to deal with this? For example, some children's asthma worsens when they have a viral infection such as a cold. Using an asthma diary might be helpful with this.
- Avoiding factors that act as triggers? The aim in managing exposure to triggers is to prevent asthma attacks and to promote normality in the life of the child and family.
- Administering medicine efficiently and effectively? Inhaling medication is not an easy skill to master and the use of inhalers and spacer devices needs to be demonstrated and practised.

Adherence with the asthma medication regime might, on occasion, be problematic for the child and family for the following reasons.

- The full cooperation of the child is required to administer inhalers successfully.
- The child might be reluctant to be seen to be taking medication, and therefore to be seen to be different from their peers.

Part

III

- The family might find it difficult to fit the regime of drug administration into their daily life.
- The family might not fully understand the reasons the drug has been prescribed and may feel dubious about its effects.
- In a disorder such as asthma where the child is often perfectly well between attacks, it may be difficult for the family to appreciate the reason for using a 'preventer' medicine when the child has no symptoms.

Conclusion

On completion of this chapter you will have become more aware of the special needs of the children and families being cared for by healthcare professionals. You should be able to use this knowledge to enable you to participate in implementing child-friendly, family-centred care in any healthcare environment. Having considered some of the many key aspects of caring for children, you should recognise the importance of sick children being cared for by appropriately educated and qualified staff who have a greater depth of knowledge and understanding of the differing needs of children and their families.

References

Abramson, M. J., Puy, R. M. and Weiner, J. M. (1999) 'Allergen immunotherapy for asthma', *Cochrane Review* 3.

Advanced Life Support Group (2000) *Advanced Paediatric Life Support: The practical approach*, 3rd edn, London, BMJ Books.

Anderson, E. S., Peterson, S. A. and Wailoo, M. P. (1990) 'Factors influencing body temperature of 3–4 month-old infants at home during the day', *Archives of Disease in Childhood* 65, 1308–10.

Asthma UK (2004) *Where Do We Stand? Asthma in the UK today*, London, Asthma UK.

Beevers, G., Lip, G. and O'Brien, E. (2001) *ABC of Hypertension* 4th edn, London, BMJ Books.

Bloxham, N. (2006) 'Pulse oximetry' in Glasper, E. A. McEwing, G. and Richardson, J. (eds), *Oxford Handbook of Children's and Young Peoples Nursing*, Oxford, Oxford University Press.

Bloxham, N. and Kelsey, J. (2008) 'Peripheral intravemous therapy', in Kelsey, J. A. and McEwing, G. (eds), *Clinical Skills in Child Health Practice*, Edinburgh, Churchill Livingstone.

British Thoracic Society (BTS) (1997) *The British Guidelines on asthma management*, Thorax 52.

BTS and Scottish Intercollegiate Guidelines Network (SIGN) (2008) *British Guideline on the Management of Asthma: A national clinical guideline* [online] http://www.sign.ac.uk/pdf/sign101.pdf (accessed 12 December 2008).

Caldwell, C. (1998) 'Management of acute asthma in children', *Nursing Standard* 12(29) (8–14 April), 49–54.

Camargos, P. Castro, R. and Feldman, J. (1999) 'Prevalence of symptoms related to asthma among schoolchildren in Campos Gerais, Brazil', *Pan American Journal of Public Health* 6(1) (8–15 July).

Cates, C. and FitzGerald, M. (2001) 'Asthma', *Clinical Evidence* 5, 1011–27.

Chandler, T. (2000) 'Oxygen saturation monitoring', *Paediatric Nursing* 12(8), 37–42.

Cross, S. (1999) 'Better care for people with asthma', *Nursing Standard* 13(46) (4–10 August), 51–4.

De Bisschop, C., Guenard, H., Desnot, P. and Vergeret, J. (1999) 'Reduction of exercise-induced asthma in children by short, repeated warm ups', *British Journal of Sports Medicine* 33(2) (April), 100–4.

Frankes, M. (1997) 'Asthma in the emergency department', *Journal of Emergency Nursing* 23(5) (October), 429–38.

Frew, A. J. and Holgate, S. T. (2005) 'Respiratory medicine', in Kumar, P, and Clark, M. (eds), *Clinical Medicine*, 6th edn, London, Elsevier.

Glasper, E. A. (2002) 'Contemporary issues in the care of sick children and their families', *British Journal of Nursing* 11(4), 248–56.

Global Initiative for Asthma (GINA) (2007 updated) 'Global strategy for asthma management and prevention', NHLBI/WHO Workshop Report, Bethesda: National Institutes of Health, National Heart, Lung, and Blood Institute [online] http://www.ginasthma.org (accessed 12 December 2008).

Harrop, M. (2003) 'Respiratory and cardiovascular problems', in Barnes, K. (ed.), *Paediatrics: A clinical guide for practitioners*, London, Butterworth Heinemann.

Hockenberry, M. Wilson, D., Winkelstein, M. and Kline, N. (2003) *Wong's Nursing Care of Infants and Children*, Missouri, Mosby.

Holliday, L. and Kierulff, C. (2008) 'Administration of medicines', in Kelsey, J. and McEwing, G. (eds), *Clinical Skills in Child Health Practice*, London, Elsevier.

Hunter, S. (1995) 'The use of steroids in asthma treatment', Nursing Standard (9, 38, 14–20) (June) 25–7.

Jordan, S. and White, J. (2001) 'Bronchodilators: implications for nursing practice', *Nursing Standard* **15**(27) (21 March), 45–55.

Kaur, B., Anderson, H. R., Austin, J., Burr, M., Harkins, L., Strachan, D. and Warner, J. O. (1998) 'Prevalence of asthma symptoms, diagnosis, and treatment in 12–14-year-old children across Great Britain (international study of asthma and allergies in childhood, ISAAC UK)', *British Medical Journal* 316, 118–24.

Kieckfeler, G. and Ratcliffe, M. (2004) 'Asthma', in Allen, P. and Vessey, J. (eds), *Primary Care of the Child with a Chronic Condition*, 4th edn, Missouri, Mosby.

Lane, E. (2006a) 'Assisting with taking a blood sample' in Glasper, E. A., McEwing, G. and Richardson, J. (eds), *Oxford Handbook of Children's and Young Peoples Nursing*, Oxford, Oxford University Press.

Lane, E. (2006b) 'Assisting with cannulation and cannula care', in Glasper, E. A., McEwing, G. and Richardson, J. (eds), *Oxford Handbook of Children's and Young Peoples Nursing*, Oxford, Oxford University Press.

Magnus, P. and Jaakkola, J. (1997) 'Secular trend in the occurrence of asthma among children and young adults: critical appraisal of repeated cross sectional surveys', *British Medical Journal* 314, 1795–803.

McClowry, S. G. and McLeod, S. M. (1990) 'The psychological responses of school age children to hospitalization', *Children's Health Care* **19**(3), 155–60.

McCowan, C., Neville, R. G., Thomas, G. E., Crombie, I. K., Ricketts, I. W., Cairns, A. Y., Warner, F. C., Greene, S. A. and White, E. (1998) 'Effect of asthma and its treatment on growth: four-year follow up of cohort of children from general practices in Tayside, Scotland', *British Medical Journal* 316, 668–72.

Meadow, R. and Newell, S. (2002) *Lecture Notes on Paediatrics*, 7th edn, Oxford, Blackwell Science.

Morgenstern, B. and Butani, L. (2004) 'Casual blood pressure measurement methodology', pp. 77–96 in Portman, R. (ed.), *Paediatric Hypertension*, New Jersey, Humana Press.

Newacheck, P. and Halfon, N. (2000) 'Prevalence, impact and trends in childhood disability due to asthma', *Archives of Paediatrics and Adolescent Medicine* 154, 287–93.

National Institute Clinical Excellence (NICE) and National Collaborating Centre for Womens and Children's Health (NCCWCH) (2007) *Feverish Illness in Children: Assessment and initial management in children younger than 5 years*, clinical guideline, Royal College of Obstetricians and Gynaecologists [online] http://guidance.nice.org.uk/CG47/guidance/pdf/English (accessed 16 August 2007).

Oddy, W. H., Holt, P. G., Sly, P. D., Read, A. W., Landau, L. I., Stanley, F. J., Kendall, G. E. and Burton, P. R. (1999) 'Association between breast-feeding and asthma in six-year-old children: findings of a prospective birth cohort study', *British Medical Journal* 319, 815–19.

Office for National Statistics (ONS) (2004) *Asthma and allergies: Decrease in hospital admissions in 90s* [online] http://www.statistics.gov.uk/cci/nugget.asp?id=722&Pos=1&ColRank=1&Rank=192 (accessed 24 December 2008).

Rudolf, M. and Levene, M. (1999) *Paediatrics in Child Health*, Blackwell Science, Oxford.

Rydstrom, I., Dalheim-Englund, A., Holritz-Rasmussen, B., Moller, C. and Sandman, P. (2005) 'Asthma: quality of life for Swedish children', *Journal of Clinical Nursing* 14, 739–49.

Sharek, P. J. and Bergman, D. A. (2000) 'Beclometnasone for asthma in children: effects on linear growth', *Cochrane Review* 1.

Sabina, I., Von Mutius, E., Lau, S., Bergmann, R., Niggerman, B. et al (2001) 'Early childhood infectious diseases and the development of asthma up to school age: a birth cohort study', *British Medical Journal* 322, 390–5.

Shaheen, S., Sterne, J., Songhurst, C. and Burney, P. (2000) 'Frequent paracetamol use and asthma in adults', *Thorax* 55, 266–70.

Simon, C., Everitt, H. and Kendrick, T. (2005) *Oxford Handbook of General Practice*, 2nd edn. Oxford, Oxford University Press.

Simpson, A. B., Glutting, J. and Yousef, E. (2007) 'Food allergy and asthma morbidity in children', *Paediatric Pulmonology* **42**(6), 489–95.

Strachan D. P. (1999) 'The epidemiology of childhood asthma', *Allergy* **54**(49), 7–11.

Swallow, V. M. and Jacoby, A. (2001) 'Mothers' evolving relationships with doctors and nurses during the chronic childhood illness trajectory', *Journal of Advanced Nursing* **36**(6), 755–64.

Syers, S. (2008) 'Physical assessment', in Kelsey, J. A. and McEwing, G. (eds), *Clinical Skills in Child Health Practice*, Edinburgh, Churchill Livingstone.

Taylor, J., Muller, D., Wattley, L. and Harris, P. (1999) *Nursing Children Psychology: Research and practice*, 3rd edn, Cheltenham, Stanley Thornes.

Wolf, F. M., Guevara, J. P., Grum, C. M. Clark, N. M. and Cates, C. J. (2003) 'Educational interventions for asthma in children', *Cochrane Reviews* 1.

Zureik, M., Neukirch, C., Leynaert, B., Liard, R,. Bousquet, J. and Neukirch, F. (2002) 'Sensitisation to airborne moulds and severity of asthma: cross sectional study from European Community respiratory health survey', *British Medical Journal* 325, 411–18.

Websites

British Thoracic Society: www.brit-thoracic.org.uk

National Asthma Audit 1999/2000: www.asthma.org.uk

National Institute of Clinical Excellence: www.nice.org.uk

For temperature measurement, go to the thermometry page at: www.graduateresearch.com/thermometry/theory.htm

Part

III

Chapter

22

Care of the adolescent

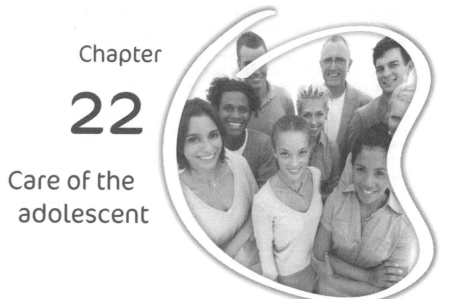

Michael Cooper, Alan Glasper and Chris Taylor

 Links to other chapters in *Foundation Studies for Caring*

 Links to other chapters in *Foundation Skills for Caring*

W Don't forget to visit www.palgrave.com/glasper for additional online resources relating to this chapter.

Introduction

This chapter explores general adolescent healthcare and development before moving on to look at the issues surrounding eating disorders (specifically anorexia nervosa). It also discusses healthcare policy relating to the care of adolescents within the National Health Service (NHS). The scenario relates to a young person with an eating disorder and traces their experiences through various institutional and noninstitutional environments, looking at the effectiveness of different intervention strategies. Anorexia nervosa is used to illustrate the complex interplay between the process of adolescence and a major psycho/physiological disorder.

Learning outcomes

This chapter will enable you to:

- outline the physical parameters of adolescent transition from childhood to adulthood
- investigate healthcare policy for young people in different settings
- consider the health of young people with health problems as they go through transition from child to adult services
- discuss how young people can be involved in shaping their health service and care
- review the rising tide of alcohol abuse among young people and the potential associated health risks
- describe the psychological developmental journey through adolescence
- outline the principal theories of the causation of anorexia nervosa
- differentiate between anorexia nervosa and other causes of weight loss and anorexia

- explore the impact of illness on the adolescent developmental sequence
- identify the physiological and psychological implications of extreme low weight
- describe nursing interventions required to reach and maintain physiological integrity
- understand a patient's desire not to gain weight
- recognise and respond therapeutically to a patient's strategies for food avoidance/excess
- discuss how personal and professional belief systems impact on the giving of care
- discuss the nature of a therapeutic relationship with emotionally distressed clients
- explore and debate the legal and ethical issues involved in treatment interventions.

Part

III

Concepts

- Physical and psychological development
- Healthcare policy
- Patient involvement in healthcare
- Transition
- Physical and psychological assessment
- Causation, theoretical issues, personality traits, co-morbidity, family systems

- Mental health issues in a paediatric environment
- Health education: diet, alcohol abuse, exercise, healthy body weight, body image
- Psychological care: managing manipulation, emotional distress, the therapeutic encounter

- Moral and legal implications of nursing people with eating disorders
- Professional values, social and personal narratives
- Issues around continuing service provision

Healthcare policy for young people

A number of key documents inform and influence policy and practice in adolescent healthcare:

- *Bridging the Gaps: Healthcare for adolescents* (RCPCH, 2003)
- *Adolescent Health* (BMA, 2003)
- *National Service Framework for Children, Young People and Maternity Services* (DH, 2003)
- *Every Child Matters* (DFES, 2003).

The first published chapter of the *National Service Framework for Children*, 'Standards for hospital services' was published in 2003 ahead of the other standards, and advocates child-centred services that consider the whole child, not simply the illness. Seeing the whole child also means recognising that health protection and promotion, and disease prevention, are integral to the young person's care in any setting. In exploring child-centred care it is recognised that the child exists within the context of a family, school, friends and local community. Children and young people have rights, and treatment is a partnership. Respecting the role of parents is seen as a significant part of providing services for children. Prevention and health promotion are also seen as a fundamental question of attitude which looks beyond the immediate treatment of the presenting problem.

The remaining chapters of the *National Service Framework for Children, Young People and Maternity Services* published the following year (DH, 2004) set out core standards that develop the principles further. Safeguarding and promoting the welfare of children and young people is one of the core principles. The emphasis is on promoting health and well-being, identifying needs and intervening early, centring services around the young person and their family, supporting families and carers, and the young person's transition to adult services.

Youth Matters (DfES, 2005) is now the government's key policy document for improving the lives of young people in England. This policy is aimed at:

- making services more responsive to what young people and their parents want
- balancing greater opportunities and support with promoting young people's responsibilities
- making services for young people more integrated, efficient and effective
- improving outcomes for all young people, while narrowing the gap between those who do well and those who do not
- involving a wide range of organisations from the voluntary, community and private sectors in order to increase choice and secure the best outcomes
- building on the best of what is currently provided.

In 1998 Russell Viner and Mark Keane completed a piece of work on behalf of the children's charity Action for Sick Children, also entitled *Youth Matters: Evidence-based best practice for the care of young people in hospital*. This policy document specifically concentrated on the care young people should receive in hospital environments. They showed that there were and still are a range of problems facing young people in healthcare settings:

- The commissioning and provision of care to adolescents in hospital is poor.
- Only 10 per cent of health authorities in the United Kingdom have specifications for adolescent physical health.
- Only 40 per cent have specifications for adolescent mental health.
- The dispersal of adolescents throughout different speciality wards caters for the convenience of medical staff, not the needs of patients.
- The colocation of all adolescents within a dedicated adolescent unit within a hospital is best practice.
- Adolescent in-patient units should be established in most district general hospitals in the United Kingdom.
- 15 adolescent beds are needed for each 250,000 population.
- Only 8 per cent of health authorities contain adolescent provider units in their hospitals.
- Adolescent units are cost-effective and provide the best-quality care for adolescent patients.
- The psychosocial and developmental needs of young people are very different from those of children and adults.
- The common needs of adolescence unite sick young people more than the particular needs of their disease separate them.
- Adolescent units will free up adult beds in areas of need.

- Young people aged from 12 to 19 should be cared for in dedicated adolescent in-patient units.
- Young people with major psychiatric diagnoses such as psychoses or anorexia nervosa should be managed in specialised adolescent mental health units.
- Obstetric cases are best managed in obstetric units.
- Adolescent-friendly hospitals should provide:
  - overall care
  - psychosocial aspects of care
  - education and vocational training
  - transition to adult care
  - health education and promotion.
- There should be hospital-wide policies in adolescent units and other departments such as emergency departments and other ambulatory care facilities.
- Planning of units must include representatives of young people.
- There should be clear operational policies and flexible admission age groups.
- Adolescent units must have 'house rules' for the conduct of young people.
- There must be flexible visiting.
- There must be patient involvement in decision making.
- Self-care should be a priority.
- In staffing an adolescent unit there should be:
  - a designated consultant
  - specially educated staff (the skill-mix will include social workers, psychologists, child psychiatry, physiotherapists (PTs), occupational therapists (OTs), dieticians, recreation workers, teachers and nurses with a mix of qualifications)
  - an appropriate ratio of male and female staff.
- The education of young people in hospital is critical to their future. This must include information technology (IT) with wireless access to allow young people ready access to the internet and, importantly, email.
- There should be transition policies.

Since the publication of Viner and Keane's work, the Royal College of Paediatrics and Child Health (RCPCH) has published a subsequent policy, *Bridging the Gaps: Healthcare for adolescents* (2003) in which it indicated that adolescents between the ages of 10 and 20 make up 13–15 per cent of the total population of the United Kingdom, and among minority ethnic communities the proportion is considerably higher.

Adolescence is considered a time when patterns of health behaviour and the use of services are developed, and these tend to be continued during adult life. Importantly the Royal College report highlights that in contrast to all other age groups, mortality among young people has not fallen significantly over the last 50 and more years. This is because the main causes of mortality among young people are accidents and self-harm, with a worrying recent rise in suicide among young men.

Morbidity among the young mainly arises from chronic illnesses and mental health problems, with the likelihood of long-term adverse consequences if they are not handled well. Additionally there is a crucial relationship between physical, mental and social health. The Royal College report shows that:

- Young people have specific health needs, many of which remain unmet.
- For most adolescents their parents remain key providers of healthcare and they require support in this task.
- Young people say that there are barriers to their effective use of both primary and secondary healthcare services, including lack of information and difficulties in achieving low-visibility access for confidential issues. Furthermore services are not seen as youth friendly because of:

Part

III

- concerns about confidentiality for those under 16
- lack of expertise and continuity of care by professionals
- failure to respect the validity of young people's views
- young people in hospital having to be accommodated either in a children's ward or with a population they regard as elderly.

The Royal College believes that health services must pay greater attention to the special needs of young people if they wish to improve the emotional, psychological and physical health of the population. They consider that the views and needs of young people should be taken into account at all stages of planning and delivery of health services for adolescents, and that health strategies must address the particular needs of adolescents, particularly in relation to sexual health, substance abuse, mental health and accident prevention.

Chrysalis into butterfly: The physical stages of adolescent development

The emergence of the young adult or adolescent from the body of the child they once were is a period of the lifecycle in which there is a complex landscape of biological, psychological and social factors. Combined, these cause significant transformations in the individual's personal development (Hauser, Powers and Noam, 1991). As with the butterfly as it emerges from the chrysalis, the changes are profound. Not since the first year of life will the human being have undergone such rapid growth in their physical, psychological, emotional, social and moral development.

The term 'puberty' signifies the period of rapid physical growth and sexual maturation that indicates the start of adolescence. Puberty is triggered by a chain of hormonal effects which cause a number of physical changes. In females:

- Breasts develop (the average age for appearance of breast buds is 10–11 years, with a range between 9 and 11½ years).
- The hips become more rounded.
- The menarche (the first menstrual period). Menarche usually occurs two years after the appearance of breast buds, with a critical weight of 45 kg or 17 per cent body fat required before menarche begins. This is an important point to remember in girls with eating disorders.
- The appearance of pubic hair usually follows about two to six months after breast development. However, in about one-third of girls the initial appearance of pubic hair is first.
- Pubic hair develops from none to sparse and downy, more coarse and curly, denser, curled and finally adult in quality, with spread of hair to the thighs.
- There is often an increase in normal vaginal discharge associated with uterine development.
- Since the middle of the nineteenth century, the age at which menarche occurs has been declining in western countries. This is probably attributed to the results of better nutrition, the decline in infectious diseases and better healthcare generally (Kelsey and McEwing, 2006).

In males:

- Enlargement of penis and testes occurs at about 12 years of age, with slow growth of pubic hair at about the same time, and approximately one year later, accelerated growth of the penis.
- Spermarche (first ejaculation of live sperm). Ejaculation occurs about 1½ years after the accelerated growth of the penis begins.
- Nocturnal emissions.
- Body and facial hair usually appear about two years after the beginning of pubic hair growth.

- The lowering of the voice occurs quite late in puberty.
- Some changes also occur to the male breasts. This includes an enlargement of the areola. There may also be some general enlargement but this usually disappears within a year or so. Gynaecomastia, or enlargement of the male breast during puberty, can be acutely embarrassing for boys who suffer this.

Other physical changes that occur during puberty in both males and females include:

- Growth of the internal organs, including the lungs and heart. This increases physical endurance. Boys are able to take in more air in one breath due to their increased shoulder and chest size. The systolic blood pressure (BP) rises at an accelerated rate during puberty, and the pulse rate decreases.
- The lymphoid system including the tonsils and adenoids decreases in size, improving asthma, in some young people.
- The growth of the skeletal system is reflected in limb growth. Boys' longer growth period is reflected in their greater height and longer arms and legs, although they can be significantly smaller than their female peers, as girls enter puberty first while boys typically do not do so for a further two years.
- The extremities grow first, followed by neck, hip, chest, shoulder, trunk and depth of chest. This gives rise to the comic-book caricature of the long-legged gangly appearance of teenage boys, with trousers and sweaters that never fit the limbs as well as the body properly.
- Muscle mass increases in boys and girls. For girls this peaks at menarche then slows. However for boys it continues, resulting in a higher lean body mass in boys.
- Adolescence is a time of continued brain growth. There is no actual increase in number of neurons but growth of the myelin sheath continues until at least puberty, enabling faster neural processing which corresponds with the development of cognitive abilities.
- During the pubertal growth spurt the rate of growth can double. The final 20–25 per cent of linear growth is achieved. This can be as much as 12.5 cm in a peak year. Girls gain an average of 5–20 cm in height and 7–25 kg in weight. Boys gain 10–30 cm in height and 7–30 kg in weight.

> **(a) Learning activity**
>
> Read the Royal College of Psychiatrists (2004) booklet on *Surviving Adolescence*.

Part III

> **(e) Evidence-based practice**
>
> Clift, Dampier and Timmons (2007) report a study on young people's experiences of being admitted as an emergency to children's wards. Despite the often-cited negative aspects of care delivery, the young people in this sample (six of them) were quite positive about their admission. However the areas considered by the young people to be in need of improvement included ward facilities, strategies employed by healthcare professionals to help young people achieve sufficient sleep and rest, and importantly peer support while in hospital.

Overview of adolescent psychological development

> **(a) Learning activity**
>
> Before reading on it might be helpful for you to jot down your current understanding of anorexia nervosa.

Among the dominant ideas about adolescence is that as well as being a period in human development linked to biological markers, it involves transitions which can be seen as stages, in which the central task is establishing identity. Erikson (1965) describes the adolescent task, or crisis, as identity versus confusion. There is a search for identity, that is, as a separate self, but always in relation to others.

A simple definition for adolescence that acknowledges the developmental stages is:

> The period of transition from childhood to adulthood that can be divided into early (11–14 years), mid (15–17 years) and late (18–21 years).
>
> (RNAO, 2002)

Clearly individuals negotiate these stages in their own time and in their own way, but it is still helpful to work with conceptual models of the process. Many such models take a staged approach, starting with the pre-adolescent and continuing the process of change through to postadolescence (La Voie, 1994).

Jacobs (1998) looks at adolescence in three stages, which we can adapt for our purposes as:
- early adolescence and sexuality (relates to intimacy)
- middle adolescence: authority and independence (relates to individuation)
- later adolescence: faith and responsibility (relates to moral development and life values).

The first stage outlined by Jacobs could be linked to changing patterns of intimacy and attachment. The second stage outlined relates to individuation, the process of becoming who we are. This involves renegotiating a self-concept less dependent on our parents' construction of who we are and more reliant on peers and role icons. The final stage relates to developing beliefs and moral values. This is often a time of intense interest in what is right and wrong, fair and unfair, true and not true.

There is however a view that suggests that the dilemma of adolescence has been overplayed, and that we are perhaps looking for unnecessary trouble by defining it as a life stage that by its very nature involves serious conflict and upheaval. More recent thinking suggests there is much less necessary difficulty and much more continuity from the child that was, through adolescence to the adult that will be. It is considered that most adolescents negotiate this period of life transition with relatively little major disruption or sustained high-risk behaviour (Offer, 1987, cited in Burt, 2002).

Although for most the period of adolescence might be relatively uneventful, healthcare settings are likely to see more of young people involved in high-risk behaviours. These high-risk behaviours are linked to mental health problems, low self-esteem and dysfunctional families (BMA, 2003).

From a professional point of view, we should take as much account of the adolescent's developmental stage as we would of the developmental stage of a younger child. If we want to be helpful and respectful we need to go to where they are. This is the starting point of any helping relationship.

Learning activity

Reflect on illness and its relationship to your own journey through adolescence. This could be an illness you suffered from, or one that affected a friend or relative. How did it influence you and your peers?

Young people in transition

Recent policies from the Department of Health (DH, 2006b) and the Royal College of Nursing (RCN, 2007) suggest that a named person or coordinator works with young people with ongoing health needs, their families and all agencies, to plan for transition to adult services. Furthermore transition clinics should operate in both paediatric and adult services to ensure the seamlessness of the process. Young people in healthcare transition to adult services are the concern of all health service professionals, and yet it is this arena of clinical care, which is at the juxtaposition of child, adult, mental health and learning disabilities practice, which is proving to be contentious.

The transition of young people from children's to adult health services is now an important issue in contemporary healthcare in the United Kingdom. This is because children who would have died in early childhood from a range of life-limiting diseases such as cystic fibrosis are now with modern medical care surviving into adult life. Despite this Fiorentino and colleagues

(1998) have shown that young disabled people experience a poor handover to adult services. Child healthcare in children's units generally ceases at 18 and sometimes 16 years of age, and the impetus to improve this element of policy noncompliance is primarily to provide safe and effective transition to adult services.

Transition planning in the health service for young people with medical conditions must secure optimal health for the young person. Failure to achieve this can have severe consequences on the educational, social and psychological development of the young person. Additionally the financial implications of not doing this can only impact negatively on the Exchequer and the taxpayer. Therefore young people should be supported to make the transition to adulthood healthcare in terms of their education, health, development and well-being. To do this young people must be enabled to take responsibility and be able to make informed choices.

It is important to remember that the highs and lows of being an adolescent are exacerbated for young people with chronic health problems. All healthcare professionals should appreciate the reality that a poor transition to adult health services increases the risk of noncompliance to treatment regimes, and for the young person this can be manifest in morbidity, mortality, and adverse social and educational outcomes. The healthcare policies discussed earlier illuminate the evidence based on best practices which show that well-planned and implemented transition from child to adult services improves all these outcomes, but crucially this success depends on close collaboration between the two services. Both these arms of the health service need to recognise that transition is a process and not a single healthcare event. The paediatrician, nurse, dietician and other healthcare professionals who have looked after a child and family with a chronic health problem cannot simply say, 'Farewell, have a good life' when the child reaches 18, and hand over care to an adult team. Hospitals should be places to foster good transition, and where the relationship between child and adult services are seamless.

Benchmarked good practice suggests that staff in both child and adult settings should develop robust care policies or procedures for young people about to experience transition. Families should be given transition packs and thus empowered to navigate their way through the differing world of adult services. Importantly a named transition coordinator should be appointed to monitor how the young person and family develop the skills to function independently in this different world of adult healthcare. When young people and their families are being prepared for this journey of transfer to adult medial teams, it should be stressed that they are at an age where noncompliance may be an issue. It should therefore be mandatory for NHS trusts to conduct regular audits of the transition process, and importantly monitor nonattendance at outpatient clinics by young people to prevent their being lost in the transition process.

Part
III

(a) Learning activity

In your interprofessional learning group, conduct an informal audit of how well your hospital arranges transition for young people using the audit tool in Table 22.1. Use the five-point scale to award an overall score for your hospital.

Table 22.1 **Policy audit for specific transitional care**

There is no plan for transition of young people to adult services.	There is a plan for transition of young people to adult services without the resources to implement the plan.	There is a plan for transition of young people to adult services with resources within the paediatric service to implement the plan but difficulty identifying appropriate adult services to transfer to.	There is a plan for transition with resources allocated in the paediatric and adult area and transition clinics running in both settings but without a named person/coordinator.	A named person/coordinator works with young people with ongoing health needs, their families and all agencies, to plan for transition to adult services. Transition clinics operate in both the paediatric and adult services.
1	2	3	4	5

In your groups consider the evidence (please discuss the presence or lack of evidence). Specifically consider the following. When you have been in clinical placement in a hospital or elsewhere:

- Do staff refer to *Transition: Getting it right* (DH, 2006b) and the RCN *Lost in Transition* policies (RCN, 2007), and are copies of these policies available in clinical areas?
- Have you seen a transitional care policy or procedure, or transition packs for families?
- Is the policy updated?
- Is there a named transition coordinator?
- Do young people and their families know the name of transition coordinator?
- Do young people and their families know the date when the move to adult services will occur?
- Have the young people developed the necessary skill set to function independently in an adult clinic?

- Have the adult services to which young people are to be transferred been identified?
- Is there a pre-transition meeting between the family and the child and adult team?
- Is there an ongoing audit of transition process in place?
- Is there an audit of nonattendance or poor compliance?
- Look for areas of good practice such as:
- Are all 12+ year-olds offered 'air-time' with doctors, nurses or other healthcare professionals on their own when they attend outpatients?
- Are all competent 14+ year olds offered copies of letters written about them?
- Are adolescent unit facilities are available in the healthcare setting?

The serious lack of inpatient adolescent facilities in many NHS trusts belies the reality that the common shared needs of young people unite them more than their medical diagnosis separates them. It is perhaps because of this poor understanding of the needs of young people with chronic health ailments that a good working knowledge of transition should be part of the healthcare student curriculum for all fields of practice. It is only through the students of today, who will be the registered nurses of tomorrow, that we can begin to more fully champion the rights of young people as they endure the right of passage that is healthcare transition.

Involving young people in healthcare

The Commission for Patient and Public Involvement in Health (CPPIH) which was established in January 2003 to solicit the views of healthcare consumers was abolished on 31 March 2008 and replaced by local involvement networks (LINks). These networks purport to give all citizens a bigger voice in shaping their local health and social services. The demise of CPPIH and the introduction of LINks was designed to give more power to local communities to help them have a greater say in the design of service configurations.

a) Learning activity

In your learning group consider how successful the whole initiative of patient and public involvement has been in reflecting the views of young users of health services.

Wicke and colleagues (2007) point out that children and young people are still not as fully involved in decisions about their healthcare as is mandated in a range of government healthcare policies. For example standard 7 of the *National Service Framework for Children, Young People and Maternity Services* (DH, 2003) and *Standards for Better Health* (DH, 2006a) are quite explicit in emphasising the need for NHS trusts to engage with patients and members of the public in developing services. Despite this Coles and colleagues (2007), in an audit of compliance with this standard, found that involvement of children and their families in service planning was at a low level of development. Hill and colleagues (2004) point out the reality that children and young people are some of the highest users of state services and yet their voice is rarely sought and many initiatives are designed, delivered and evaluated by adults. Additionally Doran, Drever and Whitehead (2003), in analysing the data from the 2003 census, confirmed that the previous estimates of between 10,000 and 50,000 young carers had been taken too lightly, and that the real figure was closer to 114,000, with recent press reports putting it as high as 175,000 or more. Clearly young people are both in receipt of care and major deliverers of care to others. It is therefore crucial that healthcare professionals such as nurses begin to take a more proactive stance in seeking this group's view in determining not only what a really good hospital for children and young people should be like, but also what services they need to function effectively. You might want to refer back to Chapter 8 on Healthcare Governance for more on this.

First-hand information from young people can be invaluable in helping NHS institutions respond to consumer views. Although there are some important areas of existing consultation with children and young people, LINks have been introduced to help strengthen the system that enables sections of the community such as the 11 million children who live in England to influence the care they receive. The function of LINks is to enhance the small voice that children and young people have had thus far in the health service in determining the shape of their future health services.

The rising tide of alcohol abuse among young people

W

The Alcohol Health Alliance was officially announced on 13 November 2007 under the auspices of the Royal College of Physicians (www.rcplondon.ac.uk/alcoholalliance/). It consists of 21 relevant bodies including the RCN, all of which are concerned at the rising medical toll of alcohol misuse among children and young people.

This is particularly important for healthcare professionals who work with young people because alcohol use among children is increasing year on year. The alliance is attempting to reduce the damage to health caused by abuse of this drug through health promotion. It is also calling for better regulation of the drinks industry. Although there is no doubt that were alcohol to be invented tomorrow it would be a prescription-only drug, society has to accept that its very existence in some parts of the world is an indication of man's quest for a mood-enhancing substance which dates back a very long time. However, historically the consumption of alcohol was not an everyday occurrence for most human beings, but was reserved for feast days and holidays. In some modern cultures alcohol consumption has become part of everyday life.

W

Against this backdrop of rising alcohol consumption it is not hard to see why children become aware of alcohol at an early stage of their development. The Information Centre is an NHS special health authority (www.ic.nhs.uk) which provide provides among other things national statistical knowledge to underpin health and social care. It has been estimated that the average 12-year-old's weekly pocket money entitlement will buy up to 17 units of alcohol, and the Information Centre's research suggests that consumption of alcohol among boys who had drunk some during the previous week rose from eight units in 2000 to 12 units in 2006. In girls the figure rose from five units to eight over the same period. The Alcohol Alliance believes that not enough is being done to protect children's health from the harmful effects of alcohol: it claims that 13 children a day are hospitalised by the effects of alcohol misuse.

Robson (2001), in a review of alcohol misuse among children, has discussed the pivotal position that parents have as role models for children. He suggests that sensible drinking by parents in the home and elsewhere might be an important criterion in protecting children against alcohol misuse Worryingly this paper also confirms that much alcohol is consumed by children in their own homes. An investigation by the *Independent on Sunday* (Owen, 2007) revealed that children as young as 10 are spending significant periods receiving healthcare interventions ranging from residential rehabilitation to specialist counselling as a result of their drinking. The number of children hospitalised because of alcohol rose by a third between 1995/6 and 2005/06, from 3,870 to 5,281 (Owen, 2007). Worryingly there has been a 62 per cent increase in 12–14-year-olds needing alcohol treatment (Alcohol Health Alliance, 2007). These statistics do not reflect those children admitted to emergency departments for alcohol-related injuries: Robson (2001) cites a tenfold increase from 20 to 200 children admitted to the Alder Hey Children's Hospital in Liverpool between 1985 and 1996.

All healthcare professionals should be concerned about the rising numbers of young people who are consuming large quantities of alcoholic beverages, causing them to need treatment in hospital. Owen (2007) has suggested that girls make up nearly 60 per cent of all hospital admissions for alcohol misuse. This is perhaps not surprising given that young girls' celebrity role models are frequently and prominently featured in the media suffering from the ill-effects of alcohol consumption.

So what can healthcare professionals do to help tackle the rising tide of morbidity caused by alcohol abuse?

You need to be conscious of the role of parents, and how they can positively influence their children's development as they progress through the stages of childhood, culminating in that final transition between childhood and adulthood. If young people are particularly vulnerable to the pernicious influence of alcohol it is important that parental roles are not underestimated. Only in working with parents and their young children can the embers of later alcohol abuse be extinguished, allowing young people to make responsible decisions about alcohol in the future. The statistics quoted above are a damning indictment of how society has neglected the toll of alcohol on children's and young people's health.

a Learning activity

Consider in your interprofessional learning group: in your working lifetime, do you think it will become common to see young people developing critical end-stage liver disease warranting transplantation (similar perhaps to the effects of type 2 diabetes in children who are obese)?

Adolescent mental health: the context of care

Working with adolescents is considered challenging, as they have needs that differ from both children and adults, yet they often receive their healthcare in environments with either children or adults. If we add to this issues of emotional distress or mental health, things seem to move beyond many children's nurses' perceived areas of expertise or competence. Interpreting the government-led policy and legislative aspirations in terms of prevention, health promotion, rights and the child within the context of the family presents particular challenges when nursing a young person with an eating disorder.

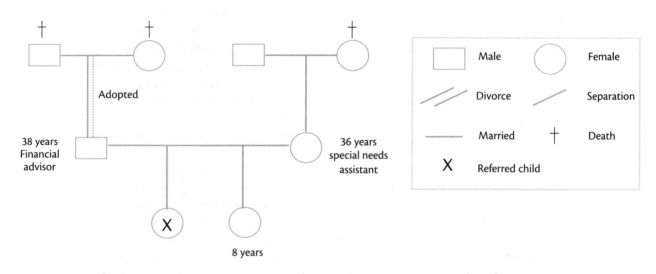

Figure 22.1 A family genogram

Genograms and family trees

The challenge of organising information about family members has led to the development of family trees (or genograms), as a way to record significant information in formats that are accessible and usable for clients and therapists alike.

Family trees are maps providing a picture of family structure over several generations, with schematic representation of the main stages of the family lifecycle. They are a useful adjunct in both assessment and treatment. They give a concise, graphic summary of the family's current composition, and can be extended to include dates, marriages, separations, health, occupations, relationships and important points from individuals' past histories.

> **(a) Learning activity**
>
> In your learning group take time to explore what other assessments and assessment tools may be used when working with young clients and their families.

Eating disorders

> **[S] Scenario: introducing Anna**
>
> Anna, who is 12 years old, lives with her parents, younger sister and elder brother, in a detached family house which they own. Anna's father James (38) has recently changed his job from postman to financial adviser, allowing him to spend more time at home with the family. Her mother
>
> Jenny (36) is a part-time special needs assistant. Anna is reported by her parents to have a difficult relationship with her 8-year-old sister Elle. Her maternal grandfather lives close by and visits frequently.

Depending on the diagnostic criteria, eating disorders other than anorexia are considered as subdiagnostic categories of anorexia. Anorexia, or anorexia nervosa (both are names for the same condition) is a complex condition with controversial theories of causation. It is characterised by serious loss of weight, which is self-induced by food avoidance, exercise and purging. It is best known as a disorder of adolescent girls and young women, but also occurs in boys and men.

Eating disorders take on a special significance before puberty and in adolescence. In adolescence there is a critical growth period during which the young person physically develops, and if this is missed, the young person is unable to catch up with growth development at a later stage. (See Chapter 11 on hydration in relation to 'catch up'.) Therefore, when anorexia nervosa occurs during these critical periods, there is a certain urgency for professionals to treat it promptly. One of the primary aims of such interventions is to help the young person to reach a healthy weight and thereby not miss their critical growth period.

The term 'eating disorder' covers a wide spectrum of conditions characterised by psychological and behavioural disturbances associated with weight, food and eating. In her review of recent developments in anorexia Rachel Bryant-Waugh (2006) explores the problems of diagnosis. The diagnostic criteria for anorexia continue to be a matter for debate, and they remain difficult to apply to younger individuals (Nicholls, Chater and Lask, 2000). 'Eating disorders' has often been used to refer to two specific conditions, anorexia nervosa and bulimia nervosa, and they remain significant health problems in childhood and adolescence. However there has been dissatisfaction with this definition, and there is good evidence that a large number of patients of all ages fall into a 'not otherwise specified' category of eating disorder. There is also debate about the scope for improvement in the patient's condition. It is important to be mindful of these issues when exploring the diagnostic criteria.

Eating disorders can be viewed as psychological illnesses in which distress is somatised, or expressed in disordered eating behaviours. Palmer (2006) reviewing anorexia nervosa, suggested that although it is about 130 years since anorexia was first clearly described, its management and treatment remain unsatisfactory. Anorexia nervosa has the highest mortality rate of any psychiatric disorder, and yet this most lethal of psychiatric disorders is considered the Cinderella of research (Morris and Twaddle, 2007).

Eating disorders and males

Eating-related problems are common in adolescence. In the United States Croll and colleagues (2002) suggest that every second girl and every third boy has a transient eating problem, of which 10 per cent continue into adulthood. Eating disorders are generally seen as a women's issue, and this has led to men being under-represented in empirical studies, although of every ten individuals clinically diagnosed with an eating disorder, one is male (Ousley, Cordero and White, 2008). The course and outcome of eating disorders are remarkably similar in both boys and girls (Eliot and Bake, 2001).

Although both males and females are sensitive to body image and to sociocultural issues, some researchers suggest that males are can be more sensitive to these issues (DeBate et al, 2008; Hatmaker, 2005). There are also indications of increased vulnerability around issues of sexual identity in males, with gay males seen to be twice as at risk as the general population (Hatmaker, 2005). It is therefore important to be mindful of young men in relation to eating disorders, as the incidence is increasing. Anorexia is not the only eating disorder males suffer from: issues of body image can be expressed in a desire for extreme muscularity of physique.

Other types of eating disorders occurring in this age range may be related to:
- food avoidance emotional disorder (FAED)
- selective eating
- restrictive eating
- food refusal
- dysfunctional dysphagia
- appetite loss secondary to depression.

The prevalence of anorexia nervosa is thought to vary from 0.5 per cent to 1 per cent among the adolescent population.

Diagnosis of anorexia nervosa

Increasingly, there is an international consensus on the criteria for diagnosing mental and behavioural disorders. There are two major classification systems:
- the International Classification of Diseases (ICD-10) (WHO, 1994)
- the Diagnostic and Statistical Manual of Mental Disorders (DSM-IV-TR) (APA, 1994).

DSM-IV and ICD-10 have many similarities in their definitions of anorexia nervosa. Although they both use the criteria of weight loss, body image distortion, amenorrhoea and so-called weight phobia, there are differences in the way they define these. Both define weight loss as a weight 15 per cent below that expected for age and height, but ICD-10 refers to Quatlets Body Mass Index as one way of defining that expectation. Both systems consider the special situation of pre-pubertal patients who fail to meet expected growth targets. ICD-10 has further advantages in that it covers 'self-induced loss of weight', and links body image distortion to the main theme of psychopathology: the fear of becoming obese.

Both the syndrome and the spectrum character of eating disorders make it clear that there are atypical cases of anorexia nervosa that do not fulfil the complete sets of criteria listed in the two major systems of classification.

Using the ICD-10 system the following eating disorder diagnoses are possible:
- anorexia nervosa (F50.0)
- atypical anorexia nervosa (F50.1)
- bulimia nervosa (F50.2)
- atypical bulimia nervosa (F50.3)
- overeating, with other psychological disturbances (F50.4)
- vomiting, with other psychological disturbances (F50.5)
- other eating disorders (F50.8)

- eating disorder, unspecified (F50.9).

Using the DSM-IV system, there are other possibilities:
- anorexia nervosa (307.1): restricting type
- anorexia nervosa (307.1): binge eating/purging type
- bulimia nervosa (307.51): purging type
- bulimia nervosa (307.51): non-purging type
- eating disorder not otherwise specified (EDNOS) (307.50).

Numerous research studies have focused on the issue of those who tend to develop eating disorders. They are more common in women than men, but in children, boys appear to be over-represented compared with the proportion of males seen in adults. It has been suggested that eating disorders are more common in social classes 1 and 2, and a number of high-risk groups have been identified including dancers and fashion models. There is increasing evidence that eating disorders are less restricted than previously thought in their occurrence across different cultural and ethnic groups.

> **a Learning activity**
>
> In your learning group consider what factors might contribute to the development of an eating disorder.

The precise aetiology of eating disorders remains obscure, but is probably multifactorial. Lask and Bryant-Waugh (2000) suggest that an eating disorder does not occur at a particular moment. Rather it develops over time, with some causative factors being in place since birth, others emerging in early life, and yet others much later.

We can consider the aetiology of eating disorders under the following headings:
- biological factors: genetic, endocrine, temperament, personality traits
- sociocultural factors: thinness, media, gender, prejudice against obesity
- familial factors: dysfunctional interaction and communication, abnormal eating, attitudes and behaviour
- psychological factors: stress, adaptation to life events, self-image.

It seems that a genetic disposition is necessary, but not enough in itself for the development of the disorder, and that anorexia is found in families with perfectionist and competitive traits, and possibly autistic spectrum traits. The disorder is usually precipitated as a coping mechanism against developmental challenges, transitions, family conflicts and academic pressures, for example, although it can be found without apparent precipitants in families that appear to be functioning well (Morris and Twaddle, 2007).

Findings suggest that the course of anorexia nervosa is characterised by high rates of partial recovery and low rates of full recovery, while the course of bulimia nervosa is characterised by higher rates of both partial and full recovery (Herzog, Sacks and Keller, 1993).

Eating disorders and the nursing role: the nurse's beliefs

> **a Learning activity**
>
> What do you believe about people with anorexia? How might what you believe right now influence the care you give?

Nursing young people with an eating disorder creates particular challenges in the delivery of care. It is vital that nurses understand the psychological profile of anorexic patients, and know how to overcome the difficulties this can create in forming a therapeutic relationship, otherwise anorexic patients may well continue to be seen as 'difficult' patients with a self-induced illness, which will prevent therapeutic care (George 1997: 902). It has been suggested that some of the difficulties experienced in nursing anorexic young people are related to the nurse's belief system.

Part III

How a nurse delivers care, their attitudes and behaviours constitutes their *therapeutic style* (Cooper, 2005). The key elements of an effective therapeutic style have been identified (Ramjan, 2004) as:

- trust and commitment
- accurate empathy, unconditional positive regard and genuineness
- honesty and support
- confidentiality.

Since the seminal work *The Unpopular Patient* (Stockwell, 1972), it has been acknowledged that a nurse's beliefs profoundly influence the care they give. The importance of the professional's belief system in the delivery of care is central to the quality of the care given. With relation to nurses, Cooper and Glasper (2001) also emphasise the importance of the nurse's belief system in influencing their therapeutic style. They suggest that the nurse's beliefs are affected by commonly accepted 'tribal stories'. That a patient is unpopular as identified by Stockwell (1972) is an example of a tribal story. Such collective beliefs, they suggest, remain unchallenged by the reflective process. Each professional group might have shared tribal stories or unique stories within their 'tribe' or professional group. Here is an example:

> Sometimes when I am working with an anorexic person I feel it is all a waste of time. My skills could be better used looking after somebody who has a real illness. We are very busy here. There is not the time to give these people what they need. Anyway, they should be looked after somewhere else. This is not the place for them. They are always manipulative, and they tell lies. I came into professional practice to look after children with real illnesses, not these people. Anyway, even if I had time, I would not know what to say. Even if you do speak to her, she won't answer.

Learning activity

Think about the possible consequences of a belief system for the way a professional worker delivers care and a young person responds. What could help professionals change the way they think?

Bodycombe-James (2000) identified a number of research studies over the years after Stockwell's original work, suggesting a definite pattern in the types of patient who are considered unpopular, and supporting Stockwell's general findings. Her own small study of nurses' attitudes showed that children were described in negative terms if they were uncooperative. Deviant behaviour was also viewed very negatively, and made the child unpopular. Her conclusions also suggested that toddlers were generally more popular than adolescents.

If the views of the nurses Bodycombe-James spoke to were representative of the wider group, then young adolescents with eating disorders are likely to be viewed negatively. Further support for this comes from the work of King and Turner (2000). They identify core values as one of the themes emerging from the study of nurses working with adolescent females with anorexia. These young people challenge nursing core beliefs, leading to emotional turmoil and frustration in the nurse. Resolution occurs through a process of repositioning the young person's situation in relation to core beliefs. These beliefs may have to be expanded or changed to meet the new situation. The change of perspective, in order to promote quality care, can be seen as an element of the therapeutic encounter. Wright (2001) suggested that nurses who believe that the patient with an eating disorder is not responsible for the development of the disorder are more effective in giving care. Another important belief identified was that the carer has to believe their intervention can help the patients achieve a positive outcome. Many nurses can find it hard to do so.

(e) Evidence-based practice

It has already been established that there is a paucity of research to guide the treatment of anorexia nervosa (Palmer, 2006; Morris and Twaddle, 2007). However, there is high-quality research on the effects of starvation to guide the management of care (Morris and Twaddle 2007).

The National Institute for Clinical Evidence (NICE) website offers guidelines based on category three evidence, which is perhaps the best evidence base offered at present. Those aspects of the guidelines that focus on children and adolescents make a number of suggestions, the most important of which are:

- Treatment, dietary education and meal planning should normally involve family members, and patients should be offered family interventions that directly address the eating disorder. Patients should be offered individual appointments separate from those with their family members or carers.

- The need for inpatient treatment and urgent weight restoration should be balanced against educational and social needs. Inpatient treatment should be within a reasonable distance from home to allow contacts to be maintained and be age appropriate.
- Feeding against the will of the patient should only be done in the context of the Mental Health Act 1983 or the Children Act 1989.

(a) Learning activity

Work out Anna's body mass index (BMI) before reading on. For a reminder refer to Chapter 10 on Nutrition (Table 10.1).

[S] Scenario continued

The doctor who interviews Anna on admission makes these notes on her history and presenting complaints:

Anna's BMI is now 11.8. Risk assessment: A BMI < 12.0 carries a very high risk independently of other variables.

It is also well reported that the rapidity of weight loss as well as other features such as the inability to rise unaided from squatting, abnormal blood test results, circulatory failure and low core body temperature should all form part of a physical risk assessment risk assessment (NICE, 2004).

Anna has always been 'faddy' about food. At the age of 5 she complained about the amount of butter on her toast. Over the last year she has progressively cut out foods, including chocolate, meats, fats and dairy products. Daily, she only eats dry toast, one jacket potato without the skin, and tuna. She took over cooking six months ago when her mother injured her hand. As her mother's hand improved, food avoidance became more obvious.

Exercise: up until admission to hospital, she attended ten dancing classes per week, participating in six different dancing styles, plus practice and exercise. She admits to a constant, overriding urge to dance or exercise, and difficulty in keeping still. Prior to admission, she was doing 100 sit-ups before breakfast.

Mood low and she has diminished concentration. The only time she smiles is when she is dancing.

Apathy and fatigue – has stopped socialising outside school. She spends her spare time alone in her bedroom, possibly exercising.

Abdominal pain, constipation and headaches. Complains that when she eats, she feels bloated and feels 'like her ribs are going to burst open'.

She is not happy with what she sees when she looks in the mirror. She has a distorted body image and denies knowing her weight. Feels that her tummy and thighs are too fat.

She hates drawing attention to herself. Anna is unhappy with her appearance and her perceived lack of ability. She has difficulty in standing up for herself. She has been exploited by her classmates, and been forced to do their homework for them.

She verbalises how 'horrible' she is.

Difficulty in dropping off to sleep, and wakes early.

Puberty – had been developing breasts, but this has slowed recently. She has not yet reached menarche.

Part

III

a Learning activity

In your learning group discuss your understanding of menarche and what influences it.

S Scenario continued

The doctor's further notes comment:

Personality traits
- Always slightly obsessional, and a perfectionist.
- Quiet, unassertive demeanour.
- Spends twice the recommended time on homework, and is still unhappy with her results.
- Has very few close friends, particularly dislikes boys. She chose a secondary school out of her catchment area to avoid contact with boys.
- Is one of the brightest pupils in the school, highest achiever in her year.
- Acknowledges she eats to please others, not herself.

a Learning activity

In your learning group consider how Anna's personality traits compare with those most commonly associated with the anorexic position.

S Scenario continued

The doctor's further notes comment:
Family history

Father: Disrupted attachments. His biological father was killed when he was aged 2 years. His mother was unable to care for him owing to a severe depression. He was subsequently accommodated in a children's home until he was 10 years old. He had no further contact with his mother. He was then fostered until aged 18 years, when his foster parents divorced. There has been no further contact. He has a foster sister but has no contact with her. No history of any illnesses.

Mother: Has two sisters and a brother. They live locally but have limited contact. Father is alive and well and visits every fortnight; not a close relationship, however. Her own mother died six years ago of lung cancer. Admits to having been very close, and still misses her. She frequently visits the grave. Anna's mother denies ever having an eating problem, but she says she watches what she eats. Her weight has never been above 51 kg. She has had a recent operation on her hand.

a Learning activity

Think about how the information on Anna in the scenario might have been collected. What particular skills would a healthcare professional need to develop to gain such personal and sometimes potentially painful admissions? (See Chapter 5 on communication.)

Attachment

Attachment behaviour is defined simply as any form of behaviour that results in a person attaining or retaining proximity to a preferred individual. Attachment is an overall term referring to the state and quality of an individual's attachment. Broadly, attachment can be divided into secure and insecure attachments. Attachment behaviour is triggered by separation or threatened separation from the attachment figure.

Attachment and attachment behaviour are based on an attachment behavioural system, a model of the world in which the self and significant others and their relationships are represented. The ability to form focused, permanent and emotionally meaningful relationships with specific others is one of the most important acquisitions of the infancy period.

The attachment an infant makes to its mother has a powerful influence over its subsequent development. Attachment describes the infant's predisposition to seek proximity to certain people and be more secure in their presence. Ideally, the infant will make a secure attachment, but patterns differ, and some infants' attachments are characterised by insecurity or ambivalence. The attachment patterns are already established at a year old, and remain constant throughout the lifecycle. These early patterns can repeat themselves in later relationships (Bowlby, 1969/1980). Disruptions in the first years of life because of inconsistent or inadequate care, or poor parenting skills, may lead to a failure to develop a secure attachment. There is a general assumption that the mother is likely to be the primary care giver in the first years of life, but changing patterns of family life mean this is not necessarily the case.

In adolescence a secure attachment shows itself in increasing autonomy and the capacity to evaluate life experiences in a helpful way. Insecure attachments will manifest in a dismissing approach to relationships. Other individuals with insecure attachments will be preoccupied, with relationships that are entangled and enmeshed, while yet others will be disorganised (Howe et al, 1999). Each of these relational styles will influence the relationship the nurse can make with the young person.

(a) Learning activity

- List the factors that might affect attachment.
- Take time to discover which authors and theories inform the concept of attachment.
- Consider how Anna and her family members might be described in terms of their attachment behaviours.
- Consider how, as a professional worker, working directly with the young person and their families, you can assist in promoting secure patterns of attachment between parents and their infants.

(S) Scenario continued

Here are more case notes on Anna and her family.

Family dynamics

There have been longstanding marital problems, recently felt to have been directed towards Anna by her father. Her mother has thought of divorce, but has been threatened that she will have no house or money. It is apparent that there is an alliance between the mother and Anna, and between her father and Anna's sister.

Her father is now 38 years old and is a financial advisor. He has recently changed his occupation from a postman, having studied at evening classes, and as a consequence is around more. He is described as being authoritative, unsympathetic, detached, and rarely giving praise. He tends to 'fly off the handle', and can go for many weeks without speaking to the family. Anna believes he prefers her younger sister and she is jealous

of their shared interests in football and television. He and Elle have similar personalities.

Anna also feels anorexia is 'her own fault'.

Her mother is 36 years old and works part-time as a special needs assistant. She is a youthful, petite woman, who has sometimes been mistaken for Anna's sister. There is a restrictive but affectionate style of parenting. Her mother finds remaining detached and tolerating her daughter's distress around eating and restricting exercise very difficult. She has an enmeshed relationship with her daughter, and she admits to being very close to her own mother who died six years ago. Both often talk about her and frequently visit her grave together.

Anna's sister is 8 years old and Anna describes her as a 'tomboy and messy'. She is outgoing, independent and makes friends easily. They often argue and fight, although previously they were close. They appear to have no positive feelings for one another.

Anna's developmental history

Uncomplicated pregnancy, birth weight 6 lb 10 oz.

Difficult delivery – face presentation with severe moulding.

Initially spent 24 hours in a special care baby unit (SCBU).

Her mother described her as a 'whinging baby' who never slept.

Little support from her husband.

Anna required constant attention so that her mother was constantly tired, and felt there was something wrong with the baby.

Anna did not sleep through the night until aged 4 years.

Breast-fed for six months, took to solids well.

She was always a 'faddy' eater and her mother was frequently concerned.

Grew below 50th percentile, but within normal limits.

Anna attended play school from the age of 3 years, with no separation difficulties.

She tended to be quiet with few friends, solitary play.

Infants' school: aged 5 years.

Quiet, hardworking, conscientious.

Few close friends, teased by boys, and found them 'disgusting'.

Measles aged 4 years. No other childhood illnesses or operations.

Coped well when her sister was born, with no sibling rivalry.

a Learning activity

- What was Anna's birth weight expressed in kilograms?
- Check out your understanding of percentiles. (Refer to Chapter 19, page 363.) An understanding of the developmental and family history might assist the current assessment.

- Before reading on, consider how the factors outlined in the scenario may have impinged on Anna. You may like to discuss this with a colleague to share your ideas. You might hold different views which would broaden your perspective.

The scenario information shows that there is a possibility that Anna was genetically predisposed to developing a psychiatric problem:

- Her father's disrupted attachments might have interfered with his parenting ability.
- Anna has always had a close relationship with her mother. This might have intensified at the time of her grandmother's death, perhaps coinciding with increasing marital disharmony, which has been noticeable since her father's change of occupation.
- The combination of tension at home, possible enmeshment with her mother, perceived criticism from her father, sibling rivalry, school pressure, poor peer relations and excessive exercise at the time of early puberty, might have contributed to the onset of an eating disorder now.

Enmeshment

The term 'enmeshment' comes from the family systems theory tradition (Von Bertalanffy, 1968). It refers to a condition where two or more people weave their lives and identities around one another so tightly that it is difficult for either one of them to function independently. The result is that the behaviour of one family member has an immediate and marked effect on those with whom that person is enmeshed. It is a state without adequate or healthy boundaries (for further descriptions of boundaries, see Minuchin, 1974).

The opposite, extreme way of relating, detachment or disengagement, is a condition where people are so independent in their functioning it is difficult to establish how they are related and function together. Healthy relationships are thought to occur in the space between enmeshment and detachment.

a Learning activity

Reflect on how your own family history might influence the assessment process if you were the professional doing the assessment.

Treatment for anorexia

Treatment for anorexia involves a multidisciplinary approach including medical supervision, nutritional counselling and mental health intervention.

> **a) Learning activity**
>
> How would you describe Anna's current weight? Refer to her BMI. What is your own BMI?

> **s Scenario continued**
>
> Anna's primary nurse, having read the doctor's notes and having made a nursing assessment, creates a care plan for her.

> **a) Learning activity**
>
> Before reading on think what you would include in Anna's care plan. Try to consider the rationale for every action, as if you were explaining it to a more junior colleague, or to Anna or her mother. You may like to use a tool such as the activities of daily living as a checklist (see page 521).

Anna's admission treatment plan

Problem	Action
Excessive activity	Strict bed rest, to remain in a cubicle Observe for exercising Gentle activities – e.g. puzzles Can make telephone calls

Treatment rationale

Excessive exercise can exacerbate physical complications and lead to injury; however, total restriction is unhealthy and unlikely to be successful (Lask and Bryant-Waugh, 2000: 290).

Problems encountered in practice

Anorexics feel compelled to exercise and will go to great lengths to increase activity, and also have a constant need to maintain movement. In a busy ward it is difficult to keep up the level of observation and supervision needed to restrict this. A further complication of bed rest is an increased risk of osteoporosis. Therefore strict bed rest should only be used in a limited way, when the advantages outweigh the disadvantages.

> **a) Learning activity**
>
> In your learning group, identify the challenges or possible risks in imposing a regime of bed rest. Consider physical as well as psychological functions.

> **c Professional conversation**
>
> Jo, a staff nurse on the unit where Anna is being treated, comments, 'As a staff nurse in this unit I feel it is important to develop an understanding of the strategies clients might use, and why. Initially, they may have started exercising in pursuit of fitness or for pleasure, but as the activity becomes increasingly compulsive and demanding, it becomes a danger to their health, and often leads to further social isolation. The additional gain that Anna receives from such excessive exercise may be a defence against having to think about worries and fears. Other strategies that I have observed include standing by an open window, and wearing minimal

clothing in order to induce shivering, thereby increasing energy output. Therefore it is important to establish a realistic regime and provide other diversionary activities as a defence against anxiety.'

Anna's treatment plan continued

Problem	Nursing action
Low body weight	Monitor by weighing twice weekly, pre-breakfast. Empty bladder prior to weighing. Weigh in bra and pants.

Treatment rationale

This serves two functions. The first is to reassure the patient that they will not be allowed to get fat (Akridge, 1989), and the second is to monitor the effectiveness of the treatment programme. The young person's need to control their weight must be relinquished (Lask and Bryant-Waugh, 2000: 274).

Weight gain can also significantly improve their mental state. An individual diet programme gives a common goal that assists consistency of care. Sometimes a target weight strategy is employed; however, Lask and Bryant-Waugh (2000: 274) suggest that a target weight might become an obsessive preoccupation with both the client and staff, increasing potential conflict. They do suggest that there should be a goal in mind.

Problems encountered in practice

This is often viewed as the most difficult area, as it confronts the patient's fears directly. The enforcement of a feeding regime, including nasogastric feeding if necessary, causes conflict amongst staff. The view might be taken that such enforcement is force-feeding and therefore an infringement of the patient's rights. Legal and ethical issues must be considered here. Issues around how and when to feed, and the patient's potential dependence on this passive feeding regime, have to be explored.

Discussion of possible solutions

The ethical issues should be discussed with the treatment team. An individual, graded re-feeding plan is negotiated with the dietician.

(a) Learning activity

Remember to jot down phrases that might need following up, for example 'individual, graded re-feeding plan'. What does this mean precisely and how is it 'negotiated with the dietician'? What skills does the dietician need in order to work therapeutically with Anna? It may be useful for you to try to spend some time with a dietician, although you should aware that their clients or patients will not always welcome an observer.

Each meal and snack is supervised. The treatment team taking charge at this stage can be seen by the client as helpful. Such a structure could be seen in terms of Winnicott's (1986) concept of 'holding'. It can also be suggested that the staff need 'holding' as well, in order to contain the anxiety generated in the patient, and by the strategy. Consistency among the multidisciplinary team is essential to avoid the potential of manipulation and division. This is seen as a function of supervision.

(a) Learning activity

For your learning group find out in practice what strategies are used to ensure a consistent approach to care. Debate these with your fellow group members.

How do the staff in your practice area support each other? You may like to discuss your findings with various colleagues who work in different practice environments.

It is possible to use other methods for monitoring the effectiveness of the treatment programme, including pelvic ultrasound. This serves the function of helping to determine healthy weight by measuring the size of the ovaries and uterus (Lask and Bryant-Waugh, 2000: 175).

Anna's treatment plan continued

Problem	Action
Maintain hygiene	Daily baths, showers and dental care.

Treatment rationale

This serves the function of containing the patient's anxiety and encouraging normal healthy daily activities of living and self-care.

Problems encountered in practice

Malnutrition and associated depression can reduce the patient's motivation for self-care. Poor peripheral circulation can cause problems with dry skin, chilblains and occasionally gangrene. Dental caries can result from acid erosion if there is excessive vomiting. If there are any self-harming behaviours, for example cutting or scratching, these will need to be addressed.

Learning activity

As a student healthcare professional, consider what your immediate actions might be if you came upon a patient who is self-harming. Where would you find support to manage the situation appropriately?

Discussion of possible solutions

Encourage and support daily self-care. As weight increases, so will motivation. There is a need to be aware of possible depression.

Anna's treatment plan continued

Problem	Action
Monitor physical state	Four-hourly observations: temperature, pulse, respiration and blood pressure. Bed rest, or activity as allowed. Accurate fluid intake/output chart. Accurate food intake chart. Quilt and socks to be used.

Treatment rationale

Because of Anna's poor physical state, poor peripheral circulation and loss of subcutaneous body fat, frequent observation of her medical state is essential. Postural hypotension on standing could lead to injuries from osteoporosis if she fell. There is a potential for cardiovascular complications and susceptibility to cardiac arhythmias, owing to electrolyte imbalances.

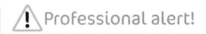 Professional alert!

Very emaciated patients can deteriorate suddenly, developing severe infections which lead to systemic failure.

Learning activity

Check out your knowledge on postural hypotension and cardiac arhythmias as a result of electrolyte disturbance.

Why is Anna at particular risk of osteoporosis? How might this affect her in later years?

Part

III

Problems encountered in practice

Patients like Anna tend to be resistant to being disturbed, as these patients do not see themselves as ill.

Discussion of possible solutions

Management and monitoring of the patient's physical state is a key nursing responsibility. Exact recordings of physical status, dietary intake and output are of special importance.

Summary of Anna's treatment

Problem	Action
Diet	Quarter portions + BD Ensure Plus supplement. Supervision during and half-hour after meals. Meals to include foods from each group – carbohydrate, fats, protein. The patient can identify three food dislikes, which are not to be changed once chosen. No low-calorie foods/drinks. All changes to be decided by the dietician.

(a) Learning activity

In your learning group find out how intake and output for patients with an eating disorder are recorded. Is this different from such recordings in other practice areas? You may find it useful to discuss the challenges of recording such information accurately.

(a) Learning activity

Consider your ability to assist in choosing appropriate foods from the three groups for balanced meals. Refer to Chapter 10 on nutritional assessment and needs to check out your knowledge.

S Scenario continued

Over time there are some changes to Anna's treatment plan:

One week later the only changes are:
- Some weight loss, 27 kg.
- Diet – meals increased to half portions.
- Medication – lactulose.

Two weeks later:
- Hygiene – hair can be washed once weekly.
- Diet – full portions + overnight nasogastric feeds as there is further weight loss.
- Anna's parents are allowed to stay for meals as long as they are able to remain detached and do not undermine nursing efforts with feeding.

Three weeks later:
- Anna is struggling with full portions.
- She complains of abdominal pain, and being constipated.

At this point Anna is transferred to the adolescent psychiatric unit.

Anna is readmitted six months later. She had reached her target weight of 43 kg prior to discharge. She is discharged ten days later, after a weight loss of 5.5 kg. She is now only eating quarter of an orange, one piece of pasta, and diluted Diet Coke daily. Anna feels life is not worth living.

⚠ Professional alert!

Anorexia nervosa has a high co-morbidity with other mental health problems, particularly depression and attempted suicide (Halvorsen, Anderson and Heyerdahl, 2004).

S Scenario continued

On her readmission to the unit, the staff restart Anna on the original plan with quarter-food portions and nasogastric feeding. Anna is refusing all oral intake except sips of water. She agrees to drink 100 ml water hourly or she would require additional intravenous fluids. Her oral intake improves, and she returns to the psychiatric unit as a day patient six days later.

a **Learning activity**

Think about the risk of hospital acquired infection in Anna's case.

S **Scenario continued**

Anna is readmitted three months later. She had been attending as a day patient at the psychiatric unit, but has not eaten or drunk for five days. She collapsed, and it is a very difficult admission.

Sixteen days later Anna's weight has increased to 34.4 kg. Once her physical state is stable, she could be transferred back to the adolescent unit. There is the need to introduce a small oral intake, to reintroduce the concept of feeding.

Twenty-two days later, Anna's weight has increased to 35.2 kg, and she is transferred back to the psychiatric unit.

a **Learning activity**

Anna has made some progress in her treatment and is gaining weight. She is still very distressed at her weight and still has difficulty eating. Think about the possible risks to her. What other agencies might be involved in managing future care?

In your interprofessional learning group:
- Discuss how anorexia nervosa might be situated within the wider social discourses of both women and men in society.
- Explore and debate the legal and ethical issues involved in treatment interventions.

Conclusion

The majority of adolescents with anorexia nervosa will recover or improve sufficiently to obtain a good quality of life. A significant number will go on to develop a severe form of the disorder or further serious mental health problems (Crisp et al, 1992). A recent outcome study has suggested that in a cohort of 51, 82 per cent had no eating disorder at follow-up but almost half (41 per cent) had one or more psychiatric diagnoses, with depression and anxiety being the most common (Halvorsen et al, 2004).

The most commonly observed psychiatric problems, even in those who have recovered from their eating disorder, include depression, anxiety disorders, obsessive compulsive disorder, and drug and alcohol misuse (Steinhausen, Rauss-Mason and Seidel, 1991). Two-thirds, or even more, of former patients accomplish employment and normal educational careers, but only a minority enter marriage or a stable relationship. Later work by Steinhausen (2002) supported the earlier findings, concluding that the later years of the twentieth century did not see an improvement in outcome, and there was still a relatively poor prognosis in terms of mental health.

Some authors, for example Herzog, Sacks and Keller (1993), claim that a younger age of onset is predictive of a better outcome, and other studies (Bryant-Waugh et al, 1996) have shown no significant correlation between age of onset and outcome.

However, eating disorders in all age groups represent the severe end of psychiatric morbidity, having an adverse effect in virtually all areas of life, and not infrequently leading to a premature death. Mortality rates are as high as 22 per cent in some samples, although results are variable (Lucas, Duncan and Piens, 1976).

There is evidence to show that specialist treatment can result in a better outcome for patients than nonspecialist treatment (Crisp et al, 1991), but access to specialist units remains problematic and most patients are cared for in primary and secondary care settings. However, contrary findings from Burls, Gold and Meads (2001) suggest that outpatient care had slightly better results in some areas. Recent thinking tends to favour intensive interventions on an outpatient basis rather than inpatient admission where possible, and it is argued that resources should reflect that pattern (NICE, 2004). In terms of the evidence base, it is fair to say

Part
III

that as yet the relative effectiveness of care strategies for the person with anorexia is unclear. There is an indication that specific focused family work can be effective, but more research needs to be done. Professionals can, however, contribute to improved care for these patients by increasing their awareness and knowledge in this challenging area.

> **(a) Learning activity**
>
> Consider how the information that you have gained from this chapter may impact in a range of settings on your care of patients who may experience difficulties with eating.

References

Akridge, K. (1989) 'Principles and practice: anorexia nervosa', *Journal of Obstetric, Gynaecologic and Neonatal Nursing* 18, 25–30.

American Psychiatric Association (APA) (1994) *Diagnostic and Statistical Manual of Mental Disorders* (DSM-IV-TR), Washington, DC, APA.

Bertalanffy, L. von (1968) *General Systems Theory: Foundations, development, application*, New York, Braziller.

British Medical Association (BMA) (2003) *Adolescent Health*, London, BMA.

Bodycombe-James, M. (2000) 'Paediatric nurses' enjoyment of caring for sick children', I Glasper, E. A. and Ireland, L. (eds), *Evidence-Based Child Health Care: Challenges for practice*, Basingstoke, Palgrave Macmillan.

Bowlby, J. (1969/1980) *Attachment and Loss*, Vol. 1, London, Hogarth.

Bryant-Waugh, R. (2006) 'Recent developments in anorexia nervosa', *Child and Adolescent Mental Health* 11(2), 76–81.

Bryant-Waugh, R., Hankins, M., Shafran, R., Lask, B. and Fosson, A. (1996) 'A prospective follow up of children with anorexia nervosa', *Journal of Youth and Adolescence* 25(4), 431–7.

Burls, A., Gold, L. and Meads, C. (2001) 'How effective is outpatient care compared to inpatient care for the treatment of anorexia nervosa? A systematic review', *European Eating Disorders Review* 9 229–41.

Burt, M. R. (2002) 'Reasons to invest in adolescents', *Journal of Adolescent Health* 31(6, suppl. 1), 136–52.

Clift, L., Dampier, S. and Timmons, S. (2007) 'Adolescents' experiences of emergency admission to children's wards', *Journal of Child Healthcare* 11(3), 195–207.

Coles, L., Glasper, E. A., FitzGerald, C., Le Fluffy, T., Turner, S. and Wilkes-Holes, C. (2007) 'Measuring compliance to the NSF for children and young people in one English strategic health authority', *Journal of Children's and Young Peoples Nursing* 1(1), 7–15.

Cooper, M. (2005) 'Principles of therapeutic style', in Cooper, M., Hooper, C. and Thompson, M. (eds), *Child and Adolescent Mental Health Theory and Practice*, London, Hodder Arnold.

Cooper, M. A. and Glasper, E. A. (2001) 'Deliberate self-harm in children: the nurse's therapeutic style', *British Journal of Nursing* 10(1), 34–40.

Crisp, A. H., Callender, R. J. S., Halek, C. and Hsu, L. K. G. (1992) 'Long-term mortality in anorexia nervosa; a twenty-year follow up of the St Georges and Aberdeen cohorts', *British Journal of Psychiatry* 161, 104–7.

Crisp, A. H., Norton, K., Gowers, S. et al (1991) 'A controlled study of the effect of therapies aimed at adolescent and family psychopathology in anorexia nervosa', *British Journal of Psychiatry* 159, 325–9.

Croll, J., Neumark Sztainer, D., Story, M. and Ireland, M. (2002) 'Prevalence and risk and protective factors related to disordered eating behaviors among adolescents: relationship to gender and ethnicity', *Journal of Adolescent Health* 31(2) (August), 166–75.

DeBate, R., Lewis, M., Zhang, Y., Blunt, H. and Thompson, S. H. (2008) 'Similar but different: sociocultural attitudes towards appearance, body shape dissatisfaction and weight control behaviors among male and female college students', *American Journal of Health Education* 139(5) (Sept/Oct), 296–302.

Department for Education and Skills (DfES) (2003) *Every Child Matters*, green paper, London, The Stationery Office. (2005) *Youth Matters*, London, The Stationery Office.

DfES (2007) *Aiming High for Children: Supporting families*, London, DfES.

Department of Health (DH) (2003) 'Standard for children and young people in hospital,' *National Service Framework for Children, Young People and Maternity Services*, London, HMSO.

DH (2004) *National Service Framework for Children, Young People and Maternity Services*, London, HMSO.

DH (2006a) *Standards for Better Health*, London, The Stationery Office.

DH (2006b) *Transition: Getting it right for young people*, London, The Stationery Office.

Doran, T., Drever, F. and Whitehead, M. (2003) 'Health of young and elderly informal carers: analysis of UK census data', *British Medical Journal* 327, 1388.

Eliot, A. O. and Bake, C. W. (2001) 'Eating disordered adolescent males', *Adolescence* 143, 535–43.

Erikson, E. (1965) *Childhood and Society*, Harmondsworth, Penguin.

Fiorentino, L., Datta, D., Gentle, S., Hall, D. M. B., Harpin, V., Phillips, D. and Walker, A. (1998) 'Transition from school to adult life for physically disabled young people', *Archives of Disease in Childhood* 79, 306–11.

George, L. (1997) 'The psychological characteristics of patients suffering from anorexia nervosa and the nurses role in creating a therapeutic relationship', *Journal of Advanced Nursing* 26, 899–908.

Halvorsen, L., Andersen, A. and Heyerdahl, S. (2004) 'Good outcome of anorexia nervosa after systematic treatment: intermediate to long-term follow up of a representative country sample', *European Child and Adolescent Psychiatry* 13, 295–306.

Hatmaker, G. (2005) 'Boys with eating disorders', *Journal of School Nursing* 21 (December), 329–32.

Hauser, S. T., with Powers, S. I. and Noam, G. G. (1991) *Adolescents and Their Families: Paths of ego development*, New York, Free Press.

Hay, I. and Asman, A. F. (2003) 'The development of adolescents' emotional stability and general self-concept: the interplay of parent, peers, and gender', *International Journal of Disability, Development and Education* 50(1), 77–91.

Herzog, D. B., Sacks, N. R. and Keller, M. B. (1993) 'Patterns and predictors of recovery in anorexia nervosa and bulimia nervosa', *Journal of the Academy of Child and Adolescent Psychiatry* 32,

835–42.

Hill, M., Davis, J., Prout, A. and Tisdall, K. (2004) 'Moving the participation agenda forward', *Children and Society* 18, 77–96.

Howe, D., Brandon, M., Hinings, D. and Schofield, G. (1999) *Attachment Theory, Child Maltreatment and Family Support*, Basingstoke, Macmillan.

Hurrelmann, K. and Engel, U. (eds) (1989) *Adolescence: International perspectives*, Berlin, De Gryter.

Jacobs, M. (1998) *The Presenting Past: The core of psychodynamic counselling and therapy*, Buckingham, Open University Press.

Kelsey, J. and McEwing, G. (2006) 'Physical growth and development in children', in Glasper, A. and Richardson, J. (eds), *A Textbook of Children's and Young Peoples Nursing*, Edinburgh, Churchill Livingstone.

King, S. J. and Turner, S. (2000) 'Caring for adolescent females with anorexia nervosa: registered nurses perspective', *Journal of Advanced Nursing* 32(1), 139–47.

La Voie, J. C. (1994) 'Identity in adolescence: issues of theory, structure and transition', *Journal of Adolescence* 17, 17–28.

Lask, B. and Bryant-Waugh, R. (2000) *Anorexia Nervosa and Related Eating Disorders in Childhood and Adolescence*, 2nd edn, Hove, Psychology Press, pp. 290–2.

Lucas, A., Duncan, J. W. and Piens, V. (1976) 'The treatment of anorexia nervosa', *American Journal of Psychiatry* 133, 1034–8.

Minuchin, S. (1974) *Families and Family Therapy*, Cambridge, Mass., Harvard University Press.

Morris, J. and Twaddle, S. (2007) 'Anorexia nervosa clinical review', *British Medical Journal* 334, 894–8.

National Institute for Clinical Excellence (NICE) (2004) *Eating Disorders: Core interventions in the treatment and management of anorexia nervosa, bulimia nervosa and related eating disorders*, National clinical practice guideline CG9, London, British Psychological Society/Gaskell.

Nicholls, D., Chater, R. and Lask, B. (2000) 'Children into DSM don't go, a comparison of classification systems in childhood and early adolescence', *International Journal of Eating Disorders* 28, 317–24.

Ousley, L. E., Cordero, D. and White, S. (2008) 'Eating disorders and body image of undergraduate men', *Journal of American College Health* 56, 6.

Owen, J. (2007) 'Children and alcohol: Britain's deadly cocktail', *Independent*, 4 November [online] http://news.independent.co.uk/health/article3127405.ece (accessed 22 December 2008).

Palmer, R. (2006) 'Come the revolution: revisiting the management of anorexia nervosa', Advances in *Psychiatric Treatment* 12, 5–12.

Ramjan, L. M. (2004) 'Nurses and the "therapeutic relationship": caring for adolescents with anorexia nervosa', *Journal of Advanced Nursing* 45(5). 495–503.

Registered Nurses Association of Ontario (RNAO) (2002) 'Enhancing healthy adolescent development: nursing best practice guideline', Toronto, Canada, RNAO [online] www.rnao.org (accessed 22 December 2008).

Robson, J. W. (2001) 'Alcohol misuse', *Archives of Disease in Childhood* 84, 95–7.

Royal College of Nursing (RCN) (2007) *Lost in Transition: Moving young people between child and adult services*, London, RCN.

Royal College of Paediatrics and Child Health (RCPCH) (2003) *Bridging the Gaps: Healthcare for Adolescents*, London, RCPCH.

Royal College of Psychiatrists (2004) *Surviving Adolescence: A toolkit for parents* [online] http://www.rcpsych.ac.uk/mentalhealthinfo/youngpeople/adolescence.aspx (accessed 7 December 2008).

Steinhausen, H. C. (2002) 'The outcome of anorexia nervosa in the 20th century', *American Journal of Psychiatry* 159, 1284–93.

Steinhausen, H. C., Rauss-Mason, C. and Seidel, R. (1991) 'Follow up studies of anorexia nervosa: a review of four decades of outcome research', *Psychological Medicine* 21, 447–54.

Stockwell, F. (1972) *The Unpopular Patient*, RCN, London.

Taylor, J. and Muller, D. (1995) *Nursing Adolescents: Research and psychological perspectives*, Oxford, Blackwell Science.

Viner, R. and Keane, M. (1998) *Youth Matters: Evidence-based best practice for the care of young people in hospital*, London, Action for Sick Children.

Wicke, D., Coppin, R., Doorbar, P. and Le May, A. (2007) 'Every child matters, but what matters to them? Using teenager's views to shape health services', *Journal of Children's and Young People's Nursing* 1(3), 129–36.

Winnicott, D. (1986) *Holding and Interpretation: Fragment of an analysis*, London, Hogarth Press and Institute of Psychoanalysis.

World Health Organization (WHO) (1994) *The International Classification of Diseases (ICD-10)*, Copenhagen, WHO.

Wright, S. (2001) 'Eating disorders: why do nurses choose this field?' *Nursing Times* 97(46), 37–8.

Part

III

Chapter

23

Care of the adult – surgical

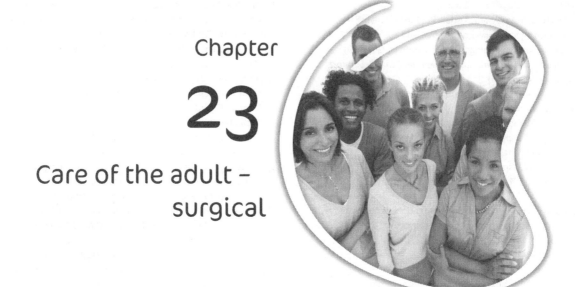

Kevin Hambridge and Gill McEwing

Links to other chapters in *Foundation Studies for Caring*

Links to other chapters in *Foundation Skills for Caring*

W Don't forget to visit www.palgrave.com/glasper for additional online resources relating to this chapter.

Introduction

Colorectal cancer (CRC) is the second most common cause of cancer death in the United Kingdom. In England and Wales 30,000 new cases are diagnosed in each year (Kumar and Clark, 2005), and Scotland has one of the highest incidences of CRC in the world (41 per 100,000 in men, 29 per 100,000 in women) (Clinical Outcomes Working Group, 2000). Approximately half of those diagnosed will die from the disease. The incidence of colorectal cancer is increasing. One reason for this is the ageing population, and like many other cancers, the incidence of CRC increases sharply with age. The incidence in young people is very low and usually linked to hereditary factors. In people of 45–55 years the incidence is 25 per 100,000, but it is ten times greater in people of 75 years and over (NICE, 2005). The most common age for presentation is 60–65 years.

Causative factors include low intake of dietary fibre, high meat (Sweet, 2002) and fat intake, obesity (Murphy et al, 2000) and long-term smoking (SIGN, 2005). Protective factors include high consumption of fruit and vegetables, increased fibre intake, exercise, hormone replacement therapy and aspirin or NSAIDs (Longmore et al, 2007). There is also a genetic link. The survival rate after diagnosis is now approximately 45 per cent at five years, and at this stage most patients appear to be cured (NHS Scotland, 2003). These improvements have been linked with early diagnosis and the standardised management of the disease. Early diagnosis is only possible if there is early recognition of symptoms by the patient.

This chapter follows the journey of a patient presenting with symptoms of CRC, from their diagnosis in primary healthcare, through their treatment in secondary healthcare, until their discharge home.

Learning outcomes

The chapter will enable you to:

- be aware of the causes, presentation, treatment and prognosis of CRC
- explain the investigations involved in the diagnosis of CRC
- outline some nursing models and frameworks of care
- understand the health promotion and education issues related to CRC
- outline the role and function of the pre-admission clinic
- identify the purpose and areas of risk assessment involved in the admission of a patient to hospital
- understand the role of the nurse and other members of the healthcare team in the care of a patient receiving surgery
- outline the role of the nurse in the admission of a patient to hospital
- outline the role of the nurse in preparation for surgical intervention
- outline the role of the nurse when transferring a patient to theatre
- outline the role of the nurse in the immediate postoperative period
- outline the role of the nurse when recovering a patient from surgery
- outline the role of the nurse in preparing for discharge of the patient
- recognise the need for psychological support in caring for a patient experiencing surgery for cancer.

Concepts

- Health promotion
- Health education
- Primary care
- Family care
- Communication
- Nursing theory
- Preparation for surgery
- Risk assessment
- Recovery from surgery
- Discharge from hospital

The bowel or large intestine is made up of two main sections, the colon and the rectum. About two-thirds of tumours develop in the colon – this affects men and women equally – and the remaining third develop in the rectum, which is more common in men (SIGN, 2005). Most of these tumours develop from small polyps which are often present for ten or more years before they become malignant. Although the disease progresses slowly, about a third of patients present as an emergency, often after they have experienced symptoms for weeks or months.

Diagnosis of the disease is straightforward, and established usually by a sigmoidoscopy or colonoscopy. The difficulty is in deciding whether to refer the patient for investigation and access to diagnostic facilities. In 1999/2000 one-third of patients waited more than three months for their first hospital appointment after being referred by their GP (NICE, 2005). The government produced guidelines in July 2000 that if the GP suspects CRC, the client should be seen by a specialist within two weeks (Thompson et al, 2003).

To improve the survival rates, guidelines have been produced (NICE, 2005b; SIGN, 2005). The aims of the national guidelines are to reduce the incidence of CRC and encourage early diagnosis. Delay in diagnosis of CRC can occur at three points: delay by the patient in presenting to the GP, delay in referral by the GP, or delay by the hospital in either establishing a diagnosis or treating the disease. The survival rate is directly related to recognition and treatment of the disease (Hobbs, 2000). Consistency in referral patterns and disease management should improve survival. The key recommendations of the NICE guidelines include a rapid referral for endoscopy for all patients suspected of CRC, and that patients should be cared for by a specialist multidisciplinary team (NICE, 2005b).

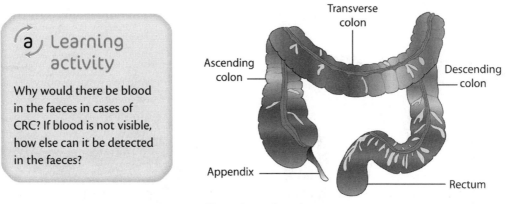

Figure 23.1 The colon

The presentation of CRC varies depending on the site of the disease. If the colon in the left side of the abdomen is affected (this involves the descending colon, sigmoid colon or rectum), the clinical signs include bleeding and mucus passed rectally, altered bowel movements, and in 60 per cent of cases a mass can be felt rectally. The presentation of right-sided bowel cancer (involving the ascending colon or parts of the transverse colon) include weight loss, falling haemoglobin and abdominal pain (Longmore et al, 2007).

S Scenario

The GP informs James that he needs to be investigated fully, and that there is a possibility he might have bowel cancer. She reassures him that he will be referred to the local hospital for rapid investigation, and he should be seen within the next two weeks. The GP faxes the urgent referral form to the hospital, and confirmation of its arrival is sent back to ensure that the fax has not been lost.

Statistically every GP in the United Kingdom will see one new case of CRC each year (Hobbs, 2000). The NHS Executive has now published guidelines for urgent referral for patients suspected of cancer (DH, 2000). For colonic tumours, it is recommended that the patient has a computed tomography (CT) scan of the abdomen, chest and pelvis. For a rectal tumour, it is recommended that the patient has a magnetic resonance imaging (MRI) scan of the pelvis, CT scan of the abdomen and chest, and an ultrasound scan looking for lower tumours that are localised. For an anal tumour, the patient is referred to a centralised specialist (www.cancerimprovement.nhs.uk/bowel, 9 October 2007).

S Scenario continued

Ten days later James is seen in outpatients at the hospital by the colorectal surgery doctor. The doctor discusses his history and symptoms with him, and following a physical examination agrees that further investigations are required. A endoscopy will be arranged.

Three main methods are effective in the primary diagnosis of CRC: endoscopy, double contrast barium enema and CT pneumocolon. The success of each method depends on adequate bowel preparation (SIGN, 2005). CRC is usually seen through an endoscope (colonoscope or sigmoidoscope). The whole large bowel can be seen using a colonoscope and a flexible sigmoidoscope, which can reach deep enough into the bowel to detect about 60 per cent of tumours. These instruments allow a clear view of the tumour and can also be used to remove polyps or take samples of tissue for biopsy. CT or MRI is necessary to assess the extent of the tumour (Kumar and Clark, 2005). A new form of imaging, virtual colonoscopy, is now being adopted in an increasing number of units.

Part

III

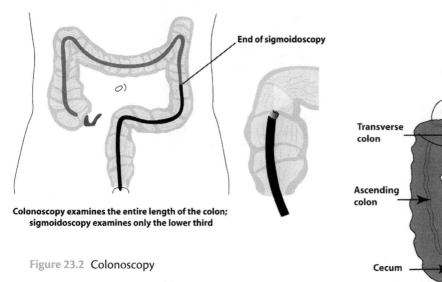

Colonoscopy examines the entire length of the colon;
sigmoidoscopy examines only the lower third

Figure 23.2 Colonoscopy

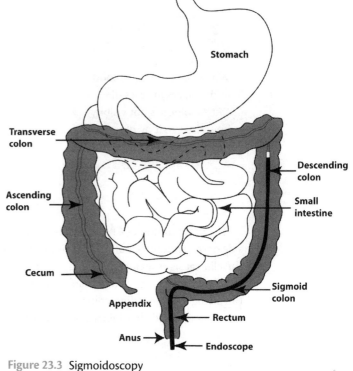

Figure 23.3 Sigmoidoscopy

Pathophysiology

There are five main sites of CRC. They are the caecum and ascending colon (15 per cent), transverse colon (10 per cent), descending colon (5 per cent), sigmoid colon (25 per cent) and rectum (45 per cent) (Longmore et al, 2007). Patients usually survive for approximately three years after diagnosis. The degree to which the cancer has spread will determine the type and effectiveness of treatment and the ultimate prognosis. The spread of the disease is usually defined in terms of Dukes stages. There are four stages in this classification:

A cancer localised within the bowel wall
B cancer penetrating the bowel wall
C cancer in lymph nodes
D distant metastases.

However a new and more precise method of classification is also being introduced, termed TNM classification, which is based on the depth of tumour invasion (T), lymph node involvement (N) and metastatic spread (M).

Approximately 55 per cent of patients present with advanced CRC (Dukes stage C or D), where the cancer has spread to the lymph nodes, metastasised to other organs, or is so locally invasive that surgery to remove the primary tumour alone is unlikely to be sufficient for cure (http://www.cancerhelp.org.uk).

W

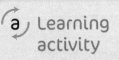

Learning activity

Look up the TNM staging and identify the differences from Dukes staging.

The treatment for malignant tumours of the sigmoid colon is a sigmoid colectomy. Anastomosis is achieved during the first operation using staples. The intention is for the operation to provide a cure. Radiotherapy is generally only used pre-operatively or postoperatively for rectal tumours. Chemotherapy is only used in tumours with Dukes staging C or D, but studies are taking place to assess any benefits to patients with Dukes stage B tumours (Longmore et al, 2007).

S Scenario continued

James will require admission to hospital. In other words, he is moving from primary to secondary care.

Nursing models

Nurses work in both the primary and secondary care services, and the care they provide is organised using models and structures that are designed to fit the requirements of the individual patient at that time. *Nursing theory* is the knowledge that is used to support nursing practice. It involves a range of interconnected subjects that can be applied to practice (Colley, 2003). This knowledge comes from experiential learning and research. Nursing is a relatively new science, and most of the theory of nursing has been produced in the last 30 years. Not all the theories support each other.

Nursing models are a combination of theories and concepts which provide a framework for nurses to assess, plan, implement and evaluate the care they give. By using nursing theories nursing practice can be explored, and research can be directed to fill any gaps in knowledge (Siviter, 2004).

Nursing is evolving from the biomedical model, where the nurse primarily provided the care prescribed by the doctor. This model is based mainly on pathophysiology and the treatment of disease, and does not take into account the psychological, social or cultural differences between individual patients. Even Florence Nightingale recognised that patients were individuals, and she believed it was the nurse's responsibility to adapt the environment to enable the patient to have the best possible opportunity of recovery.

The major nursing theorists to propose models for nursing include Virginia Henderson's definitions of nursing, Imogene King's general system's framework, Betty Neuman's systems model, Dorothea Orem's self-care framework, Hildegard Peplau's theory of interpersonal relations and Calista Roy's adaptation model, but these are only a sample of those who developed theoretical models for nursing. Some models were developed for specific areas of practice, such as Anne Casey's model for children's nursing (Casey, 2007), and others seemed to fit certain specialities better than others, such as Roy's model for mental health and Orem's for rehabilitation nursing. Individual models have different perspectives when providing care for the patient, Orem's model provides a patient-centred approach which has been seen to be relevant to the care of older people (Glasson et al, 2006), and Roper, Logan and Tierney's model focuses on the nurse meeting the patient's individual needs. A *nursing framework* is a structure used to organise the care given to the patient. This can be based on one or several models (Siviter, 2004).

Learning activity

Look up some of the models listed in Table 23.1 and decide which patient group might respond best to each approach of nursing. Which model would suit James Osborne's visit to hospital?

Part

III

Table 23.1 Models for nursing

Virginia Henderson's definitions of nursing	http://www.stti.iupui.edu/library
Imogene King's general system's framework	http://www.nurses.info/nursing_theory_person_king_imogene.htm
Betty Neuman's systems model	http://www.neumansystemsmodel.com/
Dorothea Orem's self care framework	http://www.muhealth.org/~nursing/scdnt.html
Hildegard Peplau's theory of interpersonal relations	http://publish.uwo.ca/%7Ecforchuk/peplau/hpcb.html
Calista Roy's adaptation model	http://www2.bc.edu/~royca/
Roper, Logan and Tierney Elements of nursing: a model for nursing based on a model of living	http://www.sandiego.edu/nursing/theory/roper.txt

There has been some disapproval of nursing models because the structure of the model prevents the nurse from being flexible and intuitive when trying to meet the patient's needs (Tierney, 1998). This has been exacerbated by the creation of prewritten plans of care, for example for a patient experiencing a myocardial infarction or cholycystectomy, which impose standard care for all patients experiencing these conditions regardless of age, gender, social, emotional or lifestyle differences.

Organisation of nursing care and care pathways

The nursing process is a framework for organising individualised nursing care. It involves four stages: assessment, planning, implementation and evaluation (Richards and Edwards, 2003). The intention of the nursing process is to enable continuity of care by thorough documentation of information, to provide continuous observations and ensure effective interventions. However there has been a lot of criticism of the nursing process approach to care, as it imposes rigid constraints on practice, and is cumbersome and outdated (Walsh, 1997).

Most models result in the creation of a care plan which is used to determine the nursing care given to an individual patient. An essential component is that the goals are measurable to enable care to be evaluated and then improved upon.

Critical pathways, or integrated care pathways, are multidisciplinary approaches to care that are being developed. They provide care that is cost-effective, patient-focused, multidisciplinary and collaborative (Herring, 1999). They can be used to translate national evidence-based guidelines into local protocols, and encourage the application of the guidelines in clinical practice. Many care pathways have been developed, and national users' groups exist to give advice and support their use (Campbell et al, 1998). Other benefits suggested are that they improve team work, reduce duplication and improve documentation, with continuous records of care (Norris and Briggs, 1999). However little research has been done to evaluate whether care pathways improve the quality of patient care (De-Luc, 2000). These care plans detail the essential steps in the care of patients with a specific clinical problem, and describe the expected progress of the patient. They are based on desired patient outcomes within an agreed timeframe, utilising known resources for each patient group.

General pre-admission assessment

In many hospitals, before admission to the surgical ward the patient is contacted and invited to attend the pre-admission unit or clinic (PAC) for pre-operative assessment. The timing of this visit varies between hospitals.

Scenario continued

James is informed that he will receive an appointment to attend the PAC. He asks the doctor why this is necessary.

C **Professional conversation**

Lucy, a student nurse, has her first clinical placement on the surgical unit. She has been assigned to the PAC and asks Teena, a staff nurse, to explain the functions of the clinic.

Teena explains, 'We like to bring patients in so we can identify any potential anaesthetic difficulties, to improve safety and quantify risks. It also gives a chance to start putting together information to begin planning postoperative care. We have a discussion with the patient and their relatives to help reduce fear and anxiety (AAGBI, 2001). Research shows the PACs have a good effect. They lead to a reduction in patient cancellations and length of stay, because they give us an opportunity to plan patient needs before they are admitted to hospital (Beck, 2007).'

The functions of PACs include (Beck, 2007):
- assessing the patient's fitness for the anaesthesia
- undertaking a physical examination
- writing up the patient's medical history, including their current health status and medications prescribed
- carrying out the 'clerking' procedure in advance of admission, including a nursing assessment using a framework such as the 'activities of daily living', and beginning discharge planning
- performing investigations and clinical scores using local guidelines or NICE guidelines
- information sharing – written data about anaesthetics, risks such as pressure ulcers and so on, and an opportunity for the patient to ask questions.

a **Learning activity**

Investigate the advantages for both the care team and the patient of attending a PAC.

The type and number of tests the patient will have depends on (NICE, 2003):
- their health status – determined by their blood pressure, pulse rate, body mass index (BMI), illnesses they have had previously, medicines they are prescribed and any history of health problems in their family
- their age – the need for specific tests can increase with age
- the type of surgery – more tests may be needed if they are having major surgery.

a **Learning activity**

The pre-admission nurse will undertake many important tasks including the monitoring of blood pressure, pulse, temperature and respirations. Find out why this is necessary.

Part

III

S **Scenario**

James undergoes an admission assessment, which involves the nurse asking him a series of questions relating to his:
- personal details
- religious needs
- occupation
- relevant medical/surgical history

- allergies to food, drugs, topical agents or metal (Scott et al, 1999)
- current medication
- discharge assessment – type of house, facilities at home, carers, transport arrangements and current involvement with social services (if any).

Figure 23.4 shows examples of the forms used for pre-admission assessments.

PRE-ADMISSION/ADMISSION

Patient Name:	Admitting Nurse:
Date of Birth:	Date:
Hospital Number:	Time:
Consultant:	Signature:

Baseline Observations:

Temp	Pulse	Resps	BP	O2 Sats	BMI

Risk Assessments (circle then specify action taken/intervention in multidisciplinary evaluation):

CJD	Blood Borne Virus	Latex Allergy	DVT
Yes / No	Low / Medium / High	Yes / No	A / B / C

Pressure Ulcer	Manual Handling	Nutrition	Falls
High / Moderate / Low	Yes / No	Low / Medium / High	High / Moderate / Low

Discharge Assessment (specify action taken for any areas of concern on care pathway):

Where does the patient live? House / Flat / Bungalow (circle) / Other...................................	
If the patient lives in a flat, what floor?	
Is lift available?	Yes / No (circle)
Are there steps into the house?	Yes / No (circle)
How many?	
Does accommodation have stairs?	Yes / No (circle)
How many?	
Is there a handrail?	Yes / No (circle)
Is the bathroom upstairs?	Yes / No (circle)
Is there a toilet downstairs?	Yes / No (circle)
Is there a walk-in shower?	Yes / No (circle)
If applicable how ill the proposed treatment affect the patient's ability to use these facilities post discharge?	
Will patient be discharged to their home address?	Yes / No (circle)
Is equipment required for discharge?	Yes / No (circle)
If yes specify arrangements made:	
Is the patient a carer themselves for others at home?	Yes / No (circle)
Who will be the patient's carer after discharge?	
Are potential carer(s) able to look after the patient's discharge needs?	Yes / No (circle)
Does the patient have suitable transport arrangements for transport home from hospital?	Yes / No (circle)
Does the patient currently use community services?	Yes / No (circle)

Details of specialist referral: e.g. **Community Nurse, Occupational Therapist:**

Specialist	Contact Name and Number	Date Arranged	Date to Commence

Long Stay Surgery
Trial V2 Issued August 2007/Review August 2008
Page 3 of 19

Figure 23.4 (a) Example of pre-admission assessment forms

PRE-ADMISSION/ADMISSION

Patient Name:	Admitting Nurse:
Date of Birth:	Date:
Hospital Number:	Time:
Consultant:	Signature:

Assessment of Self Care Needs (identify problems and needs and individualise the care pathway accordingly):

Breathing:

Smoker? Yes / No (circle)   Number per day.................

Hydration:

Alcohol intake units per week...............

Nutrition:

Special dietary requirements communicated to catering staff? Yes / No (circle)

Sensory Status:

Contact lenses / Glasses / Hearing Aids (circl⌐

Hygiene / Skin Condition:

Communication:

Language Spoken...................................

Mobility:

Sleep and Rest:

Elimination:

Psychological Well-Being:

Pain and Discomfort:

Options with regard to the management of pain discussed? Yes / No (circle)

Patient Controlled Analgesia (PCA)

The following factors should be considered when it is anticipated the patient will be using PCA. If any of the following apply, the Anaesthetist should be informed as it will assist in the decision as to whether the patient is suitable for PCA. Advice given should be recorded in the pathway.

☐ Increased risk factors due to age (>75 years)	☐ Physical disability e.g. arthritis	☐ Emergency admission
☐ Mental impairment/ confusion	☐ Neurological problems	☐ Pregnant or breast feeding
☐ Cardiovascular history	☐ Contraindications due to medication (current or planned e.g. hypnotics/sedatives	☐ Patient's choice (doesn't wish to use PCA)

Figure 23.4 (b) Example of pre-admission assessment forms

Part

III

It is imperative for the nurse to assess the patient's home circumstances and commence discharge planning at this point. Although discharge planning should be a 'process and not an isolated event' (DH, 2003), evidence suggests that discharge planning is usually suboptimal and haphazard (Audit Commission, 2000).

It is also important that the nurse conducts an assessment of the patient's care needs, which will provide information for the first stages of the nursing process or care pathway. This involves the identification of problems and needs in relation to:

- Breathing – do they smoke? Do they suffer from asthma?
- Hydration – what is their alcohol intake per week, and normal fluid intake?
- Nutrition – are there any special dietary requirements?
- Sensory status – do they wear contact lenses, glasses and/or a hearing aid?
- Hygiene/skin condition.
- Communication abilities.
- Mobility.
- Sleep and rest.
- Elimination.
- Psychological well-being.
- Attitude to pain and discomfort, including their suitability for patient-controlled analgesia.

An anaesthetic assessment of the patient is also made by the anaesthetist. The purpose of this is to assess and optimise their fitness before surgery. Behar (2007) states that this should include a medical history and physical examination, including an airway assessment and measurement of vital signs.

S Scenario continued

The staff note in James's 'Preoperative tests' booklet (NICE, 2003) that his surgery is classified as Grade 4 (major) and his ASA grade is Grade 1, meaning that he is a 'normal healthy patient'. This assessment then dictates which type of tests he will require in preparation for surgery.

---

a Learning activity   W

Find out what the NICE Guidelines suggest for James at http://www.nice.org.uk/nicemedia/pdf/CG3NICEguideline.pdf.

Risk assessment

It may also be prudent at this stage for the nurse to assess the patient for the various risks they might be exposed to during hospitalisation. This is achieved by performing various risk assessments using recognised evidence-based tools and scoring systems. These can include a manual handling assessment, a pressure ulcer risk assessment, a deep vein thrombosis risk assessment, a nutritional assessment and a falls assessment.

A manual handling assessment is essential in order that any equipment that is required to reduce manual handling risks for the patient and the practitioner is utilised (MHO Regulations, 1992).

It is imperative that a pressure ulcer risk assessment is completed in order to assess the patient's risk of developing a pressure ulcer during their hospital admission. Pressure ulcer risk assessment tools are used to assist in making decisions regarding the prevention of pressure ulcers. This is because pressure ulcers, formally called pressure sores, cost the National Health Service (NHS) approximately £1.4–2 billion per year (Bennett, Dealey and Posnett, 2004), and the incidence of pressure ulcers can be as high as 18 per cent of hospital patients (EPUAP, 2002). Pressure ulcers can affect bony prominences including the heels, sacrum, buttocks, elbows, shoulders, toes, and can occur on the fingers while measuring pulse oximetry, and less frequently on patients' lips, nose, mouth, ears and skull. It is crucial that a measurement tool that numerically predicts the degree of risk of an individual developing a pressure ulcer is used. It is equally important that the chosen risk assessment tool demonstrates validity and reliability in order to predict those patients at potential risk.

Examples of pressure risk assessment tools include the Norton Scale (1962: see Morton, McLarena dn Exton-Smith, 1985), which has four risk areas to consider. The Waterlow Assessment (1985; see Waterlow, 1991) assesses the degree of risk in many important aspects, and gives guidance of useful equipment. This is the most widely used tool in the United Kingdom. Finally there is the Braden Scale (1985; see Braden and Bergstrom 1987) which has been used mostly in the United States, and shows greater sensitivity than the others.

There are NICE guidelines (2005a) for pressure ulcer prevention, which can be used to direct the practitioner. They state that:

- The first assessment should happen within six hours of patient contact, and assessment should be ongoing thereafter.
- Patients at risk should be repositioned frequently so that less than two hours is spent in the same position. Additionally, suitable aids and equipment for positioning and mobilising the patient should be used.
- There is scope for self-care: that is, the patient can be taught how to redistribute their weight and perform passive movements while they are bedbound.
- It is essential that the patient's nutrition is assessed and support given as appropriate. Thus, a Malnutrition Universal Screening Tool assessment (Bapen, 2003) should be completed.
- Based on the degree of pressure ulcer risk, it may be important for a pressure-relieving device to be used. This can include a foam mattress or a low air loss bed.

⟦S⟧ Scenario continued

James's BMI is 27, but he has lost about 5 kg recently and his skin is healthy.

(a) Learning activity   W

Look up the Waterlow Assessment chart and decide what risk level James is at pre-operatively. Visit http://www.judy-waterlow.co.uk/downloads/Waterlow%20Score%20Card-front.pdf, or read Chapter 10 in the companion skills volume.

Do you think pressure area care needs to be commenced for James?

Part

III

A **deep vein thrombosis (DVT) risk assessment** is important, and should be completed in order to assess the patient's risk of venous thrombo-embolism during hospitalisation (Welch, 2005). Nurses a have prime role in prevention of DVT, and DVT risk assessment should be an integral part of admission assessment. The House of Commons Health Committee (2005) stated that up to 25,000 people die per year in England as a result of venous thrombo-embolism formation. Once the degree of DVT risk is ascertained, by the use of a recognised risk assessment tool such as the Autar DVT scale (Autar, 2003), nursing care should be planned and implemented as part of the patient's individualised care plan or care pathway in order to prevent DVT. Based upon their degree of risk, the patient could be measured and fitted with anti-embolism stockings which mimic the calf muscle pump action. They can be advised on how and when to mobilise, how to perform limb exercises, and given breathing exercises which help venous return. They could also be prescribed anticoagulant therapy or intermittent pneumatic compression.

(a) Learning activity

Look up the Autar DVT Risk Assessment Scale and determine James's DVT risk.

A **nutritional risk assessment** is normally also completed. This is necessary at admission to hospital to identify any malnutrition and enable any necessary care to be implemented. It is also important to assess whether the patient is at risk of malnutrition during their hospital stay. Nutrition is often a low priority in healthcare, and malnutrition can happen easily, but it can also be prevented. This is important because clinical outcomes can be improved with optimum nutrition.

Malnutrition 'means bad nutrition and applies to any condition in which deficiency, excess or imbalance of energy, protein or other nutrients adversely affects body function and/or clinical outcome' (RCP, 2002). Because malnutrition in the hospital setting has been a problem for many decades, with up to 70 per cent of patients being malnourished on discharge from hospital (RCP, 2002), initiatives to improve nutrition have been advised and implemented. These include:

- *Essence of Care* (DH, 2003b): 'fundamental and essential aspects of care'
- *NSF for Older People* (DH, 2001) (highlighted nutritional care)
- 'Better hospital food' programme (NHS Estates, 2001)
- NICE guidelines (2006).

The NICE guidelines (2006) relating to nutrition emphasised that care should be 'patient centred', taking into account 'individual patients' needs', using 'informed decisions' about food, working in 'partnership', utilising effective 'communication' skills, based upon 'evidence-based practice' and 'culturally appropriate'. Healthcare organisations should provide education and training for staff, work in a multidisciplinary manner and use specialist nurses in the field of nutrition.

The risk assessment tool that the nurse can use in order to assess James's degree of malnutrition risk is the Malnutrition Universal Screening Tool (BAPEN, 2003), which follows five steps:

1 Obtain a BMI score and convert it to a tool score.
2 Note the percentage of any unplanned weight loss and give this a score.
3 Establish any acute disease effect on nutrition and give this assessment a score.
4 Add the scores for steps 1, 2 and 3 to obtain the overall risk of malnutrition.
5 Use management guidelines, evidence-based practice and local policies to develop a plan of care for the client's hospital stay.

ⓐ Learning activity

Revisit the MUST screening tool on p. 180 and determine whether James is at risk.

A further assessment might be carried out to determine whether the patient has a latex allergy. This is because 1 per cent of the general population are allergic to latex (Charous et al, 2002), and latex is commonly used in hospital settings during universal precautions (particularly for gloves).

Psychological preparation of the patient

Preparation of the patient psychologically for surgery can also be an important role of the pre-admission nurse. This includes information relating to the theatre experience in order to help to reduce the patient's anxiety, and reduce the physical risks of surgery (Hughes, 2002).

Attending the PAC can provide many benefits for the individual patient and also for the healthcare organisation. These improvements include reducing the length of hospital stay for the patient, improving the psychological well-being of the patient, reducing dependence on healthcare for the patient after discharge, a reduction in readmission rates, a reduced mortality rate, greater patient satisfaction with the service and increased patient knowledge about their condition (Spilsbury and Meyer, 2001).

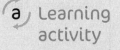

t ☆
Practice tip

A patient diagnosed with suspected CRC might have bowel preparation in order to cleanse the bowel pre-operatively. This may involve the patient being prescribed a strong laxative such as Picolax to clear the bowel. It is imperative that the patient is informed of the importance of drinking plenty of fluids in order to reduce the risk of dehydration, and to omit certain foods at a recommended time.

Learning activity

Look up the guidelines for Picolax in the British National Formulary (BNF).

Admission to hospital

S   Scenario continued

James and Emma arrive for James's admission to the ward. There are many nursing activities during the pre-operative period in order to prepare him physically and psychologically for theatre. He is shown around the ward to make him aware of the environment, and the call bell system is explained to him. All this helps to reduce anxiety.

On admission, a designated nurse should complete his assessment, or alternatively review the assessments that have been conducted in the PAC. The nurse is responsible for documenting accurate information upon which care can be based. The care pathway requires the nurse caring for the patient to sign the form after each span of duty, stating the care given. If James is taking any medications these will be recorded, and the medications will be stored for safe-keeping.

Figure 23.5 shows some typical admission assessment forms.

On admission the nurse should place two identification bracelets on the patient, one on the wrist and the other on another limb such as the ankle, as it will be a necessary to check their identity throughout the hospital stay: for example when administering any medication and when entering theatre. Two identity bracelets are used in case one is removed when a cannula is inserted (Scott et al, 1999). A wrist band stating the patient's known allergies is also a prudent measure to ensure that the risk of the patient being exposed to a known allergen is reduced.

Even though the patient has had observations recorded in the PAC, baseline observations should be re-recorded including the pulse, blood pressure, oxygen saturation level and temperature.

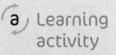

Learning activity

Discuss with a colleague how you think James might be feeling at this time.

The patient will also require pre-operative education and information. As long ago as 1975, Hayward argued that the lack of information given to patients pre-operatively resulted in negative outcomes postoperatively. Hughes (2002) states that giving information in an effective way can help to reduce the patient's anxiety levels, reduce the patient's pain levels and reduce the risk of postoperative complications. This information giving must be reinforced at regular intervals. The majority of patients who are admitted to hospital with CRC are suffering a degree of anxiety, having presented to the GP with what might have seemed a minor ailment, which has quickly led to arrival in hospital knowing they have cancer (Alexander et al, 2006). Research has demonstrated that a diagnosis of cancer is considered to be a confrontation with death (Rasmussen and Elverdam, 2007). This rapid change of circumstances might not have given the patient time to prepare psychologically for the experience.

The nurse admitting the patient needs to adopt a sensitive supportive approach,

Part

III

CARE PATHWAY
Long Stay Surgery

Addressograph Label:		Prefers to be Known as:
		Age:
		Room No:

	Next of Kin/Contact Person:
	Address:
Telephone Number:	
	Day Time Contact Number:
Date/Time of Admission:	Night Time Contact Number:

Instructions for Use of Pathway

It is the responsibility of the member of staff who carries out the care to initial the relevant box to indicate that the intervention has been carried out or the outcome achieved. The member of staff allocated to care for the patient must sign the large signature box **on every shift** ensuring that any variances are described with action taken and outcomes documented in evaluation notes. Actions required to meet individual or medical needs must be added to the pathway. Please ensure that each day is actually dated and each sheet has the patient details completed. Written notes recorded in the multidisciplinary evaluation section must be accompanied by the date and time (using the 24 hour clock) that the entry is made and must be signed.

This pathway is intended as a guide for patient care and is not a substitute for clinical judgement.

Signature of all staff involved in the patient's care (AHPs, Medical, Nursing Staff):

Print Name	Initials	Designation	Signature

Figure 23.5 (a) Admission assessment

PRE-ADMISSION/ADMISSION

Patient Name:	Admitting Nurse:
Date of Birth:	Date:
Hospital Number:	Time:
Consultant:	Signature:

Assessment of Self Care Needs (identify problems and needs and individualise the care pathway accordingly):

Breathing:

Smoker? Yes / No (circle)   Number per day.................

Hydration:

Alcohol intake units per week...............

Nutrition:

Special dietary requirements communicated to catering staff? Yes / No (circle)

Sensory Status:

Contact lenses / Glasses / Hearing Aids (circl·

Hygiene / Skin Condition:

Communication:

Language Spoken....................................

Mobility:

Sleep and Rest:

Elimination:

Psychological Well-Being:

Pain and Discomfort:

Options with regard to the management of pain discussed? Yes / No (circle)

Patient Controlled Analgesia (PCA)

The following factors should be considered when it is anticipated the patient will be using PCA. If any of the following apply, the Anaesthetist should be informed as it will assist in the decision as to whether the patient is suitable for PCA. Advice given should be recorded in the pathway.

☐ Increased risk factors due to age (>75 years)	☐ Physical disability e.g. arthritis	☐ Emergency admission
☐ Mental impairment/ confusion	☐ Neurological problems	☐ Pregnant or breast feeding
☐ Cardiovascular history	☐ Contraindications due to medication (current or planned e.g. hypnotics/sedatives	☐ Patient's choice (doesn't wish to use PCA)

Part III

Figure 23.5 (b) Admission assessment

PRE-ADMISSION/ADMISSION

Patient Name:	Admitting Nurse:
Date of Birth:	Date:
Hospital Number:	Time:
Consultant:	Signature:

Intervention	Initial
Contraindications for procedure have been identified and appropriate action taken	
Patient aware of pre-operative fasting times i.e. 6 hours food and 3 hours fluids prior to admission	
Patient aware of expected length of stay	
Discharge assessment shows no adverse factors for planned length of stay	
Patient orientated to room and surroundings	
Patient demonstrates understanding of use of call bell	
Results of pre-operative investigations indicate suitability for surgery	
Understanding of written information for consent confirmed	
Actions to deal with identified risks have been taken as specified within multidisciplinary evaluation	
Baseline observations repeated on admission to ward and recorded on observation chart if patient pre-assessed	
Patient consents to the use of PR analgesia if applicable	
Patient consents to use of bed rails following procedure	
Valuables stored: Yes / No (circle)	
Additional self care needs (specify if applicable):	

Date/Time	Multidisciplinary Evaluation	Signature/Designation

Figure 23.5 (c) Admission assessment

allowing time for them to express their fears, and for the nurse to give clear explanations of the preparation for surgery and postoperative experience. This preparation should involve the family where possible. A study by Mohan and colleagues (2005) investigating nurses' experiences caring for cancer patients in general wards revealed that they considered the work emotionally demanding, and that they felt they did not have the specialist knowledge, the time or the appropriate environment to provide quality care and support these patients and their families. There is evidence that patients with cancer should be cared for on specialist cancer wards, as the nurses would have the knowledge and skills to communicate and give appropriate psychological support to them (McCaughan and Parahoo, 2000).

S | Scenario continued

In the discussion with the nurse, Emma asks what will happen next, how long her husband will be in hospital, and how long the operation will take. She also wants to know when they will know the results and whether it has been successful.

---

a | Learning activity

Discuss with a colleague what else Mr and Mrs Osborne might ask, and what the answers to these, and the questions mentioned, should be.

The patient might also be reviewed by other members of the healthcare team, such as a physiotherapist, an anaesthetist, the colorectal nurse and a member of staff from theatre on a pre-operative visit. Risk assessments commenced in the PAC can be revisited, such as deep vein thrombosis risk assessment, pressure ulcer risk assessment, nutritional assessment and manual handling risk assessment, and any preventive measures put into place. The nurse should make sure the patient is aware of the expected length of their stay, and discuss any issues relating to a smooth discharge home.

Pre-operative care

Pre-operatively, the surgeon who will be performing the operation ensures that the patient has given their informed consent for the required operation (DH, 2001). This involves giving the patient a full explanation of what the operation entails and any potential complications. The patient has an opportunity to ask questions, and should then be willing to sign the consent form (Alexander et al, 2006).

a | Learning activity   **W**

Look up further information on informed consent, to establish who can and cannot give consent and in which circumstances, by referring to DH (2001a):

http://www.dh.gov.uk/en/
Publicationsandstatistics/Publications/
PublicationsPolicyAndGuidance/DH_4006757.

The patient then needs to be prepared physically for theatre. This involves skin preparation of a shower, wash or bath and removal of any rings, watches or necklaces (Alexander et al, 2006). They will be nil by mouth with regards food for six hours and water/clear fluids for two hours (Brady, Kinn and Stuart, 2003). This is to ensure they have an empty stomach to reduce the risk of vomiting and inhalation (O'Callaghan, 2002). Because of the length of time being nil by mouth, the patient should be offered mouth care as this is an 'essential nursing procedure' which should be an 'integral' part of hygiene (Xavier, 2000). Their bed will be prepared for transfer to theatre, which may involve a theatre canvas or equivalent for transferring them from the bed to the theatre trolley in the anaesthetic room and recovery area. They should be encouraged to pass urine (micturate) before theatre and before sedatory premedication is administered.

The nursing documentation, hospital notes, blood results, x-rays, CT scans and any other relevant medical information pertinent to the patient are collated. They are informed when to prepare physically for theatre and apply the theatre clothing. The nurse then completes the theatre checklist, which includes items such as:

- accuracy of identity bracelet – corresponds with patient records
- allergies checked against wristband
- consent form signed by patient, anaesthetist and surgeon
- any false teeth have been removed
- ascertaining whether the patient has a bridge/crown

Part

III

- whether contact lenses have been removed
- voided urine
- operation site is marked
- operation site is prepared
- x-ray and test results available
- time patient last ate documented
- time patient last drank documented
- date of last anaesthetic documented
- make-up/nail varnish removal where appropriate.

Figure 23.6 shows an example of this pre-procedure care checklist. Once the checklist has been completed, the sedatory premedication can be administered. The patient should then be encouraged to remain in bed until collection by the theatre staff in order to reduce the risk of falling.

PRE-PROCEDURE CARE

Patient Name:
Date of Birth:
Hospital Number:
Consultant:

Pre-Procedure Check List			
	Yes (✓)	No (✓)	Not Applicable (✓)
Accuracy of identity bracelet confirmed			
Identity bracelet corresponds to patient records			
Allergies checked against wrist band and patient records			
Consent form signed by patient, Anaesthetist and Consultant			
False teeth removed			
Bridge/Crown present			
Contact lenses removed			
Jewellery removed (wedding ring taped)			
Make up / nail varnish removed			
Voided Urine			
Operation site marked			
Operation site prepared			
Prosthesis/Metalwork present			
X-rays and test results available			
Pre-medication given at			
Time patient last ate:			
Time patient last drank:			
Date of last menstrual period (ask patient if she could be pregnant if applicable):			
Date of last anaesthetic			
Ward Nurse Signature	Date:		Time:
Escort Nurse Signature	Date:		Time:
Anaesthetic Practitioner Signature	Date:		Time:

Long Stay Surgery
Trial V2 Issued August 2007/Review August 2008
Page 6 of 19

Figure 23.6 Pre-procedure care checklist

Transfer to theatre

It is important to inform the patient, and their relatives if present, that they may be in theatre for between two and four hours. Based upon the local policy and guidelines of the organisation, the nurse may escort the patient to theatre. On arrival in theatre the patient is greeted by the theatre staff, and patient details are confirmed from the hospital notes and the theatre list. Staff must ascertain that a consent form has been completed and the patient has given their informed consent for the operation. The theatre staff examine the theatre checklist to ensure it has been completed fully and that any blood results, x-rays and other pertinent test results are available. The patient should be given a full explanation of all the procedures they will experience as a way of reducing anxiety (Hughes 2002). The theatre staff should try to create a calm, relaxed and quiet environment. It might be hospital policy that the ward nurse stays with the patient until they are fully anaesthetised (Dougherty and Lister, 2006).

(C) Professional conversation

Lucy, the student nurse, is going to accompany James into the anaesthetic room. She asks Teena, the staff nurse, to explain the role of the nurse in the anaesthetic room, and what will be happening to the patient. Teena explains, 'Skilful communication is very important because this is a stressful time for the patient and accurate information is necessary to ensure safety. As the nurse you need to make sure the documentation is correct, the consent form will be checked, the procedure verified with the patient, allergies checked and that any premedication prescribed has been administered.'

'The anaesthetic will be administered by an anaesthetist,' Teena continues, 'a throat pack will be inserted and the eyes will be taped shut to prevent damage to the cornea. Working in conjunction with the anaesthetist the operating department practitioner will ensure that the airway is maintained and James is positioned safely for anaesthesia, a manual handling risk assessment is made and James is moved correctly, the diathermy plate is applied and an intravenous cannula is inserted.'

The patient will be anaesthetised, intubated (a tube is passed via the mouth or nose through the trachea) and taken into the operating theatre. The consent form is checked again, the procedure verified and allergies rechecked.

Throughout the surgical procedure intravenous fluids are administered if prescribed, blood loss is measured and vital signs are monitored. A urinary catheter is inserted and urine output monitored. As the patient is at risk of developing hypothermia because they will have a large area of skin exposed for a relatively long period of time in a cool operating theatre, steps are taken to help maintain their body temperature, such as warming intravenous fluids (Scott et al, 1999).

The patient is positioned to enable the surgery to be performed. Manual handling risk reassessment and pressure ulcer risk reassessment are continued. Pressure-relieving devices may be used because of the increased risk of sores developing because of immobility, pressure, effects of anaesthetic (hypotension or hypothermia) and unconsciousness (Scott and Buckland, 2005).

The circulatory and metabolic changes that take place during surgery increase the patient's risk of developing pressure sores (NICE, 2005a). Any damage is not always apparent at the time of the operation, and becomes visible hours or days later (Scott et al, 1999), therefore prevention strategies need to be employed. Changing position may not be an option so specialised theatre mattresses or overlays may be used.

DVT is most likely to occur if there is a damaged epithelium, slow blood flow and hypercoagulable blood. These factors are known as Virchow's triad (Alexander et al, 2006). All patients undergoing surgery have an increased risk of DVT, especially those having major abdominal surgery. Many patients undergoing surgery for CRC are placed in the lithotomy position which further increases the chance of DVT. Pneumatic compression boots or Flotron boots are used as a preventive measure. The intermittent compression pushes blood from the smaller blood vessels into the deeper vessels and into the femoral veins. The increased blood flow reduces venous stasis and flushes out locally activated clotting factors. The compression decreases vessel distension, lowering the risk of injury to the endothelial layer.

> **S** | **Scenario continued**
>
> During James's operation, because he is at risk of developing DVT, intermittent compression boots are applied throughout the operation.

Table 23.2 Glossary of key terms

Endothelial layer	The layer of flat cells lining the closed spaces of the body such as the inside of blood vessels, lymphatic vessels, the heart, and body cavities.
Femoral vein	The largest vein in the groin. It passes, together with the femoral artery, beneath the inguinal ligament to enter the abdomen and form the external iliac vein. The femoral vein is one portion of the venous system that carries blood from the lower extremity back to the heart.
Locally activated clotting factors	Damage to blood vessel walls exposes subendothelium proteins, mainly collagen, present under the endothelium. When this happens coagulation begins. Primary homeostasis and platelets immediately form a plug at the site of injury.
Vessel distension	Enlargement or ballooning effect of the vessel.
Venous stasis	Congestion and slowing of circulation in veins due to blockage by either obstruction or high pressure in the venous system, usually best seen in the feet and legs.

The patient's recovery from anaesthetic

> **S** | **Scenario continued**
>
> Following surgery James is kept in the recovery area until the immediate effects of the anaesthetic have worn off. He should be able to maintain his own airway, and his observations should be stable before he returns to the ward (Alexander et al, 2006).

Scoring systems have been devised in order to assess a patient's suitability and safety for leaving the recovery area and returning to the ward. Examples of these include the post-anaesthesia discharge scoring system (PADSS) (Chung, 1995) and the Aldrete system (Aldrete, 1998). As with other scoring systems the patient in recovery is given a score related to an assessment or observation which the nurse makes. This can include the patient's vital signs, nausea and vomiting, pain levels, any bleeding, consciousness and colour. When the patient has scored a specified number following the assessment, this gives the nurse a more objective opinion of when they are suitable for discharge from the recovery care.

ANAESTHETIC ROOM CARE

Patient Name:		Date:
Date of Birth:		Time into Anaesthetic Room:
Hospital Number:		Anaesthetic Room Practitioner:
Consultant:		Signature:

Intervention	Initial
Patient positioned safely for anaesthesia	
Consent form checked	
Procedure verified with patient	
Allergies checked	
Intravenous cannula inserted	
Medication administered prior to surgery as prescribed	
Intravenous fluids administered as prescribed	
Vital signs monitored and within normal limits	
Anaesthetic administered by Consultant (specify type):	
Airway maintained. Type of airway used (specify):	
Throat pack inserted Yes / No (circle)	
Eyes taped Yes / No (circle)	
Manual handling risk assessed. Correct techniques for moving patient adopted and specified in multidisciplinary evaluation. Patient transferred to theatre	

Date/Time	Multidisciplinary Evaluation	Signature/Designation

Peripheral IVI	X
IV Cannulae	C
ECG Electrodes	■
CVP	Z
Arterial Line	O
BP Cuff	B
Pulse Oximeter	H
Diathermy Plate	●
Temperature Probe	▲
Other	

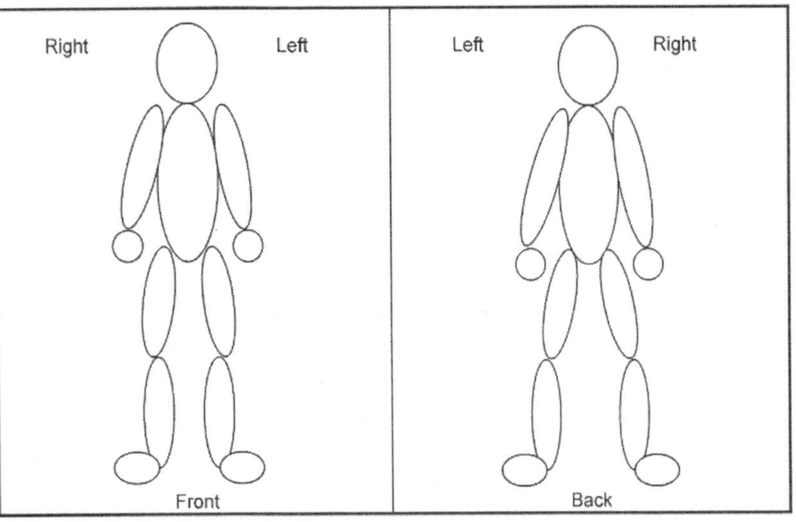

Right   Left   Left   Right   Front   Back

Figure 23.7 Anaesthetic room care

CARE DURING PROCEDURE

Patient Name:		Date:	
Date of Birth:		Time Entering Theatre:	
Hospital Number:		Theatre Practitioner:	
Consultant:		Signature:	

Intervention	Initial
Patient positioned safely during procedure (specify position):	
Consent form checked	
Procedure and operative side verified	
Allergies checked	
Manual handling risk assessed	
Correct techniques for moving patient adopted: Patslide / Lift / Self (circle)	
Table attachments used (specify):	
Pressure sore risk assessed: High / Medium / Low (circle)	
Pressure area relieving devices used (specify):	
Venous foot pumps applied: Yes / No (circle)	
Patient Warming Device Yes / No (circle)	
Skin Preparation (specify):	
Tourniquet: Left Arm Right Arm Time On (specify): Pressure mm/Hg Left Leg Right Leg Time Off (specify):	
Irrigation fluid use (specify):	
Intravenous fluids/blood transfusion maintained	
Catheter inserted (give details including name of person inserting catheter):	
Packs (specify):	
Drains (specify): Sutured Yes / No (circle)	
Blood loss measure and recorded on fluid balance chart	
Skin Closure (specify):	
Dressings (specify):	
Infiltration (specify):	
Implants Yes / No (circle and specify details on following page)	
Type of specimens taken (specify): Number of specimens taken (specify):	
Diathermy plate removed and site shows no adverse skin reactions	
Throat Pack Removed: Yes / Not applicable	
Procedure Performed (specify):	
Patient transferred to recovery	

Figure 23.8 Care during procedure

Table 23.3 **The main areas of concern immediately following surgery**

Airway	When the endotracheal tube is removed it is essential to maintain a patent airway. This may involve suctioning. Ensure nothing is obstructing the airway, such as the tongue, a foreign body, blood, secretions, vomit or laryngeal spasm. Position the patient in the semi-prone or lateral position, tilt the head backwards and pull the mandible forwards to help achieve this. A Guedel airway can be used and left in position. This will be expelled by the patient when reflexes return (Alexander et al, 2006).
Breathing	Respiratory assessment is performed, involving the patient's rate, depth, rhythm, noises and bilateral movement. There is a potential for hypoventilation caused by opiates or anaesthetic inhalations or hyperventilation caused by anxiety, pain or shock. The patient may receive prescribed oxygen via a face mask in order to break down anaesthetic gases and prevent chest infections. Aspiration pneumonia can occur if the patient vomits while regaining consciousness, therefore suction equipment should be readily available.
Level of consciousness	The patient's consciousness level will be continually monitored and they will be orientated to time and place. Bedrails can be used for patient safety if considered necessary.
Circulatory status	Observations should be made every five minutes on: • skin colour • skin perfusion, checked by estimating the capillary refill time • pulse – tachycardia may occur due to pain, hypovolaemia, anaesthetic drugs, septicaemia, fear, fluid overload • blood pressure: there might be hypotension caused by hypovolaemia, effects of analgesia, or hypertension, as a result of pain, anxiety, some anaesthetic drugs.
Wound	The recovery nurse will be made aware of the surgical procedure undertaken and will observe the wound for swelling, haemorrhage, **haematoma**, bleeding or large **serous** ooze; Any drains will be observed for the amount and nature of blood and serious fluid loss.
Temperature	Body temperature will be observed to identify any hypothermia caused by **vasodilation**, exposure in theatre, large amounts of IV fluids or any **pyrexia** caused by infection or blood transfusion reaction.
Fluid balance	The patient's fluid balance is monitored continually, maintaining totals of input via an intravenous infusion/blood transfusion and output via a urinary catheter, drains and nasogastric tube. Reduced urine from the urinary catheter can be the result of obstruction of catheter, inadequate output because of low **systolic pressure**, hypovolaemia or dehydration, The cannula site should be checked frequently to ensure correct positioning and flow. Sips of water may be allowed as required. If the patient is nil by mouth for a period of time, mouthcare will be need to be performed.
Pain	The patient is provided with pain relief, which will have commenced in theatre and is administered on a continual basis. In surgical trauma pain is worsened by fear, anxiety and restlessness (Alexander et al, 2006), therefore the patient should be reassured as they regain consciousness. The patient may have patient-controlled analgesia or an epidural.
Nausea and vomiting	Postoperative nausea and vomiting is a potential factor caused by opiates, hypotension, abdominal surgery or pain – therefore prescribed anti-emetics may be administered as required or **prophylactically** (Alexander et al, 2006).
Manual handling risk assessment	Correct techniques must be used when moving the patient.
Pressure ulcer risk assessment	Preventive measures should be continued. The patient's position should be changed regularly based on the pressure ulcer risk assessment.
DVT	Stockings and/or intermittent compression boots may be used.
Communication	Good communication is essential to reduce the patient's anxiety and assist in their regaining their awareness of what is happening. Hearing is the first sense to return, and verbal reassurance should be given to the patient that the operation is completed and they should be told where they are.
Documentation	Accurate and thorough documentation should be provided to ensure safety and continuity of care – procedure details, current status, treatments and medical orders should all be recorded clearly.

Part

III

Table 23.4 Glossary of key terms 2

Patent	Open
Capillary refill time	Capillary refill is the rate at which **blood** refills empty **capillaries**. It can be measured by pressing a **fingernail** until it turns white, and taking note of the time needed for colour to return once the nail is released. Normal refill time is less than 2 seconds. The capillary refill time (CRT) is a common measure of **peripheral perfusion**.
Haematoma	A collection of blood in tissue under the skin or in an internal organ as a result of injury to the tissue or organ, or to an abnormal bleeding tendency.
Hypovolaemia	A state of decreased **blood** volume.
Perfusion	The process of nutritive delivery of **arterial blood** to a **capillary** bed in the **tissue**
Prophylactic	A drug or agent that is given to prevent infection, disease or condition.
Pyrexia	A condition characterised by an abnormally high core body temperature, caused by an imbalance between heat production and heat loss.
Serous	Serous fluid is thin watery fluid like serum, a clear liquid that can be separated from clotted blood.
Systolic pressure	Peak pressure in the arteries, which occurs near the beginning of the cardiac cycle when the **ventricles** are contracting.
Tachycardia	Rapid heart rate.
Vasodilation	Refers to the widening of **blood vessels** resulting from relaxation of **smooth muscle** cells within the vessel walls.

When the patient has met the criteria for leaving the recovery unit, the ward area is contacted and the patient is transferred to the ward. It is important that the recovery nurse remains with the patient during their time in recovery. When transferring the patient back to the ward nurse, they must hand over any specific postoperative instructions. Observations must be taken and recorded immediately before discharge from the recovery unit.

> **S** Scenario continued
>
> James has made the initial recovery from the anaesthetic and is ready to be returned to the ward.

Postoperative care

> **a** Learning activity
>
> Discuss with a colleague the purpose of postoperative care.

Preparations must be made to receive the patient back from theatre: their bedspace and the immediate environment readied, and all the necessary equipment put in place: typically a drip stand, oxygen mask and suction apparatus. There is a handover from the theatre staff, who should inform the nurse exactly what operation the patient has had performed, the recovery care, any potential complications, the pain relief given, the present fluid balance and any specific postoperative instructions.

The nurse should communicate effectively with the patient in order to orientate them to the ward environment and as a way of assessing the quality of their airway patency. The nurse should then commence a systematic assessment of the patient.

RECOVERY CARE

Patient Name:	Date:
Date of Birth:	Time Entering Recovery:
Hospital Number:	Recovery Practitioner:
Consultant:	Signature:

Observations on entry into recovery:

BP	Temp	Pulse	Resps	SAO2	O2 Flow

Intervention	Initial
Patient's airway maintained. Time airway removed (specify):	
Patient positioned in accordance with comfort and to prevent complications.	
Manual handling risk assessed Correct techniques for moving patient adopted and specified in multidisciplinary evaluation	
Vital signs recorded at 5 minute intervals and within normal limits	
Oxygen administered as prescribed	
Pressure sore risk assessed: High / Medium / Low (circle)	
Pressure area relieving devices used (specify):	
Venous foot pumps in situ and functioning	
Epidural/PCA infusion maintained at prescribed rate with no adverse effects	
Patient does not appear distressed by pain or nausea	
Cannula site patent and secure	
Intravenous fluids/blood transfusion administered at prescribed rate with no adverse effects	
Wound drains patent/amount and nature and amount of drainage monitored	
Operative site clean and dry	
Sips of water tolerated as desired	
Patient is safely recovered from anaesthetic as evidenced by level of consciousness	
Patient's colour is perfused	
Patient is able to move four extremities	
Patient demonstrates 'usual' breathing pattern	
Progress reviewed by Anaesthetist	

Observations of Discharge from Recovery:

BP	Temp	Pulse	Resps	SAO2	O2 Flow

Procedure details, current status, treatments and medical orders handed over to ward nurse	
Patient transferred to ward (specify time):	

Figure 23.9 Recovery care

Part
III

POST-OPERATIVE CARE

| Patient Name: |
| Date of Birth: |
| Hospital Number: |
| Consultant: |

Signature of Nurse Responsible for Care			
	Date	Time	Signature
am			
pm			
night			

Intervention	Initial		
	am	pm	nt
Post-operative observations stable compared to baseline (state frequency of recordings on observation chart)			
Pain is controlled to the patient's satisfaction (level of pain and interventions recorded on MEWS chart)			
Epidural/PCA infusion maintained at prescribed rate with no adverse effects			
Nausea is controlled			
Oxygen is administered as prescribed			
Wound remains clean and dry with dressing intact			
Wound drain is patent and drainage is monitored			
Manual handling risk assessed Correct techniques for moving patient adopted and specified in multidisciplinary evaluation			
Pressure sore risk assessed: High / Medium / Low (circle)			
Pressure area relieving devices used (specify):			
Measures to prevent DVT are in place (specify):			
Intravenous fluids administered at prescribed rate with no adverse effects			
Oral fluids (as permitted) tolerated			
Diet (as permitted) tolerated			
Cannula site patent and secure			
Patient has passed urine and output is satisfactory			
Additional self care needs (specify if applicable):			

Figure 23.10 Postoperative care

Assessing the airway

There are many ways in which the airway might be compromised postoperatively (Walker, 2003). These include foreign objects, vomit, bronchospasm, a blocked or poorly positioned artificial airway and an anaphylactic response to drugs or an allergen. Therefore, it is essential that the nurse assesses the patient's airway in order to ensure adequate oxygen amounts are able to enter the lungs for oxygenation purposes. If the airway is occluded in any way, then immediate action should be taken to rectify this predicament. This may involve the insertion of an artificial airway, the chin lift technique to open up the airway, or positioning the patient in a lateral or semiprone position.

a Learning activity

Find out the accurate positioning of patients to assist in the provision of a good airway. Make sure you can perform the chin lift technique.

The nursing care of a surgical patient is mainly concerned with assessment and observation, and often in the postoperative period this is based on routine and regular observations. The traditional pattern for the assessment of vital signs is every 15 minutes for the first hour, then hourly for four hours, reducing to four-hourly over the next 12 to 24 hours (Zeitz, 2005).

There appears to be little written evidence on best practice for frequency and period of time to record vital signs following surgery (Zeitz and McCutcheon, 2003).

Table 23.5 Glossary of key terms 3

Bronchospasm	A sudden constriction of the muscles in the walls of the **bronchioles**.
Anaphylactic	An **acute systemic** (multisystem) and severe **allergic** reaction.
Occluded	Blocked.

Respiratory assessment

Once the patient's airway has been established, their breathing status should be assessed and continually monitored. This is in order to determine the adequacy of the gaseous exchange of oxygen and carbon dioxide. The aspects of breathing that should be regularly assessed include the rate of breathing, the rhythm, the depth, any noises, and the oxygen saturation level.

The 'normal rate' of breathing is between 10 and 17 breaths per minute (Moore, 2007). If the patient's breathing rate is above 18 breaths per minute (tachypnoea) or below ten breaths per minute (bradypnoea), this assessment should be reported and acted upon very swiftly. The 'rhythm' of breathing is another imperative assessment to make. The nurse should assess that the patient's breathing is equal, bilateral and symmetrical (Ahern and Philpot, 2002) and also observe for any breathing difficulty.

Table 23.6 Glossary of key terms 4

Auscultation	The technical term for listening to the internal sounds of the body, usually using a **stethoscope**. It is performed for the purposes of examining the **circulatory system** and **respiratory system** (**heart sounds** and **breath sounds**), as well as the **gastrointestinal system** (bowel sounds).
Cyanosis	A blue colouration of the **skin** and **mucous membranes** due to the presence of deoxygenated **hemoglobin** in **blood vessels** near the skin surface.
Hypoxaemia	A deficiency in the concentration of dissolved oxygen in **arterial** blood.
Hypoxia	A deficiency in oxygen.
Pulse oximetry	A **noninvasive** method allowing the monitoring of the **oxygenation** of a patient's **hemoglobin**.
Rales	Rales, crackles or crepitations, are the clicking, rattling or crackling noises heard on auscultation of (listening to) the **lung** with a **stethoscope** during **inhalation**.
Stridor	A high-pitched sound resulting from turbulent air flow in the upper airway. It may be inspiratory, expiratory or present on both inspiration and expiration.
Vasoconstriction	The narrowing of the blood vessels resulting from contraction of the muscular wall of the vessels, particularly the large **arteries**, **arterioles** and **veins**.

The depth of the patient's breathing should be assessed, as should any noises being made. The breathing should be regular and effortless. The patient's skin should be observed to identify any **cyanosis**, which can occur when the oxygen saturations of arterial blood drops below 85 per cent (Ahern and Philpot, 2002).

The patient's **pulse oximetry** should be monitored to established the percentage of haemoglobin that is saturated with oxygen. The patient will be receiving prescribed oxygen therapy at a prescribed rate, for a prescribed amount of time in order to maintain their oxygen saturation levels above 95 per cent. This will sustain satisfactory levels of oxygenation and will prevent **hypoxia** and **hypoxaemia**. Potential problems with recording accuracy associated with oxygen saturation reading include peripheral **vasoconstriction**, if the patient is shivering, if dried blood is present and if the probe is dirty (Walsh, 2002). Additionally, pressure ulcers on fingers have been identified in patients with oxygen saturation readings, so it is imperative that the probe is moved to different digits at regular intervals.

The rationale for observing the patient's breathing regularly postoperatively is to identify any potential signs of inadequate ventilation. These can include hypoventilation, slow, shallow breathing, respiratory **stridor** indicated by a large wheeze, restlessness, increased heart rate and cyanosis, rales detected by auscultation and any audible gurgling respiration or excessive secretions (Walsh, 2002).

Circulatory assessment

It is crucial that the patient's cardiovascular system is monitored on a regular basis postoperatively in order to identify potential complications swiftly. These can include haemorrhage, types of shock, dehydration or fluid overload.

The patient's skin colour should also be monitored; it should be pink and warm. If their skin is observed as pale and cool this could be an indication of reduced peripheral perfusion (blood reaching the skin), and it is then wise to perform a capillary refill time measurement. This is performed by the nurse by pressing the fingertip against the skin for 5 seconds. The skin colour should blanch and then should return to normal within 2 seconds. If the refill time is more than 2 seconds it could mean reduced peripheral perfusion (Jevon 2007).

The patient's vital signs, including pulse, respiration, BP and temperature, should probably be monitored every 15 minutes for the first hour, then hourly for four hours, then four-hourly. The nurse should be aware of local guidelines regarding observations and frequency.

Subbe and colleagues (2001) describe a modified early warning system which is used in their care setting in order to identify patients in the early stages of deterioration. The nurse assesses and scores the patient's BP, pulse, respiratory rate, temperature, conscious level and urine output. Also known as a 'track and trigger' system (Oakey and Slade, 2006), this is used to identify and assess unwell hospital patients and allows health professionals to look for trends in the patient's physiology. Subtle changes that might otherwise be missed lead to a changing score which may indicate that the patient's condition is deteriorating.

> **ⓐ Learning activity**   W
>
> Look up an early warning system scoring chart at http://www.ihi.org/IHI/Topics/ PatientSafety/SafetyGeneral/Tools/ ColourBandedEarlyWarningObservationChart.htm

Level of consciousness

On return to the ward it is prudent to assess the patient's orientation to their surroundings and their responsiveness. This is in order to detect altered levels of consciousness, which can be caused by cerebral hypoperfusion (reduced blood flow to the brain) or hypoxia (Hughes, 2004) or drugs (Ahern and Philpot, 2002) such as anaesthesia, sedation or analgesics. Any changes to their consciousness should be reported and recorded.

Body temperature

The patient's temperature should be recorded regularly in order to identify hypothermia or pyrexia. An abnormal temperature can indicate the presence of an infection, a deteriorating patient and disorders of the patient's thermoregulatory function (Carroll, 2000).

Pain control

It is important to assess the patient's pain. Pain should be assessed using a recognised, evidence-based assessment tool based upon the scales described by Mackintosh (2005). These include the verbal ratings scale, the visual analogue scale, the verbal analogue scale and the numerical rating scale. One purpose of this is to determine the effectiveness of pain relief.

The patient might have been given a patient-controlled analgesia (PCA) system or an epidural infusion. A PCA is a system whereby the patient self-administers a determined small dose of morphine intravenously (Mackintosh, 2007). In an epidural infusion, a catheter is inserted into the patient's epidural space and a combination of opioid analgesia (a chemical substance that has a morphine-like action in the body) and/or anaesthetic drugs is delivered in a predetermined dose via a syringe driver. The combination of exceptional pain relief and negligible side-effects provides high patient contentment with epidural analgesia compared with other methods of relieving pain (Weetman and Allison, 2006).

Fluid balance

It is essential that the patient's fluid balance is monitored on a continual basis. They will be at risk of fluid and **electrolyte imbalance** for many reasons, such as dehydration caused by bowel preparation, an **infiltrated cannula**, poor fluid prescription and inappropriate postoperative fasting (Anderson, 2003; Hughes, 2004).

It is important to assess the patient's condition and to keep an accurate record of output and intake. Depending on hospital protocol regarding the operation, the patient might be nil by mouth or allowed some fluids orally. Intake can be from oral intake (if permitted) or from prescribed intravenous infusion. Common intravenous fluids which could be administered include 0.9 per cent sodium chloride, 5 per cent dextrose and Hartmann's solution.

Output from the patient can be from any wound drains, vomitus or nasogastric tube aspiration and urine from a catheter. An accepted normal urine output is 1.5–2 litres within 24 hours or 1 ml per kg per hour (Ahern and Philpot, 2002). It is important to identify a poor urine output as this is an early indication of a deteriorating patient. Smith (2000) suggests that a minimum urine output should be >0.5ml/kg /hour. It is important for a student nurse to report poor urine output so that an effective treatment strategy is commenced swiftly in order to prevent renal failure from occurring.

Table 23.7 Glossary of key terms 5

Electrolyte imbalance	The chemicals in the bloodstream regulate important functions in the body. When dissolved in water these chemicals are electrolytes: they separate into positively and negatively charged ions. The body's nerve reactions and muscle function are dependent on the proper exchange of these electrolyte ions outside and inside cells. Electrolyte imbalances can develop by excessive ingestion, diminished elimination of an electrolyte, diminished ingestion or excessive elimination of an electrolyte.
Infiltrated cannula	Infiltration occurs when the infusion cannula is no longer fully in the vein.

Wound care

It is important for the nurse to perform wound care. This involves checking the dressing for oozing, checking the wound for complications and monitoring any drain output. It is necessary to establish whether the patient has any barriers that would impede wound healing and try to correct them. This can include poor nutrition, obesity and diabetes (Watret and White, 2001). Complications of the wound which should be observed for include wound infection, haemorrhage, haematoma, dehiscence and sinus formation.

Risk assessments

The nurse should revisit the risk assessments for the patient, including the manual handling assessment and the pressure ulcer risk assessment. If the degree of risk has changed postoperatively, the nurse should be aware of the associated evidence-based care involved. Additionally, the patient's care plan or care pathway will guide the nurse regarding how much the patient can mobilise. It is common practice for the patient to remain on bed rest on the day of the operation.

Part

III

Patient name					Hospital number		Date		
INTAKE (ML)					**OUTPUT (ML)**				
Time	ORAL		INTRAVENOUS		URINE		NASO-GASTRIC		DRAIN
	Volume taken	Total	Volume started	Total	Volume measured	Total	Volume measured	Total	Vol	Total
0100										
0200										
0300										
0400										
0500										
0600										
0700										
0800										
0900										
1000										
1100										
1200										
1300										
1400										
1500										
1600										
1700										
1800										
1900										
2000										
2100										
2200										
2300										
2400										

Figure 23.11 Fluid balance chart

> **a Learning activity**
>
> Discuss with a colleague how James's risk assessment might have changed.

Hygiene

The patient's hygiene requirements need to be assessed and any assistance given as required, while promoting the patient's independence. This may include assisting the patient to wash their hands and face, or provision of mouth care. A healthy oral status is essential for patient comfort and general contentment (White, 2000). It is essential that the nurse provides individualised nursing care relating to oral hygiene, involving a toothbrush and research-based products (Evans, 2001).

> **a Learning activity**
>
> Discuss with your mentor how a patient's mouth should be assessed and the provision of oral care.

Medications

It may be necessary to administer medicines to the patient. These medicines might be in relation to any previous medical conditions they suffer from, or related to the operation. They could include analgesia (a PCA or epidural analgesia as previously stated), prescribed oxygen therapy, anti-emetic medication or antibiotics. These medicines should be administered strictly adhering to local guidelines of medicines management as well as the safe principles of administering medications (NMC, 2002a).

Nausea and vomiting

Postoperative nausea and vomiting may be an issue for the patient following the operation. It is imperative that the nurse assesses and monitors this situation and administers anti-emetics if required. Factors which may increase the patient's risk of having postoperative nausea and vomiting include having abdominal surgery (Habib and Gan, 2001), reduced oral intake (Kenny and Rowbotham, 1992) and the type of anaesthetic used (Larsson and Lundberg, 1995).

> **a Learning activity**
>
> Investigate other factors that might cause postoperative nausea and vomiting.

Documentation

The nurse must ensure that as well as giving nursing care which is evidence-based, this care is thoroughly documented. This documentation within the care plan, care pathway, risk assessment forms, patient evaluation and drug chart should be in line with the guidelines issued by the NMC (2002b). Hence, the documentation should be 'factual', 'accurate', and a 'full account of your assessment and the care you have planned and provided'.

The days following the operation

The length of the postoperative period will depend upon the patient's individual progression and recovery from the operation and individual differences in practice within care settings. This will be a time of recuperation for the patient, continuous observation of their condition and promotion of independence.

The patient will increase their activity daily, and equipment that has aided their recovery will be gradually removed by the nurse when the need for it has ceased. This will involve removing the patient's nasogastric tube usually when the patient has bowel sounds, has no nausea or vomiting and is drinking adequate amounts of fluid to satisfy their requirements. The patient may have restricted fluid and food for a few days postoperatively until the peristaltic action of their bowel recommences adequately. This should mean that the patient is eating normally by postoperative day 4 or 5, depending on their progression. This also means that the intravenous infusion is discontinued when it is no longer required.

(e) Evidence-based practice

Following gastrointestinal surgery it is traditional to fast the patient until bowel function has returned, which is usually approximately five days (Ng and Neill, 2006). The rationale for this was the fear of postoperative complications such as prolonged **ileus, anastomotic breakdown**, bowel obstruction and **aspiration pneumonia**. Fasting with nasogastric suction is thought to reduce nausea, vomiting and abdominal distension and to allow healing time for the **anastomosis** (Lewis, 2001). However these symptoms occur more commonly in upper gastrointestinal surgery (Silk and Gow, 2001). A review of the literature by Ng and Neill (2006) found that early oral feeding was safe and well tolerated, and resulted in a shorter period of ileus and reduced hospitalisation time.

Table 23.8   Glossary of key terms 6

Anastomotic breakdown	When the join between two parts of the bowel breaks apart.
Anastomosis	The connection of two structures. It refers to connections between **blood vessels** or between other tubular structures such as loops of **intestine**.
Aspiration pneumonia	An acute, chemical lung injury resulting from the inhalation of gastric contents.
Ileus	A disruption of the normal propulsive **gastrointestinal** motor activity from nonmechanical mechanisms.
Peristaltic action	The wavelike muscular contractions of the intestine or other tubular structure that propel the contents onward by alternate contraction and relaxation.

The urinary catheter which has been in situ since theatre will also be removed, once its role in assisting fluid balance measurements has diminished. It will be imperative that the nurse ensures the patient is able to pass urine satisfactorily following the removal of the catheter. The PCA system or the epidural analgesia infusion will be removed when it has been assessed that the patient's pain levels can be controlled on oral analgesia. If the patient has a drainage tube from their wound area, this is removed using an aseptic technique when its role of removing serous fluid and blood loss has ceased.

(S) Scenario continued

James is recovering steadily from his operation. He has been receiving prescribed oxygen continually via a mask or nasal prong since his return to the ward from theatre.

Any delivery of oxygen should be for a prescribed period of time. Then, in consultation with the anaesthetist, the patient's need should be assessed, which can be aided by the monitoring of their oxygen saturations on air. Once it is no longer required it is discontinued.

From the first day postoperation the patient should be assisted out of bed and mobilised for short distances. This can be assisted by the physiotherapist, and the level of mobility will increase daily as the patient recuperates.

The wound dressing should stay intact for several days. This will depend on the hospital's policy for wound management. At the appropriate time it is removed using an aseptic technique and the wound redressed with a suitable evidence-based type of dressing.

The patient will have to be advised that postoperatively when their bowels are used, they may have urgency, diarrhoea and loose stools. This can take several months to settle down (www.surgerydoor.co.uk, 2007).

(a) Learning activity

Look up the physiological process of wound healing. Contact the tissue viability nurse to find out the hospital wound management policy.

> **a Learning activity**
>
> What are the potential complications postoperatively which the nurse will be trying to identify and prevent?

Preparing for discharge

The length of time spent in hospital has reduced over recent years, which has increased the importance of preparing the patient to return home.

> **S Scenario continued**
>
> James's good recovery has continued, and he is now ready to be discharged home.

> **a Learning activity**
>
> Discuss with a colleague why the length of hospital stay has been reduced in recent years.

Planning the patient's discharge should begin before hospitalisation for planned surgery. Evidence shows that patients who receive accurate and relevant information are less likely to require support following discharge (Williams, 2007). Studies have revealed that following gastrointestinal surgery patients require information on wound and pain management, activity level, nutrition and possible complications, and that verbal information supported by written advice is the most beneficial (Williams, 2007).

Before going home any medications the patient will need to continue following discharge, such as mild analgesics, will be discussed with them. A small supply of medications will be provided by the hospital pharmacy with written advice for their administration. Advice will be given by the nurses on how to care for the wound and how to recognise any signs of infection. Dietary advice will be provided by the hospital dietician, and supported by written nutritional advice leaflets.

The patient should also be given information before discharge regarding the importance of resting, since for a period of time following discharge they will feel tired and weak. It might be several months before the patient has fully recovered. They can be advised, for example, to rest between periods of light activity for the first few weeks, and not lift anything, garden or mow the lawn for six weeks postoperatively. It is also imperative that the patient does not drive until they are able to perform an emergency stop. They should also be encouraged to check their insurance policy as it may contain a clause about driving after operations. They can return to normal activity after three months as far as driving, sexual relations and heavier work are concerned (www.surgerydoor.co.uk,nd).

The patient might have sutures or clips which need removal at around seven to ten days. This can be done in the outpatients department, by a district nurse or at the GP surgery by the practice nurse. The patient will be asked to return to the outpatients department when the histological report of the removed part of the bowel is available, and this will be discussed with the consultant (or junior doctor) and the colorectal nurse.

The colorectal nurse will have an important role to play in the ongoing care of the patient and supporting the family. Following surgery for CRC a repeat colonoscopy should be performed every three years, and the client's carcinoembryonic antigen measured every three months (Kumar and Clark, 2005).

An increasing number of people survive cancer, but the knowledge that they have had cancer has an impact on their lives. Cancer disrupts the individual's time and life perspective. People tend to put a greater value on their time, and prioritise how and with whom they wish to spend their time. It is important that patients who survive cancer are given support from specialist nurses to enable them to re-establish their lives (Rasmussen and Elverdam, 2007).

Part III

> **(a) Learning activity**
>
> Discuss with a colleague how James's diagnosis of cancer might affect his wife and children, and their relationships.

Conclusion

The exact cause of CRC is unknown. There are some genetic links, so either genetic mutations or genetically inherited diseases such as adenomatous polyps predispose to the condition. Other conditions such as ulcerative colitis and Crohn's disease can also increase the risk. The incidence of CRC strongly suggests links with a sedentary lifestyle, overeating and diets high in meat, especially red and processed meat. Other factors are thought to reduce the risk, include a diet high in fibre and exercise. Therefore health promotion has an important role in prevention of this disease.

CRC is common in the United Kingdom. If it is detected in its early stages the prognosis is improved. The more advanced the cancer, the less chance the treatment will be curative, but it can slow the progress of the disease. To improve early detection, health education services are attempting to foster greater awareness of the early signs of the disease.

Survival rates have improved, but half the patients who have undergone what was hoped to be curative resection for CRC will relapse and eventually die within five years from local recurrence or metatases. This is caused by micro metatases invisible at the time of surgery, and the risks are higher in Dukes stage C (50 per cent) and stage B (30 per cent) (Cassidy et al, 2006). But if the cancer is treated early, before it has spread to other organs, the chances of a full recovery are about 80 per cent.

This chapter has looked at the journey of a patient from primary care, diagnosis, admission to hospital for surgery, followed by recovery from the operation until discharge home. The care required throughout this journey has been discussed and supported with appropriate evidence.

References

Ahern, J. and Philpot, P. (2002) 'Assessing acutely ill patients on general wards', *Nursing Standard* **16**(47), 47–54.

Aldrete, J. A. (1998) 'Modifications to the post anaesthesia score for use in ambulatory surgery', *Journal of Perianaesthesia Nursing* **13**(3), 148–55.

Alexander, M., Fawcett, J. and Runciman, P. (eds) (2006) in *Nursing Practice: Hospital and home the adult*, 3rd edn, Edinburgh, Churchill Livingstone, pp. 129–31.

Anderson, I. (2003) *Care of the Critically Ill Surgical Patient*, 2nd edn, London, Arnold.

Association of Anaesthetists of Great Britain and Ireland (AAGBI) (2001) *Pre-Operative Assessment: The role of the anaesthetist.* London, AAGBI.

Audit Commission (2000) *Inpatient Admissions and Bed Management in NHS Acute Hospitals*, London, HMSO.

Autar, R. (1996) 'Nursing assessment of clients at risk of deep vein thrombosis: the Autar DVT scale', *Journal of Advanced Nursing* **23**(4), 763–70.

Autar, R. (2003) 'The management of deep vein thrombosis: the Autar DVT risk assessment scale revisited', *Journal of Orthopaedic Nursing* **7**(3), 114–24.

Beck, A. (2007) 'Nurse-led pre operative assessment for elective surgical patients', *Nursing Standard* **21**(51), 35–8.

Behar, J. (2007) 'Anaesthesia: introduction and preoperative assessment', *Student British Medical Journal* 15(January), 1–44.

Bennett, G., Dealey, C. and Posnett, J. (2004) 'The cost of pressure ulcers in the UK', *Age and Aging* 33, 230–5.

Braden, B. J. and Bergstrom, N. (1987) 'A conceptual schema for the study of aetiology of pressure ulcers', *Rehabilitation Nurse* **12**(1), 8–12.

Brady, M., Kinn, S. and Stuart, P. (2003) 'Pre-operative fasting for adults to prevent peri-operative complications', *Cochrane Reviews* 4, art. no. CD004423.

Breeze, J. (?date) 'Colorectal cancer', *Nursing Times* 97(39), pp?.

British Association for Parenteral and Enteral Nutrition (BAPEN) (2003) *The Malnutrition Universal Screening Tool (MUST)*, Maidenhead, BAPEN.

Campbell, H., Hotchkiss, R., Bradshaw, N. and Porteous, M. (1998) 'Integrated care pathways', *British Medicial Journal* 316, 133–7.

Carroll, M. (2000) 'An evaluation of temperature measurement', *Nursing Standard* **14**(44), 39–43.

Casey, A. (2007) 'Partnership model of nursing', in Glasper, E., McEwing, G. and Richardson, J. (eds), *Oxford Handbook of Children's and Young People's Nursing*, Oxford, Oxford University Press.

Cassidy, J., Bissett, D., Spence, R. and Payne, M. (2006) *Oxford Handbook of Oncology*, 2nd edn, Oxford, Oxford University Press.

Charous, B. L., Blanco, C., Tarb, S., Hamilton, R. G., Baur, X., Beechold, D., Sussman, G. and Yunginger, J. W. (2002) 'Natural rubber latex allergy after 12 years: recommendations and perspectives', *Journal of Allergy and Clinical Immunology* 109, 31–4.

Chung, F. (1995) 'Recovery pattern and home readiness after ambulatory surgery', *Anaesthesia and Analgesia* **80**(5), 896–902.

Clinical Outcomes Working Group I2000) *Clinical Outcome Indicators Report* [online] http://www.crag.scot.nhs.uk/committees/croc/coi00.htm (accessed 9 February 2009).

Colley, S. (2003) 'Nursing theory: its importance to practice', *Nursing Standard* **17**(46), 33–7.

De-Luc, K. (2000) 'Care pathways: an evaluation of their effectiveness', *Journal of Advanced Nursing* **32**(2), 485–96.

Department of Health (DH) (2000) *Referral Guidelines for Suspected Cancer*, London, DH [online] www.dh.gov.uk/PublicationsAndStatistics/Publications/PublicationsPolicyAndGuidance/PublicationsPolicyAndGuidanceArticle/fs/en?CONTENT_ID=4008746&chk=jtslsg (accessed 9 August 2008).

(DH) (2001a) *Reference Guide to Consent for Examination or Treatment*, London, HMSO [online] http://www.dh.gov.uk/en/Publicationsandstatistics/Publications/PublicationsPolicyAndGuidance/DH_4006757 (accessed 10 December 2008.

DH (2001b) *National Service Framework for Older People*, London, DH.

DH (2003b) *Essence of Care: Patient-focused benchmarks for clinical governance*, London, DH.

DH (2003a) *Discharge from Hospital: Pathway, process and practice*, London, HMSO.)

Dougherty, L. and Lister, S. (2006) *The Royal Marsden Hospital Manual of Clinical Nursing Procedures*, 6th edn, Oxford, Blackwell.

European Pressure Ulcer Advisory Panel (EPUAP) (2002) 'Summary report on the prevalence of pressure ulcers' *EPUAP Review* **4**(2), 49–57.

Evans, G. (2001) 'A rationale for oral care', *Nursing Standard* **15**(43), 33–6.

Glasson, J., Chang, E., Chenoweth, L., Hancock, K., Hall, T., Hill-Murray, F. and Collier, L. (2006) 'Evaluation of a model of nursing for older patients using participatory action research in an acute medical ward', *Journal of Clinical Nursing* 15, 588–98.

Habib, A. and Gan, T. (2001) 'Combination therapy for post operative nausea and vomiting: a more effective prophylaxis', *International Journal of Ambulatory Surgery* **9**(2), 59–71.

Hayward, J. (1975) *Information: A prescription against pain*, London, RCN.

Herring, L. (1999) 'Critical pathways: an efficient way to manage care', *Nursing Standard* **13**(47), 36–7.

Hobbs, R. (2000) 'ABC of colorectal cancer: the role of primary care', *British Medical Journal* 321, 1068–70.

House of Commons Health Committee (2005) *Government Response to the House of Commons Health Committee Report on the Prevention of Venous Thrombolism in Hospitalised Patients*, London, HMSO.

Hughes, E. (2004) 'Principles of post operative patient care', *Nursing Standard* **19**(5), 43–51.

Hughes, S. (2002) 'The effects of giving patients pre-operative information', *Nursing Standard* **16**(28), 33–7.

Jevon, P. (2007) 'Measuring capillary refill time', *Nursing Times* **103**(12), 26–7.

Kenny, G. and Rowbotham, D. (eds) (1992) *Postoperative Nausea and Vomiting*, London, Synergy Medical Education.

Kumar, P. and Clark, M. (2005) *Clinical Medicine*, 6th edn, Edinburgh, Elsevier.

Larsson, S. and Lundberg, L. (1995) 'A prospective survey of postoperative nausea and vomiting with special regard to incidence and relations to patient characteristics, anaesthetic routines, and surgical procedures', *Acta Anesthesiologica Scandinavica* 39, 339–45.

Lewis, S. J., Egger, M., Sylvester, P. and Thomas, S. (2001) 'Early enteral feeding versus "nil by mouth" after gastrointestinal surgery: systematic review and meta-analysis of controlled trials', *British Medical Journal* 323: 773.

Livingstone, J. (1993) 'Role of pre-admission clinics in general surgical unit: a 6 month audit', *Annals of the Royal College of Surgeons of England* **75**(3), 211–12.

Longmore, M., Wilkinson, I., Turmezei, T. and Cheung, C. K. (2007) *Oxford Handbook of Clinical Medicine*, 7th edn, Oxford, Oxford University Press.

McCaughan, E. and Parahoo, K. 2000 'Medical and surgical nurses' perceptions of their level of competence and educational needs in caring for patients with cancer', *Journal of Clinical Nursing* **9**(3), 420–8.

Mohan, S., Wilkes, L., Ogunsiji, O. and Walker, A. (2005) 'Caring for patients with cancer in non-specialist wards: the nurse experience', *European Journal of Cancer Care* **14**(3), 256–63.

Moore, T. (2007) 'Respiratory assessment in adults', *Nursing Standard* **21**(49), 48–56.

Murphy, T., Calle, E., Rodriguez, C., Kahn, H. and Thun, M. (2000) 'Body mass index and colon cancer in a large prospective study', *American Journal of Epidemiology* **152**(9), 847–54.

Mackintosh, C. and Elson, S. (2008) 'Chronic pain: clinical features, assessment and treatment', *Nursing Standard* **23**(5), 48–56.

National Institute of Clinical Excellence (NICE) (2003a) *Preoperative Tests: The use of routine preoperative tests for elective surgery*, Clinical Guideline 3 [online] http://www.nice.org.uk/nicemedia/pdf/CG3NICEguideline.pdf (accessed 23 December 2008).

Ng, W. Q. and Neill, J. (2006) 'Evidence of early oral feeding of patients after elective open colorectal surgery: a literature review', *Journal of Clinical Nursing* 15(6), 696–709.

NHS Estates (2001) *Better Hospital Food* [online] www.betterhospitalfood.com (accessed 23 December 2008).

NHS Scotland Information and Statistics (2005) *Key Health Topics: Cancer: facts and figures: colorectal (or large bowel) cancer* [online[www.isdscotland.org/isd/3348.html (accessed 9 February 2009).

NHS Executive (date) *Referral Guidelines for Suspected Cancer* [online] http://www.nice.org.uk/pdf/cg027niceguideline.pdf (accessed 23 December 2008).

NICE (2003b) *Routine Tests Carried out Before a Planned Surgical Operation*, London, NICE.

NICE (2004) *Improving Outcomes in Colorectal Cancer* [online] http://www.nice.org.uk/guidance/CSGCC/?c=91496 (accessed 9 February 2009).

NICE (2005a) *The Prevention and Treatment of Pressure Ulcers: Quick reference guide*, London, NICE.

NICE (2005b) *Referral Guidelines for Suspected Cancer*, London, NICE.

NICE (2006) *Nutrition Support in Adults*, Clinical guidance 32, London, NICE.

Nursing and Midwifery Council (NMC) (2002a) *Guidelines for the Administration of Medicines*, London, NMC.

NMC (2002b) *Guidelines for Records and Record Keeping*, London, NMC.

Norris, A. C. and Briggs, J. S. (1999) 'Care pathways and the information for health strategy', *Health Informatics Journal* 5, 209–12.

Norton, D., McLaren, R. and Exton-Smith, A. N. (1985) *An Investigation of Geriatric Nursing Problems in Hospital*, Edinburgh, Churchill

Part

III

Livingstone.

O'Callaghan, N. (2002) 'Pre-operative fasting' *Nursing Standard* **16**(36), 33–7.

Oakey, R. J. and Slade, V. (2006) 'Physiological observation track and trigger system', *Nursing Standard* **20**(27), 48–54.

Pan-Birmingham Cancer Network (2006) *Sigmoid Colectomy: Your operation explained* [online] www.birminghamcancer.nhs.uk (accessed 1 May 2007).

Rasmussen, D. and Elverdam, B. (2007) 'Cancer survivors' experience of time: time disruption and time appropriation', *Journal of Advanced Nursing* **57**(6), 614–22.

Richards, A. and Edwards, S. (2003) pp. 24–5 in *A Nurse's Survival Guide to the Ward*, London, Churchill Livingstone.

Royal College of Physicians (RCP) (2002) *Nutrition and Patients: A doctor's responsibility*, London, RCP.

Scott, E. M. and Buckland, R. (2005) 'Pressure ulcer risk in the perioperative environment', *Nursing Standard* **20**(7), 74–86.

Scott, E., Earl, C., Leaper, D., Massey, M., Mewburn, J. and Williams, N. (1999) 'Understanding perioperative nursing', *Nursing Standard* **13**(49), 49–54.

Scottish Intercollegiate Guidelines Network (SIGN) (2005) *Management of Colorectal Cancer*, Guideline number 67, Edinburgh, SIGN.

Silk, D. and Gow, N. (2001) 'Postoperative starvation after gastrointestinal surgery', *British Medical Journal* 323, 761–2.

Siviter, B. (2004) pp. 38–49 in *The Student Nurse Handbook: A survival guide*, Edinburgh, Bailliere Tindall.

Smith, G. (2000) *Alert: Life threatening events, recognition and treatment*, University of Portsmouth.

Spilsbury, K. and Meyer, J. (2001) 'Defining the nursing contribution to patient outcome: lessons from a review of the literature examining nursing outcomes, skill mix and changing roles', *Journal of Clinical Nursing* **10**(1), 3–14.

Subbe, C. P., Kruger, M., Rutherford, P. and Gemmel, L. (2001) 'Validation of a modified early warning score in medical admissions', *International Journal of Medicine* **94**(10), 521–5.

Surgery Door (nd) 'Sigmoid colectomy' [online] www.surgerydoor. co.uk/so/detail2.asp?level2=Sigmoid-Colectomy (accessed 1 May 2007).

Sweet, M. (2002) 'Eating meat more than 10 times a week almost doubles chances of bowel cancer', *British Medical Journal* 324, 1544.

Thompson, M. R., Heath, I., Ellis, B. G., Swarbrick, E. T., Faulds Wood, L. and Atkin W. S. (2003) 'Identifying and managing patients at low risk of bowel cancer in general practice', *British Medical Journal* 327, 263–5.

Tierney, A. (1998) 'Nursing models: extant or extinct?', *Journal of Advanced Nursing* 28(1), 77–85.

Turnbull, D., Farid, A., Hutchinson, S., Shorthouse, A. and Mills, G. H. (2002) 'Calf compartment pressures in the Lloyd-Davies position: a cause for concern?' *Anaesthesia* **57**(9) (September), 905–8.

Walker, J. (2003) 'Care of the post operative patient part 1', *Professional Nurse* **18**(11), 615–16.

Walker, J. (2003) 'Post operative care part 2', *Professional Nurse* **18**(12), 673–4.

Wallis, M. (2001) 'Deep vein thrombosis: clinical nursing management', *Nursing Standard* 15(18), 47–57.

Walsh, M. (1997) 'Will critical pathways replace the nursing process?' *Nursing Standard* **11**(52), 39–42.

Walsh, M. (2002) *Watsons' Clinical Nursing and Related Sciences*, London, Balliere Tindall.

Waterlow, J. (1991) 'A policy that protects', *Professional Nurse* 6(5), 258–64.

Watret, L. and White, R. (2001) 'Surgical wound management: the role of dressings', *Nursing Standard* **15**(44), 59–69.

Weetman, C. and Allison, W. (2006) 'Use of epidural analgesia in post-operative pain management', *Nursing Standard* **20**(44), 54–64.

Welch, E. (2005) 'The assessment and management of venous thromboembolism', *Nursing Standard* **20**(28), 58–64.

Wellington Hospital GI Unit (nd) 'Flexible sigmoidoscopy' [online] http://www.thewellingtongiunit.com/diagnostic-flexible-sigmoidoscopy.asp (accessed 9 December 2008).

White, R. (2000) 'Nurse assessment of oral health: a review of practice and education' *British Journal of Nursing* **9**(5), 260–6.

Williams B. (2007) 'Supporting self-care of patients following general abdominal surgery', *Journal of Clinical Nursing* 1–9.

Xavier, G. (2000) 'The importance of mouth care in preventing infection', *Nursing Standard* 14(18), 47–51.

Zeitz, K. 2005 'Nursing observations during the first 24 hours after a surgical procedure: what do we do?' *Journal of Clinical Nursing* **14**(3), 334–43.

Zeitz, K. and McCutcheon, H. (2003) 'EBP – to be or not to be, this is the question!' *International Journal of Nursing Practice* 9, 272–9.

Websites

Cancer Help: http://www.cancerhelp.org.uk

Early warning system scoring chart :
http://www.ihi.org/IHI/Topics/PatientSafety/SafetyGeneral/Tools/ColourBandedEarlyWarningObservationChart.htm

Malnutrition Universal Screening Tool: http://www.bapen.org.uk/pdfs/must/must_full.pdf

NHS Cancer Services Collaborative 'Improvement Partnership' bowel cancer section: http://www.cancerimprovement.nhs.uk/View.aspx?page=/tumour_groups/bowel.html

Waterlow Assessment chart: http://www.judy-waterlow.co.uk/downloads/Waterlow%20Score%20Card-front.pdf

Legislation

Manual Handling Operations Regulations (1992) UK Government Statutory Instructions No 2793.

Chapter

24

Care of the adult – medical

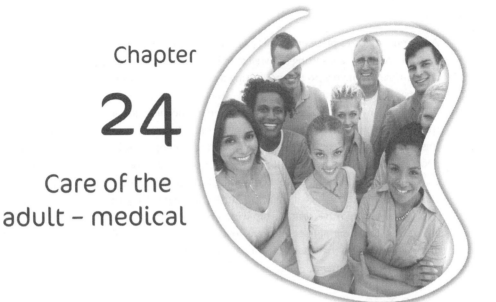

Margaret Chambers, Adele Kane and Kathryn Tattersall

(with thanks to Janet Dean and Paula Shobbrook)

Links to other chapters in *Foundation Studies for Caring*

Links to other chapters in *Foundation Skills for Caring*

W Don't forget to visit www.palgrave.com/glasper for additional online resources relating to this chapter.

Introduction

Adult nursing takes place in a variety of settings – in the community, in patients' own homes and in residential care settings, as well as in hospital wards and outpatient departments. Using an example of a man who is experiencing a chest disorder, this chapter illustrates the context of nursing adult patients.

While many adult patients are admitted to hospital for investigative procedures and treatment, many of these are now available on a daycase basis. It is generally accepted that this is more convenient and less stressful for many people, and it is widely documented that people do prefer this service (McMillan, 2005). Ambulatory care also enables cost-effective use of limited resources and reduced waiting lists (Oakley, 2005). Such an approach to patient care poses a particular challenge for nurses, however. They must be able to establish an effective and supportive relationship with a number of patients in a stressful situation, often in a very limited time. Nurses must ensure that patients receive high-quality holistic care while in the unit, but also that their communication skills promote continuity of care once patients have left the department.

Learning outcomes

This chapter will enable you to:

- outline the advantages and disadvantages of ambulatory care for investigative procedures for patients, carers and healthcare professionals
- analyse the importance of interprofessional communication and discuss ways in which this could be enhanced
- explore the legal and professional issues of information giving, confidentiality and informed consent in adult nursing
- identify and discuss key aspects of respiratory assessment

- identify the health risks associated with smoking, and discuss strategies which may help patients to stop smoking
- discuss the pathophysiological effects of lung cancer, and identify implications for nursing care
- describe the preparation required for a patient undergoing fibre-optic bronchoscopy and list the potential complications of the procedure
- identify strategies that may help reduce patient anxiety
- discuss discharge planning following ambulatory care.

Concepts

- Information giving
- Health risks
- Informed choice
- Diagnostic interventions
- Informed consent
- Invasive procedures

- Role of nurse
- Ambulatory care
- Holistic care
- Emergency care
- Assessment
- Patient safety

- Monitoring
- Infection control
- Evaluation
- Anxiety
- Nursing judgements
- Trust

- Advanced practice
- Sedation
- Evidence-based care
- Malignant
- Chronic illness
- Benign

> ### (a) Learning activity
>
> Consider in your learning group what is meant by holistic nursing, and identify the problems in providing holistic care in the ambulatory setting.

Holistic care is described as care incorporating multiple dimensions including physical, emotional, social and spiritual aspects of the person (Govier, 2000), while the term *ambulatory care* is defined as 'health services provided on an outpatient basis to those who visit a hospital or clinic and depart after treatment on the same day' (Mosby, 2006). The provision of holistic care in the ambulatory setting presents the nurse with a number of challenges, and requires the enhancement of communication skills (Rogan Foy and Timmins, 2004). The development of a therapeutic relationship is central to the provision of holistic care, but ambulatory care has reduced the time available for this development to take place (Rogan Foy, and Timmins 2004). Even so, opportunities for nurses to provide holistic care in the daycare setting do arise, and patients have cited the significance of the nurse's emotional presence as fundamental to this process (Costa, 2001). So even though ambulatory care is characterised by a rapid turnover of patients and short patient episodes, it is essential that nurses engage with patients in a meaningful way so that the development of an empathetic, therapeutic relationship can be established and all patient needs can be met.

[S] Scenario: Introducing Peter Stevens

Peter Stevens is 58 years old, divorced and works as a roofer. He lives in a first-floor council owned flat with his adult daughter Julie, who has a three-month-old baby. He has smoked since the age of 15, preferring to roll his own, and continues to do so, although recently he has cut down from 4 to 2 ounces of tobacco a week. He drinks alcohol occasionally and does not own a car, using public transport, with his daughter giving him lifts when she can.

Peter has been well apart from occasional upper respiratory tract infections and a 'smoker's cough' in the morning for some years. He became unwell six weeks ago, when he developed a 'flu-like' illness and became lethargic. He also noticed a painless hoarseness of his voice. After a week he visited his general practitioner (GP), who advised him to increase his fluid intake and to take paracetamol for the headache and shivers. He

also arranged for an outpatient chest x-ray at the local hospital.

Peter then developed pain in his chest and back, which was made worse by lying down and unrelieved by taking the paracetamol. He returned to his GP and reported the pain. The GP contacted the hospital and arranged for the x-ray that day. He referred Peter to a medical consultant specialising in respiratory disease for assessment of his x-ray and clinical condition within the week. He was seen in the outpatients department a few days later. The consultant suspected carcinoma of the bronchus and organised blood and pulmonary function tests. Peter was asked to attend outpatients again for a fibre-optic bronchoscopy. After ten days he was asked to attend the day unit of the local hospital for a fibre-optic bronchoscopy.

[a] Learning activity

Visit an outpatients clinic or talk to a nurse working in the area. How does the clinic nurse's role differ from that of the ward-based nurse?

Patients' experience of ambulatory care depends on the preparation and advice they receive from the nurse. Good communication is at the heart of good nursing, and the ability to communicate well is even more important during short patient episodes. The importance of preparation for procedures cannot be over-emphasised, and should begin from the moment the patient consults their GP and in the outpatients clinic. Information supplied in the outpatients clinic is fundamental to the successful preparation of the patient for surgical and investigative procedures.

t☆ Practice tip

Many information leaflets have been written to help health professionals prepare patients for investigative procedures. If they are to prove beneficial to patients it is important that they are used appropriately:

- Leaflets should be used in addition to and not instead of verbal information.
- Select an appropriate leaflet, in the correct language, and ensure that the patient can read it or that someone is available to read it to them.
- Provide the leaflet well before the procedure, to allow time for assimilation of the information.
- Ensure that the patient knows who can answer any questions and how to contact them.
- Highlight or mark crucial information such as the need to refrain from food and drink or not to drive following procedures, for additional emphasis.

Part
III

a) Learning activity

Take a careful look at some of the information leaflets available in your practice area. Bring in a selection to your learning group, and consider how effective they would be for a variety of patient groups: for example, a person with a learning disability, a person who has a visual impairment or someone whose first language is not English.

Bronchoscopy

a) Learning activity

What is a bronchoscopy? You may find it useful to look up or review the anatomy of the respiratory tract. Consider your response before reading on.

A bronchoscopy is an endoscopic view of the trachea-bronchial tree (Gardner, 2005; Mosby, 2006). There are two types of bronchoscopy, rigid and flexible fibre-optic. Rigid bronchoscopy is usually performed under a general anaesthetic, normally for the relief of airway obstruction (Gardner, 2005), while a flexible fibre-optic bronchoscopy allows direct, detailed examination of the larynx, trachea and bronchi. The latter procedure is tolerated well by the majority of patients (although particular care should be taken when examining critically ill, hypoxic or asthmatic patients), and does not require a general anaesthetic. Instead the patient is sedated and the larynx and upper airways are anaesthetised prior to insertion of the bronchoscope (Gardner, 2005). The procedure is usually performed by a doctor with specialist training, although more recently nurse practitioners have been trained to carry out endoscopic procedures.

a) Learning activity

Find out whether there are there any nurse endoscopists practising in your clinical area. Consider the professional implications for nurses who choose to advance their clinical practice in this way.

A bronchoscopy may be diagnostic or therapeutic. Most are performed to investigate a suspected diagnosis, often of lung cancer as in Peter Stevens's case. Therapeutically bronchoscopy can be used to remove foreign bodies or excess secretions from the airways, to control bleeding points and to allow direct treatment of tumours (Belli, 1999).

a) Learning activity

Try to organise a visit to an endoscopy unit to observe some procedures. (If this is not possible, watching a video is a good alternative.) This will enable you to respond more accurately to patients' questions when preparing them for their procedures. Observe what other endoscopic procedures are performed.

Principles of care

Preprocedural preparation

- Before the procedure the patient is starved (nil by mouth) to reduce the risk of aspiration of the stomach contents into the lungs if the patient should vomit (Gardner, 2005).
- A written informed consent is obtained.
- The patient is sedated using an intravenous drug, and the mucosa of the nose and throat are sprayed with a local anaesthetic agent to reduce discomfort (Gardner, 2005).

The procedure

- The bronchoscope is passed through the nose or mouth, via the vocal cords into the tracheobronchial tree.
- Coughing is suppressed by local anaesthetic spray through the bronchoscope as the procedure progresses.
- Any abnormal tissue seen can be sampled by taking a biopsy, or a brush can protrude from the end of the bronchoscope and sweep off some of the superficial mucosal cells to collect them in a specimen jar.
- Sputum specimens can also be collected.
- During the procedure the patient's condition is continually monitored by the clinician performing the procedure and by the assisting nurse.

Postprocedural care

- Once the procedure is completed patients are encouraged to rest to allow the effects of any sedation to wear off, and they are observed for any signs of complications.
- Patients must remain 'nil by mouth' until their swallowing reflex (which is depressed by the local anaesthetic) returns to normal, usually two to four hours after the procedure.
- As the effects of the sedation may persist for many hours, patients are not allowed to drive home.

Lung cancer

Lung cancer is the commonest form of malignant disease in the western world (Ferlay et al, 2007), and the second commonest cancer diagnosed in the United Kingdom (Cancer Research UK, 2008). Around 90 per cent of lung cancers in men and 83 per cent in women are thought to be caused by smoking or through indirect exposure (passive smoking) (Cancer Research UK, 2008). Other causes are thought to include exposure to radioactive materials, radon gas, chemicals and asbestos (Cancer Help, 2008). The risk of contracting lung cancer is directly related to the duration and intensity of the smoking (Cancer Research UK, 2008). The risk of lung cancer in smokers is 15 times that of life-long nonsmokers (Doll et al, 2005), so a patient like Peter, a heavy smoker for 43 years, is at high risk.

Lung cancer is an umbrella term which includes several different tumours arising from different cells in the respiratory tract. There are two main types. Around 20 per cent are small cell lung cancers (SCLC) and around 80 per cent are non-small cell lung cancers (NSCLC) (Cancer Research UK, 2008). Small cell carcinomas are highly malignant. They can divide and spread (metastasise) very rapidly, whereas non-small cell tumours (including adenocarcomas, squamous cell and large-cell carcinomas) are slower growing (Quinn, 1999). However, generally the prognosis for patients with lung cancer is very poor. Only 7 per cent of patients will still be alive five years after diagnosis (Cancer Research UK, 2008).

Cigarette smoking has been linked to all types of lung cancer, but adenocarcinoma – the commonest type in non-smokers (Subramanian and Govindan, 2007) – is rising in incidence probably because of the increased use of low-tar cigarettes (Franceschi and Bidoli, 1999). It is important to identify which type of tumour the patient has, as both treatment and prognosis vary from type to type (NICE, 2005). Occasionally a lung tumour may be benign (without the capacity to spread to other parts of the body as malignant tumours can), but this is rare.

One of the difficulties in improving the survival of patients with lung cancer is the lack of an effective screening procedure to detect the disease at any early stage when curative treatment may be possible (Day, 1998; Kosco and Held-Warmkessel, 2000). The identification of biomarkers for early detection and treatment is therefore a priority (Hirsch and Lippman, 2005). Often, as with Peter, by the time the patient seeks medical advice the disease is well established and curative treatment is not possible (ICHSC and RCP, 2006).

> **t** ☆
> ## Practice tip
>
> Many patients are reluctant to admit the extent of their smoking habit, and initially underestimate the amount they smoke when questioned. A nonjudgmental approach is essential.

Part

III

a Learning activity

What symptoms might occur with this condition that would make a person ask for an appointment with a GP?

Signs and symptoms that are suggestive of lung cancer include haemoptysis or any of the following persistent symptoms (lasting more than three weeks) (NICE, 2005):

- cough
- pain in the chest, neck or back
- dyspnoea
- weight loss
- hoarseness
- finger clubbing
- cervical superclavicular lymphadenopathy (swollen glands in the neck).

Some patients suffer with hoarseness, which is caused by paralysis of one of the vocal cords, rendering normal speech impossible. The paralysis is caused by the tumour damaging the left recurrent laryngeal nerve as it passes through the chest to supply the left vocal cord (Hoffman, Mauer and Vokes, 2000).

A doctor may suspect lung cancer if a patient presents with such signs and symptoms, particularly if the patient is a smoker, or has been exposed to other causative agents. To confirm the diagnosis, a chest x-ray is performed which will reveal the presence of a tumour but not its type. To identify the exact nature of the tumour, cells must be obtained from the growth for histological examination, either from biopsy specimens (usually obtained via a bronchoscopy), or from sputum specimens, as tumour cells are shed into the sputum (Schrieber and McCory, 2003). Once the cell-type of the tumour has been identified, treatment can be offered.

The treatment available for lung cancer depends on several factors including the type and position of the tumour, the extent of metastatic disease and the physical condition of the patient. Surgery, radiotherapy and/or chemotherapy can be used, either as potentially curative treatment or as palliation in an attempt to improve the quality of the patient's remaining life by reducing the severity of the symptoms (Claxton, 1999; Dest, 2000).

Public health

Health of the Nation (DH, 1992)

Lung cancer was one of the target areas identified in the *Health of the Nation* white paper by the Conservative government in 1992. The aim was to reduce lung cancer death rates by 30 per cent in men under 75 and 15 per cent in women under 75 by the year 2010. The following preventive measures were advocated:

- health education on the effects of smoking
- helping people not to start smoking
- helping people to stop smoking
- protecting nonsmokers from passive smoking
- preventing occupational exposure to causative agents.

Saving Lives (DH, 1999a)

When the Labour government came to power in 1998, it reviewed the previous Conservative government's health strategies and subsequently produced a white paper, *Saving Lives: Our healthier nation* (DH, 1999a). This was presented as an

a Learning activities

- What were the other target areas identified in *Health of the Nation* (DH, 1992)?
- Many smokers are aware of the potential health risks associated with smoking but they continue to smoke. Why? You may like to discuss this with friends and colleagues who smoke and consider the range of responses. Compare these with smokers' comments later in the chapter.

action plan to tackle poor health. The key agenda is to improve the health of everyone, but improve the health of the worst off in particular. The plan is focused on the main causes of early death:

- cancer
- coronary heart disease and stroke
- accidents
- mental illness.

Targets were established for priority areas by the year 2010:

- Cancer: to reduce the death rate in people under 75 by at least 20 per cent.
- Coronary heart disease: to reduce the death rate in people under 75 by at least 40 per cent.
- Accidents: to reduce the death rate by at least 20 per cent and serious injury by 10 per cent.
- Mental health: to reduce the death rate from suicide and undetermined injury by at least 20 per cent.

Saving Lives placed more emphasis on people taking responsibility for their own health through physical activity, better diet and stopping smoking. It was proposed that this would be supported by:

- NHS Direct, a nurse-led telephone helpline and internet service providing advice and information on health
- health skills programmes for people to help themselves and others
- expert patient programmes to help people manage their own illnesses.

> **a Learning activity**
>
> This white paper underpins the political development of the health service today. The executive summary provides an overview of the key points. Access and read it (website details are in the references at the end of the chapter).

Smoking kills (DH, 1999b)

Another 1999 white paper, *Smoking Kills*, outlined proposed government action aimed at reducing the number of smoking-related deaths in the United Kingdom, and in particular to reduce smoking by children and pregnant women (see page 484). These actions include (DH, 1999b):

- a ban on tobacco advertising
- increased support for those wishing to stop via GP services, including a limited supply of nicotine replacement therapy for some
- priority attention to pregnant women who smoke
- additional funding to reduce cigarette smuggling
- enforcement of legislation related to underage sales and proof of age cards to protect young people.

Choosing Health (DH, 2004)

The government published a further white paper, *Choosing Health: Making healthier choices easier*, in November 2004. This set out the ways in which it would make it easier for people to make healthier lifestyle choices. *Choosing Health* focuses on six key priorities:

- tackling health inequalities
- reducing the numbers of people who smoke
- tackling obesity
- improving sexual health
- improving mental health and well-being
- reducing harm and encouraging sensible drinking.

The emphasis is placed on success being driven by the public becoming engaged in the improvement of their own health. With regard to smoking, the aim was to reduce adult smoking rates from 26 per cent (in 2002) to 21 per cent or less by 2010, working on the principle that 70 per cent of smokers want to quit.

The government identified a number of 'big wins', or policies to support the public in their quest for healthier lifestyles. Those related to smoking cessation were identified as:

- support for smoking cessation (stop smoking services)
- reducing the exposure to secondhand smoke (a staged approach to ending smoking in public places)
- reducing tobacco advertising and promotion
- national smoking communication campaigns and education
- reducing the availability of illicit and smuggled tobacco and underage sales.

On 1 July 2007 the smoke-free law (Health Act 2006) was implemented, making it against the law to smoke in virtually all enclosed and substantially enclosed public places and places of work. It has been illegal to sell tobacco to young people under the age of 18 years since 1 October 2007. More information and tips about quitting smoking can be found at http://gosmokefree.nhs.uk.

Smoking: the health risks

Smoking is a major health risk – 'the single greatest cause of illness and premature death in England today' (DH, 2004) – and nurses have an important role in helping patients to give up smoking or not take up smoking.

As well as lung cancer, smoking causes other tumours: cancer of the mouth, nose, larynx oesophagus, pancreas, bladder, cervix and leukaemia. It also causes emphysema, bronchitis, chronic obstructive pulmonary disease, arteriosclerosis, peptic ulcers and infertility. Female smokers are at higher risk of osteoporosis, spontaneous abortion and of giving birth to low-birthweight babies (Burgess, 1994). There is also increasing concern about the health effects of passive smoking – breathing in other people's tobacco smoke. People who live with smokers or work in smoky atmospheres for significant periods of time incur significant risk (Britton, 2005), and several thousand people a year are thought to die from lung cancer as a result of passive smoking (Cancer Research UK, 2008). Even low-level passive smoking can cause illness. Asthma can be triggered by passive smoke (Britton, 2005), and children are at particular risk because they have little or no choice over their personal exposure to passive smoke. This leads to many children being admitted to hospital every year (Leung, Ho and Lam, 2004).

Despite the general knowledge that smoking is bad for your health, in 1999 28 per cent of adults, approximately 13 million people in the United Kingdom, were smokers (DH, 1999b). In 2006 this figure had fallen to 22 per cent (ONS, 2006). Most smokers are introduced to the habit in their teens (McCarron et al, 2001). There are many reasons that people begin or continue to smoke, including curiosity, peer pressure, anticipating adulthood, rebelliousness and role models. Once established as a behaviour, smoking becomes a habit and addiction to nicotine can result, making it difficult to stop.

Smoking is related to social class, being more prevalent in lower socioeconomic classes (as defined by the Registrar General) (Harwood et al, 2007). For example, in 2005 29 per cent of manual workers smoked compared with 19 per cent of nonmanual workers (Goddard, 2006). This clearly has implications for the targeting of health education, screening and healthcare provision. There is also concern that the downward trend in smoking, which has been evident since the 1960s, is now levelling out, and increasing numbers of young people are starting to smoke (DH, 1999b). According to the National Youth Information Agency (2008), a quarter of Britain's 15-year-olds (girls and boys) are smokers.

a Learning activity

Visit your local health promotion library and investigate the ways in which the nurse can support smokers who wish to give up smoking: for example, nurse-led smoking cessation clinics.

In your learning group, consider what health education activities could be undertaken by nurses and other healthcare professionals to prevent the uptake of smoking in the first place.

The NHS Executive (1998) has issued guidance on the commissioning of cancer services, and indicates areas of good practice related to reducing the incidence of smoking. Primary prevention of smoking is felt to be crucial, and strategies include school-based prevention programmes, mass media campaigns, restrictions on cigarette sales to minors, and the banning of cigarette advertising and sponsorship. Increasing taxation to increase the price of tobacco products might also reduce smoking levels. However, given the higher incidence of smoking among those of low income, price rises might simply increase financial hardship.

It is vital to remember that giving up smoking is a very difficult process. This is also true for healthcare professionals who smoke, and they should be encouraged and supported to become nonsmoking role models (Sarna et al, 2005).

e Evidence-based practice

Several smoking cessation interventions have been shown to be effective (Lancaster et al, 2000):

- brief advice from a healthcare professional
- nicotine replacement therapy with advice
- advice and support to pregnant women.

Current evidence suggests that other strategies may be less effective, including:

- use of antidepressant and anxiety-reducing drugs
- behavioural therapy such as aversive conditioning
- acupuncture
- hypnosis
- self-help materials such as booklets and pamphlets.

Nurses need to be fully informed of the physiological, psychological and social causes and effects of smoking to enable them to function effectively as health educators, as nurses often interact with smokers in both hospital and community settings. The risk of developing lung cancer diminishes after stopping smoking, becoming apparent after about five years. If people who have been smoking for many years stop, even well into middle age, they can avoid most of their subsequent risk of lung cancer (Peto et al 2000). In addition, *reduction* in smoking has been shown to lessen the risks of contracting lung cancer (Godtfredsen, Prescott and Osler, 2005). However, the risk of a former smoker remains greater than that of a non-smoker, even 30 years after stopping (Ebbert et al, 2003).

a Learning activity

How effective could you be in supporting a patient, friend or relative who wanted to stop smoking? Survey your area to find any additional support groups available to your patients/clients.

Part III

c Professional conversation

Jane Phillips, ward manager, comments, 'Peter Stevens has been smoking for many years and would probably find it very difficult to stop, particularly now when he is very anxious regarding his state of health. If he has lung cancer, it could be argued that it is too late for him to stop. The damage to his health is already done, and if it is one of the pleasures in his life, would it not be kinder to allow him to continue to smoke for the limited time he has left?

'There are however other issues to consider. If Peter does have lung cancer, the best chance for curative treatment would be surgery, and if it is possible to operate on him, stopping smoking six weeks prior to the operation can make a significant difference in terms of morbidity and mortality. Passive smoking might also be having detrimental effects on the health of his daughter and granddaughter. It might be too late for Peter, but not for those living with him.'

S Scenario continued

Peter Stevens arrives at the day unit with his daughter at 10 am, where his named nurse welcomes him. He is escorted to a private room for assessment of his current situation. As instructed, he has taken nil by mouth since midnight in preparation for the bronchoscopy – he last ate 16 hours ago and last drank 10 hours ago.

a Learning activity

Locate the 'nil by mouth policy' for your unit. How current is it? What evidence is there to support the policy? What are the dangers of prolonged fasting prior to anaesthetic or procedures requiring sedation?

Patients who are to receive a general anaesthetic should not eat or drink prior to the procedure to ensure that the stomach is empty, in order to prevent aspiration should vomiting occur while the patient is unconscious. Patients who are undergoing procedures that might cause vomiting (such as bronchoscopy) require similar precautions, particularly if they are to be sedated and may be unable to protect their own airway.

Research has shown that not eating or drinking for four hours is sufficient to ensure an empty stomach, and that clear fluids can be given up to three hours pre-operatively with no ill effects (Rowe, 2002), Keeping patients nil by mouth for prolonged periods causes dehydration and discomfort, and can significantly affect the patient's nutritional status. Nursing research undertaken by Hamilton-Smith (1972) identified ritualistic nursing practices which resulted in patients being starved for much longer than necessary. For example, all patients on the morning theatre list were kept nil by mouth from midnight, regardless of the scheduled time of their surgery. A study by Chapman (1996), undertaken 24 years later, identified similar issues, and even more recently Woodhouse (2006) showed that while nurses were aware of the rationale for pre-operative fasting and acknowledged the importance of evidence-based practice, they were nevertheless unaware of up-to-date studies in the area. This raises concerns that the results of nursing research are not having an impact on some areas of clinical practice, and that interventions regarding fasting times are ritualistic (Woodhouse, 2006).

It is important to ensure that patients are treated individually, and starved for the minimum time, to guarantee safety while reducing discomfort. Peter Stevens arrived for his bronchoscopy having eaten nothing for 16 hours and drunk nothing for 10 hours. This would suggest that either he had been given inappropriate, standardised instructions, or he did not understand the instructions he had been given. This is not good care.

S Scenario continued

Peter has a persistent cough and is expectorating green sputum (no haemoptysis), particularly in the morning. He is dyspnoeic on exertion, and has a very hoarse voice. His vital signs and blood test results are within normal limits for a man of his age. His chest x-ray is abnormal, revealing according to the radiologist's report, 'a left upper lobe mass, with consolidation and collapse', and his pulmonary function tests are abnormal, suggesting obstructive disease.

He is still suffering chest and back pain, of a sharp, stabbing nature. His GP has now prescribed diclofenac orally, which has been only partially effective. Peter identifies pain as his major problem.

Despite his quiet, hoarse voice, Peter is able to communicate effectively. He does not speak unless spoken to, and tends to respond as briefly as possible. He is cooperative but appears very anxious. When questioned, he admits that he is concerned about the investigation itself, and also about his diagnosis. He is aware that his x-ray is abnormal, and thinks this may be the result of 'infection, pneumonia, cancer or anything'. He feels that he is in limbo: 'The worst bit is not knowing. It's probably not to do with the fags – actually I'm sure it's not. Whatever, it doesn't really matter, I just want rid of it.'

He says that he feels optimistic it will soon be all over. He is not aware – although the healthcare professionals are – that his x-ray is highly suggestive of a large central obstructing tumour, probably malignant, which clinically is inoperable, and is already causing recurrent laryngeal nerve damage.

Part

III

Learning activity

Should Peter Stevens have been told that he probably has cancer? Consider the pros and cons before reading on. If he should be told, when should this be done and by whom?

It can be very difficult for healthcare professionals to decide when it is appropriate to reveal information regarding the diagnosis to patients. The principles of autonomy and individuality, enshrined in the *Code of Professional Conduct* (NMC, 2008), would indicate that patients are entitled to information about their condition. The amount and type of information that should be disclosed is also a matter of sensible and responsible judgement (Thompson et al, 2006). In the early stages of investigation of a health problem there may be many potential diagnoses to be eliminated, and it might not be helpful to discuss all of them fully with the patient, as confusion and anxiety could result. Once a definite diagnosis has been reached, it is crucial for Peter to be fully informed, so he can make rational decisions about possible treatments, if he chooses to accept any.

Peter is clearly aware of the possibility that he has cancer, and that this could be related to smoking, although he dismisses this. If he asks directly, 'Have I got cancer?' it would probably be most appropriate to tell him that this is quite possible, but until the results of the bronchoscopy are known, it is not certain. He should also be reassured that the results will be made known to him as quickly as possible, and that he (and his daughter if he wishes) will have the chance to discuss them with the doctor.

If he does not ask, it may be because he is not yet ready to deal with this possibility, and it would be reasonable to tell him that the bronchoscopy will be able to reveal the cause of his symptoms, without mentioning cancer at this stage.

Lack of information is a major cause of dissatisfaction amongst patients with cancer (NHS Executive, 1998), and it is important to be aware that the quality of communication between patients and health professionals can influence concordance with advice or treatment (Vermeire et al, 2001). Thus the appropriate delivery of accurate information, at the right time, in the best available environment, is a crucial part of Peter Stevens's care.

Assessment

When a patient arrives in the day unit, the nurse's responsibility is to undertake a focused assessment of their condition. During the assessment, patients are informed why the questions are being asked, and their queries are then answered in plain language. The time available for this is limited, so it is imperative that the appropriate information is acquired. The accuracy of the data obtained depends upon the patient's ability to communicate information and the nurse's skill to perceive it correctly (Stafrace, 1998). In order to do this the patient must have the nurse's full attention, which means allowing time away from other distractions. This may be achieved by pulling the bed curtains around the bed area, or using an empty room or assessment area, which also provides privacy for the patient.

Practice tip

Remember that bed curtains provide only visual privacy. Conversations behind the curtains can very easily be overheard. Patient confidentiality must always be considered.

Learning activity

Well-developed communication skills are vital to good nursing practice. Before reading on, consider the factors that may hamper effective communication skills.

Factors that may get in the way of effective communication include:

- patient anxiety about their condition, procedures and the environment
- lack of privacy
- use of professional jargon

- pressure of time (which may be real or imagined)
- lack of 'listening' skills (Rogan Foy and Timmins, 2004)
- lack of formal training in communication skills (Buchanan, 1995).

a Learning activity

Consider your own communication skills, both verbal and nonverbal. How effectively do you feel you communicate? A visit to your library or a literature search will demonstrate an enormous amount of information to help you.

S Scenario continued

Before beginning the assessment Jane, the nurse, should greet Peter by name and introduce herself to him and Julie, and explain what exactly is going to happen. It is also important for Jane to check that neither of them have any immediate needs which should be satisfied before continuing with the assessment.

t Practice tip

Before assessing any patient, gather all the available information and make sure you have read the medical notes and referral letter so that you are aware of the clinical history and can ask the most relevant questions. To save time, you can copy relevant data on to nursing records, but remember to check with the patient that the details are still correct!

c Professional conversation

Bob Jenkins, charge nurse, comments, 'Effective communication pathways between the primary care team and the hospital-based professionals are essential to effective care, and evidence suggests that current systems are somewhat lacking! Poor interprofessional communication can lead to inadequate symptom control, duplication of effort and wasted time, resulting in frustration and distress for patients and their families. In particular, communication between hospitals and GPs cause difficulties (NHS Executive, 1998).

'In some hospitals, computer-based information systems enable information to be accessed quickly and passed from outpatient to hospital-based departments.'

a Learning activity

Find out which information systems are in place in your areas of practice, and ensure that you can use them effectively. Identify as many communication pathways as possible.

How is information relayed to the primary care team following investigative procedures? How long does it take? Can you suggest any improvements to the current system?

The nursing assessment should include the gathering of important biographical information to ensure that all the patient's records are accurate, a review of the patient's social situation, and both psychological and physiological assessments of the patient's current health situation.

The key information required may be summarised as follows:

- Is this the patient intended to have the procedure?
- Is there any psychological or physiological reason that this bronchoscopy should not be performed?
- Can the patient be discharged safely once they have recovered from the procedure?

If there is any cause for concern, this should be communicated to the endoscopist and the rest of the care team, as the procedure may need to be postponed or cancelled if the difficulties cannot be resolved quickly.

Psychological assessment

S Scenario continued

The nurse will need to ask Peter whether he understands why he has come for a bronchoscopy, and what is involved. Asking what he has already been told by his GP, the outpatient nurses and the consultant can be very revealing. Personal knowledge and level of understanding can be assessed and any important knowledge deficits can be identified. This will also give the nurse an opportunity to answer any questions that Peter or his daughter might have about the procedure, and to assess his ability to give a genuinely informed consent. Although his arrival in the day unit implies his consent, written consent is required and consent can be withdrawn at any time. He might have changed his mind or be too confused or distressed to continue.

Informed consent

Before an invasive procedure such as a bronchoscopy, the person who is going to carry out the procedure is legally obliged to obtain the patient's consent. Failure to do this might result in legal action against the bronchoscopist for battery (Dimond, 2008). However, obtaining the patient's consent involves more than simply asking them to sign the appropriate form. There are a number of legal and ethical principles to be observed.

Consent can be either implied or expressed. Implied consent is assumed when patients take actions that imply they agree to a procedure. Peter has arrived at the hospital ready to undergo bronchoscopy. This could be regarded as implied consent to the procedure. Implied consent is often regarded as adequate for minor procedures, such as measuring blood pressure, but it is usual practice to ensure expressed consent for more complex procedures.

Expressed consent may be either verbal or written. Verbal consent is often used when administering an injection or taking a blood sample, and it is quite valid in law (Medical Protection, nd). Written consent is usually obtained for complex procedures, especially where there is some risk involved. It is not required in law that consent must be written, but it is generally regarded as good practice (Dimond, 2008). In the event of legal action, it is much easier to prove that consent has been expressed if documentary evidence can be produced.

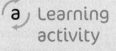 **Learning activity**

Before reading on, revisit Chapter 4 and consider what is meant by the term informed consent. Discuss this in your learning group.

Every adult must have the mental capacity to consent or refuse treatment. Specific criteria are used to decide whether an adult does or does not have the capacity to consent.

a Learning activity

With reference to the Mental Capacity Act (2005), identify the criteria that determine that an adult does not have the mental capacity to consent to treatment.

Regardless of whether the consent is written or verbal, some criteria must be satisfied if the consent is to be valid:

Part

III

- The patient must be able to understand what is going on and what they are consenting to.
- The consent must be voluntary. There must be no coercion either from healthcare professionals or from relatives and friends.
- The consent must not be obtained by deceit. Questions asked by the patient regarding the treatment must be answered truthfully.
- The consent must be informed. Informed consent recognises patients' rights to autonomy and self- determination, enabling them to make valid choices regarding the acceptance or refusal of treatment (Sims, 2008).

> **a ⟳ Learning activity**
>
> Visit the Department of Health website and obtain the guidance on consent in various groups, such as competent adults, adults with mental health problems or learning disabilities, and adolescents under the age of 18 years.
>
> Consider the nurse's role in obtaining consent, then refer to Sims (2008).

> **s ⟲ Scenario continued**
>
> At the start of the interview, the nurse noticed that Peter was very anxious. Most patients are anxious when they arrive in hospital for either treatment or investigation, and addressing this issue is an important aspect of nursing care. While it is accepted that some anxiety is inevitable, it may be possible to reduce levels of anxiety and help the patient to feel more at ease in an alien environment.

> **a ⟳ Learning activity**
>
> Before reading on consider the causes of Peter's anxiety.

Nurses must be able to recognise anxiety, and this can be manifest in a number of ways:

- Patients might freely admit that they are anxious, or they might be very quiet and withdrawn, or very talkative. They might appear to be aggressive.
- Physical signs can suggest anxiety, such as tachycardia, hypertension, tachypnoea, heightened startle response, or symptoms such as sweating, urinary frequency, abdominal discomfort and increased perception of pain (Chambers, 2008).
- Sometimes there is disordered cognitive functioning, such as difficulty in concentrating and remembering, and misunderstandings (Spear, 1996).

> **a ⟳ Learning activity**
>
> Review the effects of the autonomic nervous system and its links to the physical manifestation of anxiety.

The effects of anxiety and stress, initiated by the excitement of the autonomic nervous system and the release of noradrenaline and stress hormone, are (Curtis, 2000; Barker, 2007):

- tachycardia and palpitations
- raised blood pressure
- raised respiration rate
- pupil dilation
- constriction of blood vessels in the skin
- palmar sweating
- tension in the muscles
- decreased activity in the gastrointestinal activity
- feelings of discomfort in the stomach ('butterflies').

In the longer term it can lead to:

- headaches
- hypertension
- indigestion
- anorexia
- cardiovascular disorders
- cancer
- death.

> **a ⟳ Learning activity**
>
> Consider the implications of the physical and cognitive effects of anxiety for the assessment process.

Various techniques can be used to support an anxious patient (Chambers, 2008):

- Cognitive interventions such as providing accurate information, in an appropriate form, have been shown to reduce anxiety (Rogan Foy and Timmins, 2004). It is important to provide the amount of information that the patient is ready to accept.
- Behavioural intervention such as relaxation techniques, including controlled breathing or guided imagery, can be helpful.
- Sensory interventions such as reducing noise and light levels, the use of massage, aromatherapy, warm baths or music.
- Pharmacological interventions such as anxiolytic drugs which can be used on a short or long-term basis.

(e) Evidence-based practice

It is generally accepted by the nursing profession that giving patients information can be helpful in reducing their anxiety levels, and research supports this view (Beddows, 1997; Radcliffe, 1993). In a small-scale study conducted in a day surgery unit, nine out of ten trained nurses identified patient empowerment and anxiety reduction as their reasons for providing information (Reid, 1997). Less popular responses (50–80 per cent) included meeting the patient's needs, providing reassurance, to prepare patients for the unknown and to encourage patient choice. Other reasons were to satisfy personal accountability, encourage compliance, comply with the Patients' Charter (DH, 1991) and avoid litigation. Interestingly, none of the sample group felt that giving information contributed to ease of discharge, which is clearly a key aspect of daycare patient management.

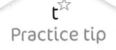

t☆ Practice tip

Anxiety can be communicated interpersonally, and maintaining a calm, confident and professional approach can be very helpful when dealing with anxious patients.

(a) Learning activity

What techniques could be helpful in reducing Peter's anxiety while he is attending the bronchoscopy suite?
You may want to read Chapter 5 in the companion skills volume.

One simple and inexpensive way to reduce anxiety during outpatient bronchoscopy is the use of music. In 1995 Dubois, Barter and Pratter, using a prospective randomised trial, demonstrated a significant reduction in anxiety levels in a sample of 21 patients who were played calming music throughout the procedure. Anxiety levels were assessed by means of physiological parameters (heart rate, blood pressure and oxygen saturation) and patients' self reports. The control group, who did not hear any music (two patients), were found to be more anxious. The research also demonstrated that staff undertaking the bronchoscopies were unable to assess accurately the level of distress experienced by patients during the procedure. A study by Hayes et al (2003) also showed that patients awaiting gastro-enteroscopy also benefit from listening to music for 15 minutes prior to their procedures.

Physiological assessment

Pain

It is important to assess pain early in any assessment procedure, as a patient in pain is unlikely to be able to communicate in a relaxed and effective manner. When pain is a significant problem, this should be relieved whenever possible before continuing with the assessment.

Peter is troubled with pain, and his current analgesic regime is not very effective. His medication should therefore be reviewed, and he should be given appropriate advice on how to obtain further support in his pain management (for further details see Chapter 15 on pain management).

Many patients who are taking analgesic medication regularly are concerned when asked to be 'nil by mouth' for a procedure, as they may miss several doses of their analgesia and suffer serious pain as a consequence. It is often possible for 'nil by mouth' patients to continue with pain relief, swallowing the medication with the smallest amount of plain water possible. If this is not possible, alternative routes can be used to administer pain relief: sublingual, rectal or injected drugs can be prescribed. It is important that pain control issues are discussed with the patient when procedures are planned, in order that the appropriate treatment can be organised and the patient kept fully informed.

Several measurements can be taken to assess the patient's physiological status. Temperature, pulse, respiration and blood pressure are recorded prior to the procedure, and the results provide a crucial 'baseline' against which comparisons can be made during the procedure and in the recovery phase. These are essential for the early recognition of any deterioration in the patient's condition during and after the procedure (Kenward, Hodgetts and Castle, 2001). Any major abnormality in the initial reading may result in the postponement of the bronchoscopy. It is therefore vital that the measurements are taken and recorded accurately.

> t ☆
> ## Practice tip
>
> All patients undergoing invasive procedures will require temperature, pulse, respiration and blood pressure (BP) recordings, but some patients may need additional monitoring, depending on their underlying physical condition.
> For example, a patient with diabetes will also need capillary blood glucose measurements.

In order to avoid hypoglycaemia, insulin-dependent diabetic patients must be given an infusion of 5 per cent dextrose along with a sliding scale insulin administration, and patients whose diabetes is controlled by oral medication should normally omit their medication when 'nil by mouth' (Wood, 2005).

> **a** Learning activity
>
> How are capillary blood glucose levels measured?
> Consider what problems could arise if a diabetic patient needs to be 'nil by mouth' in preparation for bronchoscopy.

Temperature

Disorders of body temperature may indicate that the patient has an infection, their condition is deteriorating, or that they have a problem with their thermoregulation. Traditionally the temperature is recorded orally in the sublingual pocket of the mouth, with the lips sealed. This may be difficult for patients who are dyspnoeic and mouth breathing, or confused. In these cases the axilla should be used as an alternative.

> **a** Learning activity
>
> What is the normal range of oral temperature for an adult? Is the range different for axillary recording?

Normal body temperature is maintained between 36 and 37.5 °C, but may vary by as much as 0.6 °C according to the site chosen for measurement. The axillary temperature lies at the lower end of the normal range (Jamieson, McCall and Whyte, 2002).

> **a** Learning activity
>
> There are a number of temperature measuring devices. Find out which of these are available in your clinical area, and check that you know how to use them all to obtain accurate results.

Pulse

The pulse may be recorded using an electric monitoring device or may be palpated manually. The most accessible, and therefore most commonly used, site for palpation is the radial pulse (Docherty and Coote, 2006; Higgins, 2008). Before measuring the pulse allow the patient to rest, so that the pulse rate is not artificially elevated by physical exertion (Docherty, 2002). Take note of the rate, rhythm and volume of the pulse over one minute.

> ### (a) Learning activity
>
> What is the normal range of the pulse rate in an adult? What is meant by the terms 'tachycardia' and 'bradycardia'? Suggest three other sites that may be used to palpate arterial pulse rates.

Blood pressure

Blood pressure is a measure of the force that blood exerts on the blood vessel walls, and is usually measured in millimetres of mercury (mmHg), using a sphygmomanometer or electronic monitoring device. Mercury sphygmomanometers are being phased out because of the health hazards of mercury. However should an electronic device be used it is important to follow the manufacturer's instructions in order to achieve an accurate recording (Jamieson et al, 2002).

Systolic blood pressure represents the maximum pressure of the blood against the walls of the arteries, caused by contraction of the ventricles when pushing blood into the aorta.

Diastolic blood pressure represents the minimum pressure of the blood against the vessel walls when the ventricles are at rest (Dougherty and Lister, 2004).

> ### (e) Evidence-based practice
>
> It is often assumed that nurses record blood pressure accurately. However, research has indicated that there is a lack of knowledge regarding its measurement, and the procedure was performed incorrectly by a large percentage of those surveyed (Gillespie and Curzio, 1998).

Systolic blood pressure is estimated by inflating the cuff while palpating the brachial or radial artery, and noting the systolic pressure when the pulsations stop. The British Hypertension Society has made recommendations for good practice when recording blood pressure. In preparation the nurse should provide an explanation of the procedure to the patient.

1   The patient should be seated for at least five minutes, relaxed and not moving or speaking.
2   Position the patient correctly, supporting the arm and ensuring the upper arm is at the same level as the heart.
3   Ensure that tight or restrictive clothing is removed from the arm.
4   Use an appropriately sized cuff so that the bladder covers 80 per cent of the circumference of the upper arm.
5   Apply the cuff evenly and smoothly on the arm, with the tubing exiting from the top of the cuff, ensuring that the centre of the bladder covers the brachial artery.
6   Position the manometer within 3 ft of the patient and at the operator's eye level.
7   Place the diaphragm of the stethoscope gently over the point of maximum pulsation of the brachial artery.
8   Do not tuck the diaphragm under the edge of the cuff.
9   Inflate the cuff to approximately 30mmHg above the palpated systolic blood pressure.
10   Deflate the system at 2–3 mmHG per second or per heart beat.
11   Systolic pressure is measured when a minimum of two clear repetitive sounds are heard, and the diastolic blood pressure is measured at the point when the sounds can no longer be heard.
12   The measurement should include a recording of the blood pressure to the nearest 2mmHG, the arm used and its position.

Part

III

Ensure that the earpieces of the stethoscope are the right way round, otherwise you will hear nothing! Have them pointing towards your nose.

Do not be alarmed if the patient is hypertensive and had has tachycardia. Check in the notes and compare with the measurements taken in the outpatients' clinic.

For more information go to http://www.bhsoc.org/how_to_measure_blood_pressure.stm.

Blood pressure is recorded before an investigation or surgery in order to assess the patient's normal range and act as a baseline for the assessment of the patient's cardiovascular status following the procedure (Jamieson et al, 2002).

Respiration

Many patients undergoing bronchoscopy will have respiratory symptoms, and they may well have abnormalities of their respiratory rate, depth and rhythm. It is still very important to observe their respiration, as very severe abnormalities might have developed recently, and a baseline for comparison during and after bronchoscopy is essential. A full respiratory assessment is not appropriate at this time, but it is helpful to be aware of how such an assessment may be conducted.

> **a Learning activity**
>
> Review the physiology of blood pressure in a good anatomy and physiology textbook. Why is it important to record the blood pressure prior to an investigation such as a bronchoscopy?

> **t Practice tip**
>
> When observing respiration, make sure that patient does not realise what you are doing. If the patient knows that you are watching them breathe, they will instinctively take voluntary control of their breathing. A good tip is to observe respiration while holding the patient's wrist, encouraging them to think that you are still counting their pulse rate.

> **a Learning activity**
>
> Review the control of respiration in a physiology text. Why might Peter's breathing be abnormal?

Smoking causes paralysis of the cilia of the lung, reduces the elasticity of the bronchioles and causes thickening of the alveoli. This reduces the capacity for gaseous exchange to take place, causing a rise in the levels of carbon dioxide in the blood, resulting in an increase in respiratory rate. In addition the cancer developing in the lung further reduces the lung's capacity for gaseous exchange.

Respiratory assessment involves the actual observation of respiration and information related to coughing, sputum production, haemoptysis and dyspnoea. If a patient is particularly breathless, closed questions that can be answered with a 'yes' or a 'no' will avoid further distress. It is also important to remember that respiratory assessment cannot be separated from cardiovascular assessment, as the two systems are closely interrelated.

A psychosocial history will reveal factors that might affect respiratory function. Note if the patient has any allergies or occupational exposure to asbestos, coal dust, gas fumes or other potential toxins. Ask whether the patient smokes, or has smoked in the past, and if so, how many and for how long.

The presence of a cough is significant, and the nature of the cough should be evaluated. Listen and try to identify the character of the cough. Is it:

- dry and hacking, which might indicate viral infection, early congestive cardiac failure or nervousness?
- loose and productive, which might indicate possible problems in the peripheral bronchi and lung parenchyma (the essential active cells of the lung tissue)?
- appearing to stem from the upper airways, which may be indicated by a loud harsh stridor or audible wheeze?
- chronic and productive, which might indicate pulmonary disease?
- painful (if so, note the type and position of the pain)?

Factors exacerbating the coughing should be explored. For how long has the cough been noticed, and what factors make it worse or better? A recent onset of coughing for a few days is suggestive of infection, but a cough getting progressively worse over weeks or months is suggestive of carcinoma (NICE, 2005; BTS, 2006).

In addition it important to know the nature of any sputum that is being expectorated, particularly the frequency, amount and colour. Is it:

- thick yellow or green, or flecked with blood, which might indicate bacterial infection?
- rusty coloured, which might indicate bacterial pneumonia?
- frothy, liquid white or pink, indicating pulmonary oedema?
- bloody, which could indicate pulmonary embolism or cancer of the lung causing erosion of a blood vessel?

Also determine whether there is any haemoptysis, and ascertain the colour, amount and the frequency of it.

The patient must be assessed for any signs of breathing difficulty or dyspnoea. This might be acute or chronic, and any factors that could exacerbate the breathlessness should be established. For example:

- Is the breathlessness related to exertion or positioning?
- Has the breathlessness become suddenly or progressively worse?
- What could the patient do a year ago or a month ago that they are unable to do now?
- Is the dyspnoea more severe at night, and can the patient lie down without undue distress?

This last factor is important for the bronchoscopy procedure, as it will determine whether the patient will be able to tolerate the semi-recumbent position normally used.

Physical examination

Once the history has been taken a physical examination is performed. When assessing respiratory function, it is important to observe the chest. Therefore the patient needs to remove the outside clothing so that the chest movements can be seen clearly (Moore, 2007).

Many respiratory abnormalities can be witnessed when assessing chest movements. Observe the rate, pattern and depth of respiration. The normal resting respiratory rate of the adult is 12–16 inspirations per minute, with expiration taking approximately twice as long as inspiration. Assess the patient for abnormal breathing patterns, or uneven rhythm or respiration. Compare the movements on both sides of the body, noting any difference in the shape or symmetry of the chest, and the use of accessory muscles, which may be demonstrated by the use of the scalene, sternomastoid and pectoralis muscles when breathing (Chapman et al, 2005; Simpson, 2006).

The colour of the skin may be an indicator of respiratory status. Central cyanosis (that is, blue discoloration seen in the mucous membranes of the mouth and lips) is associated with low arterial oxygenation, which may be the result of inadequate ventilation. Agitation, drowsiness confusion and impaired consciousness indicate hypoxaemia (Jevon and Ewens, 2001).

Pulse oximetry

This is a very useful noninvasive monitoring technique for measuring the haemoglobin oxygen (SpO2) saturation. It can make a valuable contribution to the respiratory assessment of the patient, and gives a reflection of the amount of oxygen available in the tissues (Moyle, 2002). However it should be noted that other indicators of respiratory function such blood CO_2 levels

t☆

Practice tip

A persistent cough can be one of the earliest signs of a lung tumour. It is often overlooked by people who smoke, who might have had 'smoker's cough' for some time. When assessing patients, always remember to ask them whether the cough has changed in any way.

t☆

Practice tip

Always let the patient rest before physical examination, so that observations recorded are reliable and not affected by physical exertion.

Part

III

and acid base are not measured by pulse oximetry, which should therefore be considered as part of the holistic assessment of the patient and other tests such as arterial blood gases (Booker, 2008).

A probe placed on the finger or earlobe indicates the presence of oxy-haemaglobin present in the capillary blood, which is displayed on a monitor. Normal values of oxygen saturation in adults vary between 96 and 99 per cent. However, this may be less than 90 per cent in patients with chronic lung disease and it is important to note that this may be normal for them. In all cases a low SpO2 needs further investigation by blood gas analysis (Bateman and Leach, 1998). Pulse oximetry provides rapid 'real time' information about the onset of some pulmonary complications, making it invaluable during a bronchoscopy as well as many other procedures. However to interpret the reading correctly, it is important to note if the patient is receiving oxygen therapy, and to understand the limitations of the recordings.

(e) Evidence-based practice

Pulse oximetry is widely used in many clinical situations as it is noninvasive and easy to establish. However research undertaken by Stoneham, Savile and Wilson (1994) identified a significant lack of knowledge of the basic principles of pulse oximetry amongst nurses and junior doctors, and both groups made serious errors when interpreting the readings.

Several factors that will result in inaccurate readings. The most important of these is that no direct indication of a patient's ventilation can be obtained by pulse oximetry, which measures oxygenation only. Thus it is possible for a previously well-oxygenated patient to have a satisfactory oximetry recording after they have actually stopped breathing.

When using a finger probe for pulse oximetry, abnormal readings may be obtained if:

- the patient has poor circulation in their fingers
- the patient has cardiac dysrhythmias
- the probe is not positioned correctly (Booker, 2008)
- the patient is wearing nail varnish (Hughes and Pride, 1999), although more recent studies suggest that nail varnish may not affect the readings in healthy patients (Rodden et al, 2007)
- the patient has dark skin pigmentation (Feiner, Severinhous and Bickler, 2007)
- the patient is shivering (Hughes and Pride, 1999)
- overhead light is excessive (Hughes and Pride, 1999).

t☆ Practice tip

When using any sort of monitoring equipment, ensure that you have received adequate instruction in its use and that you are sufficiently knowledgeable to use it safely.

Once the assessment is completed, any concerns should be discussed with the bronchoscopist, who will then decide whether to proceed or not. In addition to physiological and psychological concerns that the assessing nurse may wish to discuss, organisational issues must be considered. The lack of a suitably experienced bronchoscopist, lack of adequate staff, lack of facilities to deal with any emergency that might arise (pneumothorax, haemorrhage, cardiopulmonary arrest) and inability to provide safe postprocedural care remain absolute contraindications to the procedure (Belli, 1999). The results of the blood tests and pulmonary function tests undertaken in the outpatients clinic must also be considered.

a Learning activity

Find out more about the blood tests normally performed prior to bronchoscopy (haemaglobin level, full blood count, urea and electrolytes levels, clotting screen). Why are they required? Arrange to visit a pulmonary function laboratory to learn more about the tests and watch them being performed. Perhaps you could undertake the pulmonary function tests yourself under supervision.

S Scenario continued

The nurse prepares Peter for bronchoscopy and his written consent is obtained. His nose and throat are sprayed with Lidocaine and he is sedated with intravenous Alfentanil (an opiod analgesic). The bronchoscopy is then performed.

Applied pharmacology

a Learning activity

Before reading on, find out as much as you can about the drugs Lidocaine and Alfentanil, and revisit your knowledge about oxygen.

Lidocaine

Lidocaine is a local anaesthetic agent, and because it is a useful surface anaesthetic (BMA/BPS, 2007), it is used during bronchoscopy to reduce discomfort caused by introduction of the bronchoscope and to suppress the cough reflex, while the trachea and bronchi are examined. A Lidocaine solution is sprayed into the nose and throat before the procedure, and additional doses are administered through the bronchoscope as the procedure progresses. Lidocaine is effectively absorbed via the mucous membranes and has a rapid onset. The effects last for one and a half to two hours.

Patients who have had their throats sprayed with Lidocaine will not be able to swallow normally until the effects of the drug have worn off. It is therefore important to protect their airways by ensuring that they remain 'nil by mouth' until this happens.

Alfentanil

Alfentanil is an opioid analgesic which, when used intravenously, has a very rapid onset (1–2 minutes: BMA/BPS, 2007) and short duration of action. It is therefore very useful during short, invasive procedures, to ensure that the patient is pain free and relaxed during the procedure and can recover rapidly afterwards.

As with all opioids, respiratory depression can occur, and close observation of respiratory effort is crucial. Naloxone, an opiate antagonist which acts as a respiratory stimulant, can be used to reverse the depressant effects, but serious respiratory compromise will require resuscitation and assisted ventilation.

Any drug that causes respiratory depression must be used with extreme caution in any patients who have a respiratory problem, such as Peter.

Oxygen

Oxygen is commonly used in hospitals and is generally regarded as safe. However it must be remembered that high concentrations of oxygen (above 24–28 per cent) can adversely effect the respiratory drive of some patients with chronic lung disease. Prolonged use of high concentrations of oxygen causes collapse of the alveoli (Jevon and Ewens, 2001). It should therefore be used with caution, as prescribed and monitored (O'Driscoll, Howard and Davison, 2008). Oxygen also supports combustion and is therefore a major fire hazard.

Part
III

a Learning activity

How is oxygen prescribed in your area?
Examine all the different methods of oxygen
administration.

Oxygen is usually administered nasally to patients
undergoing bronchoscopy in order to ensure that the
passage of the bronchoscope does not result in hypoxia.
Oxygen saturation levels are monitored by pulse
oximetry throughout the procedure.

The role of the nurse in endoscopy

The nurse has two main roles when assisting with a procedure such as endoscopy. The first
is the care and monitoring of the patient. This includes the preparation of the patient, care
throughout the procedure and postprocedural care, including preparation for discharge. A
key dimension of the nurse's role is allaying the patient's anxiety throughout the procedure.
This may be achieved through effective verbal and nonverbal communication. The second
important aspect of the role is to assist the endoscopist to perform the procedure correctly
and safely. This includes preparing, maintaining and assisting with the equipment, handling
specimens and ensuring accurate record keeping (NMC, 2007).

Maintenance of equipment

The equipment used for all endoscopic procedures needs to be maintained in good working
order to ensure that the investigations are performed safely and effectively. Specific guidelines
are followed for inspection of the bronchoscope, and relevant training is required to ensure
the correct care and maintenance of the equipment. The nurse needs to be familiar with the
preparation of the bronchoscope, which should be inspected before use to check for faults. If
there are any suspected abnormalities, the instrument should not be used. After use, correct
cleaning, disinfection and storage are essential, and detailed nursing knowledge of the correct
procedure is required. The introduction of the Control of Substances Hazardous to Health
(COSHH) legislation by the Health and Safety Executive (1999) has had an impact on the
cleaning of endoscopic equipment.

a Learning activity

What are the procedures followed for this process in your
endoscopy unit?
   Familiarise yourself with the infection control policy in
your area. Are there recommendations for bronchoscopic
procedures?

What is meant by universal precautions?
   How is a risk assessment for COSHH carried out in your
area of practice, and who is responsible for undertaking it?

Assisting with the bronchoscopy procedure

The nurse assisting with the bronchoscopy procedure should be aware of the complications
that could arise during the procedure and be familiar with the emergency procedures to
follow should complications occur.

Before assisting with the bronchoscopy it
is important to determine the purpose of the
procedure in order to ensure the proper preparation of the equipment such as specimen pots and
pathology request cards. Chest x-rays are required
to locate any lesion. Often anterior–posterior and
lateral chest x-rays are needed, so it is important
that these are available.

a Learning activity

Consider the difference between an anterior–
posterior chest x-ray and a lateral chest x-ray. Why
might both be needed? You may find it useful to
visit your local radiography department to discuss
this with the radiographer.

The results of a clotting screen (to ensure that the patient has normal coagulation time) will also be required.

During the procedure, the flexible bronchoscope is passed into the mouth or nose and into the upper airways. Supplementary oxygen can be administered as required, and the nurse may have to assist with suctioning secretions out of the mouth using an oropharyngeal sucker.

Care of the patient during the procedure

Patients may be extremely anxious about the procedure, and be in need of psychological support. Explaining what is happening to them at every stage can reduce their anxiety and increase cooperation (Richardson, Adams and Poole, 2006). They need to be reassured that they will be able to breathe normally through the bronchoscope. The patient must be monitored continuously throughout the procedure.

> **ⓐ Learning activity**
>
> Before reading on, make a list of the observations you would make of a patient undergoing a bronchoscopy and why.

The minimal level of observation should include:

- level of consciousness
- response to the procedure (for example pain, dyspnoea)
- response to any drugs administered
- levels of oxygenation determined by pulse oximetry
- respiratory rate and depth
- blood pressure and any changes in cardiac status.

Specimens and record keeping

Accurate record keeping is essential to ensure continuity of care and to provide a baseline for reference when making discharge decisions. Documentation should include the patient's condition during the procedure, with observations of blood pressure, pulse, respiration and oximetry recorded. Any biopsies that were taken and the tests requested should also be recorded.

> **ⓐ Learning activity**
>
> Revisit the guidelines of the Nursing and Midwifery Council in respect of record keeping (NMC, 2007).

> **t☆ Practice tip**
>
> When collecting biopsies, check that the patient details are accurate on the specimen pot and the request card and that the spelling is correct. Make sure that you use a date of birth, address and hospital number as well as the name to avoid confusion. It is a good idea to label the specimen pots before the procedure, especially if several biopsies are taken.

Complications of bronchoscopy

> **ⓐ Learning activity**
>
> Consider and list the complications that might occur following this procedure, before reading on.

The complications of bronchoscopy are rare, but include (Chapman et al, 2005):

- respiratory depression
- pneumonia
- pneumothorax
- airway obstruction
- laryngospasm
- cardiac dysrhythmias/ arrest
- pulmonary oedema
- systemic infection
- haemorrhage
- nausea and vomiting
- hypotension
- drug reactions
- perforation of the trachea
- aspiration.

(a) Learning activity

List the patient monitoring techniques that you already know about. Could they be used to detect such complications?

(s) Scenario: Problems during bronchoscopy

A patient is undergoing bronchoscopy and you are the assisting nurse. The procedure has progressed normally and the patient's observations have been stable throughout: pulse 78 bpm, and blood pressure 140/80 mmHg. The endoscopist decides to take a biopsy of a suspected tumour, which is a routine test. After this has happened, you notice that the blood pressure has suddenly dropped to 70/40 mmHg and the pulse has risen to 120 bpm. What does this alert you to?

At this point the endoscopist notes that there is a large amount of fresh blood pooling in the lung. The patient coughs and a large volume of bright red blood is visible, quickly covering the pillows. What do you think has happened?

You summon help and prepare the resuscitation equipment while the endoscopist maintains the patient's airway with suctioning. The patient is given intravenous fluids and blood and his condition stabilises. He is taken for surgery.

The cause of this incident was a major end-bronchial bleed following biopsy of a highly vascular tumour.

(a) Learning activity

Consider the following:

- Are you aware of the physiological markers of major haemorrhage?
- What are the resuscitation procedures in your area?
- What is the location of the resuscitation equipment in your area? Is it regularly checked to ensure that drugs and equipment are not out of date and the equipment is working properly?

It is your responsibility as the designated nurse to be able to answer 'yes' to all of the above.

When a cardiac arrest occurs in hospital, nurses are most likely to be the first on the scene. It is therefore essential that nurses are able to diagnose a cardiac arrest, know how to summon help, and how to initiate basic life support when required (Soar and Spearpoint, 2005). Evidence suggests that a significant number of healthcare professionals are ineffective when performing cardiopulmonary resuscitation. Poor underpinning knowledge and lack of practice leading to lack of confidence have been reported, resulting in reduced levels of competence. Lack of practice results in rapid deterioration of psychomotor skills. There is evidence that if staff are well trained, resuscitation occurs more rapidly, which increases the chance of patient survival. Although theoretical knowledge is important, it is crucial to practise life-support skills regularly using a mannequin, preferably in a simulated arrest scenario (Soar and Spearpoint, 2005).

(t) Practice tip

Attend basic life support training regularly, at least every six months, and keep updating your psychomotor skills!

Patient discharge

The completion of a daycase procedure requires the timely and appropriate discharge of the patient. Recovery may be divided into three stages (Lugay et al, 1996):

- Early recovery, when the patient has emerged from the anaesthesia and sedating drugs, and is able to open their eyes and protect their own airway.
- Intermediate recovery, when the patient is ready to go home, can stand and walk unaided, and their vital signs have been stable for one hour.
- Full recovery, when the patient has resumed their normal daily activities, for example going to work and driving.

Liaison with the patient's GP, practice nurse or district nurse is essential to ensure continuity of care. It is important that key information reaches the healthcare professionals who will be responsible for the patient by the quickest and most reliable route. If the procedure has not gone as planned, it may be necessary to speak directly to a member of the primary care team before the patient leaves the hospital.

To ensure the patient has reached the intermediate recovery stage, the following points should be considered:

- Is there any evidence of physiological or psychological complications arising from the procedure?
- If the patient's throat has been anaesthetised, has their swallow reflex returned to normal?
- Does the patient know whom to contact and how if any problems arise?

Any patient who has been sedated for a procedure may well suffer some loss of memory, so information given in the immediate post-procedure phase will need to be supplemented with written information, or the repetition of information to a relative or friend.

- Does the patient have access to a telephone and can they use it? (Regular observation in the postprocedural phase enables the rapid detection of immediate complications, but some problems can be delayed, for instance slow bleeding and infection.)
- Does the patient have appropriate transport and an escort home?
- Does the patient understand the next stage of their care? Do they need to see their GP or return to outpatients? If so, when?

> ### t ☆
> ### Practice tip
>
> Discharge planning should begin at or before admission to ensure good continuity of care. Questions relating to the safe discharge of the patient should be answered before the procedure or before the patient is admitted. If the patient's safety is likely to be compromised after discharge, the procedure cannot go ahead.

Part

III

> ### (a) Learning activity
>
> Who takes responsibility for the discharge of patients in your endoscopy unit?

Research designed to identify an optimal method for determining when to discharge safely patients who have undergone endoscopic procedures after conscious sedation (Lugay et al, 1996) posed the question, 'Is it possible to predict which patients will suffer pre-discharge or post-discharge complications following an endoscopic procedure?'

Although this was a limited study, results suggest a close correlation between intraprocedural occurrences and postprocedure complications. Thus any patient who experiences intraprocedural events requires closer postprocedural monitoring. Also, there is evidence that age is predictive of length of time in recovery, with older patients taking longer to recover than younger patients. Thus it would seem logical to organise procedures to ensure that older patients are examined earlier in the day, so there is enough time for them to recover fully prior to discharge.

It may not be possible to give the patient accurate diagnostic information following a bronchoscopy. Even if a tumour has been seen, the exact nature of the tumour is unconfirmed until results from biopsies are available. Many patients will therefore face a period of anxiety and uncertainty awaiting results. At this very stressful time, patients are often not in contact with health professionals, and rely on family and friends for support. It may be helpful to give patients and their families information regarding potential sources of support, such as patient support groups, telephone helplines and nurse specialists. Evidence suggests that such services are well used if the patients are aware of them. One study revealed that a nurse specialist in Glasgow received an average of eight calls per referred patient (Fennerty, Reid and O'Donnell, 1996).

It is also helpful to remind the patient that they can contact their GP or practice nurse for advice and support whenever they need it, ensuring that they have the relevant contact information.

---

a Scenario: Peter Stevens's story continued

Peter's bronchoscopy is completed uneventfully. Biopsy specimens are obtained and dispatched for pathological analysis. After a period of supervised recovery and a final nursing assessment, he is allowed to leave the hospital, accompanied by his daughter Julie.

Peter commented afterwards, 'It was all right actually. I was pretty worried about it before I came in, but to be quite honest, I don't really remember much about it! I was glad to have my daughter with me. She asked all

the questions: you know, what happens next, when will we know anything? The nurses were very good. They kept explaining things. I remember being thirsty, and having to wait for a drink, and my throat was a bit sore for a couple of days, but nothing to really bother about.

'The worst thing is still not knowing – they just said I have to wait for the results. I really want to know what's going on now.'

---

a Learning activity

Reflect on what you have learned while studying this scenario, perhaps by reviewing the learning outcomes and concepts at the beginning of the chapter. In particular consider what you gained while visiting an endoscopy unit to observe a procedure, and in discussion with the endoscopy staff.

The key professional considerations related to this procedure are transferable to many investigative procedures and treatment protocols:

- patient safety
- reducing patient activity
- effective interprofessional communication
- effective use of resources.

Write a reflective account of your learning experience for inclusion in your personal portfolio. Identify how your learning in these key areas has developed.

Conclusion

In reading this chapter and participating in the prescribed activities you should have fully appreciated the parameters of adult healthcare and the complexities of where this care is delivered. In examining the scenario of the patient you have been able to consider both how contemporary care is delivered in various settings, and how healthcare professionals work together for the benefit of the patients and their families. In addition to understanding the holistic needs of patients, you should have gained an appreciation of the importance of communication at every step of the care experience.

a Learning activity

Consider in your learning group what is meant by holistic nursing, and identify the problems in providing holistic care in the ambulatory setting.

References

Barker, S. (2007) *Vital Notes for Nurses: Psychology*, Oxford, Blackwell.

Bateman, N. and Leach, R. (1998) 'ABC of oxygen', *British Medical Journal* 317, 798–801.

Beddows, J. (1997) 'Alleviating pre-operative anxiety in patients: a study' *Nursing Standard* 11(37), 35–8.

Booker, R. (2008) 'Pulse oximetry', *Nursing Standard* 22(30), 39–43.

British Hypertension Society (BHS) (nd) 'How to measure blood pressure' [online] http://www.bhsoc.org/how_to_measure_blood_pressure.stm (accessed 23 February 2009).

British Medical Association and British Pharmaceutical Society (BMA/BPS) (2007) *British National Formulary*, London, BMJ Publishing/RPS Publishing.

British Thoracic Society (2006) 'Guidelines for managing cough' [online] www.brit-thoracic.org.uk (accessed 5 February 2009).

Britton, J. (2005) 'Passive smoking and asthma exacerbation', *Thorax* 60, 794–5.

Buchanan, M. (1995) 'Enabling patients to make informed decisions', *Nursing Times* 91(18), 27–9.

Cancer Help (2008) Information for cancer patients [online] http://www.cancerhelp.org.uk (accessed 2 May 2008).

Cancer Research UK (2008) General information on cancer [online] http://info.cancerresearchuk.org (accessed 2 May 2008).

Chambers, M. (2009) 'Anxiety', in Glasper, E., McEwing, G. and Richardson, J. (eds), Foundation Skills for Caring, Basingstoke, Palgrave Macmillan.

Chapman, A. (1996) 'Current theory and practice: a study of pre-operative fasting', *Nursing Standard* 10(18), 33–6.

Chapman, S., Robinson, G., Stradling, J. and West, S. (2005) *The Oxford Handbook of Respiratory Medicine*, Oxford, Oxford University Press.

Claxton, D. (1999) 'Diagnosing, detecting and treating lung cancer', *Nursing Times* 95(20), 44–6.

Costa, M. (2001) 'The lived perioperative experience of ambulatory surgery patients', *AORN Journal* 74 (6), 877–81.

Curtis, A. J. (2000) *Health Psychology*, London, Routledge.

Department of Health (DH) (1991) *Patient's Charter*, London, HMSO.

DH (1992) *Health of the Nation: Key areas handbook – cancers*, London, DH.

DH (1999a) *Saving Lives: Our healthier nation*, London, DH [online] http://www.archive.official-documents.co.uk/document/cm43/4386/4386-01.htm (accessed 8 February).

DH (1999b) *Smoking Kills*, London, DH.

DH (2004) *Choosing Health: Making healthier choices easier*, London, DH.

Dest, V. (2000) 'Lung cancer', *Registered Nurse* 63(5), 32–8.

Dimond, B. (2008) *Legal Aspects of Mental Capacity*, Oxford, Blackwell.

Docherty, B. (2002) 'Cardiorespiratory physical assessment for the acutely ill: Part 1', *British Journal of Nursing* 11(11), 750–8.

Docherty, B. and Coote, S. (2006) 'Monitoring the pulse as part of track and trigger', *Nursing Times* 102(43), 28–9.

Doll, R., Peto, R., Boreham, J. and Sutherland, I. (2005) 'Mortality from cancer in relation to smoking: 50 years observation on British doctors', *British Journal of Cancer* 92(3), 426–9.

Dougherty, L. and Lister, S. (eds) (2004) *The Royal Marsden Hospital Manual of Clinical Nursing Procedures*. 6th edn, Oxford, Blackwell.

Dubois, J., Barter, T. and Pratter, M. (1995) 'Music improves patient comfort level during outpatient bronchoscopy', *Chest* 108(1), 129–30.

Ebbert, J.O., Yang, P., Vachon, C. M., Vierkant, R. A., Cerhan, J. R.,

Folsom, A. R. and Sellars, T. A. (2003) 'Lung cancer risk reduction after smoking cessation: observations from a prospective cohort of women', *Journal of Clinical Oncology* 21(5), 921–6.

Feiner, J. R., Severinhous, J. W. and Bickler, P. E. (2007) 'Dark skin decreases the accuracy of pulse oximeters at low oxygen saturation: the effects of oximeter probe type and gender', *Anesthesia and Analgesia* 105(6 supp.), S16–S23.

Fennerty, A., Reid, A. and O'Donnell, M. (1996) 'A named nurse programme for the care of patients with lung cancer', *Thorax* 51(supp. 3), A57.

Ferlay, J., Autier, P., Boniol, M., Heanue, M., Colombet, M., Colombet, S. and Boyle, P. (2007) 'Estimates of the cancer incidence and mortality in Europe in 2006', *Annals of Oncology* 18(3), 581–92.

Franceschi, S and Bidoli, E (1999) 'The epidemiology of lung cancer', *Annals of Oncology* 10(supp. 5), S3–S6.

Gardner, E. (2005) 'Care of the patient requiring thoracic surgery', pp. 265–87 in Pudner, R. (ed.), *Nursing the Surgical Patient*, 2nd edn, Edinburgh, Elsevier.

Gillespie, A. and Curzio, J. A. (1998) 'Blood pressure measurement: assessing staff knowledge'.*Nursing Standard* 12(23), 35–7.

Goddard, E. (2006) *General Household Survey: Smoking and drinking among adults 2005*, Newport, Office for National Statistics.

Godtfredsen, N., Prescott, E. and Osler, M. (2005) 'Effect of smoking reduction on lung cancer risk', *Journal of the American Medical Association* 294(12), 1505–10.

Govier, I. (2000) 'Spiritual care in nursing: a systematic approach', *Nursing Standard* 12(14), 32–6.

Hamilton-Smith, S. (1972) *Nil By Mouth: A descriptive study of nursing care in relation to pre-operative fasting*, London, Royal College of Nursing.

Harwood, G. A., Slasberry, P., Ferketich, A. K. and Wewers, M. E. (2007) 'Cigarette smoking, socioeconomic status and psychosocial factors: Examining a conceptual framework', *Public Health Nursing* 24(4), 361–71.

Hayes, A., Buffum, M., Lanier, E., Rodahl, E. and Sasso, C. (2003) 'A music intervention to reduce anxiety prior to gastrointestinal procedures', *Gastroenterology Nursing* 26(4), 145–9.

Higgins, D. (2008) 'Patient assessment: Part 5, measuring pulse', *Nursing Times* 104(11), 24–5.

Hirsch, F. R. and Lippman, S. M. (2005) 'Advances in the biology of lung cancer chemoprevention', *Journal of Clinical Oncology* 23(14), 3186–97.

Hoffman, P. C., Mauer, A. M. and Vokes, E. E. (2000) 'Lung cancer', *The Lancet* 355(9292) , 479–85.

Hughes, J. M. and Pride, N. B. (1999) *Lung Function Tests: Physiological principles and clinical application*, London, W. B. Saunders.

Information Centre for Health and Social Care and RCP (2006) *National Lung Cancer Audit: Report for the audit period 2005*, December.

Jamieson, E. M., McCall, J. M. and Whyte, L. A. (2002) *Clinical Nursing Practices*, 4th edn, Edinburgh, Churchill Livingstone.

Jevon, P. and Ewens, B. (2001) 'Assessment of a breathless patient', *Nursing Standard* 15(16), 48–53.

Kenward, G., Hodgetts, T. and Castle, N. (2001) 'Time to put the R back in TPR', *Nursing Times* 97(40), 32–3.

Kosco, P. and Held-Warmkessel, J. (2000) 'Lung cancer – can early detection become a reality in the 21st century?' *American Journal of Nursing* (April supp,), 13–7.

Lancaster, T., Stead, L., Silagy, C. and Sowden, A. (2000) 'Effectiveness of interventions to help people stop smoking: findings from the Cochrane library', *British Medical Journal* **321**(7257), 355–8.

Leung, G. M., Ho, L. M. and Lam, T. H. (2004) 'Second hand smoke exposure, smoking hygiene and hospitalisation in the first eighteen months of life', *Archives of Pediatric and Adolescent Medicine* 158, 687–93.

Lugay, M., Otto, G., Kong, M., Mason, D. and Wilets, I. (1996) 'Recovery time and safe discharge of endoscopy patients after conscious sedation', *Gastroenterology Nursing* **19**(6), 194–200.

McCarron, P., Davey Smith, G., Okasha, M. and McEwen, J. (2001) 'Smoking in adolescence and young adulthood and mortality in later life: prospective observational study', *Journal of Epidemiology and Community Health* 55, 334–5.

McMillan, R, (2005) 'Day surgery', pp. 119–220 in Woodhead, K. and Wicker, P. (eds), *A Textbook of Perioperative Care*, Edinburgh, Elsevier Churchill Livingstone.

Medical Protection (nd) Consent information [online] http://www.medicalprotection.org/uk/factsheets/consent-basics (accessed 5 February 2009).

Mosby (2006) *Mosby's Pocket Dictionary of Nursing, Medicine, and Professions Allied to Medicine*, 5th edn, London, Mosby.

Moyle, J. (2002) *Pulse Oximetry*, London, British Medical Journal Books.

National Institute for Clinical Excellence (NICE) (2005) *Lung Cancer: The diagnosis and treatment of lung cancer*, Clinical guidance 24, London, NICE.

National Youth Information Agency (2008) General information [online] http://www.youthinformation.com (accessed 2 May 2008).

Nursing and Midwifery Council (NMC) (2007) *Record Keeping*, London, NMC.

NMC (2008) *Code of Professional Conduct*, London, NMC.

Oakley, M. (2005) 'Day surgery', pp. 35–43 in Pudner, R. (ed.), *Nursing the Surgical Patient*, 2nd edn, Edinburgh, Elsevier.

O'Driscoll, B., Howard, L. and Davison, A. (20080 'Guideline for emergency oxygen use in adult patients', *Thorax* 63(suppl. vi), 1–73.

Office for National Statistics (ONS) (2006) *General Household Survey 2006: Smoking and drinking among adults 2006*, Newport, ONS.

Peto, R., Darby, S., Deo, H., Silcocks, P., Whitely, E. and Doll, R. (2000) 'Smoking, smoking cessation and lung cancer in the UK since 1950:combination of national statistics with two case-controlled studies' *British Medical Journal* **321**(7257) 323–9.

Radcliffe, S. (1993) 'Pre-operative information: the role of the ward nurse' *British Journal of Nursing* 2 (6), pp. 305–9.

Reid, J. (1997) 'Meeting the informational needs of patients in a day surgery setting – an exploratory level study', *British Journal of Theatre Nursing* 7(4), 19–24.

Richardson, C., Adams, N. and Poole, H. (2006) 'Psychological approaches for the nursing management of chronic pain, Part 2', *Journal of Clinical Nursing* 15, 1196–202.

Rodden, A. M., Spicer, L., Diaz, V. and Steyer, T. (2007) 'Does fingernail polish affect pulse oximeter readings?' *Intensive and Critical Care Nursing* 23, 51–5.

Rogan Foy, C. and Timmins, F. (2004) 'Improving communication in day care settings', *Nursing Standard* **19**(7), 37–42.

Rowe, J. (2002) 'Preoperative fasting is it time for a change?' *Nursing Times* 96(17, supp.),14–15.

Sarna, L. Bialous, S. A., Wewers, M. E., Froelicher, E. S. and Danao, L. (2005) 'Nurses, smoking and the workplace', *Research in Nursing and Health* **28**(1),79–90.

Schrieber, G. and McCory, D. C. (2003) 'Performance characteristics of different modalities for diagnosis of suspected lung cancer', *Chest* 123, 115S–25S.

Simpson, H. (2006) 'Respiratory assessment', *British Journal of Nursing* **15**(9), 484–8.

Sims, J. M. (2008) 'Your role in informed consent: Part 1,' *Dimensions of Critical Care Nursing* **27**(2), 70–3.

Soar, J. and Spearpoint, K. (2005) 'In hospital resuscitation', in *Resuscitation Guidelines*, Resuscitation Council (UK).

Spear, H. (1996) 'Anxiety', *Registered Nurse* (July), 40–5.

Stafrace, J. (1998) 'Assessment: the key to patient safety when undergoing an endoscopic procedure', *Gastroenterology Nursing* **21**(3), 131–4.

Stoneham, M., Savile, G. and Wilson, I. (1994) 'Knowledge about pulse oximetry among medical and nursing staff', *The Lancet* **344**(12), 1339–42.

Subramanian, J. and Govindan, R. (2007) 'Lung cancer in never smokers', *Journal of Clinical Oncology* **25**(5), 561–70.

Thompson, I., Melia, K., Boyd, K. and Horsburgh, D. (2006) *Nursing Ethics*, 5th edn, Edinburgh, Churchill Livingstone Elsevier.

Vermeire, E., Hearnshaw, H., Van Royen, P. and Denekens, J. (2001) 'Patient adherence to treatment: three decades of research: a comprehensive review', *Journal of Clinical Pharmacy and Therapeutics* **26**(5), 331–42.

Wood, S. (2005) 'Nutrition and the surgical patient', pp. 71–83 in Pudner, R. (ed.), *Nursing the Surgical Patient*, 2nd edn, Edinburgh, Elsevier.

Woodhouse, A. (2006) 'Pre-operative fasting for elective surgical patients', *Nursing Standard* **20**(21), 41–8.

Further reading

Baldwin, D. R., Hummerston, S., Saha, S., Johnstone, I. E. and Crosby, V. (2008) *Giving Information to Lung Cancer Patients: Guidance for healhcare professionals discussing options for patients on the lung cancer pathway*, Nottingham, British Thoracic Society Lung Cancer and Mesothelioma Specialist Advisory Group. This document provides guidance for the delivery of a suspected or confirmed lung cancer diagnosis and discussion of subsequent treatment. There is information regarding different treatments for lung cancer, and resources which include a very useful six-step guide to the breaking of bad news.

Bassett, C. (1997) 'Medical investigations 4: bronchoscopy', *British Journal of Nursing* 6(4), 592–3. This article is part of a very useful series which provides clear and concise information about a variety of medical investigations. This information will enable nurses to explain procedures to their patients more confidently, and to provide essential pre- and post-procedure care.

Belli, M. (1999) 'Bronchoscopy', *American Journal of Nursing* **99**(7), 24AA–24DD. Another useful review of bronchoscopic procedure, which highlights contraindications to the procedure, discusses drugs commonly used and explains postprocedural care.

Burgess, L. (1994) 'An epidemic of massive proportions', *Professional Nurse* (May), 566–72. This article provides an excellent overview of the physiological, psychological and sociological effects of cigarette smoking in the United Kingdom. Thorough knowledge of this subject provides nurses with greater insight into patients' smoking habits, and may assist in the identification of effective smoking cessation strategies.

Day, J. (1998) 'Lung cancer: screen or prevent?' *Practice Nursing* **9**(5), 32–4. The lack of an appropriate screening procedure for lung cancer results in a poor prognosis, as many patients have widespread disease by the time they are diagnosed. In this article issues related to potential screening techniques are discussed, and the need to focus on primary prevention by reducing smoking is highlighted.

Moore, T. (2007) 'Respiratory assessment in adults', *Nursing Standard* **21**(49), 48–56. This is a continuing professional development (CPD) article for the Learning Zone which aims to support the understanding of respiratory physiology and the assessment of respiratory status, including the assessment of cough and sputum and the use of pulse oximetry. It includes a self-assessment questionnaire.

NHS Executive (1998) *Guidance on Commissioning Cancer Services: Improving Outcomes in Lung Cancer: The research evidence*, London: Department of Health. A fascinating document which provides an overview of the research evidence underpinning recommendations currently being made by the NHS Executive, aimed at improving the outcomes in the treatment of patients with lung cancer. The available research evidence is reviewed in seven intervention categories: prevention; access, diagnosis and staging; multiprofessional teams; communication, information and support; radical treatment for NSCLC; radical treatment for SCLC; and palliative interventions and care. Of particular interest to nursing students is the research related to smoking cessation and the role of the nurse in the multidisciplinary team.

Quinn, S. (1999) 'Lung cancer: the role of the nurse in treatment and prevention', *Nursing Standard* **13**(41), 49–54. Having provided a very useful overview of the aetiology, pathophysiology and treatment of lung cancer, this article focuses on the nurse's role in palliative care, reviewing the management of dyspnoea and emphasising the importance of addressing the patient's spiritual needs.

Wilkinson, S., Locker, J., Whybrow, J., Percival, J. and Owen, L. (2004) 'The nurse's role in promoting smoking cessation', *Nursing Standard* **19**(14), 45–52. Another useful article from the *Nursing Standard*'s CPD series. Smoking cessation strategies are discussed and various products and local support services are outlined. There is a self-assessment questionnaire.

Legislation

Control of Substances Harmful to Health (COSHH) 1999
Health Act 2006
Mental Capacity Act 2005

Websites

Help for nurses to quit smoking: http://www.tobaccofreenurses.org
Oncolink: www.cancer.med.upenn.edu
Cancer Help: www.medweb.bham.ac.uk/cancerhelp
Cancer Research: UK http://info.cancerresearchuk.org

British Association for Cancer United Patients (BACUP): www.cancerbacup.org.uk
British Lung Foundation: www.lunguk.org/index.htm
Government documents: www.doh.gov.uk

Video

Kaymed (1991) *Practical Aspects of Fibreoptic Bronchoscopy*.

Part

III

Chapter

25

Care of the older adult – community

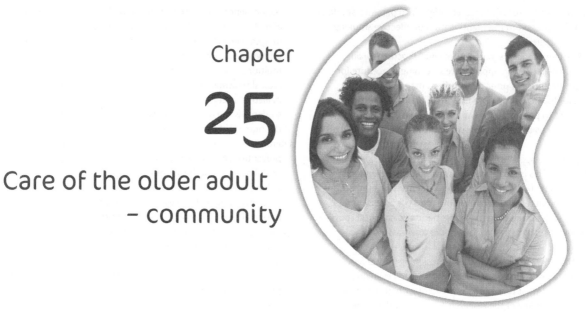

Carolyn Gibbon and
Alison Cochrane

Links to other chapters in *Foundation Studies for Caring*

Links to other chapters in *Foundation Skills for Caring*

W   Don't forget to visit www.palgrave.com/glasper for additional
online resources relating to this chapter.

Introduction

Frail elderly people within the population are now recognised as a client group with their own special needs. Although there are obviously exceptions, people generally live longer than previous generations. However, this means that some people also experience longer periods of frailty, with a consequent need for greater and more varied amounts of care. There are clearly implications for where that care is given and by whom. A number of factors need to be considered when making these decisions, and ideally the care needs of the individual should be the main determinant. However, in our current western society the decisions are increasingly being influenced by economic considerations.

This chapter explores these factors through the experience of Vera, her family and those caring for her. Vera is frail and elderly, and eventually leaves her own home to live in a nursing home. The care she receives along the way is influenced by standards discussed by *National Service Framework for Older People* (DH, 2001a) and *A New Ambition for Old Age* (DH, 2006a).

Learning outcomes

This chapter will enable you to:

- develop an understanding of the main issues related to being frail and elderly
- explore the impact of grief on individuals
- discuss the psychological and physiological effects of ageing
- explore the use and effects of pharmacology with the frail elderly
- identify the roles of the members of the community team and explore the ways in which continuity of care is maintained
- identify various tools used to assess the needs of frail, elderly people and how the findings are used to plan and evaluate care
- understand the issues related to care management within a person's own home and within a nursing and/or residential home.

Concepts

- The ageing process
- Needs and risk assessment
- Degenerative disorders in old age
- Pharmacological interventions
- Increasing dependency
- Care management

- Loss and grief associated with moving home
- Legal and ethical issues
- Bereavement – loss of spouse
- Community team
- Adaptive mechanisms

- Financial issues
- Continuing care for older people
- Social constructs in relation to older age

[S] Scenario: Vera's experience

Vera Jenkins is 87 years old, widowed for six months, and currently lives in her own three-bedroomed semi-detached house which she and George purchased when they were newly married. They have one son, Matt, whom Vera seldom sees. He is divorced with no children and lives abroad.

George was a chartered accountant; he managed their personal finances and ensured that Vera would have some additional savings set aside to supplement her state pension. Since George died, Vera has found it increasingly difficult to cope with everyday life. She has become physically frail and is experiencing mild confusion and disorientation which she finds distressing.

Defining what is meant by 'elderly' and 'frail' is not easy, as each term can be approached from a variety of perspectives. Wade (1996) points out that 70-year-olds have different needs from 90-year-olds, yet each group is classed as 'elderly'. The word 'frail' also invokes images of varying degrees of dependence. Therefore it is essential to consider the impact that the use of these terms can have.

> **a** **Learning activity**
>
> In your learning group construct your personal definitions of the words elderly and frail. Are there any gender differences in your definitions? Determine whether your ideas are supported by research. Discuss this with your fellow students.

Incidence

W

It was in 1821 that records began to be compiled in relation to how long individuals live. Currently there are 60.2 million people in the United Kingdom, of whom 5.5 per cent were aged over 85 in 2003. This was projected to rise to 7.9 per cent by 2031 (www.statistics.gov.uk). The majority are women, as women tend to live longer than men.

> **a** **Learning activity**   W
>
> Information about population trends in localities can be found at www.statistics.gov.uk. In your learning group, look at the projections for your local area. What are the implications for caring for older people?

Receiving primary care

> **S** **Scenario continued**
>
> Over the last three months social services have become involved in Vera's care following a telephone call from her neighbour, Mrs Barker. Mrs Barker has tried to help Vera by taking her a hot meal on a regular basis. This has received a mixed reception, depending on Vera's mental state and the fact that she sometimes perceives it as an affront to her pride and ability to cope. Mrs Barker believes that professional intervention is now needed, as she is only able to offer limited support because of her own family commitments.

> **a** **Learning activity**
>
> Consider how you might respond in similar circumstances; try to put yourself in Vera's shoes. Vera has been demonstrating that she is going through the grieving process. Make notes on what you understand by grieving and how it might feel (see Costello and Kendrick, 2000).

> **S** **Scenario continued**
>
> A social worker has alerted Vera's general practitioner (GP), who visits and is concerned about Vera's deteriorating condition. Vera says very clearly, 'You're not going to put me in the workhouse. I can manage.' While respecting her wishes, the GP decides to maintain close contact with social services and reassess the situation on a regular basis.

> **a** **Learning activity**
>
> What does Vera mean by the workhouse? What association do some elderly people believe exists between workhouses and healthcare? Discuss this in your learning group. Read Webster (2001), chapters 2 and 3.

S Scenario continued

Matt, Vera's son, is contacted by Mrs Barker, who thinks he ought to know what is going on. Matt contacts social services and speaks to the social worker who is managing Vera's care. He explains that although at present he is unable to fly home, he will if the situation requires it. He is keen to know whether residential care is the answer, but the social worker explains that this could only be considered in discussion with Vera, and the possibility has not yet been put to her. The social worker instigates a care package whereby a care worker provides support to Vera in her own home for a couple of hours each day.

a Learning activity

Social service provision is vast and can vary from area to area. In your learning group, arrange to collect examples of care packages from your own locality, and consider the ways in which they are able to address individual needs. Discuss this from an interprofessional perspective.

S Scenario continued

Vera is becoming even frailer and far less mobile. She is now unwilling to leave the house, so her care worker does her shopping and collects her pension. Her immobility, combined with her deteriorating mental state and reduced motivation, means that Vera spends long periods of time just sitting in her chair. As a result her troubles are compounded by the development of a small sacral pressure ulcer. The discovery of the pressure ulcer was quite by chance when the care worker noticed a stain on Vera's dress which she first associated with incontinence. The GP was informed and a healthcare practitioner, in this case a community nurse, now visits daily to dress the ulcer. The nurse has undertaken a course in prescribing and is able to choose suitable dressings, following protocols laid down by the local community trust.

The nurse has also provided pressure-relieving aids, as well as trying to encourage Vera to move around a little more. Vera has also been referred another healthcare practitioner, the community physiotherapist, who has agreed to visit to assess her mobility and see whether she requires a walking aid.

Pressure ulcers

The term' pressure ulcer' (also called a pressure sore or decubitus ulcer) is defined in Dougherty and Lister (2004) as any area of damage to the skin or underlying tissues caused by direct pressure or shearing force. They cause pain and discomfort, delay rehabilitation, and can cause disability and death.

There are four main causes of pressure sores:

- pressure
- shearing forces
- trauma or friction
- moisture.

Assessment of the risk of developing a pressure ulcer is vital, and the nurse must take into account factors such as age, nutritional status, circulatory status, mobility, dependence level and mental awareness (Collier, 2002). A number of assessment tools can be used to assist in this process. The Norton score (Norton, McLaren and Exton-Smith, 1975) is an assessment tool devised specifically for use with older people. Criteria focus on the general physical condition, the mental state, activity, mobility and incontinence, and a score is awarded for each section. A total score is then given, and the lower the score, the greater risk the patient has of developing pressure ulcers.

It is vital that attention is paid to the prevention of pressure ulcers, and Collier (2002: 929) recommends the following strategies:

- Assess the patient for risk factors.

Part

III

- Ensure regular changes of position to relieve pressure on vulnerable areas such as the heels, sacrum, elbows, or shoulders.
- Maintain cleanliness and hygiene.
- Prevent mechanical, physical or chemical injury.
- Ensure adequate nutrition and hydration.
- Promote continence.
- Ensure good body alignment.
- Use devices to redistribute pressure over pressure points.
- Inspect the skin several times a day.
- Promote mental alertness and orientation.
- Educate the patient, family and care givers in skin-care measures.

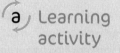 **Learning activity**

Access to the Norton score, usually printed as an aide memoire, should be readily available. Observe the tool and become familiar with the criteria for assessment.

Pressure ulcers take many different forms, and a grading system has been devised to grade the level of severity (Collier, 2002):

Grade 1   There is redness, warmth and slight erosion of the epidermis. It goes white when touched.

Grade 2   There is shallow ulceration with redness and heat, and does not blanch when touched.

Grade 3   The ulceration is deep, foul-smelling with a necrotic base.

Grade 4   The ulcer involves all layers of the skin, the underlying muscles, and may involve the bone or joints. It is deep.

All ulcers should be examined closely to determine the extent and depth of tissue involvement. They are then measured in centimetres and recorded. Regular inspection then determines the stages of healing.

The healing process has several recognised phases:

Stage 1   Inflammatory process. Cells are released to help in clot formation.

Stage 2   Granulation. Occurs in deep dermal wounds as new tissue is laid down.

Stage 3   Epithelisation. Occurs quickly in small wounds, when squamous cells migrate across the wound surface.

Stage 4   Remodelling/maturation. This stage may take from two days to two years. Vascularisation decreases, collagen matures and the appearance of the granulation tissue changes from red to white.

You can read more about pressure ulcers in Chapter 10 of the companion skills volume.

S Scenario continued

Vera has a sacral pressure ulcer that the community nurse assesses as being Grade 2. This will need treatment, and there are a number of products available, including topical agents to clean and/or protect ulcers, and dressings to assist in the healing process. The sore is treated with a hydrogel as there are some exudates. A dry dressing is placed over this, and the ulcer is checked on alternate days and the findings noted on the care plan.

a Learning activity

For more specific information on ulcers consult your local tissue viability nurse as a resource person. (You can also find out more on all the topics in this chapter from the further reading at the end of the chapter.)

S | Scenario continued

Referral to the medical consultant

The care worker and community nurse are very concerned as Vera is becoming increasingly frail and confused. The GP again visits Vera, and after spending some time talking to her, makes a referral to a consultant with a specialist interest in older people at the local district general hospital. It is hoped that the consultant will be able to establish the reason for Vera's physical and mental decline. This assessment needs to take place before considering whether Vera might be safer living somewhere other then her own home.

The GP writes a letter of referral to the consultant:

Dear Dr Smart,

Re: Mrs Vera Jenkins, 2 Holly Cottages, Castleberry, TU15 1SH. Age 87

I visited Mrs Jenkins today who is frail. She has been deteriorating both mentally and physically since the death of her husband George, six months ago from an MI. Both social services and the community nurse are now expressing concerns about her ability to manage at home. I would value your opinion regarding the cause of her deterioration. I am not convinced that this is necessarily the onset of a dementing illness, and feel the need to exclude depression in the light of her recent bereavement before any decision is taken regarding possible consideration for residential care. Mrs Jenkins is reluctant to take any form of medication and therefore no antidepressants have as yet been prescribed. I have spoken with the son who lives abroad. He is intending to return in two months time and it would be helpful if a case conference could be arranged around this time.

Presenting symptoms

Mrs Jenkins has enjoyed relatively good health over the years. Following a difficult birth, she only had the one child. It is a source of disappointment that she was unable to have more children. There have been no significant episodes of ill health.

More recently there have been considerable physical changes which have led to her current state of frailty. She is 160 cm tall but only currently weighs 52 kg, having lost approximately 13 kg since the death of her husband.

I have found Mrs Jenkins to be mildly confused and disoriented, and when spoken to she is either tearful or over-cheerful. Mrs Jenkins was distraught following George's death, but at first appeared to be coping. She has always kept herself 'tidy' but has recently started to look unkempt, and on a number of occasions has been seen wearing inappropriate clothes for the weather. One of her great interests is her garden, and this has started to look neglected. She continues to go to the local shops, but frequently returns having forgotten what she had gone for in the first place.

I look forward to hearing from you.
Dr H. Monroe, General Practitioner

How and why do our bodies alter with age?

According to Herbert (2006), past research into human ageing has emphasised loss or deterioration of function. Yet we need to adopt a more positive approach, as the majority of older people can function quite adequately in the physiological sense.

For Vera this decline has been taking place over many, many years. Vera has enjoyed good health, except for her pressure ulcer, and now she is experiencing the normal physical changes associated with the ageing process.

When considering the ageing process, a number of variables, such as good health, being a nonsmoker and exercise, must be taken into account. Whilst these variables may delay ageing, there are no guarantees. Herbert (2006) explains how in the past the interest was in looking for the 'elixir of life', but over time a greater understanding of the ageing process has developed.

Part

III

Ford and Wills (2002) note that when reviewing physiological changes, the assessment made by a healthcare practitioner is important. It takes place in three parts:

- **Interview**. This takes time because of slower functioning, reduced energy and/or memory deficits of older people. Information may need to be collected on several different occasions.
- **Observations**. Looking at the individual can reveal a great deal of information. Smell may detect unusual breath, excretory or skin odours. Touch can determine strength, flexibility, texture and temperature. Hearing is used to detect quality of speech or respirations.
- **Examination.** There should be inspection and palpation, with the findings carefully recorded.

Physiological changes

Skin

This thins and becomes less elastic, with reduced vascularity. The superficial blood vessels are less efficient in dilating and contracting to regulate body temperature. Older people are at greater risk than younger people of developing hypothermia. Wound healing is retarded, especially as feelings of heat, pressure and pain are not as acute. This can be seen with Vera and the development of her pressure ulcer.

Skeleton

Bone mass loss is greater in women than in men (Herbert, 2006), and it leads to bones becoming weaker and the vertebrae compressing, causing a loss of height. They can also change shape, and because of altered mineralisation, also change texture. Osteoporosis (bone loss) begins to take place from about 40 years of age, and is thought to be related to exercise, diet and hormonal changes. This combination leads to increased risk of bone fractures. Older people tend to lead a more sedentary lifestyle which can also lead to bone loss (Herbert, 2006).

Joints and muscles are also affected. Vera will be finding it more difficult to move about, and may even find it painful. Vera has not been eating properly, yet attention to diet, especially the need for proteins, potassium, calcium and Vitamin D, may slow this process down (Ford and Wills, 2002).

Cardiovascular

Barker (1998) notes that degenerative diseases of the heart and blood vessels are the most common effects of ageing. The work done by the heart reduces slightly with age, and thus there is a tendency for perfusion to the other body organs to be reduced (Herbert, 2006).

Currently Vera tends to sit for long periods and has periods of heightened activity when distressed. These need to be moderated so that she enjoys a balance of activity and rest.

Gastrointestinal

The gastrointestinal tract alters with age, but nutritional factors certainly have an influence. Herbert (2006) provides a comprehensive review of the impact of nutrition on the gastrointestinal tract.

Vera is currently taking an inadequate diet because of a lack of interest in food caused by her distress. Thus she is at risk of developing digestive problems, constipation and malnutrition. For useful resources with regards to malnutrition view www.uclan.ac.uk/sonic

Genitourinary

In some older people the filtration functions of the renal system slow down. Bladder capacity reduces from 500 ml to 250 ml, leading to frequency and nocturia (Ford and Wills, 2002). The generalised weakening of muscles affects the bladder, making it more difficult to empty, and can cause urine retention. For Vera a reduction in oestrogen following the menopause has caused the pelvic floor muscles to relax, leading to problems of stress incontinence or dribbling.

Special senses

Barker (1998) notes a number of issues in relation to the senses. The lenses in the eye harden with age and become increasingly opaque, leading to cataracts. The ear is affected because of loss of hairs on the cochlea and vestibule.

Taste buds degenerate with age, leading to the loss of taste perception, which in turn affects salivation, mouth cleanliness and appetite.

Vera will find diminished perception of sound, pitch and amplitude, and her balance will also be affected. This is an added problem for her.

Nervous system

This changes with age as the brain reduces in weight and response times slow down. Short-term memory may be affected, but changes are very individual and only a minority may develop dementia (Barker ,1998).

Vera will be at risk of a greater susceptibility to hazards and be less aware of pain.

Reproductive system

Testosterone reduces in men leading to hypertrophy of the prostate, slow erection and thinner pubic hair (Ford and Wills, 2002). Ovulation stops with the menopause as oestrogen production ceases. The female reproductive organs atrophy, and the vagina is less vascular and moist but more alkaline.

S Scenario continued

Vera continues to deteriorate. She needs lots of encouragement to wash and change her clothes, and she remains tearful. The consultant, having assessed Vera, has diagnosed a moderate dementia with an overlying depression. There is no doubt that George's recent death has caused Vera much distress, but Vera has also said how worried she is about her ability to remember things and cope with what seem like normal everyday activities. In fact she thinks she is going mad. The consultant has commented in his report to the GP that it is this level of insight, which is often apparent in the early stages of dementia, that is likely to be contributing to Vera's depression. He believes that Vera's willingness to talk about her loss will over time help relieve some of the effects of her depression, but he has suggested that the GP prescribe a mild antidepressant.

---

a Learning activity

In your learning group consider the differences between sadness and depression, then compare and contrast the symptoms of dementia with those of depression. You will find that some are similar while others are quite different. Why might it be important for any healthcare practitioner who visits Vera to be aware of these differences?

A number of different healthcare and social services practitioners have now become involved in Vera's well-being. It is important that the activities are coordinated so that Vera receives the best possible care and that there is no disparity or duplication in the services provided. This type of working is known under a number of different names, such as multidisciplinary, interprofessional and interagency. Barrett, Sellman and Thomas (2005: 10) state that 'the prefix multi tends to indicate the involvement of personnel from different professions, disciplines or agencies, but does not necessarily imply collaboration. The prefix inter tends to imply collaboration.'

Vera has so far had contact with the following healthcare practitioners:

- social worker
- community nurse
- occupational therapist
- general practitioner
- consultant with a special interest in older people
- community physiotherapist
- home care workers.

A care manager will be appointed to coordinate decisions that are taken to ensure that Vera receives the most appropriate care. The care manager will have had training in care management, which provides the skills to draw together the assessments made by each practitioner and formulate a plan of care. The person appointed needs to be very competent, with a high level of experience and training. Ross and Victor (2006: 177) define the care manager as 'any practitioner who undertakes all, or most of, the core tasks of care management, who may carry budgetary responsibility, but is not involved in any direct service provision'.

> **a / Learning activities**
>
> Recalling your own experience of practice in both institutional and community settings, consider the measures taken to ensure that communication remains effective between different members of the team. Which healthcare professional takes the lead role and why?
>
> Look at the action plan in *Partnership in Action* (DH, 2000) and consider how you could implement the recommendations of the NHS taskforce on staff involvement.

> **S   Scenario continued**
>
> Social services have appointed Ali, a social worker, as the healthcare practitioner who will be the care manager for Vera. Because of the increasing concerns for Vera's safety, Ali reconsiders the possibility of residential care, an option previously put forward by Matt, Vera's son. He spends time with Vera, putting forward options and providing her with information which might help her to make an informed choice. Vera is still convinced that she wants to remain in her own home, but agrees to participate in an assessment of her daily living and safety needs. A social worker is able to carry out a needs assessment, and Ali decides to use a tool based on the Clifton Assessment Procedures for the Elderly (CAPE) (Pattie and Gilleard, 1981).

The CAPE relates to four subscales which observe physical disability, apathy, communication difficulties and social disturbance. The criteria for scoring are based on zero for no assistance, 1 for some assistance and 2 for maximum assistance. However, there is some criticism of the assessment tool in relation to its validity and reliability (see Bowling, 2004).

S Scenario continued

Table 25.1 gives an extract from Vera's CAPE assessment.

Table 25.1 Vera's CAPE assessment

CAPE scale	Findings	Score
1 Bathing and dressing	Needs prompting to wash. Needs assistance with getting in and out of the bath	1
2 Walking	Walks slowly, but steadily	1
5 Disorientated	Unable to always know where she is or to find her way around	2
6 Dress and appearance	Appears dishevelled and unkempt	2

The CAPE results suggest there are high levels of dependency, with an indication of deteriorating mental health. The case manager decides to contact Matt to discuss the situation with him. Although the idea is again put to Vera, she is still reluctant to consider leaving her home.

a Learning activity

How appropriate do you think the CAPE assessment is for identifying Vera's needs? Find out what assessment tools are used by your local social services department. Consider whether they would be as suitable for assessing Vera's needs.

The case manager selected the CAPE needs assessment as being the most suitable for assessing Vera's needs, but others might prove more suitable, for example the *Single Assessment Process for Older People* (DH, 2006b). Ross and O'Tuathail (2006) provide an overview of the components of the single assessment process (SAP), explaining that this process covers the user's perspective, clinical history, health behaviour, personal care and physical well-being, the senses, mental health, relationships, safety and the environment. The assessment is conducted at four levels:

- contact assessment
- overview assessment
- specialist assessment
- comprehensive assessment.

The assessment helps to determine the plan of care that is required, and clearly is tailored to the individual.

Part

III

S Scenario continued

The immediate care plan for Vera includes increasing the amount of time the home care worker spends with her and maintaining the daily visits from the community nurse, who will keep the GP informed of developments pending the setting-up of a case conference. This will consider the best ways of meeting Vera's longer-term needs. Ali will monitor the care package, and has agreed to contact Matt. He explains that although Vera can be supported at home in the short term, her interests need to be considered with a view to longer-term care. He asks when it might be convenient for Matt to return to the United Kingdom. It is agreed to hold the case conference in two months' time. Vera is invited to attend, and time is taken to explain to her what will be discussed, the nature of the questions that she may need to consider, and the options that might arise. She is delighted to hear that Matt is coming home.

a Learning activity

In your notes about the team you should have the phrase 'case conference'. What do you understand by this? What are the differences between case management and care management?

S Scenario continued

Ali chairs the case conference to which Vera and Matt are invited. The decision to call a case conference has resulted from concerns over Vera's ability to live safely at home: it would appear impossible for her to continue living in her own home for much longer. Prior to the case conference, Ali meets with Matt and Vera to discuss some of the options. Vera is understandably distressed about any thought of possibly losing her independence and security. She is tearful at the thought of leaving the house and its associations with George.

Matt is able to reassure Vera that any move into residential care could be temporary, and may be the best short-term option. Vera admits that she has recently become distressed and frightened at night; she keeps thinking she can hear people breaking into the house. She agrees that she may feel safer with others around, at least for a while. With advice from Ali, Matt and Vera are able to visit a number of residential homes. At the one Vera

likes best, there happens to be a resident she already knows through George's work. The home also has a nursing home facility for those residents requiring such care, but currently there are no vacancies.

All the healthcare and social care practitioners involved in Vera's care are able to be present at the case conference. Occasionally it is impossible for all the practitioners to meet, and a telephone conference may take place instead. Mrs Barker has also been invited to attend part of the meeting with Vera's permission. All those present now have the opportunity to meet with Vera and Matt to discuss their assessments, review the current plan of care, and consider the longer-term implications.

The outcome of the conference is that while Vera does not require 24-hour nursing care, she does need intensive support at home with a review every six weeks. However, a nursing home is located as it seems inevitable that Vera will need this type of care sooner rather than later.

a Learning activity

Currently there is a great deal of discussion about funding social care and who will be eligible, and the government's policy on this continues to evolve. It would be useful to access the document *Securing Good Care for Older People* (Wanless, 2006) and determine what the current view is. Read the recommendations and make notes on how these could be implemented.

S Scenario continued

A more intensive care package is now instigated to fill the gap between the current situation and Vera being able to move into the nursing home. The home care worker now visits daily, for two hours in the morning and two hours in the late afternoon. She also does Vera's shopping and helps Vera wash and bathe. The Women's Royal Voluntary Service (WRVS) are also involved in delivering a hot lunch through 'meals on wheels', provided under contract with social services three days a week. Mrs Barker has agreed to provide a meal on each of the remaining days. Vera generally pays for this service herself, but sometimes she forgets and Mrs Barker has stepped in and paid the volunteer who delivers the meal.

a Learning activity

In your learning group find out about your local WRVS. Who are they, what services do they provide and how are they coordinated? What other voluntary agencies exist in your locality?

S Scenario continued

The community nurse continues to visit on a daily basis to dress the pressure ulcer, ensure Vera has taken her medication, and continually assess Vera's situation. The GP has decided to prescribe Vera the antidepressant paroxetine, 20 mg to be taken once a day in the morning, to try to lift her mood.

Part

III

> ## ⟳ (a) Learning activity
>
> The GP has prescribed Vera the antidepressant paroxetine (Seroxat). What do you understand by this? What would the healthcare practitioner who cares for Vera need to know about this medication, and why?

The effects of medication in older people

In 1992 the Royal College of Physicians (RCP) carried out a study which demonstrated that 87 per cent of people over 75 years of age were receiving regular drug treatment, and of these 44 per cent were taking three or more drugs daily. The study highlighted a number of potential problems associated with prescribing medication for older people. These include:

- A disease process might present differently, its symptoms being masked by the medication being prescribed for something else. This could lead to an incorrect diagnosis being made. For example, the use of analgesics to control pain elsewhere might mean that the chest pain associated with myocardial infarction is not recognised, or medication used to reduce inflammation might result in the absence of pyrexia in a chest infection.
- The ways in which medicines are metabolised within the body can be affected by the ageing process in a number of ways:
  - Oral medication may be absorbed more slowly.
  - Lower cardiac output may reduce the speed at which medication is transported throughout the body.
  - Effects of medication may be potentiated where plasma albumin levels are low. Many drugs bind themselves to a plasma protein like albumin. When levels are reduced the proportion of unbound medication in the plasma increases, so enhancing the effect of the drug and leading to potential overdose.
  - Many drugs are deactivated in the liver and then excreted via the kidneys. Therefore, where liver and kidney function is reduced, excretion may be slowed so that drugs might remain in the body longer and their effects are lasting.
- Where there is multiple pathology, drugs may be prescribed to alleviate a problem but their action might have an unwanted effect elsewhere which has to be counteracted by another drug. The older person with a number of different illnesses can then end up receiving a cocktail of medication where each drug counteracts or potentiates the effects of another.

> ## ⟳ (a) Learning activity
>
> Investigate the effects of ageing on the ways in which drugs are metabolised by the body. Consider these effects in relation to absorption, distribution, metabolism and elimination. A useful textbook to help you is Greenstein and Gould (2004).

> ## (c) Professional conversation
>
> **Medication concerns**
>
> June Swift, Vera's community nurse, comments, 'I am constantly on the look out for the unwanted side-effects of prescribed medication amongst the older people I visit. I need to find out what patients are currently taking as sometimes they may have been prescribed something by one doctor who is unaware that something else has been prescribed by another. Believe me, it can happen! I also check out the "over the counter" medications people are taking on top of their prescribed medication. You just wouldn't imagine what people do without realising the dangers. Local pharmacists are getting much better at spotting potential problems and give jolly good advice.
>
> 'It is not surprising that the incidence of adverse drug reactions rises with age, especially after 65 years. There are a number of reasons for this. First, there are increasing numbers of

drugs that older people need to take because they often have several different illnesses, but it's often not appreciated that the different drugs used to treat these multiple illnesses may be toxic when taken together. Second, there is often poor compliance with dosing regimes, I often find different tablets all mixed up in the same container. You really have to keep your eyes open. Third, physiological changes associated with ageing mean that dosages used for younger people may require adjusting when prescribed for an older person.

'Although I can only prescribe a limited range of medicines myself, I am well aware of the actions of those drugs regularly prescribed by doctors to older people. I do let the doctor know straightaway if I think a patient is receiving too high a dose or it is affecting them adversely. That's what professional teamwork is all about.'

Following on from their 1992 report, the RCP carried out another study in 1997 which demonstrated that people over the age of 65 receive 45 per cent of all prescriptions in the United Kingdom, indicating that polypharmacy continues to be a problem. The study was an audit of evidence-based prescribing in older people, and highlighted a number of potential problems. It made these recommendations to improve the practice of prescribing for older people:

- Allergy/sensitivity information should be recorded for every patient. If it is not known, this too needs to be documented.
- All as required (prn) drugs should have maximum frequency of administration, or a minimum period between doses, documented. This is essential for safety when prescribing.
- There is a risk of over-dosage when prescribing more than one paracetamol-containing drug. Total dosage should nor exceed 4000 mg.
- All patients in atrial fibrillation should be prescribed an anticoagulant (in the absence of a contraindication), with aspirin as second choice, for stroke prophylaxis.
- Patients with stable angina should receive aspirin as prophylaxis of coronary heart disease.
- Many older people have a history of falls, or central nervous system depression, which contraindicates the use of benzodiaxepines as a choice of sedative. Management of the source of insomnia should be sought first.

(a) Learning activities

Consider these recommendations when you read DH (2001b), particularly page 11.

Read chapter 27 in Redfern and Ross (2006) about drugs and older people, and make brief notes on particular points to be aware of, for example when giving medicines to Vera.

(S) Scenario continued

It is unclear what happened, but the neighbour Mrs Barker reported unusual isolated noises in the night. When Minna, the home care worker, arrives the next morning, Vera is wandering around the house very disoriented. She is also very cold, as though she has been up all night, which may have been the case. She is clutching one of George's jumpers. She looks as though she has been crying for some time. Minna suggests that Vera might like to go back to bed, but she refuses, so Minna wraps her in her dressing-gown and puts slippers on her feet while she telephones Ali and the community nurse.

(a) Learning activity

In your learning group place yourself in the role of a community healthcare professional such as June, the community nurse, and with the information available, make a brief assessment of the current situation. What measures would you now take to ensure Vera's safety and best meet her needs?

June discusses the situation with the GP, and agrees to meet Ali at Vera's home. She finds that Vera is experiencing interrupted sleep patterns, which could make her more at risk of falling. Wandering at night could also lead to hypothermia.

Vera is clearly becoming more and more distressed and agitated. She also appears to be unsure of where she is and the correct time of day, although Mrs Barker thinks this is worse at night.

Vera is currently totally dependent on the help provided by Minna and Mrs Barker. She appears to find it difficult to initiate or sustain a conversation, and appears to have lost interest in day-to-day events. This in turn is causing distress to Mrs Barker, who feels powerless to help her.

Ali discusses the situation with June, and carries out another assessment, called the 'mini-mental state' (Folstein, Folstein and McHugh, 1975). The maximum score on this assessment is 30 points, Vera scores very low, which appears to confirm concerns about her level of orientation and her vulnerability.

The mini-mental state assessment focuses on:

1 Orientation – time, place, person, event. (Score max. 10 points)
2 Registration – the individual is given three objects to remember, and then asked to repeat the list three times. After a short period has elapsed, they are asked to again recall the three objects. (Score max. 3 points)
3 Attention and calculation – subtracting numbers. (Score max. 5 points)
4 Recall – the person is asked to recall the three objects learned earlier. (Score max. 3 points)
5 Language – the person is asked to name a pencil and watch, give a three-stage command, and so on. (Score max. 3 points)
6 Reading – reading a sentence and doing what it states. (Score max. 2 points)
7 Three-stage command – the person takes a paper in their left (or right) hand, folds it in half and puts it on the floor. (Score max. 3 points)
8 Copying – the person is asked to copy a diagram of a pair of intersecting pentagons. (Score max. 1 point).

A telephone case conference urgently takes place to review the care package, including discussion with the GP and with Matt, Vera's son. Because all are in agreement that Vera would be at risk if she remained at home, the decision is made to transfer her to a nursing home within the next 24 hours. When this is put to Vera, rather than increasing her agitation, the news appears to have a calming effect. Even though she is unwell, it is essential that she is given the facts and that she should feel involved in her own care.

June wants to ensure that Vera has an advocate, and does not feel lost or vulnerable at a time when it feel as if all the decisions are being made without her involvement, so she makes sure that as far as she is aware, Vera's interests are taken fully into account and Vera is able to give informed consent for the move.

Part

III

a **Learning activity**

In your learning group, consider examples of where you have observed a healthcare practitioner acting as an advocate in order to ensure that a vulnerable person's interests are protected.

Healthcare practitioners provide care in a wide variety of settings, and at all times they are expected to abide by their professional codes of conduct. Nurses are bound by the Nursing and Midwifery Council *Code* (NMC, 2008), and each nurse is expected to know and understand it.

a) Learning activity

In your learning group review your own code of conduct and explore with a colleague how you could be an 'active voice' for the service user.

A number of authors have discussed how healthcare delivery is largely about power (for example see Johnson, 1997), and have identified situations where invariably the doctor has the last word. There is also a great deal of evidence to suggest that patients often feel the need to comply with a doctor's suggestion, but become distressed when they feel their own wishes are ignored. In such situations patients will often seek the help of nurses even though, paradoxically, they are often regarded as the doctor's assistant.

Informed consent is when a patient is given full information by a competent person so that they can accept or reject a course of treatment. The healthcare practitioner should be able to act as the patient's advocate in these circumstances, ensuring that the individual is provided with the information and time needed to explore the options available to them (Kendrick, 1996). All healthcare practitioners need to explore for themselves the issues around advocacy and informed consent. This is a challenging area, and case studies can be very useful for exploring your own views and for realising that there may not be any definite right or wrong answers.

S) Scenario continued

In Vera's move to Holyrood Nursing Home, she is accompanied by Ali and Mrs Barker. They are greeted by Rosalynd Shaw, the matron, and shown to a comfortable room where they can talk. Ali and Rosalynd decide to carry out a further needs assessment using CAPE (see page 514). This enables a comparison to be made against the previous CAPE assessment findings.

Table 25.2 Vera's revised CAPE behaviour rating scale findings

CAPE scale	Findings	Score
1 Bathing and dressing	Needs prompting to wash, some assistance needed to get into and out of bath	1
2 Walking	Walks slowly but steadily without aid	1
3 Incontinent of urine/faeces (day or night)	Never	0
4 In bed during the day	Never	0
5 Disoriented	Sometimes forgets where she is	1
6 Dress and appearance	Often needs prompting to select clean and/or appropriate clothes	2
7 Outside activities	Sometimes needs help crossing the road	1
8 Carries out activities in the home	Was independent until recently, now requires prompting to cook, clean and prepare food	1
9 Engages in purposeful activity	Often appears preoccupied, sits alone for long periods and tends to forget to carry out everyday tasks	2
10 Socialises with others	Has some difficulty establishing relationships	1
11 Accepting of ideas	Appears to go along easily with what is suggested	0
12 Correctly interprets what is being communicated	Usually quickly and correctly interprets what is being communicated to her	0
13 Communicates effectively	Has some difficulty being understood as speaks very quietly	1
14 Acts appropriately in relation to others during the day	Always	0

CAPE scale	Findings	Score
15 Acts appropriately in relation to others during the night	Has been found wandering at home during the night	2
16 Accuses others of doing her bodily harm	Never	0
17 Hoards apparently meaningless items	Has a large collection of paid bills in her handbag	1
18 Disrupted sleep pattern	Sometimes appears to have difficulty getting off, then wakes in the early hours	2

Source: adapted from Pattie and Gilleard (1981).

- Vera knows who she is and her age, but is uncertain which day it is.
- She is uncertain of her actual birthday, and gives a date which later turns out to be Matt's birthday.
- She knows where she is, but thinks she is visiting someone.
- She knows the name of the nearest city and the prime minister, but not the US president.
- She also knows that the national flag contains the colours red, white and blue.

The outcome of the assessment would indicate that Vera's problems largely relate to her fragile mental state and recent physical frailty. It is not entirely certain what is causing the deterioration, but there are signs associated with both an early dementing illness and the depression probably resulting from her recent bereavement. The outcome of the assessment has indicated a degree of physical and mental deterioration, some disorientation, sadness, agitation and loss of memory. The information gathered is used to develop a plan of nursing care for Vera.

a Learning activity

The nurses and other professionals in your practice area will use a philosophy or framework to guide the way in which they systematically assess, plan, implement and evaluate care. Their approach may be based around one or more models of care. Try to find out why one model is selected in preference to another. What would they describe as their philosophy of care? You will notice the term 'confusion' has not been used to describe Vera's problems. Why do you think this term is best avoided?

c Professional conversation: Models of care

Rosalynd Shaw, matron of Holyrood Nursing Home, says, 'You may be familiar with models of nursing care, but I had to sit down and think about how these might lend themselves to the nursing home situation. We looked at Roy's (1999) adaptation model of nursing where the focus is on how a patient adapts to the changed environment, change in circumstances and mental and/or physical changes. We also considered using Orem's (2001) self-care deficit model, where the emphasis is on determining what a patient can or cannot do. The aim then is to correct the deficit, through varying degrees of nursing intervention, to enable the patient to regain a higher level of independence. It is about enabling and empowering patients.

Several staff were familiar with this model, but after a lot of discussion we all eventually agreed to use the Roper, Logan and Tierney 'activities of living' model (2000). The assessment within this model has a number of similarities with the needs assessment, and it provided us with a useful framework for operating the nursing process. We then based our documentation around the model, and this seems to have served us well. The local hospitals use this, so many of the bank staff we get are already familiar with it, which ensures continuity. Having used this approach for several years, I guess we need to see whether it's still applicable or whether something else might be more beneficial. Hugo, one of our staff nurses, is currently doing a literature search.'

Taking note of the information already provided in the scenario, and using care plan documentation from your practice area, take the role of Hugo, who is Vera's named nurse. Document a nursing assessment and then construct a plan of care for Vera's first three days at Holyrood Nursing Home. Consult Walsh's (1998) book on care plans in both the community and mental health for guidance. Before you commence your plan, remember that June might have some helpful tips about that pressure ulcer, and information about the medication Vera has been prescribed.

Hugo, Vera's named nurse, identifies the following issues as problematic for Vera:

- disorientated and anxious at times, forgets to take medication, eating very little
- has some reluctance to socialise with others
- assistance is needed with hygiene and dressing
- pressure ulcer of 1 cm diameter on buttocks with scab, needing treatment
- disrupted sleep pattern.

A care plan must aim to improve the situation through a holistic approach to nursing care. It must address needs such as hygiene, dressing, nutrition, mobility and sleeping. It must also consider social needs, which in Vera's case will mean time set aside for communicating socially one to one until she feels more comfortable with other people. The whole plan will need to be reviewed on a regular basis – at least weekly – and updated as necessary.

Among those who could provide useful expertise are (in Vera's case) a bereavement counsellor and a tissue viability nurse, and also for example the occupational therapist, the community physiotherapist, the local hairdresser or a volunteer from her local church.

Figure 25.1 shows an extract from Vera's care plan.

Date:	6 June
Problem:	Disoriented in time and place
Goal:	To become reoriented to time and place by 10 June
Intervention:	Place Vera's personal items in her room
	Encourage Vera to join the other residents at mealtimes and in group discussions
	Give Vera time alone – about one hour a day
Evaluation:	11 June
	Vera recognises family photographs
	Vera enjoys lunchtime, but prefers to be on her own at breakfast
	Vera still has some difficulty with group discussions

Figure 25.1 Sample care plan

Some nursing homes use care pathways or case management rather than nursing models. What do you understand by these terms?

The care plan provided for Vera has been devised using a nursing model of care which has provided the framework for a needs assessment. The framework focuses on nursing, which fails to take account of the contribution of other care workers (Walsh, 1998). Also, there are problems associated with a multitude of written, sometimes overlapping reports, as each professional seeks to maintain their own records. To overcome this issue, care management has been introduced in the United Kingdom with a view to 'streamlining' care, improving communications, preventing overlaps between practitioners and setting standards. Care pathways are increasingly being used in nursing homes for the same reasons.

Part

III

a Learning activity

Enquire about the use of care pathways in your practice area. Does your area have a care pathways coordinator who might be able to help you with this activity? Can care pathways be adapted for use elsewhere? Do all practitioners contribute to the documentation? Revisit the *Single Assessment Process for Older People* (DH, 2006b) in order to answer some of these questions.

S Scenario continued

When Vera moves into the nursing home she is upset and slightly disoriented. Staff work hard at helping her to settle by introducing her to other residents and placing some of her personal items from home around her room. She is encouraged to eat her meals with the other residents and join them in the lounge as far as possible, but time is also set aside for her to be alone. She is encouraged to take part in the social activities but not pressurised. Perhaps surprisingly, Vera is soon found to enjoy a short game of bingo. Accompanied by Hugo, she also starts to go for short walks around the garden. She starts to talk about George, how she often used to tease him about how little he knew about plants, and he would tease her about her knowledge. Definite improvements are being noted. Although Vera makes good progress, she does not regain her appetite and loses a further 5 kg. She now weighs 46 kg.

a Learning activity

Again, take the role of Hugo. Use the information you have available to assess Vera's nutritional status and decide on the measures you would take to improve it. (Refer to Chapter 10 on nutrition.)

e Evidence-based practice

In 1998 the British Nutrition Foundation recommended estimated average requirements (EAR) , an estimate of the average requirement for energy or a nutrient for all age groups. This was updated in 2004 (BNF, 2004), when lifestyle was also taken into account. In Vera's case her requirements will also differ because of her moving into a nursing home.

Calorie intake also tends to focus on the average healthy adult, but as nutritional intake declines it becomes virtually impossible to take in adequate amounts of essential vitamins, iron, protein and calcium. Dudek (2006) states that caution should be used when adopting dietary guidelines for older people. It is vital that these guidelines are individualised because for elderly frail people, the focus is on improving the quality of life, and some of the guidelines may be inappropriate. For example, lowering fat intake may not be appropriate if the person is at risk of malnutrition. Similarly, reducing sodium intake might not necessarily be important as it would limit food choices and might make food less palatable. If older people are only moderately overweight, trying to lose weight might be a lost cause, again because of reasons already mentioned.

S Scenario continued

Here is some information Hugo has put together about Vera:

- Vera has difficulty in chewing and as her dentures do not fit properly, she finds meat difficult to eat. The dentist is making new dentures.
- Vera tends not to eat much fibre and may be at risk of constipation.
- While Vera is not too keen on fruit, she sometimes enjoys bananas and oranges.

- Because of Vera's state of mind when she first arrived at the nursing home, she was fed by a member of staff at each meal time. Gradually, she was encouraged to feed herself, and as she started to feel more sociable and independent, she joined other residents in the dinning room.
- In a reminiscence group she revealed how she and George used to enjoy a glass of sherry on a Sunday. A small glass of sherry was introduced each evening and her appetite slightly improved.

(a) **Learning activity**

From your nutritional assessment, what goals have you identified for Vera's nutrition plan, and how will these now be incorporated into the plan?

S   Scenario continued

Hugo again reports:

- It was important to ask Vera, Mrs Barker and Matt what foods Vera liked.
- It was essential to try to plan a balanced diet to facilitate weight gain.
- Help from the community dietician was very important in determining a plan.
- Nursing intervention was aimed at providing small, attractive meals high in nutrients.
- Fibre was increased as well as fluid intake to prevent constipation.
- Over time there has been a marked improvement in nutritional intake and mental state. Vera regained the 5 kg she had previously lost within a month.

(a) **Learning activity**

Improving Vera's nutritional status will also help to improve her general health. In your learning group make short notes on the terms 'health', 'health education' and 'health promotion', and discuss your interpretations.

Cowley (2006) maintains that there are five guiding principles for health strategies:

- Equity: particularly in access to the prerequisites for health, but also in healthcare provision and services.
- Participation: to affirm the right of people to define health in their own terms.
- Collective responsibility, accepting that health is primarily a social enterprise. Development at grassroots level is as significant as central policy; there should be an emphasis on multidisciplinary, collaborative actions and healthy alliances.
- 'Ecological vision' means taking full account of the impact of physical and social environments on people's health.
- There should be increasing options through policies, so that healthier choices are easier than unhealthy ones.

Statistics indicate that individuals are living longer, as are people with varying degrees of physical and/or mental dysfunction (ONS, nd). The scope for health promotion is enormous, and never more so than for older people. Health promotion aims to improve the health status of individuals and the societies within which they live. In Vera's situation, promoting health will ensure that she maintains a reasonable level of physical and mental health, which is sustained by the environment where she is now living. Many older people feel that it is a waste of time having healthcare professionals discussing how to maintain and improve their health, as they frequently believe alterations in their health are the result of 'getting old'. Yet the benefits can be huge in terms of enjoying life and being positive about the future.

Healthcare professionals need to take into account that many older people have sensory difficulties such as poor eyesight and/or impaired hearing. The memory may not be as sharp as it once was. They may be experiencing symptoms associated with a physical or mental illness. The environment will also have an impact, choice of diet may be restricted and opportunities for exercise limited. Healthcare professionals need to be conscious of any potential barriers such as holding negative attitudes about ageing, or elderly people themselves being fatalistic about their health.

S   Scenario continued

Vera does not smoke but does need to pay attention to her diet, exercise and getting enough sleep.

- Diet: the dietician was asked for advice.
- Exercise: a programme of gentle stretching exercises was drawn up increasing from gentle mobility to walks round the garden.
- Sleep: it was decided not to prescribe a mild sedative. Vera soon appeared to benefit from a combination of diet, exercise and company.

C   Professional conversation

Hugo discusses reminiscences: 'Health promotion in elderly people can be problematic as it does not always come high on the agenda in a nursing home. We have often tended to concentrate on keeping people comfortable and getting the residents involved in activities in the afternoon. Then I read an article by Granville (1996), and there were some similarities between a case mentioned and Vera, because she is a bit forgetful at times. Anyway, I talked about the article to my colleagues and we felt we could help Vera. So what we aimed to do was to promote her self-esteem, which should facilitate her friendships and social contacts, and hopefully optimise her mental health. How we set about this was to set up a reminiscence group once a week in the lounge. We also invited residents from the next-door residential home, and three of its residents now regularly attend.

'A rotating programme has been developed and it is in three parts. The first part we talk about school days, childhood, the Depression and the Second World War; the second part is about working, marriage, having children and events like the Queen's Coronation. The final part is when we talk about the years since then. This is sometimes more difficult as many of the residents have better memories of the earlier years than the later ones! We try to use old photographs, clothes, music or anything the residents can bring with them, and every couple of months we use the minibus and take them to the museum. The residents really enjoy these sessions and it is interesting to see how they become more lucid and sometimes quite animated.

'In Vera's case she found it painful to talk about children as she only had Matt. It would appear that she was unable to have any more, which must have been hard for her and George when the expectation after the war was to have children. What was fascinating though was when she talked about the garden. It seemed to take her mind off George for a little while. Her thinking is really clear. She says she once met Vita Sackville-West, the famous gardener. Vera has now become friendly with another resident, Joan, and they go out in the garden when the weather is fine. I'm so glad I found that article because we have been able to make a real difference.'

The roles of other professionals

Although Vera has now moved into a nursing home, there are a number of healthcare professionals who have a regular input into her care. You will already have a list of which personnel were involved earlier, and you will have determined what their roles were then. In the nursing home the personnel might or might not be the same; there might be more but different involvement. When considering the team, it is automatic to name the doctor, the social worker and the physiotherapist. These individuals are regarded as 'direct' carers. In a nursing home setting there is also an army of 'indirect' carers. These are the kitchen staff, cleaners, caretakers, hairdressers and many others.

Part

III

(a) **Learning activity**

In your learning groups consider who are the care workers now involved in Vera's care and how they have been prepared for their roles.

[S] **Scenario continued**

Vera appears to have settled well into Holyrood Nursing Home, but there is every indication that she might soon be able to be reaccommodated within a residential care home. Thankfully she has made good progress and appears not to require the level of nursing care originally envisaged. Vera has mixed feelings about another move, but she likes the thought of living nearer friends. Vera talks with Matt on the phone and a case conference is set for Monday week.

(a) **Learning activity**

Based on the information you have, what do you think is Matt's role in Vera's care? What support is available for Matt? Think about a family you know that has an older member living in residential care. Make brief notes on the family's role in relation to this older person.

Conclusion

Having worked through this chapter, you will have experienced many of the challenges that Vera Jenkins, her son and neighbour have had to meet. Central to the support available is been the ability of the multidisciplinary team to communicate with each other and involve Vera and others when assessing, planning and delivering the care that Vera needs, both in the community and in a residential setting.

The scenario has raised many issues that nurses working with older people need to consider. You will no doubt have been able to make comparisons with the care of older people that you have witnessed or been involved in delivering. Many decisions that older people have to make happen at a time when they are at their most vulnerable. The nurse has a duty to protect and safeguard their interests, giving an older person the time and the information that they need in order to come to a decision which could affect the rest of their lives. These can be tough decisions and they are not always appropriately managed.

Now reflect back on the outcomes set out at the beginning of this chapter, and consider how much you have learned. Think about the questions that remain unanswered and the ways in which you intend to address them.

References

Barker, K. (1998) 'The ageing process', in Marr, J. and Kershaw, B. (eds), *Caring for Older People*, London, Arnold.

Barrett, G., Sellman, D. and Thomas, J. (2005) *Interprofessional Working in Health and Social Care*, Basingstoke, Palgrave.

Bowling, A. (2004) *Measuring Health*, 3rd edn, Milton Keynes, Open University Press.

British Nutrition Foundation (2004) *Older Adults* [online] www.nutrition.org.uk/printArticle.asp?dataId+907 (accessed 5 February 2009)

Collier, M. (2002) 'Caring for the patient with a skin or wound care need', in Walsh, M. (ed.), *Watson's Clinical Nursing and Related Sciences*, 6th edn, London, Ballière Tindall.

Costello, J. and Kendrick, K. (2000) 'Grief and older people: the making or breaking of emotional bonds following partner loss in later life', *Journal of Advanced Nursing* **32**(6), 1374-1382.

Cowley, S. (2006) 'Health promotion for older people', in Redfern, S. J. and Ross, F. M. (eds), *Nursing Older People*, Edinburgh, Churchill Livingstone Elsevier.

Department of Health (DH) (2000) *Partnership in Action*, London, HMSO.

DH (2001a) *National Service Framework for Older People*, London, HMSO.

DH (2001b) *Medicines and Older People*, London, HMSO.

DH (2006a) *A New Ambition for Old Age*, London, HMSO.

DH (2006b) *Single Assessment Process for Older People*, London, HMSO.

Dougherty, L. and Lister, S. (2004) *The Royal Marsden Hospital Manual of Clinical Nursing Procedures*, 6th edn, Oxford, Blackwell.

Dudek, S. G. (2006) *Nutrition Essentials for Nursing Practice*, Philadelphia, Penn., Lippincott.

Folstein, M. F., Folstein, S. E. and McHugh, P. R. (1975) 'Mini-mental state: a practical method for grading the cognitive state of patients for the clinician', *Journal of Psychiatry and Research* 12, 189–98.

Ford, P. and Wills, T. (2002) 'Ageing and health', in Walsh, M. (ed.), *Watson's Clinical Nursing and Related Sciences*, 6th edn, London, Ballière Tindall.

Granville, G. (1996) 'Promoting health in older people', in Wade, L. and Waters, K. A. (eds), *Textbook of Gerontological Nursing*, London, Ballière Tindall.

Greenstein, B. and Gould, D. (2004) *Trounce's Clinical Pharmacology for Nurses*, Edinburgh, Churchill Livingstone.

Herbert, R.A. (2006) 'The biology of human ageing', in Redfern, S. J. and Ross, F. M. (eds), *Nursing Older People*, Edinburgh, Churchill Livingstone Elsevier.

Johnson, M. (1997) *Nursing Power and Social Judgement*, London, Ashgate.

Kendrick, K. (1996) 'The challenge of advocacy: a moral response', in Wade, L. and Waters, K. (eds), *Gerontological Nursing*, London, Ballière Tindall.

Norton, D., McLaren, R. and Exton-Smith, A. (1975) *An Investigation of Geriatric Nursing Problems in Hospital*, Edinburgh, Churchill Livingstone.

Nursing and Midwifery Council (NMC) (2008) *The Code*, London, NMC.

Office for National Statistics (ONS) (nd) Various statistics [online] http://www.statistics.gov.uk/CCI/nugget.asp?ID=6 (accessed 12 December 2008).

Orem, D. (2001) *Nursing: Concepts of practice*,4th edn, St Louis, Mo., Mosby Year Books.

Pattie, A. H. and Gilleard, C. J. (1981) *Clifton Assessment Procedures for the Elderly (CAPE)*, London, Hodder & Stoughton.

Redfern S. and Ross, F. (eds) (2006) *Nursing Older People*, 4th edn, Edinburgh, Elsevier/Churchill Livingstone.

Roper, N., Logan, W. and Tierney, A. (2000) *Elements of Nursing*, Edinburgh, Churchill Livingstone.

Ross, F. M. and O'Tuathail, C. (2006) 'Assessment of older people', in Redfern, S. J. and Ross, F. M. (eds), *Nursing Older People*, 4th edn, Edinburgh, Churchill Livingstone.

Ross, F. M. and Victor, C. R. (2006) 'Health and social care for older people in the community', in Redfern, S. J. and Ross, F. M (eds), *Nursing Older People*, 4th edn, Edinburgh, Churchill Livingstone.

Roy, C. and Andrews, H. A. (1999) *The Roy Adaptation Model*, 2nd edn, Stamford, Conn., Appleton & Lange.

Royal College of Physicians (1992) *Drugs and the Elderly*, London, HMSO.

Royal College of Physicians (1997) *Medication for Older People*, 2nd edn, London, Royal College of Physicians.

Wanless, D. (2006) *Securing Good Care for Older People* (Wanless Report) [online] www.kingsfund.org.uk/publications (accessed 21 January 2009).

Wade, L. (1996) 'New Perspectives on gerontological nursing', in Wade, L. and Waters, K. (eds), *Gerontological Nursing*, London, Ballière Tindall.

Walsh, M. (1998) *Models and Critical Pathways in Clinical Nursing*, London, Ballière Tindall.

Webster, C. (ed.) (2001) *Caring for Health: History and diversity*, 3rd edn, Milton Keynes, Open University Press.

Further reading

Bernard, M., Phillips, J., Machin, L. and Harding Davies, V. (2000) *Women Ageing: Changing identities, challenging myths*, London: Routledge. This informative book looks at the wider spectrum of women as they grow older, the challenges they meet, but more importantly, the myths that surround this ageing process. It reviews the theories and practices of ageing, and should be compulsory reading for anyone working with older women.

Department of Health (DH) (2001a) *National Service Framework for Older People*, London, HMSO. A great deal of work has already been carried out by the NHS and social services to improve care for older people. This National Service Framework (one of a series) continues the work and is important reading for students caring for older people in the community, in hospitals and the independent sector.

Health Advisory Service 2000 (HAS) (1998) *'Not because they are old': An independent enquiry into the care of older people on acute wards in general hospitals*, London, HAS. This report presents the findings of an inquiry into the care of older people on acute wards in general hospitals. The aim was to seek and bring together the views of older patients, their significant others, ward staff and managers about the care given. Fifteen recommendations are made to enhance care, including a National Service Framework for Older People.

Wade, L. and Waters, K. (eds) (1996) *A Textbook of Gerontological*

Part

III

Nursing, London, Ballière Tindall. This text is written by a number of experts in the field, and was used extensively in the development of this chapter. It is ideal for student nurses in providing them with a wide range of insights into caring for older people. The text also includes clinical discussion points and extensive references.

Websites

Age Concern: www.ageconcern.org.uk
Benefits Agency: www.dss.gov.uk/ba
British Association for Counselling: www.bacp.co.uk
British Geriatric Society: www.bgs.org.uk
British Nutrition Foundation: www.nutrition.org.uk
British Red Cross Society: www.redcross.org.uk
Citizens Advice Bureau: www.nacab.org.uk
Council for Voluntary Services: www.ncvo-vol.org.uk
Department of Health: www.dh.gov.uk
National Association of Bereavement Services: www.stjohnshospice.org.uk

National Association of Widows: www.patient.co.uk
Nursing Standard: www.nursingstandard.RCNpublishing.co.uk
Nursing Times: www.nursingtimes.net
Office for National Statistics: www.statistics.gov.uk
Population trends: www.statistics.gov.uk
Residential care: www.dh.gov.uk
Reuters Health (daily news service on health issues): www.reuters.com/news/health

Chapter

26

Mental health

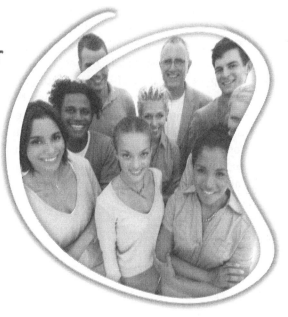

John Rawlinson

 Links to other chapters in *Foundation Studies for Caring*

2 Interprofessional learning
3 Evidence-based practice and research
4 Ethical, legal and professional issues
5 Communication
6 Culture
14 Pharmacology and medicines

25 Care of the older adult – community
27 Learning disability
32 Adult emergency care and resuscitation
35 Complementary and alternative medicine

 Links to other chapters in *Foundation Skills for Caring*

1 Fundamental concepts for skills
3 Communication
5 Anxiety
7 Breaking significant news
8 Breakaway skills
9 Patient hygiene

28 Routes of medication administration
37 Basic life support – adult
38 Clinical holding for care, treatment or interventions
40 Last offices

W Don't forget to visit www.palgrave.com/glasper for additional online resources relating to this chapter.

Part

III

Introduction

This chapter, which begins with some questions and uncertainties, is intended to help you to consider the way in which 'mental health' is understood. It uses a family-based scenario to explore the nature of mental health problems, their impact on those affected, and the responses and skills needed by practitioners and services. With reference to the developing scenario, we investigate a range of issues, mental health practice and community care. What is presented within the chapter represents the author's enquiry-led processes in considering some problems and issues in the field. You may find this and the books, journals, documents and internet resources listed at the end of the chapter useful. However, the primary learning resource should be your own process of enquiry and the sense and meaning you find on that experiential journey.

Learning outcomes

This chapter will enable you to:

- discuss the concepts of 'mental health' and 'mental illness'
- develop an empathic understanding of the experience of a person and family affected by mental ill health
- identify the characteristics of a therapeutic relationship
- identify the positive, core skills, qualities and characteristics you already have, and those you will need to develop for working with people with mental health problems

- discuss the services available for people with mental health problems and relate them to your local circumstances
- identify some key policy and legal frameworks for mental healthcare
- develop your approach to working with people with mental health problems, valuing their perception, recognising the importance of assessing potential risks and focusing on 'recovery'.

Concepts

- Mental health
- Mental illness
- Therapeutic relationships

- Depression
- Suicide and parasuicide
- Recovery

- Community care
- Mental health services
- Mental health policy and law

(a) Learning activity

Has the 'mental health' prefix simply become a euphemism for 'mental illness' or does 'mental health' have some intrinsic meaning with implications for health services? If you are following, or thinking of following, the 'mental health' nursing branch or another mental health worker course, you may also like to consider its meaning for you.

Does there seem to be a shared vision of how people's mental health problems can be understood? What is the knowledge base for mental healthcare? What could be its relationship to existing professional knowledge bases in social or healthcare professions such as nursing, social work and psychology? Consider how 'mental health' fits in with other subject areas you have investigated or studied.

(s) Scenario: Introducing the Tome family

Sabina and Barry Tome and their family live in a small house, which they own, on a former council estate in a sparsely populated rural area. They have been married for 13 years. Barry is 44 and although he is a qualified surveyor, he has had several periods of unemployment and quite a few episodes of sickness. Two years ago he was made redundant and has not worked since. Although he had some redundancy money, they now rely on Sabina's earnings in their attempts to keep up with their mortgage payments. Sabina is several years younger and works in the village shop. Between them they have three children, Sabina's daughter Cecelia who is 17 and has left home, her son Morgan who is 15 and their son Gary who is 12.

Mental health

The scenario describes a relatively typical family in Britain today. No longer does the average family consist of a husband and wife, the former who works for 40 years and the latter who looks after their children. Many marriages break up; many families realign and many families develop around different gender roles or sexual orientations. Most people can now expect periods of unemployment. In many 'normal' families, people experience mental health problems. No longer are such problems, and those who suffer from them, confined, away from society in rural asylums. We are beginning to recognise that, instead of the 'mentally ill', the 'mad', or the 'insane' being a small separate group, quite distinct from ourselves (and from whom we must be protected), mental health problems can touch any and all of our lives.

a Learning activity

With a friend or a partner in your learning group agree to spend at least half an hour together on this exercise. Talk about your experiences so far of mental health issues and identify personal experiences which may inform your understanding of the issues involved. Share together as much as you feel able, but if there are any difficult issues or experiences which you decide not to share, notice your responses and reactions internally.

Identify any personal needs you may have in respect of mental health issues and the resources or support you may call on when working through this chapter.

Uncomfortable or personal issues may be raised for any of us in this area. If you feel that exploring this personally, or working with this client group may touch on personal areas for which you do not have sufficient support, make sure that you discuss it with your learning coordinator, mentor, a friend or mental health professional.

There is no real consensus in the way in which we understand what mental health and mental illness are, or in the language we use to describe mental health problems. This may become evident both in the responses you get talking to doctors, other professionals and service users and in your reading (e.g. Goldberg and Huxley, 1992; Keen, 1999; Read, Mosher and Bentall, 2004; Tyrer and Steinberg, 2005).

a Learning activity   W

A survey of psychiatric morbidity among adults in private households was carried out in 2000 by the Office for National Statistics on behalf of the Department of Health, the Scottish Executive and the National Assembly for Wales. The information obtained is available in a searchable format at http://www.statistics.gov.uk/downloads/theme_health/psychmorb.pdf

Navigate through this to gain an overall impression of the general scale of mental health problems, or to look in more detail at the incidence of particular problems.

A survey of attitudes to mental illness has been published by the Office for National Statistics (2007) and is available at: http://www.dh.gov.uk/prod_consum_dh/

idcplg?IdcService=GET_ILE&dID=144114&Rendition=Web

Consider how attitudes may affect responses to people with mental health problems.

At the time of writing, guidance is being developed on 'Finding a shared vision of how people's mental health problems should be understood' (CSIP, 2007), available at http://www.dh.gov.uk/en/Consultations/Liveconsultations/DH_080913. Find and read this guidance and discuss the degree to which its implementation is effective.

The scale of mental health problems

(Derived from: Goldberg and Huxley, 1992; DH, 1999b; Appleby et al, 2001; Samaritans, 2007):

- About a quarter to a third of the population experience distressing psychological symptoms some time in the course of a year.
- One-quarter of routine general practitioner (GP) consultations are for people with a mental health problem.
- One in four people visit a GP with a psychological problem each year, the commonest being anxiety, depression and physical symptoms with a psychological background.
- Only 10 per cent of these problems are referred by the GP to a hospital specialist; 90 per cent of mental healthcare being provided solely by primary care.
- Mild forms of depression affect half the population at some time in their lives, although severe depression will affect only one in 100.
- Dementia affects approximately 5 per cent of the population over 65; this prevalence doubles every five years over the age of 65.
- In the United Kingdom about 5600 people die each year from suicide, as many as die from road accidents.
- Unemployed people are twice as likely to have depression as people in work.
- Children in the poorest households are three times more likely to have mental health problems than children in well-off households.
- Half of all women and a quarter of all men will be affected by depression at some period during their lives.
- People who have been abused or been victims of domestic violence have higher rates of mental health problems.
- Between a quarter and a half of people using night shelters or sleeping rough may have a serious mental disorder, and up to half may be alcohol dependent.
- Some black and minority ethnic groups are diagnosed as having higher rates of mental disorder than the general population; refugees are especially vulnerable.
- There is a high rate of mental disorder in the prison population.
- People with drug and alcohol problems have higher rates of other mental health problems.
- People with physical illnesses have higher rates of mental health problems.

Mental health services and community care policy

For about 150 years the 'mental hospital' was the main focus for the treatment and residence of those with 'mental health problems'. For much of the twentieth century, the 'asylums' were thriving, but isolated, communities, meeting virtually all the needs of both patients and (separately) staff. Little 'curative' treatment as such was available. Although much criticised and at times overused, psychoactive drugs were developed which represented the first widely available effective treatment of the symptoms of mental illness. Arguably, they also enabled the beginning of discharge into the community on a large scale. Since the description by Russell Barton in the 1950s of 'institutional neurosis' and sociological observation of 'institutionalisation' by Goffman (1961), successive governments have attempted to provide more community-based responses to mental health problems and avoid the isolating and damaging effects of hospitalisation (read the famous 'water tower' speech by Enoch Powell (1961) as minister of health). The emphasis has moved to ensuring that people experiencing mental health difficulties are treated in the least restrictive way with the minimum of disruption to their lives.

A range of community-based options for people with mental health problems has developed and mental health services have increasingly been structured around locality-based, multidisciplinary community mental health teams. Current policy (DH, 2004) includes the provision of crisis resolution services and offering home-based intervention wherever possible. This is different from community services to support people after discharge, in that it is seen as an alternative to in-patient care.

'Community care' has been presented as the ideal for many aspects of healthcare. However, this term needs further consideration as it can represent three distinct, and quite different, concepts: care in the community, care by the community and care of the community.

Care *in* the community

This simply implies that the location of care is to be within the general community, that is, in streets, towns, villages surrounded by other aspects of community life. This concept does not, however, imply any interaction or social relationship between those in care and their neighbours or the surrounding community.

Care *by* the community

This implies that those living in the community will be given care or helped and supported by others living in the local community, rather than solely by professional carers who go to their residence in order to work.

Care *of* the community

This implies that the community facilities are for the benefit of that community. There is a community identity to the services, and the residents of the community use them as needed. This would imply a range of mental health services for a locality from counselling to residential care.

It can be argued that present community care facilities are on the whole in the community, but that very little of the care is by the community. Resources limit care of the community to those who are seriously mentally ill.

(a) Learning activity

Ascertain what range of current provision is made in your locality for mental health, for people with mental health problems and by mental health services.

Which aspects of the provision represent care *in* the community, care *by* the community or care *of* the community?

How might these three different concepts conflict with one another? Consider rights, risks and resources.

Access the National Service Framework (NSF) and other key documents relevant to the implementation of mental health policy in your region. Identify the key elements of current policy that are influencing the services you are encountering.

The Labour government's direction since 1997 was outlined in *Modernising Mental Health Services* (DH, 1998). The strategy was established through the National Service Framework (NSF) for Mental Health (DH, 1999b, 2004) and the National Health Service (NHS) National Plan (DH, 2000) in England and through similar approaches elsewhere in the United Kingdom (Welsh Assembly Government, 2002, 2005; Scottish Executive, 1997, 2005). The aims of policy are (DH, 1998):

- to protect the public and provide effective and safe care for those with severe and enduring mental illness
- to meet the needs of those with mental health problems who can appropriately and safely be managed within primary health and social care
- to promote mental health in the population and help build healthier neighbourhoods.

The government's 'vision for mental health care' was summarised in *The Journey to Recovery* (DH, 2001b) and is restated with some changed priorities in the five-year review of NSF progress (DH, 2004) and urging from Professor Louis Appleby, the national director for Mental

Health, to 'break down the barriers' that can prevent people with mental health problems from rebuilding their lives in the community (DH, 2007).

Targets for mental health

In order to deal with mental health problems and the perceived inadequacies of services over many years, key targets for services and indicators are set. For the ten years 1999–2009, the NSF for Mental Health (DH, 1999b, 2004) set the standards for mental health services in England. Similar targets are also set elsewhere in the United Kingdom: Welsh Assembly Government (2002, 2005), Scottish Executive (1997, 2005).

In the NSF for Mental Health seven standards are set in order to achieve five key aims:

- Mental health promotion (Standard 1): To ensure health and social services promote mental health and reduce the discrimination and social exclusion associated with mental health problems.
- Primary care and access to services (Standards 2 and 3): To deliver better primary mental healthcare, and to ensure consistent advice and help for people with mental health needs, including primary care services for individuals with severe mental illness.
- Effective services for people with severe mental illness (Standards 4 and 5): To ensure that each person with severe mental illness receives the range of mental health services they need; that crises are anticipated or prevented where possible; to ensure prompt and effective help if a crisis does occur; and timely access to an appropriate and safe mental health place or hospital bed, including a secure bed, as close to home as possible should this be needed.
- Caring about carers (Standard 6): To ensure health and social services assess the needs of carers who provide regular and substantial care for those with severe mental illness, and provide care to meet their needs.
- Preventing suicide (Standard 7): To ensure that health and social services play their full part in the achievement of the target in *Saving Lives: Our healthier nation* (DH, 1999a) to reduce the suicide rate by at least one-fifth by 2010.

The Welsh equivalent is evident in the Welsh NSF (Welsh Assembly Government, 2002, 2005):

- Promoting social inclusion (Standard 1).
- Empowerment and support of service users and carers (Standard 2).
- Promotion of opportunities for a normal pattern of daily life (Standard 3).
- Commissioning equitable, accessible services (Standard 4).
- Delivering responsive, comprehensive services (Standards 5 and 6).
- Effective client assessment and care pathways (Standard 7).
- Ensuring a well staffed, skilled and supported workforce (Standard 8).

A wide range of **social**, **psychological** and **biological** factors has a clear link with mental health problems. This is increasingly recognised in the development of health policy (DH, 1999a; Welsh Assembly Government, 2002). Detailed research on the causes of mental illness has shown that the major risk factors for mental illness include (DH, 1999a):

- poverty, poor education, unemployment
- social isolation stemming from discrimination against people with all types of physical disabilities
- major life events such as bereavement, redundancy, financial problems, being the victim of crime
- genetic predisposition
- drug and alcohol misuse
- developmental factors such as fetal damage and injury at birth
- poor parenting.

a Learning activity

Identify relevant factors in the area in which you live or work which may affect the mental health of the local population. Where there are specific problem factors, identify any services that provide relevant help.

S Scenario continued: Barry's problems

Barry grew up living with his mother after his parents broke up when he was in his early teens. He did not have many friends at school but did reasonably well. After school he went on to a surveying course at a local college. Here, he had a more active social life, sharing a house with other male students who watched sport, drank moderately and smoked a little cannabis. He had several girlfriends before meeting his first wife, whom he married when he was 21.

In his early 20s, during his first job, he was seen as a conscientious worker, but rather quiet. He would worry about his work and sometimes became upset or preoccupied over small incidents.

His first marriage lasted five years but broke down when his wife left to live with someone else. Shortly afterwards, he had his first 'breakdown', when he disappeared from work and did not return home for several days.

Barry later described how he felt that he was unable to concentrate or work properly, everything he did went wrong and he felt that he should not be doing such a responsible job. He didn't feel able to talk to anyone, and felt that if he did, they would not be able to understand. He lacked confidence and was sure that everyone would think he was pathetic. He tended to drink a little more than usual.

Mental health and mental illness

Barry has a range of problems, some, we can understand in the same terms as we understand many of the problems in our everyday lives, such as needing money, trying to make relationships work, surviving stresses and so on.

a Learning activity

Consider the thoughts and feelings Barry described. Try to imagine how you might respond if you had such feelings.

S Scenario continued: Early help

Barry had not really thought of his problems as being 'mental health' problems. He and his wife had been to Relate, but this mainly focused on sorting out their separation and he did not feel able to talk in any depth about how he felt. He had some friends who were supportive, but did not really know how to help him when he withdrew. Some had suggested seeing a doctor, but he did not think that would help. He didn't feel

that his drinking was a problem. Eventually, as a result of going to Occupational Health at work, he was referred to a counsellor. Counselling focused on listening to him, giving him space and time to identify and address some of the problems he was having in everyday life. He didn't feel there were any great revelations, but he finished the sessions and was able to return to work and pick up the threads again.

a Learning activity

Find out about the differences between counselling and psychotherapy.

Find out what facilities are available in your area for access to counselling and psychological therapies.

Consider what sorts of care might have been options for Barry in your locality.

S Scenario continued: Recognition of problems in primary care

Barry continued working, changing his job several times and in his early 30s, he met and married Sabina and also took a managerial role in a small property development company owned by a friend. He enjoyed the challenge at first, although he found the financial insecurity of the company very worrying, especially as they soon had little Gary to care for.

In his mid-30s, there was a period when he became more and more preoccupied with his worries and felt that he was not able to live up to the expectations of the company, Sabina and the responsibilities of being the father of a young child. He stayed off work and started to spend most days in bed or in front of the television. Sabina, desperate, called the GP.

After a missed appointment, the GP asked Mike, a community mental health nurse (CMHN) to visit Barry. Mike saw him at home where Barry told him he felt tired all the time and had no energy. He felt that it wasn't worth him going to work as he believed that would only 'screw things up'. When Mike talked to Sabina, she said that he had been like this for a couple of weeks: he had no interest in her, the children or in eating, and seemed to blame himself for everything that was wrong in their lives. Barry had told Sabina that she would be better of without him.

Mike spent about an hour and a half with Barry, who seemed rather morose and withdrawn. As well as trying to engage Barry as much as he could in conversation, Mike completed a number of written assessments with him.

Barry agreed that Mike should return later in the week.

Assessment

What do we need to know in order to provide Barry with support? How could we assess:

- Barry's feelings, thoughts and perceptions?
- the feelings of other members of the family?
- what they want and need?
- the level or severity of their distress?
- his safety and the degree of risk that he might attempt suicide?
- the needs of others?

Approaches to assessment in mental health have been well discussed by Barker (2004).

a Learning activity

Find out what approaches to assessment and what assessment tools are used by professionals in your local mental health services.

In particular ascertain the approach to the assessment of mood and the assessment and management of risk.

To what extent is the client or service user's perspective incorporated into the assessment?

a Learning activity   **W**

Access 'NHS choices' at http://www.nhs.uk/ and explore the 'Map of Medicine Healthguides' including the depression care pathway at http://healthguides. mapofmedicine.com/choices/map/depression1.html)

Access the National Institute for Clinical Excellence (NICE) guideline for 'management of depression in primary and secondary care' (NICE, 2004, amended 2007) at: http:// www.nice.org.uk/guidance/index.jsp?action=byID&o=10958

Explore the 'stepped model' described in the NICE guideline and 'care pathways' and consider the relationship between life problems and health problems.

How is depression recognised in primary care?

Explore the differences between responses in primary care and the need for secondary care.

S Scenario continued: Initial treatment in primary care

Mike discussed Barry's problems with the GP, who agreed with Mike's formulation that Barry was suffering from a mild to moderate depression.

Mike, who had undergone a course of postqualifying training in cognitive behavioural therapy (CBT), agreed that he would start working with Barry using CBT techniques to address some of the issues Mike had picked up on assessment.

Barry saw Mike for an initial two appointments at home, but agreed that he would continue for a further six sessions at the local health centre, which was a short walk from Barry's home. Together, they explored some of the thoughts and feelings that Barry had about himself, and although initially Barry had reservations, he found that he started to follow the approach as Mike explained it and in addition to reviewing a number of aspects of his life, found that he felt better and was able to return to work after the fourth session.

After the final session, they agreed to meet once more after a further month and then only if Barry needed to make contact with the GP again.

Therapeutic relationships

Mental health practitioners need to be able to form such relationships with people such as Barry, who may have problems, attitudes, thoughts, feelings or behaviour which make relationships more difficult. Practitioners need to be self-aware, recognising their own contribution to the development of relationships

C Professional conversation

Mike, a community mental health nurse covering a large rural area, comments, 'Many of the 35 people on my case load have social problems which it is difficult for me to help them with. About 30 per cent have other problems such as drink or drugs, but it is difficult to get help for them from other services because of their mental health problems. With many of them, I have built up a therapeutic relationship over quite long periods of time and have been the only consistent professional helper they trust.

'I've known Barry on and off for some years now, although he hasn't been on my case load all that time. Sometimes he can be quite difficult; however, I really try to understand what is going on for him. I know that he does not see me quite as a friend; so that, while he expects me to be "on his side" and support him, he also trusts me to be honest and tell him what I think when there are aspects of his problems he is not seeing. I have been able to use the skills I have gained to work with him and have helped him recognise and identify problems before they get too bad, and help him modify the thoughts he has that contribute to how bad he feels. Sometimes he will share a particular problem and I help him to find his own solution. Although this doesn't always work, I have got to know him and I think we get on well enough so that if they do need help, I'm now usually the first person he or Sabina contacts and I can intervene before things get too bad.'

Characteristics of a therapeutic relationship

Carl Rogers is usually credited with identifying and describing a set of conditions that should exist for effective therapeutic work (Rogers, 1951):

- **accurate empathic understanding and responding,** that is, the helper strives not only to understand how the world and their problems and situation are perceived by the client, but communicates this endeavour to the client
- **acceptance or respect, also sometimes termed 'nonpossessive warmth' or 'unconditional positive regard'**, that is, the client is not made to feel that they must please

the helper or show gratitude and that the helper will not judge or be shocked by their situation, thoughts or behaviour

- **genuineness, sincerity or congruence**, that is, the helper is what they appear to be and is open in and about the relationship.

Since the work of Rogers, these principles have been widely incorporated into approaches to counselling, therapy and 'client-centred' approaches to mental health practice. A key skill in all these approaches is 'active listening'. This means an emphasis which focuses on paying attention to what the client is saying, showing them that you are listening and understanding and helping to clarify the meaning of what they are saying.

Elements of active listening include:

- questioning: enabling the client to talk freely in response to open questions
- clarifying, checking, understanding; sorting out confusion or ambiguity and encouraging the client to be specific and focus on important aspects
- responding: to verbal and nonverbal cues in the client
- noticing and being aware: not only of what is expressed, but also what is not expressed
- reflecting: mirroring back to the client either the sense and content in, or the feelings behind, what he/she is saying
- paraphrasing: listening to what the client is saying and putting the essential meaning into other words
- summarising: bringing together the main ideas and feelings at the end of or during a conversation.

(a) Learning activity

Next time you are talking to a mental health service user about his or her experience, notice the degree to which you are 'actively listening'.

How would the other person know that you are paying attention?

t☆ Practice tips

When you interact with clients, such as during an interview or assessment, consider the following:

- Remember that the emphasis is on listening, not talking.
- Avoid probing unnecessarily – don't 'interrogate', that is, ask too many questions. Is it an appropriate question – or are you are just being curious?
- Where possible ask open rather than closed questions, which allow the client to explore and develop their feelings/thoughts.
- Try not to ask 'why' questions: 'what', 'how', 'when', 'who' etc. questions are usually more helpful, enabling the client to be more specific about the situation, rather than trying to rationalise feelings, or explain situations that they do not understand.

- Avoid asking leading questions, otherwise the client explores your perspective rather than their own.
- Do you have permission to talk in the way you are? Be sensitive – take cues from the client.
- Don't go deeper than you can handle. You have a responsibility to ensure that you are working within the limits of your competence. Ask yourself whether you are the appropriate person to deal with a difficult issue, or whether counselling or therapy might be needed.
- If you don't have time for the answer don't ask the question.
- Time the questions appropriately for the situation and stage of interview.
- Try to allow the person to make the decisions rather than simply to give advice.

- Notwithstanding the above, don't dogmatically refuse to give advice, or avoid prescribing action, sometimes they may be the most appropriate and sensible things to do. Similarly, giving information, education and so on may be important interventions.
- Try not to judge or blame, or use 'shoulds' and 'oughts', which reflect your frame of reference, not the client's.
- Try not to invalidate what the client feels by suggesting that what they feel is inappropriate, silly or that they feel, or should feel, something else.
- Don't say that you're 'sure that it will be all right' when you aren't! You may not be able to make it all better!

Helping interventions

John Heron (2001) suggested that in any helping roles such as nursing, teaching, social work, medicine, there are broadly six different intervention strategies. These he divided into two groups.

John Heron's six categories of intervention

AUTHORITATIVE INTERVENTIONS

In which the practitioner tends to be dominant, assertive, interventionist.

- **Prescriptive interventions:** seek to direct the behaviour of the client (such as giving advice, suggesting).
- **Informative interventions:** Seek to impart knowledge, meaning or information not available to the client (such as giving information, interpreting).
- **Confronting interventions:** Seek to raise the awareness of the client about some limiting attitude or behaviour of which he is unaware (such as challenging inconsistencies, giving feedback). It is important to be supportive when confronting.

FACILITATIVE INTERVENTIONS

In which equality is more evident in the relationship and the role of the client is enhanced (Heron, 2001):

- **Cathartic interventions:** Seek to enable the client to discharge painful emotion, primarily grief, fear, anger or embarrassment (by laughing, crying, storming and so on).
- **Catalytic interventions:** Seek to facilitate self-discovery, self-directed learning and problem solving in the client (such as client-centred questioning and approaches).
- **Supportive interventions:** Seek to affirm the worth and value of the client's person, qualities, attitudes or actions (such as touch, validating the worth of the client).

(a) Learning activity

Think about the following questions and discuss this with your learning group before moving on to the next section:

What qualities would you identify as important for someone working with people with mental health problems?

To what extent do you consider you have these qualities?

What different qualities do you perceive in the array of professional groups involved in mental healthcare? Which qualities do they share?

At the heart of mental health work, and particularly mental health nursing, is the ability to form a helpful or 'therapeutic' relationship. A mental health nursing review in 1994 identified this as the first of the core skills of mental health nursing (Butterworth, 1994).

(e) Evidence-based practice

Skills of mental health nursing

'It is the combination of these particular skills, together with the values and practice common to the nursing profession as a whole, which provides the unique expertise of mental health nurses enabling them to:

- establish a therapeutic relationship which rests in a respect for others and a skilled therapeutic use of self
- sustain such relationships over time and respond flexibly to the changing needs of those with mental health problems

- construct, implement and plan a care programme
- provide skilled assessment, ongoing monitoring
- make risk assessments and judgements
- monitor the dosage, effects and contra indications of medication
- detect early signs of deteriorating mental health including potential self-harm and suicide risk, worsening physical conditions and potential threats to others

- prioritise work in order to respond to those most in need
- collaborate with all members of the multidisciplinary team
- network effectively, setting appropriate boundaries to professional input
- manage the therapeutic environment, determined by clear awareness of such issues as safety, dignity and partnership.'

(Butterworth, 1994)

A dozen years later, another review (DH, 2006) has identified 'best practice capabilities'.

(e) Evidence-based practice

Mental health nursing – from values to action

The best practice capabilities for mental health nurses (DH, 2006):

'1.1 Promote a culture that values and respects the diversity of individuals, and enables their recovery.

2.1 Use a range of communication skills to establish, maintain and manage relationships with individuals who have mental health problems, their carers and key people involved in their care.

2.2 Promote physical health and well-being for people with mental health problems.

2.3 Promote mental health and well-being, enabling people to recover from debilitating mental health experiences and/or achieve their full potential, supporting them to develop and maintain social networks and relationships.

2.4 Work with individuals with mental health needs in order to maintain health, safety and well-being.

3.1 Work collaboratively with other disciplines and agencies to support individuals to develop and maintain social networks and relationships.

3.2 Demonstrate a commitment to the need for continuing professional development and personal supervision activities, in order to enhance the knowledge, skills, values and attitudes needed for safe and effective nursing practice.'

The Sainsbury Centre for Mental Health (2001) identified a framework of 67 core 'capabilities' which need to be developed by all mental health practitioners if mental health services are to achieve the standards identified in the NSF for Mental Health.

(e) Evidence-based practice

The Sainsbury Centre for Mental Health (2001) core capabilities

Ethical practice

The values and attitudes necessary for modern mental health practice

Knowledge

Policy and legislation
Mental health and mental health services

Process of care

Effective communication and partnership, comprehensive assessment, care planning and review, supervision and continuing professional development (CPD), clinical and practice leadership.

Interventions

Evidence-based: medical and physical care; psychological; social; practical; mental health promotion.

Applications (to specific NSF/NHS Plan service settings)

Primary care
Community-based care coordination (CMHTs)
Crisis Resolution and Early Intervention
Acute in-patient care
Assertive outreach
Continuing care and day centres, residential and vocational programmes
Services for people with complex and special needs (e.g. dual-diagnosis and personality disorders).

The National Institute for Mental Health (NIMHE) has also taken this on by identifying ten 'essential capabilities shared by all mental health workers' (NIMHE/SCMH/NHSU, 2004).

e Evidence-based practice

The ten essential shared capabilities for mental health practice (NIMHE/SCMH/NHSU, 2004)**:**

1 **Working in partnership.** Developing and maintaining constructive working relationships with service users, carers, families, colleagues, lay people and wider community networks. Working positively with any tensions created by conflicts of interest or aspiration that may arise between the partners in care.

2 **Respecting diversity.** Working in partnership with service users, carers, families and colleagues to provide care and interventions that not only make a positive difference but also do so in ways that respect and value diversity, including age, race, culture, disability, gender, spirituality and sexuality.

3 **Practising ethically.** Recognising the rights and aspirations of service users and their families, acknowledging power differentials and minimising them whenever possible. Providing treatment and care that is accountable to service users and carers within the boundaries prescribed by national (professional), legal and local codes of ethical practice.

4 **Challenging inequality.** Addressing the causes and consequences of stigma, discrimination, social inequality and exclusion on service users, carers and mental health services. Creating, developing or maintaining valued social roles for people in the communities they come from.

5 **Promoting recovery.** Working in partnership to provide care and treatment that enables service users and carers to tackle mental health problems with hope and optimism and to work towards a valued lifestyle within and beyond the limits of any mental health problem.

6 **Identifying people's needs and strengths.** Working in partnership to gather information to agree health and social care needs in the context of the preferred lifestyle and aspirations of service users, their families, carers and friends.

7 **Providing service user-centred care.** Negotiating achievable and meaningful goals, primarily from the perspective of service users and their families. Influencing and seeking the means to achieve these goals and clarifying the responsibilities of the people who will provide any help that is needed, including systematically evaluating outcomes and achievements.

8 **Making a difference.** Facilitating access to and delivering the best quality evidence-based, values-based health and social care interventions to meet the needs and aspirations of service users and their families and carers.

9 **Promoting safety and positive risk taking.** Empowering the person to decide the level of risk they are prepared to take with their health and safety. This includes working with the tension between promoting safety and positive risk taking, including assessing and dealing with possible risks for service users, carers, family members and the wider public.

10 **Personal development and learning.** Keeping up-to-date with changes in practice and participating in life-long learning, personal and professional development for one's self and colleagues through supervision, appraisal and reflective practice.

Part

III

a Learning activity

From your initial contact with NICE guidelines, you will have noticed that cognitive behavioural therapy (CBT) is an important first line treatment (not only for depression as in Barry's case). CBT skills are therefore important skills to be developed in the mental health workforce.

Access some of the many guides, books, websites and self-help manuals on CBT and clarify for yourself the main tenets and approaches of CBT.

Scenario continued: secondary care

As Barry approached 40, he once again started to feel low. Sabina recognised the same signs, but Barry ignored her warnings. As he had done once before, he disappeared and Sabina contacted the police and reported him missing. After two days, he was found by a postal operative early in the morning wandering near the local common. He was rather dishevelled and incoherent and did not seem to know where he was. He had marks on his arms and neck, but would or could not say where he had been or what he had been doing. The local police tried to take Barry home, but he refused to go with them saying he had important things to do. The police were concerned and, using their powers under the Mental Health Act, took him to a place of safety to be seen by a mental health professional.

Legal issues

The legal aspects of mental healthcare are determined both by statute and common law. Of the former, the most relevant for mental health workers are the Mental Health Act 1983 and Mental Capacity Act 2005. At the time of its enactment the Mental Health Act 1983 was seen as liberalising legislation, but over the years it has increasingly been seen as in need of reform. The demand for reform was reinforced by a series of highly publicised mental health inquiries into homicides by mentally ill people (Reith 1998). After a prolonged review process between 1999 and 2007, during which the balance between individual liberty and public safety was hotly debated and consensus difficult to achieve, the Mental Health Act 1983 was finally amended by the Mental Health Act 2007 to reflect better the needs of a more community-oriented mental health service.

C) Professional conversation

Barry, a mental health service user, comments, 'I've been in hospital several times including "under section", when they wouldn't let me leave hospital and insisted on me having treatment. I admit things had been getting on top of me, but I had a lot of problems to deal with. On top of not feeling right, struggling with my work and worrying about my family, them putting me in hospital against my will upset me. I suppose I might have done away with myself at one point, but mostly I think I would have been OK.

'I can see that I must have been quite difficult to handle and some staff, like Helen, the ward manager have been quite strict, but fair. The social workers and nurses have tried to explain my rights and the legal situation, even though I didn't really take it in. But there were some staff who made things worse by not listening to me, or trying to play down the problems I was having.'

a) Learning activity

The Mental Health Acts 1983 and 2007

The Mental Health Act 1983 (as amended by the Mental Health Act 2007) makes provision for people suffering from a mental disorder to be given care which they may not think they need, but is deemed necessary for their health or safety or for the protection of other people.

The Mental Health Act is a piece of legislation all mental health workers need to be familiar with.

On your own, or with your learning group, find out more about the current Mental Health Act:

- How is 'mental disorder' defined?
- What is the role of various mental health professionals in bringing about care under the Mental Health Act?
- What is the role of the police under the Mental Health Act in a situation like Barry's?
- Under the Act what options are open to mental health professionals working with Barry at this difficult point?

Ascertain how far the reform of mental health legislation has now been implemented.

S   Scenario continued: Hospital care

Barry is offered admission to hospital. However, the approved mental health professional who assesses him feels that in his present state he is a significant risk to himself, and suggests to him that he is admitted voluntarily to hospital. This he declines and the Mental Health Act is used to bring him in to hospital for assessment. He is admitted under the Mental Health Act to an acute psychiatric ward within a large district general hospital. Initially he refuses to accept that he has to remain there for assessment, refuses treatment and insists that he wants to leave.

After a further assessment interview, the clinician responsible for his care in hospital feels that he should have some antidepressant medication to help his mood lift, so that he can again have further psychological intervention and to reduce his time in hospital. He remains in hospital for two weeks, gradually becoming more sociable, after which, following a special meeting to discuss what help and support he might need after leaving hospital, he is discharged home. Because after further assessment he is no longer seen as a risk to himself, he is also discharged from his Mental Health Act section. He feels better, but is rather shaky and uncertain about his future and agrees to resume therapeutic work with Mike.

a   Learning activity

Find out more about the secondary care services in your area including access to, and the roles of, crisis teams, gateway workers, home treatment teams and acute in-patient units.

If your reading of material on the Mental Health Act 1983 has not yet covered them, on your own, or with your learning group, find out and discuss more about the current Mental Health Act:

- admission for assessment
- admission for treatment
- admission in an emergency
- clinicians' and nurses' 'holding power'
- discharge meetings.

If you have the opportunity, talk to some of the service users about their experience of the treatment they have received. Identify the helpful and unhelpful aspects of the treatment and care as they have experienced it.

c   Professional conversation

Helen, a deputy ward manager on an acute in-patient unit, says, 'As in general wards, the patients we have are here for shorter periods of time often only during the acute period of their illness. About half of our patients are detained under the Mental Health Act. Making helping relationships with people, within an environment which they have not chosen, can be very demanding, but is also very rewarding. For me that is the most challenging part of the job – establishing trust and genuine helping relationships with people who are hard to engage with.

'Barry and I had had our ups and downs. When he was first admitted here, having been suicidal, he was upset, anxious and withdrawn. Although he knows me better now, as he had been "sectioned" it was particularly difficult to establish a collaborative relationship for the first part of his admission.

'It was helpful to be able to see him with Mike, the community mental health nurse [CMHN], with whom he seems to have established a good relationship.'

Diagnoses and depression

Increasingly there is an international consensus on the criteria for diagnosing mental and behavioural disorders (although not about causation). There are, however, two major classification systems: the *International Classification of Diseases* (ICD-10) (WHO, 1992) and the *Diagnostic and Statistical Manual of Mental Disorders* (DSM-IV-TR) (APA, 2000). Chapter V of ICD-10 lists 'Mental and behavioural disorders' the categories for which are shown in Table 26.1.

Table 26.1   Categories in ICD Chapter V

F00–F09	Organic, including symptomatic, disorders
F10–F19	Mental and behavioural disorders due to psychoactive substance abuse
F20–F29	Schizophrenia, schizotypal and delusional disorders
F30–F39	Mood (affective) disorders
F40–F48	Neurotic, stress-related and somatoform disorders
F50–F59	Behavioural syndromes associated with physiological disturbances and physical factors
F60–F69	Disorders of adult personality and behaviour
F70–F79	Mental retardation
F80–F89	Disorders of psychological development
F90–F98	Behavioural and emotional disorders with onset usually occurring in childhood and adolescence
F99	Unspecified mental disorder

Source: WHO ICD-10 1992.

a) Learning activity   W

Find out attitudes to diagnostic classification systems by mental health professionals with whom you have contact.

Which professionals base their approach on a diagnosis? On what concepts, frameworks, models and ideas do others base their ideas about mental health problems?

Read the ICD-10 diagnostic criteria (or consult the equivalent section in DSM-IV-TR) and ascertain the way in which the criteria which define depression and other 'mental and behavioural disorders' are organised.

See ICD-10 classification of 'Mental and Behavioural Disorders' (WHO, 2007) online: http://www.who.int/classifications/apps/icd/icd10online. How might these criteria apply to Barry's experiences?

Diagnosis of depression

> In typical mild, moderate, or severe depressive episodes, the patient suffers from lowering of mood, reduction of energy, and decrease in activity. Capacity for enjoyment, interest, and concentration is reduced, and marked tiredness after even minimum effort is common. Sleep is usually disturbed and appetite diminished. Self-esteem and self-confidence are almost always reduced and, even in the mild form, some ideas of guilt or worthlessness are often present. The lowered mood varies little from day to day, is unresponsive to circumstances and may be accompanied by so-called "somatic" symptoms, such as loss of interest and pleasurable feelings, waking in the morning several hours before the usual time, depression worst in the morning, marked psychomotor retardation, agitation, loss of appetite, weight loss, and loss of libido. Depending upon the number and severity of the symptoms, a depressive episode may be specified as mild, moderate or severe.
>
> (WHO, 1992)

The detection of depression in primary care is an important priority, and increasingly primary care professionals are developing skills and tools to identify depression. An example is the Edinburgh Postnatal Depression Scale used by midwives with women following childbirth where there is a known increased risk of depression.

Edinburgh Postnatal Depression Scale (EPDS)

Ten statements score 0–3 (*or 3–0) relating to the past seven days (Cox, Holden and Sagovsky, 1987):

1 I have been able to laugh and see the funny side of things.
2 I have looked forward with enjoyment to things.
3 *I have blamed myself unnecessarily when things went wrong.
4 I have been anxious or worried for no good reason.
5 *I have felt scared or panicky for no good reason.
6 *Things have been getting on top of me.
7 *I have been so unhappy that I have had difficulty sleeping.
8 *I have felt sad or miserable.
9 *I have been so unhappy that I have been crying.
10 *The thought of harming myself has occurred to me.

Treatment interventions for people with depression

A range of different treatment options is advocated for helping people with depression (NICE, 2007: 200):

- 'Watchful waiting': in mild depression, the patient may not need or want treatment and may recover with no intervention.
- General care:
  - help/advice with sleep, anxiety management and hygiene care
  - structured exercise programme
  - physical care and illness management.
- Psychosocial:
  - six to eight sessions over 10 to 12 weeks of CBT
  - support and a therapeutic alliance
  - problem solving
  - coping with distress, panic
  - offering information and other sources of help and resources.
- Pharmacological intervention:
  - selective serotonin reuptake inhibitor (SSRI), as effective as tricyclic antidepressants but less likely to be discontinued because of side-effects.
- Computerised CBT.
- Guided self help.

Suicide and attempted suicide

As we have seen earlier in recognising the incidence of mental health problems, some 5600 people in the UK commit suicide each year (Samaritans, 2007). The prevention of suicide has therefore assumed a high priority in government targets for mental health services through the NSFs and the Suicide Prevention Strategy for England (DH, 2002). There tend to be two foci:

- reducing suicide in the general population
- preventing suicide by those already in contact with mental health services.

The National Confidential Inquiry into Suicide and Homicide by People with Mental Illness, now based in the University of Manchester, has an ongoing role in researching and monitoring the latter. Although each suicide is a shock for those close to the individual, suicide rarely occurs 'out of the blue'.

Part

III

(e) Evidence-based practice

Of people who commit suicide (Williams and Morgan, 1996; Appleby et al, 2001):

- 90 per cent have been judged (retrospectively) to have some form of mental disorder
- 66 per cent consulted their GP in the previous month
- 60 per cent give some advance warning
- 33 per cent express clear suicidal intent
- 24 per cent were in contact with mental health services in the previous year
- 11.5 per cent were in contact with services in the previous week.

Of course it is very easy to discover these circumstances retrospectively. Clearly we need to be able to develop some ideas which will help us identify risk prospectively. Some clear patterns are evident, and should be considered in order to guide practice.

(e) Evidence-based practice

Groups at risk of suicide (Appleby et al, 2001; Samaritans, 2007):

- males (male:female about 3:1, but this varies between ethnic and cultural groups (e.g. ratio 2.8:1 in England and Wales, 2.6:1 in Scotland, 3.4:1 in Northern Ireland and 4.5:1 in Republic of Ireland), however, it is more common in Asian women than Asian men
- the elderly and young men
- divorced/widowed/single
- social class i or v.
- specific occupations (such as farmers, doctors, vets, pharmacists, dentists, nurses, pilots)
- those living alone
- the socially isolated or those in rural communities
- the unemployed or retired
- children of suicides
- other bereavements in childhood
- people who have previously harmed themselves
- those following recent major life event or loss
- people with mental disorders:
  - depressive illness (15 per cent lifetime risk)
  - schizophrenia (10 per cent lifetime risk)
  - those who abuse alcohol or drugs (3.4 per cent lifetime risk)
  - organic disorders (such as early dementia, Huntington's disease)
  - personality disorder
- people with past psychiatric problems
- family history of affective illness
- people with a terminal illness
- those in poor physical health.

Although it is almost impossible to be certain of the intent at the time of the act of those who successfully kill themselves, this profile is a little different from those who self harm themselves with a nonfatal outcome (parasuicide).

(e) Evidence-based practice

Groups at risk of parasuicide by contrast with completed suicide:

- tend to be female (female : male approx. 3:1)
- tend to be younger
- tend to be social classes IV and V
- may have social problems (such as housing, finance, unemployment), or relationship problems (such as marital disharmony or break up)
- may be impulsive
- may be imitative.

These profiles give indications of risk among *groups*. What are needed, however, are tools and questions which can be applied to individuals. As guidance to professionals in primary care, this can sometimes be reduced to a brief list of four important questions:

(e) Evidence-based practice

Recognising suicide risk in primary care (Armstrong, 1997)**:**

1 Do you feel that life is not worth living?
2 Have you felt like acting on this?
3 Have you made any plans?
4 Have you tried before?

1 only: (no intentions, no plans, no past history) – See again, GP treats depression.

1 and 2 only: (intentions but no plans or past history) – See frequently, GP treats depression and considers 2nd referral.

1, 2 and 3 or 4: (intentions and definite plans or previous attempts) – Refer urgently, monitor closely and treat depression.

t ☆
Practice tip

Identify, and where you are participating in clinical care under supervision, utilise, the recognised risk assessment tools in use in your area. In addition, ask yourself the following questions:

- Does the person now hope that things will turn out better or change?
- Do they recognise getting some pleasure out of life?
- Do they feel hopeful on a day to day basis?
- Are they able to face the next day?
- Do they see some point in living or do they despair of going on?
- Does life feel a burden, and do they wish it would end?

- Do they wish they were dead?
- Do they think about ending their life? If so, how often?
- Have they ever acted on such thoughts?
- Do they feel able to resist them?
- How likely do they think it is that they could harm/kill themselves?
- Can they give a reassurance that they will not?
- Will they seek help if there is a crisis?
- Is there a risk to any one else?

The final question always seems to be subjective and intuitive: Do you believe the reassurances or denials you are given?

Recovery

Finally, and most positively, although this chapter could equally have begun by discussing it, let us consider the notion of recovery. Conventionally the word 'recovery' implies 'getting better' – the restoration of health following sickness, often as the result of curative intervention by professionals. However, in contemporary mental health services 'recovery' has come to mean people being empowered to manage their lives in a way that allows them to have the most fulfilling, meaningful experience possible of life and a positive sense of their own contribution to their own, their family's and their community's well-being.

Users of mental health services now want 'recovery-oriented' services: that is, services that (NIMHE, 2005):

- focus on people rather than services
- monitor outcomes rather than performance
- emphasise strengths rather than deficits or dysfunction
- educate people who provide services, schools, employers, the media and the public to combat stigma
- foster collaboration between those who need support and those who support them as an alternative to coercion
- through enabling and supporting self-management, promote autonomy and, as a result, decrease the need for people to rely on formal service and professional supports.

For more detailed understanding of the 'recovery model', see *A Common Purpose: Recovery in future mental health services*, (CSIP, RCPsych and SCIE, 2007) and read *Art of Recovery* (Heyes, 2005).

[S] Scenario continued: The current situation

In the last few years, Barry has had several more bouts of depression. This has put a strain on his marriage to Sabina and relationship with the children. However, as he has come to know the community mental health team, Barry has received help through talking to them on a one-to-one basis and with other service users in groups. He and Sabina have also been for some joint sessions to help them understand better what happens between them at times leading up to his depressions.

Both of them have experienced great stress, and at the worst, he has been suicidal and she has considered leaving. He is not currently working, but is increasingly involved in a community allotment scheme. They continue to make a life together, aware that there may be further difficult times ahead, but feeling that they do have support from mental health services and their local community.

(a) Learning activity

Consider the effect of the experience of Barry's mental health problems and the care offered has had on the life of each family member.

If you can do so in a facilitated group, adopt roles for each member of the family and, in role, discuss the experiences you have had.

Conclusion

Through the scenarios, we have followed Barry and Sabina and their family and seen the impact of mental health problems upon their lives. By considering the questions, reading and undertaking the activities, you should have developed:

- an understanding of the kind of problems and experiences they have had
- recognition of the characteristics and importance of the therapeutic relationship
- an agenda for developing the essential skills you need to learn in order to provide appropriate responses to people with mental health problems
- knowledge of the services, particularly those in your local area, which have developed to respond to the kind of problems they experience
- an understanding of the notion of 'recovery' as it is used to denote a positive experience for service users
- knowledge of the changing and evolving policies and legislative framework underpinning mental healthcare.

ⓐ Learning activity

Now that you have had opportunities to consider some of the issues raised in mental healthcare, and met some of those involved as service users, carers and mental health practitioners, how do you now feel about 'mental health'? Look back over any notes you have made and reflect on the experiences you have had. How are your ideas and attitudes changing, developing, hardening, softening etc.? In what ways will any insights you are gaining in this field influence what you do in the future?

References

American Psychiatric Association (APA) (2000) *Diagnostic and Statistical Manual of Mental Disorders* (text revised), Washington DC, APA.

Appleby, L., Shaw, J., Sherratt, J., Amos, T., Robinson, J. AND McDonnell, R. (2001) *Safety First: Five year report of the National Confidential Inquiry into Suicide and Homicide by People with Mental Illness*. London, Department of Health [online] http://www.dh.gov.uk/en/Publicationsandstatistics/Publications/PublicationsPolicyAndGuidance/DH_4006679?IdcService=GET_FILE&dID=15047&Rendition=Web (accessed 30 January 2009).

Armstrong, E. (1997) *The Primary Mental Health Care Toolkit*, London, Royal College of General Practitioners.

Barker, P. (2004) *Assessment in Psychiatric and Mental Health Nursing: In search of the whole person*, Cheltenham, Nelson Thornes.

Butterworth, A. (Chairman) (1994) *Working in Partnership: A collaborative approach to care. The report of the mental health nursing review team*, London, HMSO.

Care Services Improvement Partnership (CSIP) (2007) *Consultation on guidance on 'Finding a shared vision of how people's mental health problems should be understood'*, London, Department of Health [online] http://www.dh.gov.uk/en/Consultations/Liveconsultations/DH_080913 (accessed 30 January 2009).

CSIP, Royal College of Psychiatrists (RCPsych), Social Care Institute for Excellence (SCIE) (2007) *A Common Purpose: Recovery in future mental health services*, London, SCIE [online] http://www.spn.org.uk/fileadmin/SPN_uploads/Documents/Papers/SPN_Papers/recovery2.pdf (accessed 30 January 2009).

Cox, J. L., Holden, J. M. and Sagovsky, R. (1987) 'Detection of postnatal depression: development of the 10-item Edinburgh Postnatal Depression Scale', *British Journal of Psychiatry* 150, 782–6.

Department of Health (DH) (1998) *Modernising Mental Health Services: Safe, sound and supportive*, London, DH.

DH (1999a) *Saving Lives: Our healthier nation*, London, TSO [online] http://www.dh.gov.uk/assetRoot/04/04/93/29/04049329.pdf (accessed 30 January 2009).

DH (1999b) *National Service Framework for Mental Health. Modern standards and service models*, London, DH [online] full document: http://www.dh.gov.uk/prod_consum_dh/idcplg?IdcService=GET_FILE&dID=21839&Rendition=Web; executive summary: http://www.dh.gov.uk/prod_consum_dh/idcplg?IdcService=GET_FILE&dID=24079&Rendition=Web (accessed 30 January 2009).

DH (2000) *The NHS Plan*, London, TSO [online] http://www.dh.gov.uk/prod_consum_dh/idcplg?IdcService=GET_FILE&dID=23612&Rendition=Web (accessed 30 January 2009).

DH (2001a) *The Mental Health Policy Implementation Guide*, London, DH [online] http://www.csip.org.uk/silo/files/mh-policy-implementation-guide.pdf (accessed 30 January 2009).

DH (2001b) *The Journey to Recovery: The government's vision for mental health care*, London, DH [online] http://www.dh.gov.uk/prod_consum_dh/idcplg?IdcService=GET_FILE&dID=26519&Rendition=Web (accessed 30 January 2009).

DH (2002) *National Suicide Prevention Strategy for England*, London, DH [online] http://www.dh.gov.uk/assetRoot/04/01/95/48/04019548.pdf (accessed 30 January 2009).

DH (2004) *National Service Framework for Mental Health – Five years on*, London, DH [online] http://www.dh.gov.uk/assetRoot/04/09/91/22/04099122.pdf (accessed 30 January 2009).

DH (2006) *From Values to Action: The Chief Nursing Officer's Review of mental health nursing*, London, DH, [online] main document: http://www.dh.gov.uk/assetRoot/04/13/38/40/04133840.pdf; self-assessment toolkit: http://www.dh.gov.uk/assetRoot/04/13/40/53/04134053.pdf; best practice competencies and capabilities for pre-reg. MH nurses: http://www.dh.gov.uk/assetRoot/04/13/56/48/04135648.pdf; link to literature reviews: http://www.nursing.manchester.ac.uk/projects/mentalhealthreview (accessed 30 January 2009).

DH (2007) *Breaking Down Barriers: Clinical Case for Change. Report by Louis Appleby, National Director for Mental Health*, London, DH [online] http://www.networks.nhs.uk/uploads/07/05/200705_146906_g_n_1_breaking_down_barriers_1.pdf (accessed 30 January 2009).

Goffman, E. (1961) *Asylums*, London, Penguin.

Goldberg, D. and Huxley, P. (1992) *Common Mental Disorders: A bio-social model*, London, Routledge.

Heron, J. (2001) *Helping the Client: A creative practical guide*, 5th edn, London, Sage.

Keen, T. (1999) 'Schizophrenia: Orthodoxies and Heresies', *Journal of Psychiatric and Mental Health Nursing* 6(6), 415–24.

National Confidential Inquiry into Suicide and Homicide by People with Mental Illness (2006) *Avoidable Deaths: Five year report of the National Confidential Inquiry into Suicide and Homicide by People with Mental Illness*. Manchester, University of Manchester. [online] http://www.medicine.manchester.ac.uk/psychiatry/research/suicide/prevention/nci/reports/avoidabledeathsfullreport.pdf (accessed 30 January 2009) [summary online] http://www.medicine.manchester.ac.uk/psychiatry/research/suicide/prevention/nci/reports/avoidabledeathssummaryreport.pdf (accessed 30 January 2009).

National Institute for Clinical Excellence (NICE) (2004, amended 2007) *Depression: Management of depression in primary and secondary care* (Clinical Guideline 23), London, NICE [online] guideline (67 pp., 413 KB): http://guidance.nice.org.uk/download.aspx?o=424970; quick reference guide (16 pp., 224 KB): http://guidance.nice.org.uk/download.aspx?o=424672 (accessed 30 January 2009).

National Institute for Mental Health in England (NIMHE), Sainsbury Centre for Mental Health (SCMH) and NHSU (2004) *The Ten Essential Shared Capabilities: A framework for the whole of the mental health workforce*, London, NIMHE [online] http://www.dh.gov.uk/prod_consum_dh/idcplg?IdcService=GET_FILE&dID=3466&Rendition=Web (accessed 30 January 2009).

NIMHE (2005) *NIMHE Guiding Statement on Recovery*, London, NIMHE [online] http://213.121.207.229/upload/Recovery per cent20Guiding per cent20Statement.pdf (accessed 30 January 2009).

Office for National Statistics (ONS) (2007) *Attitudes to Mental Illness 2007: Report*, London, ONS [online] http://www.dh.gov.uk/prod_consum_dh/idcplg?IdcService=GET_FILE&dID=144114&Rendition=Web (accessed 30 January 2009).

Powell, E. (1961) 'Address to the National Association for Mental Health', in *Emerging Patterns for Mental Health Services and the Public*, London, National Association for Mental Health (NAMH).

Part

III

Read, J., Mosher, L. and Bentall, R. (2004) *Models of Madness: Psychological, social and biological approaches to schizophrenia*, London, Brunner-Routledge.

Reith, M. (1998) *Community Care Tragedies: A practice guide to mental health inquiries*, Birmingham, Venture Press/BASW.

Rogers, C. R. (1951) *Client Centred Therapy*, London, Constable.

Sainsbury Centre for Mental Health (Training and Practice Development Section) (2001) *The Capable Practitioner: A framework and list of capabilities required to implement the National Service Framework for Mental Health. (A report commissioned by the National Service Framework Workforce Action Team)*. London, Sainsbury Centre for Mental Health [online] www.scmh.org.uk/pdfs/the+capable+practitioner.pdf (accessed 30 January 2009).

Samaritans (2007) *Information Resource Pack 2007*, Slough, Samaritans.

Scottish Executive (1997, 2005) *A Framework for Mental Health Services in Scotland*, Edinburgh, Scottish Executive [online] http://www.show.scot.nhs.uk/publications/mental_health_services/mhs/index.htm (accessed 30 January 2009).

Tyrer, P. and Steinberg, D. (2005) *Models for Mental Disorder*, 4th edn, Chichester, John Wiley.

Watkins, M., Hervey, N., Carson, J. and Ritter, S. (1996) *Collaborative Community Mental Health Care*, London, Arnold.

Welsh Assembly Government (2002) *Adult Mental Health Services: A National Service Framework for Wales*, Cardiff, National Assembly for Wales [online] http://www.wales.nhs.uk/sites/documents/334/adult-mental-nsf-e.pdf (accessed 30 January 2009).

Welsh Assembly Government (2005) *The Revised Adult Mental Health National Service Framework and an Action Plan for Wales*. Cardiff, National Assembly for Wales [online] http://www.wales.nhs.uk/sites3/Documents/438/Raising%20the%20Standard%20%28english%29.pdf (accessed 30 January 2009).

Williams, R. and Morgan, H. G. (eds) (1996) *Suicide Prevention: Mental health services – the challenge confronted. A manual of guidance for the purchasers and providers of mental health care*, London, NHS Health Advisory Service.

World Health Organization (WHO) (1992) *The ICD-10 Classification of mental and behavioural disorders*, Geneva, WHO.

WHO (2007) *International Statistical Classification of Diseases and Related Health Problems*, 10th revision version for 2007 ICD-10, Geneva, WHO [online] http://www.who.int/classifications/apps/icd/icd10online/ (accessed 27 January 2008) (accessed 30 January 2009).

Further reading

Barker, P. (ed.) (2003) *Psychiatric and Mental Health Nursing: The craft of caring*, London, Arnold. A comprehensive, detailed book, in which leading writers in their fields explore in some depth core and essential aspects of mental health, illness and care.

Barker, P. (2004) *Assessment in Psychiatric and Mental Health Nursing: In search of the whole person*, Cheltenham, Nelson Thornes. A second updated edition of an earlier book, which outlines a range of approaches to assessment in mental healthcare. Although the author's humanistic, person-centred perspective is well known, it deals clearly and systematically with the appropriate theoretical underpinnings of the assessment methods.

Burnard, P. (2002) *Learning Human Skills*, 4th edn, London, Butterworth-Heinemann. A popular book on basic interpersonal skills, with a large number of exercises, by one of the most prolific writers on experiential learning.

Gamble, C. and Brennan, G. (2006) *Working with Serious Mental Illness: A manual for clinical practice*, Edinburgh, Baillière Tindall/RCN. Second edition of this almost essential, practically focused book. Although, like many of the other texts, it incorporates the theory basis, this book also provides clear guidance for everyday evidence-based practice rooted in sound psychosocial intervention skills.

Hannigan, B. and Coffey, M (eds) (2003) *The Handbook of Community Mental Health Nursing*, London, Routledge. An edited collection of core chapters outlining context, services, practice, education and research relating to community mental healthcare.

Heller, T., Reynolds, J., Gomm, R., Muston, R. and Pattison, S. (2000) *Mental Health Matters: A reader*, Basingstoke, Palgrave Macmillan. An excellent interdisciplinary collection of diverse texts put together as a reader for the Open University, School of Health and Welfare course: 'Mental health and distress: Perspectives and practice' (K257S). It covers social and historical dimensions of mental health, aimed at all involved whether service users or professionals.

Heyes, S. (2005) *Art of Recovery: A pocket guide to recovery from mental distress*, Yeovil, Somerset, Speak Up Somerset.

Norman, I. and Ryrie, I. (2004) *The Art and Science of Mental Health Nursing*, Maidenhead, Open University Press. Another comprehensive, edited collection of UK-nursing authorities, writing about their fields of expertise on key aspects of mental health, illness and care.

Rogers, A. and Pilgrim, D. (2005) *A Sociology of Mental Health and Illness*, 3rd edn, Maidenhead, Open University Press. An overview on the key issues and perspectives on mental health and illness from two leading writers and researchers in the field.

Tyrer, P. and Steinberg, D. (2005) *Models for Mental Disorder*, 4th edn, Chichester, John Wiley. A good, readable introduction to the various schools of thought about mental disorder, outlining the key concepts of the main models for understanding at the time of each edition. Ironic little cartoons add a lighter but illuminating touch.

Watkins, P. (2001) *Mental Health Nursing: The art of compassionate care*, Oxford, Butterworth-Heinemann. A compassionate, practical book detailing how to develop relationships and work therapeutically with people in distress. Drawn extensively from the humanistic tradition.

Legislation

Mental Health Act 2007 Chapter 12: http://www.opsi.gov.uk/acts/acts2007/ukpga_20070012_en.pdf

Mental Health Act 1983 Chapter 20 as now amended by the Mental Health Act 2007: http://www.dh.gov.uk/prod_consum_dh/idcplg?IdcService=GET_FILE&dID=147390&Rendition=Web

Mental Capacity Act 2005 Chapter 9: http://www.opsi.gov.uk/acts/acts2005/pdf/ukpga_20050009_en.pdf

Mental Capacity Act 2005 Chapter 9: as now amended by the Mental Health Act 2007: http://www.dh.gov.uk/prod_consum_dh/idcplg?IdcService=GET_FILE&dID=145290&Rendition=Web

Chapter

27

Learning disability

Kevin Humphrys, Tony Gilbert and Neil Jackson

 Links to other chapters in *Foundation Studies for Caring*

2 Interprofessional learning
3 Evidence-based practice and research
4 Ethical, legal and professional issues
5 Communication
6 Culture
16 Safeguarding children
17 Safeguarding adults

 Links to other chapters in *Foundation Skills for Caring*

1 Fundamental concepts for skills
3 Communication
6 Sign language
8 Breakaway skills
9 Patient hygiene

W Don't forget to visit www.palgrave.com/glasper for additional
online resources relating to this chapter.

Introduction

This chapter discusses general issues in relation to people with a learning disability through the medium of a developing scenario. You should also note that this is an important decade in the relationship between people with learning disabilities and society in general. The government white paper *Valuing People* (DH, 2001a) set out the responsibilities of government, society and public services towards ensuring that four 'Key Principles: Rights, Independence, Choice and Inclusion' enhance life chances of people with learning disabilities. *Valuing People Now* (DH, 2007a), which identifies priorities for 2008–11, has followed this. These priorities are identified as personalisation, what people do during the day, better health, access to housing and making sure that change happens. There is also synergy between these priorities and those identified for other adults that rely on support (see DH, 2005, 2006a).

The chapter is in two parts. The first part focuses on a range of issues that are important to the understanding of a learning disability. This includes an identification of what a learning disability is, its relationship with other forms of disability, key issues related to the health of people with learning disability, the importance of communication, and the role of learning disability practitioners such as the learning disability nurse.

The second part of the chapter develops around a scenario that involves a young woman experiencing health problems and abuse. The aim is to explore the issues that might arise for a young person with learning disabilities and the type of support they may receive. At the same time, it is intended that the scenario and its related exercises will enable an insight into the work of health practitioners working with people with learning disability, in particular the way in which they work with service users, carers and other professionals in the development and delivery of appropriate packages of care.

Throughout the second part of the chapter there are sets of activities, which will help in the understanding of the issues. At the same time, the scenario is illuminated through the identification of emerging questions and the use of professional conversations.

Policies pertaining to the care of people with learning difficulties can be seen visually on an innovative policy tree, available via the companion website.

W

Learning outcomes

This chapter should enable you to:

- identify key concepts in relation to supporting people with a learning disability
- develop an understanding of the relationship between health professions such as adult nursing and those professions or branches of professions that focus specifically on supporting people with learning disability in the context of caring for a person with a learning disability who becomes ill
- recognise the importance of alliances between primary and secondary healthcare workers

- recognise the importance of communication with all service users/patients as a prerequisite for good healthcare
- discover the particular importance of finding alternative ways to communicate with people who have a learning disability or to augment spoken language
- recognise the importance of anti-discriminatory practice in delivering equal healthcare to all
- understand the importance of access to generic and specialist healthcare for people with a learning disability.

Concepts

- Respect for the autonomy of people with a learning disability
- Communication with people who have a learning disability
- Health and people with a learning disability
- Working with families and carers
- Interdisciplinary working
- Definitions of disability
- Access to generic services
- Role of specialist services

a Learning activity

Before reading further, and in your interprofessional learning group consider your understanding of the term 'learning disability'. Who would you include in your list? Compare your understandings with the section entitled 'Who are people with a learning disability?'

Who are people with a learning disability?

The term 'learning disability' is currently the acceptable legal and professional term applied to a particular section of the population whose intelligence quotient (IQ) is measured as below 70. Some people within this group also experience physical and sensory disabilities or they may experience neurological conditions that are often associated with learning disability, such as epilepsy and cerebral palsy (DH, 2001a). In general, having a learning disability is usually taken to indicate that the person is experiencing some form of developmental delay, and people within this group are often identified as having special educational needs when they are children. Current estimates suggest that 169,000 people with learning disabilities aged over 20 are known users of learning disability services in England, of whom 26,000 are aged 60 or over (Healthcare Commission, 2007).

What causes learning disability?

There are three main causes of learning disability: genetic abnormality, chromosomal abnormality and environmental damage before or during birth; however, this oversimplifies the debate around classification of learning disability. The white paper *Valuing People* (DH, 2001a) provides figures for England of 210,000 people with a severe learning disability (below 50 IQ) and 1.2 million with a mild learning disability (50–70 IQ). The traditional medical/ psychological approach of using the criterion of IQ has limitations, for we know that a learning disability can be caused by a number of different factors that act on the developing brain, usually taken to mean occurring below the age of 16. These factors, including genetic, social and environmental influences, infections and trauma (Priest and Gibbs, 2004), impact to varying degrees which, when combined with the person's social position and life experiences, can result in a complex picture. This complexity is often lost in the forms of definition such as the idea of 'an arrested or incomplete development of the mind', which is used by the World Health Organization (WHO, 1993) and which is set within the Mental Health Act 1983. The most recent legal term is 'mental disorder', which is enshrined in the Mental Health Act 2007.

The Mental Capacity Act 2005 arranges for people who lack capacity to make decisions and refers to this as:

> The inability to make a decision must be caused by an impairment of or disturbance in the functioning of the mind or brain. This could cover a range of problems, such as psychiatric illness, dementia, brain damage or even a toxic confusional state and of course learning disability. Whatever the problem, it has to have the necessary effect on the functioning of the mind or brain, leading the person to be unable to make the decision.

With these points in mind a more useful guide, rather than using IQ testing, is a measure of the extent to which a person can perform a range of roles within society; that is, their social competence. The strength of this idea is that it is flexible and it does not create a hierarchy based on the level of disability, nor at the same time does it imply that needs are stable and fixed. Instead, people are assessed based on their present circumstances. For example, a person with a learning disability who manages their own affairs, but who is presently experiencing an acute illness, is considered as having high support needs for a period. In contrast a person who requires daily support, but is stable with respect to the level of support needed, might be considered as having low support needs.

The idea of support needs has been incorporated into many of the assessments that are used by professionals working with people with learning disability to measure health-related problems that impair social functioning. The ratings obtained can be used as a baseline from which to determine progress.

Historical perspective

As a group, people with a learning disability have experienced a profound shift over the last century in the way in which services have been provided. At the end of the nineteenth century and for a substantial part of the twentieth century, people with learning disabilities were viewed as a danger to society as they were believed to lack moral controls over their behaviour, and might therefore be led into crime or immoral acts. The greatest fear was that they would endlessly reproduce, leading to an overwhelming increase of the population (Gilbert, 1998). This led to a service model based on isolated residential institutions or 'colonies' which after 1948 were reclassified as hospitals. For the people who remained living at home, there was the development of large 'daytime' institutions known as training centres or day centres. The second part of the twentieth century saw the development of the 'community care' programme. This has led to the closure of many of these large institutions, and the replacement of the residential institutions by ordinary housing and the day centres by a variety of community-based activities organised through individually tailored packages of care (Wertheimer, 1996; Gilbert and Rose, 1998).

This movement of people with learning disabilities from isolated and segregated services to the use of ordinary housing and everyday work and leisure facilities has led to the concept of citizenship becoming central to the design and evaluation of packages of support (Duffy, 2006). However, obstacles remain for people with learning disabilities in meeting the potential of citizenship, many of which lie in outdated social attitudes that see individuals as dependent and incapable of making choices or decisions. It would therefore seem that the central issue for all health practitioners is to enable people with learning disabilities to become informed and make decisions about their own health and lifestyle. Visit the companion website to see a 'policy tree' illustrating how learning disability care has developed over time.

W

Disability and illness

Over the years, learning disability has been viewed as an illness; however, it is important to draw a distinction between disability and illness. Previously, the dominant model of services for people with a severe learning disability was based on large hospitals. This move brought about the medicalisation of people with a learning disability, despite the fact that learning disability itself cannot be treated medically. This led to an overemphasis on medical definitions of need, with a denial of people's emotional, educational and social needs. In recent times, it has been recognised that people with a learning disability have been further damaged by the services which were established to help them (Ryan and Thomas, 1987). This has occurred because these services tended to concentrate large numbers of people with learning disabilities together away from the general population, leading to social isolation, stigma and poor environmental conditions (Wolfensberger, 1972). Issues central to the citizenship of people with learning disabilities: rights, independence, choice and inclusion, and the resources needed to achieve them, will all depend on the dominant social attitudes at the time (Brechin and Walmsley, 1989; Redworth and Redworth, 1997).

> ### ⓐ Learning activity
>
> Check out your present understanding of the causes of learning disability. Compare your list with a colleague in your learning group and you may find that this leads to some discussion points. Consider circumstances in which you might deliver healthcare to someone with a learning disability.
>
> Write down your definition for each of the terms 'disability' and 'illness' before reading on.

Medicalisation of people with learning disabilities paralleled the medicalisation of other disabled people (Oliver, 1990). Disability per se has been defined as either a personal tragedy or the result of social oppression, and the importance of understanding the competing definitions of disability is a key activity for any serious student of the subject (Barton, 1996). Disability needs to be understood within the particular historical, social and political context of a given society and the ways in which ideas of being able in body and mind come to dominate. The effect of this is to include some sections of society, while other sections come to be excluded on the basis of difference. It also needs to be remembered that the experience of disability is impacted on by other social variables such as class, gender, race and age.

> ### a) Learning activity
>
> In your practice experience to date, have you been involved with a person with learning disability? If so, reflect on the circumstances. How was the person and family approached and cared for? It may be useful to discuss this with colleagues who have also had such an experience.

Health and people with learning disability

People with a learning disability who have health problems are no different from anyone else in the community who may become ill. They have the same rights and entitlement to comprehensive healthcare at primary, secondary and tertiary stages that meets their diverse health needs as any other person (DH, 2001a). In adulthood, there is evidence that the general medical needs of people with learning disabilities are higher than those of the rest of the population (Moss and Turner, 1995; Prasher and Janicki, 2002; Disability Rights Commission, 2006) and yet there is also evidence that people with a learning disability experience difficulty accessing healthcare (Singh, 1997; Mencap, 2004). In addition, the experiences that people with learning disabilities encounter are not always positive or appropriate to their needs (Mencap, 2007; House of Lords and House of Commons Joint Committee on Human Rights, 2008; Michael, 2008).

> ### t☆ Practice tip
>
> In order to avoid discriminatory practice take pains to learn how a person with a learning disability with whom you interact communicates. Speak to carers and/or relations to discover any preferences the person might have.

The requirement to offer healthcare equally to all has important professional and ethical implications. These arise from the principle of justice, which is concerned with the fair distribution of resources. There is some evidence of discriminatory practice occurring in generic NHS services (Mencap, 2007), which when combined with the fact that people with a learning disability have greater health needs is an issue for concern.

> ### a) Learning activity
>
> In your previous learning group activity did issues in relation to communication come into your discussion? Identify what challenges might occur. Draw up a list of a variety of communication skills and strategies that health professionals, including nurses, need to develop to communicate effectively with a range of individuals who have learning disability.

Communication

The challenge for all health practitioners when working with people who have a learning disability will be in developing the skills of specialist communication in order to negotiate health interventions (see Chapter 5 for a fuller discussion of communication). The same issues are apparent when practitioners attempt to support a service user or patient whose language and/or means of communication is one that they do not share. The responsibility here lies with the practitioner to find a suitable and appropriate means of communication in order to establish a mutual frame of reference. The same is true of supporting someone with a learning disability, for when someone has limited or no spoken language more sophisticated communication skills are required.

There are two key processes to consider here. The first is the mode of communication, which will involve a range of observational and listening skills. It will also involve taking an effective communication history from the person and/or their family or carer. This will identify the person's range of communication skills, their preferred methods of communication, likes and dislikes, the ways they express discomfort or pain, and whether they use a sign language or an electronic aid. It is also essential to identify the range of self-help skills the person has so that it is clear what they can and cannot do.

The second key process is understanding or comprehension, and this will require the practitioner to do much more than ask the person whether they understood. It is essential that the practitioner is aware of the complexity of the information or instructions they are giving to the person. For example, when explaining to a person who is continent where the ward toilets are, they need to consider whether the person understands the abstract concept of 'they are at the end of the room and then turn right', even if the person states that they have understood. It would be better to take the person and show them the toilet, and to check and repeat this activity a number of times until it is apparent that the person has understood. The same can be said about a range of instructions which might be given to people with learning disability. It is easy to assume that a person who has apparently good communication skills understands all that is said to them. Equally, a common error is to assume that a person with little speech understands little (Ferris-Taylor, 1997). The support of a learning disability nurse or a speech and language therapist might be useful at this time.

> **t**☆
> ## Practice tip
>
> If you are working with a person who has a learning disability who uses a sign system, make a note of the key signs that will help you in your with your intervention. Use the signs when communicating with them.

The role of the learning disability nurse

Learning disability nursing is 'a person centred profession with the primary aim of supporting the well-being and social inclusion of people with a learning disability through improving or maintaining physical and mental health' (Mental Health Act 2007). Nurses trained to work with people with learning disability are 'specialists in the area of learning disability itself' (Northway, Hutchinson and Kingdon, 2006). Learning disability nurses can be found in a range of settings such as specialist health services, social services and the independent sector. A range of roles has been identified by the Department of Health guidance document *Good Practice in Learning Disability Nursing* (DH, 2007b):

- health facilitation – supporting mainstream access
- in-patient services – for example, assessment and treatment and secure services
- specialist roles – in community teams.

Community nurses for people with learning disabilities will often be involved in liaison work between the primary healthcare team or with general hospital services. Regardless of the setting, one of the primary components of the development of personal autonomy is to increase a person's control over their own health. One of the key roles for community learning disability teams identified in the *Valuing People* strategy is that of health facilitator.

In a situation where the person with a learning disability is receiving healthcare from a member of the primary care team or from secondary, general or mental health services, it is not unusual for a degree of collaboration to be established between these services and the specialist learning disability services (DH, 2001a; McCray, 2003). This collaboration is often established through the nurses within each team. It follows that the nurse, in seeking to restore optimum health to the person with a learning disability who has become a patient, may need to work closely with a specialist nurse for people with a learning disability. The rationale for this alliance is that both the nurse and the nurse for people with a learning disability share the same aim of restoring optimum health. Each nurse will bring to the alliance a common understanding of health and a complementary, but different set of skills.

Therefore, in the scenario developed in the next section, one of the central issues is to identify points of collaboration between the learning disability nurse and the adult nurse. Emma, a young woman with acute medical needs and ongoing general health needs, as well as needs related to her disability, provides the focus for the discussion.

This alliance between the different healthcare professionals will enhance the skills that each of them possesses. At the same time, it should increase Emma's sense of personal autonomy and her self-esteem, which has clear implications for her mental health. The adult nurse, in seeking to care for Emma, will have to adopt communication strategies that may be new; for example, the use of sign language and 'tuning in' to Emma's particular patterns of speech and the skilled reading of her nonverbal communication. This process, of discovering the person and what is significant to them, is a fundamental aspect of nursing in any branch.

[S] Scenario – Introducing Emma

Emma Hill is 24 years old and lives at home with her mother and father who are in their early 50s. Emma's mother works as a journalist with a local paper and her father is a senior accountant with the local authority. She also has a younger brother Rick, who is 15 years old. The family live in a large, comfortable, detached house situated on the outskirts of a major city. Emma attends a local day centre.

A problem has emerged because over the last year, the standard of Emma's 'work' at the day centre which she attends Monday to Friday each week has declined and she seems agitated at times. This has led to periods where she has become aggressive and fractious. It all started to happen following an incident in the grounds at the day centre, during which she fell over. The manager of the centre (a learning disability nurse) contacted Emma's parents to express his concern. The manager seems to be most concerned about the aggressive incidents that have taken place. He has had to intervene several times between Emma and a young man in her section. Following a visit to her doctor, Emma is sent to the emergency department at the local district general hospital. She is also referred to a community specialist healthcare team for people with a learning disability because of her behaviour and because of concerns that staff at the emergency department had.

t☆ Practice tip

Try to take a comprehensive history when working with someone who has a learning disability. Alongside the account provided by the person themselves the accounts of carers and/or relations can be most helpful.

[a] Learning activity

In your interprofessional learning group:
- In order to help you picture the scenario with Emma at the day centre, it may be helpful to think about your own educational experiences. Were people with learning disabilities included in your schools or college; and if they were, how were they supported? Do you have any friends with a learning disability or friends who have a brother or sister with learning disability? If so, what is their experience of attending a day centre?
- Try to find out about statutory educational provision for people with a learning disability within your area. Does your local education department promote the education of children with learning disability within mainstream schools or does it operate separate schools for these children? What do you feel might be the advantages/disadvantages of these two different types of educational provision?
- Try to find out what courses are open to young adults with learning disabilities at the local further education colleges, and whether these lead to formal qualifications such as NVQs.

Emerging questions 1

Emerging lines of enquiry can be tested and rejected or shelved, pending the arrival of new evidence. This process can be described as one of professional speculation. The first step in the process is to be clear about what we know about a situation. We then need to consider the likely reasons for any health changes or behaviour changes. Based on this, we can test out or explore whether our assumptions are correct (hypothesis testing). In order to do this, we need to decide what new information we need.

This is an important process as a means to begin the formal assessment of the service user. It must, however, be differentiated from the expression of uninformed opinion. At this stage, we are searching for guidance about the emerging problem and possible solutions to it. To help with this we may consult professional colleagues, gain evidence from the literature, records or observations.

New behaviour can be a useful indication of a change in a person's mental or physical state. The onset of illness of any kind may be accompanied by new behaviour or an escalation of existing behaviours. It is the task of the nurse, or any health practitioner, to discover the true meaning of the new behaviour or the escalation of existing behaviours for the person exhibiting it/them, and not to ascribe meaning to the behaviours from their own or other's framework of values. This process requires the practitioner to suspend judgment and explore, with the service user, the possible meanings of the new behaviour.

In the case of people with a learning disability, behaviour is often wrongly seen only as problematic and not as a means of communication. This approach to identifying the significance of behaviour will severely limit the practitioner's ability to understand the behaviour and to intervene appropriately. The practitioner must seek to understand the significance of new behaviour, or the escalation of existing behaviours in the context of the environment and the personal circumstances in which the person finds themselves (Donnellan et al, 1988; Emerson, McGill and Mansell, 1994).

> t ☆
> ## Practice tip
>
> In formulating questions about the behaviour or health of a person with learning disabilities try to avoid stereotyping. Try to consider the person as a whole rather than just the presenting circumstances – try seeing things from their viewpoint

How might the family view Emma and her needs?

It is important to discover the role that Emma plays within the family. This can only be achieved by making an assessment not just of Emma, but also of Emma in the context of her family. One way to try to discover the myths and stereotypes that the family uses to explain things that have happened to them is to undertake a family genogram (Dallos, 1991). This can help to plot and explore family relationships in a safe and nonthreatening way. We will see later on in the chapter how the community nurse begins to explore the family as a unit and the effects it has on Emma and her needs.

Emma's perception of her needs will provide the key to successful interventions with her. The practitioner will need to discover how Emma feels about herself and how she sees herself within the family, what role she thinks she plays, how she views other family members, how she feels about the recent incident at the day centre and what she thinks her other needs are.

What is the relationship like between Emma and Rick?

The way that siblings interact in any family is of interest when trying to work with one of them. It is useful to discover and assess the significance of relationship within the family. Does Emma see herself in a protective role towards Rick or is it perhaps the other way around? Do they get on? Is there rivalry in relation to Emma's problem over and above normal sibling rivalry? How are actual or potential conflicts resolved between them, who are the peacemakers?

Who is closest to Emma at the centre? How would this be discovered?

It is important to discover who, within the day centre or any other institution that is involved with Emma, has the clearest picture of her. Discovering whom she relates with best will enable you to access good information. Treat all information as provisional at this stage, as you may find that people have myths, stereotypes and prejudices in relation to Emma. The task is to build up a comprehensive picture of Emma and the things that are significant to her. Avoid making assumptions or absorbing the assumptions of others at this stage.

Is Emma usually a happy person? Consider what behaviours you might expect to notice that would offer clues.

Before attempting to assess the extent of change in behaviour and its possible meanings, it is important to discover details about Emma's personality. Is she a happy person, is she outgoing or quiet and introspective, cautious or bold?

How has her 'new' behaviour been observed or assessed?

The first 'clue' in the scenario is the part about Emma's behaviour changing. This is important and is the logical starting point for any enquiry. Changes in behaviour are usually assessed against a known baseline or 'norm' of behaviour from an ecological or functional perspective (Donnellan et al, 1988; Emerson et al, 1994). It will be important to discover the events occurring at the point of change, and useful to find out how the change in behaviour is being monitored. Provisional hypotheses can be developed at this stage; this is a normal part of professional practice as the practitioner begins informed speculation about what might be occurring. This process is one of reflection in action, which, along with reflection on action, is the key to professional practice (Schon, 1983). Has the person become physically and or mentally ill? The 'OK' Health Check (Mathews, 1996) and/or the Mini PASS-ADD (Moss et al, 1997) could be used to help determine this. Have new events entered her life, either at the centre or at home? Has the day centre changed the routine in relation to Emma? What is the significance of the incident in the grounds of the day centre?

> **t** ☆
> ## Practice tip
> It is important to try to understand behaviour changes in the context of the environment around the person. In this case understanding family dynamics is paramount.

What is a community specialist healthcare team for people with a learning disability, who works in it and what services or interventions does it offer?

A community specialist healthcare team is a collection of professional healthcare workers and support staff situated within a local community. They receive referrals from healthcare professionals in primary healthcare and, in some cases; service users will refer themselves, usually with help from their carers. The team generally works with adults, as children are usually supported by child health services or sometimes by a specialist children's disability team. The team can offer a range of interventions from a simple health assessment to sophisticated interventions such as cognitive-behaviour therapy (Kroese, Dagnon and Loumides, 2001). On referral to the team, it meets, discusses the needs that the potential service user has, and allocates work in relation to the skill base of its members and their availability. Multidisciplinary community specialist healthcare teams are typically made up of:

- nurses for people with a learning disability
- a consultant psychiatrist
- a clinical psychologist
- an occupational therapist
- a physiotherapist
- a speech and language therapist
- a social worker who works in association with the team.

Part

III

Some members of the team may also be care managers (Biggs, 1998). Several members of the team may be part-time workers or have substantial duties elsewhere. Some may take on special advisory roles in relation to issues that arise with learning disabled people; such as incontinence, epilepsy, sexuality and mental health.

S | Scenario continued

Emma's behaviour has changed at the day centre and the standard of her work has declined. Emma's key worker has had several conversations with her to try to find out what is going on. She seemed to be agitated some of the time. She keeps asking to sit down in the 'quiet' room: some of the other staff feel her behaviour is attention seeking. Emma is seen by a learning disability nurse who visits the centre, Emma refuses consent to be examined and the nurse cannot find anything wrong with her. The learning disability nurse suggests that with Emma's consent, the parents are informed and she sees her general practitioner (GP). The manager of the day centre asks the parents to come and see him, and during an informal meeting, it is discovered that the same patterns of behaviour are occurring at home. Emma and her parents agree to see the GP.

The visit to the GP does not go well as Emma is agitated at the time and is reluctant to allow the GP to examine her. The GP eventually gains Emma's consent and cooperation to allow her to make an examination. The GP is concerned about a lack of movement in Emma's left arm, and suggests that she go to the emergency department for X-rays and further examination. The GP is also concerned about bruises on Emma's' upper arm. She refers to the fact that Emma is overweight and suggests a calorie-controlled diet. Mrs Hill agrees to this, but her husband remains quiet (see DH, 2006b). The GP suggests that a community nurse, based in the local specialist healthcare team for people with a learning disability, is asked to visit and make a full assessment of Emma's needs. She agrees to make a referral to the team.

---

a | Learning activity

In your learning group look up the concept of informed consent (DH, 2001b and Chapter 4), and consider it in relation to the examination of Emma. How does informed consent, whether implied, verbal or written, relate generally to the examination and treatment of service users or patients either in the hospital or the community?

S | Scenario continued

In order for Emma to be seen by a community nurse for people with a learning disability, her GP will normally make a referral to a community specialist healthcare team and the team will decide which of its members will assess Emma's needs and work with her. The team is located near to the health centre that Emma normally uses. The referral is processed urgently because of the GP's comments about bruising on the upper arm. Concerns are starting to emerge at this point about the possibility of abuse. Abuse or the possibility of abuse is an issue that should immediately alert practitioners to initiate protocols related to safeguarding vulnerable adults.

Emma's experience of hospital

Emma's parents take her to the general hospital and she is diagnosed as having a fractured clavicle. The recommended treatment is that she wears a sling for her

left arm and rests. The team leader of the accident and emergency department is concerned about the bruising on Emma's arms, and following urgent multidisciplinary discussion initiates safeguarding procedures.

While in the accident and emergency department, Emma asks the nurses several times to go to the toilet. She uses the sign language Makaton (Walker, 1980) to do this. The nurses do not understand what the 'funny hand signals' mean and Emma is incontinent of urine. This is atypical behaviour for her and she becomes quite agitated. The nurses are quite anxious in response to Emma, and the situation becomes tense. They discuss the situation with the parents. The nurses assume that Emma is regularly incontinent and ask the parents what kind of 'nappy' Emma wears. Both parents are extremely angry that their daughter's needs have gone unnoticed yet again. They consider making a formal complaint.

Practice tip

t ☆

If you are admitting a person with a learning disability to a general hospital ward, try to ensure that their communication system is noted as part of the admission procedure.

Learning activity

a →

In your learning group consult the Nursing and Midwifery Council (NMC) *Code of Professional Conduct* (NMC, 2008) or other regulatory body guidelines and discuss with your colleagues the extent to which the incident in the accident and emergency department was an example of discriminatory practice. At the same time, consider the following questions:

- Have you or your colleagues experienced discriminatory practice?
- What are the wider implications of excluding some people from healthcare?

S Scenario continued

Concerns about the incident at the day centre

Emma returns home but does not return to the day centre. As the Hills reflect on what has happened to Emma, they feel that the centre should have discovered that Emma was in pain soon after the incident in the grounds. In their reflection, they avoid the painful question of why they had not noticed Emma's difficulties.

They make an appointment to see the manager, and during the meeting ask to see the report of the incident in the grounds. They inform the manager that they feel that the centre failed in its duty of care to Emma in relation to the incident. The manager of the centre raises questions about the bruising on Emma's upper arms. The meeting is a tense one and the situation is left unresolved.

Emerging questions 2

Again, we need to engage in the process of professional speculation and to ground this with the emerging evidence related to Emma's health needs.

Abuse is a serious issue of general concern for all health and social care professionals. The publication of a range of reports relating to the care of people with learning disabilities in Cornwall (Healthcare Commission, 2006) and Sutton and Merton (Healthcare Commission, 2007) indicates that abusive treatment is still evident within some specialist services. In addition, there is evidence of people with learning disabilities getting worse healthcare than nondisabled people, with evidence of institutional discrimination within generic NHS services being partly responsible (Mencap, 2007). It must be remembered that this client group is one of the most vulnerable in society, so health and social care professionals need to be increasingly vigilant. For nurses the NMC *Code of Conduct* (NMC, 2008) clearly states that they have a duty to protect their service user from harm.

What is the significance of the bruising to Emma's upper arm?

The pattern of the bruising corresponds with that of being gripped tightly. On examination, it appeared that the bruises predated the incident at the day centre and may not be connected to it. The bruising may have an innocent explanation but if so that explanation must be sought and verified.

What actions and investigations should take place?

The protocol for the safeguarding of vulnerable adults should be followed.

Part

III

Should the Hills pursue the process of making formal complaints against the NHS trust and the day centre?

It needs to be recognised that all users of health and other public services have the right to complain when that service fails to meet their needs. The concept of clinical governance (DH, 1997) has been established in the NHS to ensure that people experience the highest standards of service possible. Instances such as that experienced by the Hills may be subject to an investigation or to a critical incident analysis. The purpose should be to learn from the experience and to take measures that will prevent a similar incident happening again, rather than seeking to attribute blame. Moreover, nurses need to be aware that people who complain can be labelled as difficult parents and treated with more caution than they normally would be. Information about complaining should be given to the Hills in a sensitive way.

It is important at this stage that all concerned put energy into solving Emma's problems rather than becoming defensive over the incident at the day centre and the possibility of abuse. There is a need for practitioners to acknowledge the problem but also to explore ways in which the family can place it to one side while it is being explored. This will enable the family to move on to find ways of meeting Emma's needs.

What time elapsed between the incident in the grounds of the day centre and the Hills being informed?

This is a key question and may form the basis of the Hill's complaint against the centre. Incidents of any kind should be reported promptly to those people who have a right to know about them. Mr and Mrs Hill were informed of the incident by means of a communication book two days after the incident occurred. Incidents are normally reported quickly to parents.

What action and investigation took place following the incident in the day centre?

This is another key question. The Hills will want to know that the incident was properly investigated and appropriate actions taken. The centre saw the incident as a 'minor tussle' and nothing to cause concern. Emma refused to let the visiting nurse examine her and grew quite angry. The visiting nurse expressed the view, at the time, that Emma did not appear to be injured. An incident report form was completed, but the information entered on it was minimal: it stated the time and date of the incident, and that Emma said she was pushed over by Michael, another service user at the centre.

What is the significance of the incident? Was it an isolated event or part of a pattern?

It will be important to discover Emma's perception of the incident. What meaning did it have for her? Has it happened before? Is it part of a pattern of events, and what is the relationship like between Emma and the man who 'pushed her over'? The visiting learning disability nurse failed to obtain information from Emma at the time of the incident. Emma was also quiet at home. There may be more to this incident than is at first apparent. The health practitioner will return to this.

What is the significance of the bruising? Is it an isolated event or part of a pattern?

This is a key question and one that must be answered cautiously. The injury might have an innocent explanation but the circumstances of the injury and any history of similar incidents must be discovered.

Professional conversation

Jai, the district nurse, comments, 'I am not sure about this. I know that we are supposed to support people with disabilities to be independent, but Emma is quite vulnerable in this situation. She needs plenty of rest to ensure that the fracture heals properly and the parents need to help her to understand this. I want to give clear directions to Emma's mother, but she is not the sort of woman you direct easily. I find Emma's father quite hostile. He still seems to be focusing on the incident in the hospital when Emma was incontinent instead of on her needs now and in the future. The immediate issue here is helping Emma to get over her fracture.

'As for the bruising I am not sure, I have discussed it with the GP and the specialist nurse; we need to explore it quickly but carefully.

'I am also concerned about Emma's weight and it relates directly to family eating patterns. I think the best way forward is to get the family to modify its eating habits, but I am not sure how to achieve that. I could just spell it out bluntly: "Mr Hill, in order to keep your daughter healthy she needs to change her diet. She seems to take her lead from you so what I am suggesting is that you change your eating habits … ." Well, it might work, but I don't want to get a hostile response. It might work if I try to use Emma's mum to put some pressure on Mr Hill.'

What are the implications and possible complications of Emma's fracture?

Emma's fracture is one that often occurs with a young adult of this age. It is often associated with a fall, and accidents are a key area identified in health policy (DH, 1995b, 1998). The treatment consists of relief of pain in response to symptoms, and the use of a sling or brace to keep the shoulder as immobile as possible during the period of healing. It may be helpful to encourage Emma to wear her coat with her left arm inside the coat. This will act as additional support and prevent the arm from swinging.

What does Emma understand about her weight problem?

It will be important to discover the extent to which Emma's self-image and self-awareness have developed. If she has a sense of what someone of normal weight looks like, it can be used to set targets for her and to motivate her towards achieving them.

What was her diet before going into hospital?

Her diet mirrored that of her father, as she seemed to enjoy her food and took portions that were rather larger than necessary. She drank wine with her meals and was very fond of fizzy drinks such as cola. She liked chocolate and other sweets.

What is her attitude to food?

Her attitude to food seems to be that she enjoys it and it brings her comfort when she is stressed. She enjoys snacks and has tended in the past to eat meals at irregular times. She sometimes eats according to spontaneous whims or fancies, and seems to equate food with pleasure.

What is her family's attitude to food?

Mr and Mrs Hill use food as a reward or a treat in the household. Therefore, whenever something goes well, the family will celebrate with food and if one of the children has achieved something, then food will be used as a reward. This will often take the form of an outing to a burger or pizza restaurant or a take-away. This is a pleasant experience for the family; however, the children have modelled their parents' behaviour and will look for food as a reward.

S Scenario continued

Emma's family

The family is close knit with a general stance of standing together against others. All outside views such as news on the television or radio, newspaper stories, the views of other professionals and recommendations from extended family members pass through the filter of the parents' confidently and strongly held worldview. This filter takes the form of discussion about everything in order to determine their view of whatever is at issue. The parents share a rather cynical view of life, and feel that people are generally out for themselves and what they can get. They are very concerned that their children should do well in life, and believe that Emma is as capable as Rick of achieving.

To outsiders they appear somewhat 'driven' to succeed and rather defensive, particularly in relation to Emma. They are both fiercely protective of Emma and yet determined to push her to her limit. Because of the concern that Emma generates, Rick gets much less attention from his parents and is sometimes just expected to get on with things. Rick resents this at times, although he does understand that in some way his big sister is different and needs extra help. Emma loves her family dearly and is particularly attached to her father. She tends to want to please everyone in the family, but cannot achieve this. She enjoys the discussions that take place often in the house and joins in to a certain extent. Although she uses Makaton a lot, she is developing a range of speech, and the family is encouraging this very much (see Hewitt and Ephraim, 1994).

Emma is overweight and her father is obese. The family eats 'well' and enjoys wine with their meals at the weekends. Emma's father swings from 'being on a diet' to 'eating well', and his weight goes up and down. This pattern has been established over a number of years. Mr Hill has not sought professional advice regarding his obesity as he regards this as a problem that he can solve alone. Emma's mother and father are somewhat sceptical about healthcare professionals who offer advice. They are well-informed and well-connected people, and note that professionals in the health service do not always seem to follow their own advice. This seems to reduce the effect of any advice that they are offered.

The community learning disability nurse's assessment

The community learning disability nurse makes an initial and urgent visit to the family home (on behalf of the multidisciplinary team) one evening to begin the process of a formal nursing assessment. She uses a generic (multidisciplinary) team assessment schedule to gather a range of information about Emma and her family. At the same time, she uses a specific tool designed to assess the health needs of people with a learning disability, the OK Health Check (Mathews, 1996) to determine Emma's immediate and longer-term health needs. She decides that it is appropriate that the team intervenes with the family and makes an initial attempt to prioritise Emma's needs. The community learning disability nurse initiates a discussion about the bruises found on Emma's upper arms.

Emma's priorities

1. Healing of fracture.
2. Establishing facts relating to bruises.
3. Reduction of weight to within normal limits.
4. Change of eating behaviour through changing the family's eating habits.
5. Develop ability to manage own nutrition and monitor own weight.

Priority actions

1. Ensure that the management regime in relation to the fracture is maintained (in liaison with the district nurse).
2. Take all actions in relation to safeguarding vulnerable adults guidelines.
3. Discover Emma's understanding of what has happened to her. Check her means of communication in relation to the pain and pain control. Create a pain map for her to communicate the level of pain she is experiencing (the pain map could be devised using a continuum of faces from smiling to miserable).
4. Discover the family dynamics and networks, and use these as a base for practice.
5. Explore the family's eating patterns.
6. Commence work on the family's attitudes/behaviours to food, in particular targeting Emma's father.

Ⓒ Professional conversation

Eve, specialist community nurse for people with a learning disability, comments, 'The presenting problem (fracture, admission to hospital, future maintenance) is not the only issue here. I observed hostility from dad when I went through the door. I could not get anywhere near him during the first visit. His comments that "The district nurse had already told us that" and "Don't you people talk to each other?" were being used to distract me away from the real question of how well the family has been and is meeting Emma's changing needs. I managed to keep the debate centred on the needs of Emma, and I think when I suggested that the needs of Emma in relation to her weight problem could not be separated from the behaviours of the rest of the family, I hit a raw nerve. That point was met with silence by the father, but the mother quickly said, "Yes, I think there are things we need to look at anyway." When this was said, father's nonverbal behaviour told me that he was feeling distinctly uncomfortable.

'The discussion about the bruising was difficult, and I was careful to note the nonverbal behaviour of each member of the family. The explanation given was that the man at the day centre had done it during an argument with Emma. I asked if this kind of thing had happened before and all agreed that it had not.

'I need to talk with the district nurse about the general medical issues in relation to the fracture and about diet. I think we need a joint strategy about how we tackle the wider family issues. I am concerned that the family, and in particular dad, will not listen to any advice that I have to offer in relation to Emma's learning disability. I need to make sure that her developmental needs and her health needs are being adequately met. I think I will have a talk with Emma's key worker when I am next at the day centre. It would be particularly helpful to see how the centre handles the parents; I might get some clues for a general approach or even work through the centre as "best contact". I need to find out more about the incident in the day centre. It seems logical to meet with the district nurse first to establish that I've got the priorities for Emma's medical needs in the right order and I need to find out more about issues concerned with weight reduction.

'At the same time, I will need to begin to explore Emma's referral with the other members of the community team. I will need to discuss some of the issues with my colleagues if I'm going to come up with a successful strategy here.'

Ⓢ Scenario continued

Liaison with the district nurse
The specialist community nurse for people with a learning disability (Eve) and the district nurse (Jai) met in the local surgery. The meeting had been initiated by Eve, although Jai was very happy to meet and was about to make the same suggestion when he received the telephone call. Both practitioners quickly agreed on the short-term need to help Emma's fracture to heal, and also agreed on the difficulties presented by the attitude of the parents to professional healthcare workers. They decided to adopt a joint strategy to support the family in supporting Emma (Home Office, 1998; DH, 2001a). Jai would focus on Emma and on monitoring her recovery from the fracture, and give or leave clear advice about diet, but would not enter into debate about the situation. Eve would concentrate on getting Mr Hill to realise that his eating behaviour and his scepticism about healthcare professionals may have a direct and negative effect on his daughter's health and general well-being.

Visit to the day centre and discussions with the centre manager and Emma's key worker
Eve, the specialist community nurse for people with a learning disability, met with Emma's key worker about Emma in general, rather than the incident that lead to the referral. Before initiating this meeting, she asked Emma whether she minded. The story from the day centre was one of slow but steady progress, in line with Emma's level of intellectual functioning.

The key worker said that she had also experienced hostility from Emma's parents when Emma first came to the centre. She felt that it faded over time as the centre showed its care and concern for Emma to reach her potential. The key worker took the approach with the parents of honest, open discussion. If she did not know why progress was slow in a particular area, she admitted it and did not try to bluff her way through the meeting. This partnership approach seemed to work well with the Hills, and they had even said that, for the first time in the long story of their daughter's disability, they felt respected.

Joint nursing interventions by Eve, the specialist nurse for people with a learning disability, in conjunction with Jai, the district nurse

Eve's first task was to get to know Emma through visiting her and talking with her and building up mutual trust and respect. Eve followed the model of nursing outlined by Peplau (1991), in which there are four phases:

1 Orientation.
2 Identification.
3 Exploitation.
4 Resolution.

In this process Eve focused on getting a clear picture of how Emma saw herself, what she felt were the most important things in her life and what she would like for the future. Eve used a combination of spoken language, symbols and Makaton (Walker, 1980) to talk with Emma. To help in this process, Eve looked to other members of the multidisciplinary team for support and advice. In particular, she discussed Emma with the speech and language therapist, who gave Eve advice on the most appropriate way of working with Emma in order to establish a level of communication and understanding that would enable her to put forward her feelings. This is of particular importance with abstract ideas to do with feelings or questions such as 'What would you like?'

At the same time, Eve talked to the dietician and clinical psychologist about the best way of designing a programme for Emma's weight reduction. There were three key issues here:

- What is an appropriate diet for Emma? A set of meal options was developed from Emma's known likes and dislikes. The dietician also advised that fruit or low-calorie snacks might be used as rewards. At the same time, they looked at a number of exercise options that might support the weight programme.
- The second issue related to the structure of the weight reduction programme. This had to be designed in a way that motivated Emma to continue with it while at the same time it promoted her self-esteem and a positive body image. These issues are of particular importance considering her age and emerging sexuality. All of those concerned were very conscious not to create a programme that would make Emma feel bad about herself or that would make her ill. One of the central aims of the programme was that Emma should be able to keep her own record of her programme and her achievements. It was also felt to be important that Emma should learn to manage her own rewards.
- The third issue was how to engage Emma's family in the programme. Here Eve and the psychologist worked on making Mr and Mrs Hill key players in the implementation and monitoring of the programme. They were going to suggest that Emma went swimming at least twice a week and for a good walk as often as possible. This would have health benefits for the whole family (Ewles and Simnett, 1995).

The resolution phase of the intervention with Emma and her family will come about as Emma's ability to understand and influence her environment increases. In time, she will gain a clearer understanding of the relationship between the type and amount of food she eats and her size and shape. She will begin to appreciate her developing sexuality and the pleasures and responsibilities that it brings. Her family will begin to think more about the implications of their individual behaviours and the extent to which they affect their children. In understanding this relationship, they will hopefully use this knowledge to help Emma to set and achieve goals for herself. The community nurse will gradually withdraw as the family adjusts itself. It will be important for the nurse to set some markers of change and share these with the family when change has occurred. In this way, all can see how far each has travelled.

Monitoring the situation for signs of abuse

All relevant professionals agreed a strategy in line with guidance on safeguarding vulnerable adults in order to monitor the situation with Emma.

Health promotion and health education

A referral to a specialist healthcare team, and subsequent work that involves a member of the primary healthcare team, provides a useful opportunity for health promotion and health education (DH, 1995a; McBean, 1997). Both nurses involved will have an opportunity to make a general health assessment. Working together, a comprehensive picture of Emma's health strengths and needs should emerge. This provides both practitioners, in conjunction with the family, with a starting point for health promotion and health education activities (Ewles and Simnett, 1995; DH, 1995a; McBean, 1997). The focus in the case of Emma will be around diet, exercise and sexuality. To be effective, changes in diet and exercise, aimed at the maintenance of correct weight and a balanced food intake, should be incorporated into normal daily and weekly routines.

The major issue in working with this family is that of influencing attitudes in order to change behaviour. Given that attitudes are strongly held this will not be easy. The tension between the mother and father in relation to diet can be used creatively. The two practitioners involved will probably choose to influence the father through supporting a new dietary stance that will be taken by the mother following recent events. The proposed changes need to be seen by the family as important, rather than imposed, which provides an example of partnerships as identified in *Valuing People* (DH, 2001a). Information in the form of leaflets, diet sheets, alcohol unit norms, height/weight norms should be introduced sensitively. It will be much more effective if the practitioners involved respond to requests for information rather than devising a pack and presenting it. It may be helpful to use a quasi-counselling approach (Heron, 1990) of facilitating the development of new insights about diet and lifestyle and then offering information, support and guidance towards healthy choices. (See also the discussion on communication in Chapter 5.)

Communication skills

The issue of communication skills is a general one for health practitioners in all areas of professional practice. Without communication of some kind, healthcare cannot take place. It is the duty of the practitioner to discover what is significant to the service user or patient in their care and not the other way around. It follows that the practitioner must be a skilled and active listener (Heron, 1990). Close attention should be paid to nonverbal communication, as this is perhaps the most reliable medium. Communication is not just directly with the service user or patient, but with the context in which they live and their history. In the case of Emma, it would not have been very effective to give written or verbal advice about diet. Once Emma's context was understood, it became clear that the whole family's behaviour needed to change. The issues concerning the incident in the day centre would not have emerged without Eve's ability to be creative about augmenting Emma's communication.

Communication directly with Emma was dominated by the need to understand a particular sign language. The communication about the basic elements of this sign language should have taken place during Emma's admission to the general hospital. Had Emma been from a different ethnic background, one of the important questions that would have been asked was what language she spoke. An interpreter could then be sought. With Emma, whose learning disability is obvious in her appearance, the question was not asked, the assumption made was that she could not communicate and the care that followed was, in respect of not helping her to use the toilet, negligent.

Conclusion

Working through this chapter and exploring the experiences of Emma and her family should have enabled you to gain some insight into the challenges faced by someone who is growing up with a learning disability, discovering their independence and starting to make their own

Part

III

decisions, which will shape their future. It should be clear that in a case of suspected abuse all health and social care professionals need to be involved and communication between them is vital. In the case of Emma, abuse was not proven but suspected and the key people around her have now become more watchful because of dealing with the incident.

Staff involved in Emma's care, both in the community and in hospital, needed to acknowledge and address the family's concerns about the way that Emma is being understood, treated and cared for. We have seen how a lack of insight, or limitation of skill on the part of healthcare professionals, can result in important messages being missed, and the care provided being less than adequate. There are important messages here for practitioners, which emphasise the need to liaise with, and make use of, the specialist expertise that learning disability nurses can bring to the interprofessional team. There is a particular need when a service user is faced with a new or unusual challenge, for example being admitted to a general hospital.

References

Barton, L. (1996) 'Sociology and disability: some emerging issues', in Barton, L. (ed.), *Disability and Society: Emerging Issues and Insights*, Harlow, Longman.

Biggs, S. (1998) 'Care management in community care: advantages, disadvantages and developments', in Thompson, T. and Mathias, P. (eds), *Standards and Learning Disability*, 2nd edn, London, Baillière Tindall.

Brechin, A. and Walmsley, J. (eds) (1989) *Making Connections: Reflecting on the Lives and Experiences of People with Learning Difficulties*, London, Hodder and Stoughton.

Clegg, J. A. (1993) 'Putting people first: a social constructionist approach to learning disability', *British Journal of Clinical Psychology* **32**, 389–406.

Dallos, R. (1991) *Family Belief Systems, Therapy and Change*, Buckingham, Open University Press.

Department of Health (DH) (1995a) *The Health of the Nation: A strategy for people with learning disabilities*, London, HMSO.

DH (1995b) *The Health of the Nation*, London, HMSO.

DH (1997) *The New NHS: Modern and dependable*, Cm 3807, London, TSO.

DH (1998) *Saving Lives: Our healthier nation*, London, HMSO.

DH (2001a) *Valuing People: A strategy for people with learning disabilities for the 21st century*, Cm 5086, London, TSO.

DH (2001b) *Seeking Consent: Working with people with learning disabilities*, London, TSO.

DH (2005) *Independence, Wellbeing and Choice: Our vision for the future of social care for adults in England*, London, TSO.

DH (2006a) *Our Health, Our Care, Our Say: A new direction for community services*, CM 6737, London, TSO.

DH (2006b) *Choosing Health: Making healthy choices easier*, London, TSO.

DH (2007a) *Valuing People Now: From progress to transformation*, London, TSO.

DH (2007b) *Good Practice in Learning Disability Nursing*, London TSO.

Disability Rights Commission (DRC) (2006) *Report of the DRC Formal Inquiry Panel to the DRC's Formal Investigation into the Inequalities in Physical Health Experienced by People with Mental Health Problems and People with Learning Disabilities*, London, DRC.

Donnellan, A. M., LaVigna, G. W., Negri-Shoultz, N. and Fassbender, L. L. (1988) *Progress Without Punishment: Effective approaches for learners with behaviour problems*, London, Teachers College Press.

Duffy, S. (2006) *Keys to Citizenship: A guide to getting good support for people with learning disabilities*, London, Paradigm.

Emerson, E., McGill, P. and Mansell, J. (eds) (1994) *Severe Learning Disabilities and Challenging Behaviour: Designing high quality services*, London, Chapman & Hall.

Ewles, L. and Simnett, I. (1995) *Promoting Health: A practical guide*, 3rd edn, London, Scutari.

Ferris-Taylor, R. (1997) 'Communication', in Gates, B. (ed.), *Learning Disabilities*, London, Churchill Livingstone.

Forchuk, C. and Peplau, H. E. (1993) *Interpersonal Nursing Theory*, Newbury Park, Calif., Sage.

Gates, B. (1997a) 'Understanding learning disability', in Gates, B. (ed.), *Learning Disabilities*, London, Churchill Livingstone.

Gates, B. (1997b) 'Behavioural difficulties', in Gates, B. (ed.), *Learning Disabilities*, London, Churchill Livingstone.

Gilbert, J. and Rose, S. (1998) 'Commissioning and providing services', in Thompson, T. and Mathias, P. (eds), *Standards and Learning Disability*, 2nd edn, London, Baillière Tindall.

Gilbert, T. (1998) 'Sexual health and people with learning disabilities', in Morrissey, M. (ed.), *Sexual Health: A human dilemma*, Wiltshire, Mark Allen.

Gilbert, T., Todd, M. and Jackson, N. (1998) 'People with learning disabilities who also have mental health problems: practice issues and directions for learning disability nursing', *Journal of Advanced Nursing* **27**(6), 1151–7.

Healthcare Commission (2006) *Joint Investigation into the Provision of Services for People with Learning Disabilities at Cornwall Partnership NHS Trust*, London, Healthcare Commission.

Healthcare Commission (2007) *Investigation into the Services for People with Learning Disabilities provided by Sutton and Merton Primary Care Trust*, London, Healthcare Commission.

Heron, J. (1990) *Helping the Client*, London, Sage.

Hewitt, D. and Ephraim, G. (1994) *Access to Communication: Developing the basics of communication with people with severe learning difficulties through intensive interaction*, London, David Fulton.

Home Office (1998) *Supporting Families*, green paper, London, TSO.

House of Lords and House of Commons Joint Committee on Human Rights (2008) *A Life Like Any Other? Human rights of adults with learning disability*, London, HMSO.

Kay, B., Rose, S. and Turnbull, J. (1995) *Continuing the Commitment*, London, HMSO.

King's Fund (1999) *Learning Disabilities: From care to citizenship*,

London, King's Fund.

Kroese, S., Dagnan, D. and Loumides, K. (2001) *Cognitive-behaviour Therapy for People with Learning Disabilities*, Hove, Brunner Routledge.

Mathews, D. (1996) *The 'OK' Health Check for Assessing and Planning Health Care Needs of People with Learning Disabilities*, Preston, Fairfield.

Mencap (2004) *Treat Me Right*, London, Mencap.

Mencap (2007) *Death by Indifference*, London, Mencap.

McBean, S. (1997) 'Health and health promotion – consensus and conflict', in Perry, A. (ed.) *Nursing: A knowledge base for practice*, 2nd edn, London, Arnold.

McCray, J. (2003) 'Leading interprofessional practice: a conceptual framework to support practitioners in the field of learning disability', *Journal of Nursing Management* 11, 387–5.

McNally, S. (1997) 'Representation', in Gates, B. (ed.) *Learning Disabilities*, London, Churchill Livingstone.

Michael, J. (2008) *Healthcare for All: Independent inquiry into access to health care for people with learning disability*, publisher [online] www.iahpld.org.ug/healthcare_final.pdf (accessed 26 February 2009).

Moss, S., Ibbotson B., Prosser H., Goldberg D., Patel P. et al. (1997) 'Validity of the PASS-ADD for detecting psychiatric symptoms in adults with learning disability (mental retardation)', *Social Psychiatry and Psychiatric Epidemiology* 32, 344–54.

Moss, S. and Turner, S. (1995) *The Health of People with Learning Disabilities. Report to the Department of Health*, Manchester, Hester Adrian Research Centre.

Nirje, B. (1969) 'The normalisation principle and its human management implications', in Kugel, R. and Wolfensberger, W. (eds), *Changing Patterns in Residential Services for the Mentally Retarded*, Washington, DC, Presidents Committee on Mental Retardation.

Northway, R.; Hutchinson, C. and Kingdon, A. (2006) *Shaping the Future: A vision for learning disability nursing*, Learning Disability Consultant Nurse Network, UK.

Nursing and Midwifery Council (NMC) (2008) *Code of Professional Conduct*, London, NMC.

Oliver, M. (1990) *The Politics of Disablement*, Basingstoke, Macmillan.

Peplau, H. (1991) *Interpersonal Relations in Nursing*, New York, Springer.

Prasher, P. and Janicki, M. (2002) *Physical Health of Adults with Intellectual Disability*, Oxford, Blackwell.

Priest, H. and Gibbs, M. (2004) *Mental Health Care for People with Learning Disabilities*, Edinburgh, Churchill Livingstone.

Redworth, M. and Redworth, F. (1997) 'Learning disability and citizenship: paradigms for inclusion', *Journal of Learning Disabilities for Nursing, Health and Social Care* 1(4), 181–5.

Ryan, J. and Thomas, F. (1987) *Politics of Mental Handicap*, London, Free Associated Press.

Schon, D. (1983) *The Reflective Practitioner: How professionals think in action*, New York, Basic Books.

Sines, D. and Barr, O. (1998) 'Professions in teams', in Thompson, T. and Mathias, P. (eds), *Standards and Learning Disability*, 2nd edn, London, Baillière Tindall.

Singh, P. (1997) *Prescriptions for Change: A Mencap report on the role of GPs and carers in the provision of primary care for people with a learning disability*, London, Mencap.

Wake, E. (1997) 'Profound and multiple disability', in Gates, B. (ed.) *Learning Disabilities*, London, Churchill Livingstone.

Walker, M. (1980) *The Makaton Vocabulary Language Programme*, 31 Firwood Drive, Camberley, Surrey, Makaton Vocabulary Development Project.

Watson, D. (1997) 'Causes and manifestations', in Gates, B. (ed.), *Learning Disabilities*, London, Churchill Livingstone.

Wertheimer, A. (ed.) (1996) *Changing Days: Developing new day opportunities with people who have learning difficulties*, London, King's Fund.

Wolfensberger, W. (1972) *The Principle of Normalisation in Human Services*, Toronto, National Institute on Mental Retardation.

World Health Organization (WHO) (1993) *Describing Developmental Disability: Guidelines for a multi-axial scheme for mental retardation*, 10th revision, Geneva, WHO.

Legislation

Disability Discrimination Act 1995
Mental Capacity Act 2005
Mental Health Act 1983
Mental Health Act 2007

Websites

British Institute of learning Disabilities: www.bild.org.uk
Foundation for People with Learning Disabilities: www.learningdisabilities.org.uk
In Control: www.in-control.org.uk
MENCAP: www.mencap.org.uk
National Network for Learning Disability Nurses: www.nnldn.org.uk

Part

III

Insights into care settings

Chapter

28

Rehabilitation

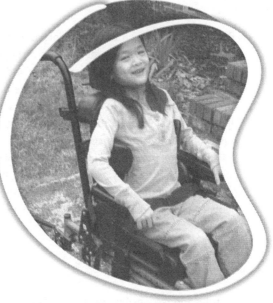

Stephen O'Connor

(with thanks to Bernard Gibbon)

Links to other chapters in _Foundation Studies for Caring_

Links to other chapters in _Foundation Skills for Caring_

W Don't forget to visit www.palgrave.com/glasper for additional online resources relating to this chapter.

Introduction

The care and management of patients at all points on the health–illness continuum incorporates the notion of caring for patients through complete episodes of illness, from the acute presentation through into postacute care and rehabilitation.

The care and management of the stroke patient is representative of the challenge to the multiprofessional team in caring for patients who have complex needs. Significant durations of in-patient care require the services of many healthcare professionals and frequently require posthospital care and management.

This chapter provides an insight into rehabilitation care, focusing on Frank Sargeant and his family who have recently experienced stroke. Its aims are to provide a grounded knowledge of stroke care, and through this illustrate key aspects of the broader context within which stroke patients are treated. It is also intended to help readers understand the experience of stroke.

Learning outcomes

This chapter will enable you to:

- understand the roles and responsibilities of the different members of the multiprofessional team
- understand the healthcare needs of the elderly
- understand the role of community rehabilitation teams
- be familiar with their role in the prevention of elderly abuse
- be familiar with the implications of the Mental Capacity Act
- identify of the physical, psychological and social needs of the patient and their carers following stroke and an awareness of the values and concepts of individual care
- apply the principles of problem solving to the planning of care, its implementation and evaluation
- be familiar with the terminology associated with stroke care and management

- appreciate the incidence and prevalence of stroke
- understand the pathophysiological basis of stroke, predisposing factors and preventative measures
- identify appropriate forms of assessment for patients following stroke and of those which can be used to monitor progress
- identify the complications of stroke and measures to prevent complications arising
- understand the impact of stroke on the person and their family
- understand the different approaches to the managerial organisation of stroke services
- identify evidence to support clinical practices.

Concepts

- Rehabilitation nursing
- Individualised care
- The nurse's role
- Problem solving
- Stroke
- Multiprofessional working

S Scenario: Frank Sargeant's experiences

Frank Sargeant collapses at his social club and on his return home appears rather incoherent. He is seen by his general practitioner (GP).

a Learning activity

Frank's GP undertakes a full medical assessment, which includes the following. In your learning group discuss what significance these might have and why:

- taking a full history
- a full physical examination
- determining any loss of consciousness
- taking blood pressure
- discussing a plan of action.

S Scenario continued

Frank is found to be hypertensive with a blood pressure recording of 190/100 mm Hg. Following further examination and the responses to questions, the GP strongly suspects that Frank has experienced a transient ischaemic attack (TIA).

a Learning activity

What is hypertension and what is a TIA? Before reading on think about what you already know about the way that blood pressure is controlled and why hypertension might rise. Think about how oxygenated blood reaches the brain and consider what might happen if this flow is obstructed in any way. As a starting point you may wish to access a physiology textbook and map out the cerebral circulation, determining both the origin and destination of the internal and external carotid arteries.

Transient ischaemic attack (TIA)

A TIA is a stroke where the neurological deficits clear spontaneously within 24 hours. This may result from emboli. Emboli that give rise to stroke have their origin in the left side of the heart or in the arteries between the heart and the brain.

Emboli formation is often associated with either valvular damage of the mitral (bicuspid) valve in the heart, which separates the left atria from the left ventricle, or damage to the semilunar valves at the opening of the aorta. This thrombotic clot known as a mural thrombus has formed on the inner wall of the ventricle, usually following a myocardial infarction. If the mural thrombus breaks away, it then becomes an embolus flowing towards the brain, until it becomes lodged as the blood vessels get smaller. The amount of damage caused will depend on the size of the vessel, the degree of obstruction and what part of the brain is denied oxygen. Sometimes emboli can be very small and the resulting effects may be only transient. Frank is thought to have experienced such a TIA.

Emboli can also form in damaged arteries, especially where arteries bifurcate, and this is frequently associated with artherosclerotic changes in which the lumen of arteries becomes reduced. When the carotid arteries are affected in this way, there is a high risk of stroke. However, an understanding of the predisposing factors leading to stroke can facilitate the development of preventative strategies.

a Learning activities

Research those causes of heart disease that might give rise to mitral valve damage. Discuss the following in your learning group:

It would seem that Frank might well have experienced a TIA. Discuss Frank's lifestyle and identify potential factors that may have given rise to this.

What is the nature and purpose of a TIA clinic?

S Scenario continued

Frank considered himself to be a fit and well 67-year-old. He retired two years ago from the light engineering factory where he started work as an apprentice toolmaker at the age of 14, 53 years before. He knows he was lucky to have stayed in work all his adult life, and puts this down to his own hard work and ability to 'fit in'; he is well aware that his children may not be so lucky, but feels strongly that they must work hard to succeed.

Frank is married. His wife Joan is 55 and is still working at the local supermarket, doing shift work as a garage receptionist. They live in their own home, which they now own after paying off the mortgage on Frank's retirement.

Frank and Joan have three children. Ken the eldest is 37, married with two children, and lives away in London. Frank and Joan are extremely proud that Ken is a successful professional; however, he rarely visits and when he does, it tends to be while on business trips and he does not bring his family. Mel is now 33, divorced, with one child. She lives locally and works shifts in a local factory, and relies on her mother for childminding. This is difficult as they both work

Part
IV

shifts and is a cause of ongoing friction between father and daughter. Billy is 30 and lives at home. He is unemployed at present, having followed his father into engineering. Billy is in a long-term relationship and plans to marry, but feels that he should not until he has a job that is secure and has prospects.

Frank's social life rotates around his local CIA social club where he has a part-time job as barman. He is also vice-chairman of the 'old folks' entertainment committee and captain of the club's first division cribbage team. Frank prides himself on the fact that he has never had a day off sick in his life and does not even know who his GP is. However, Frank smokes 40 cigarettes a day, drinks at least 50 units of alcohol a week (mainly beer), and even he accepts his wife's opinion that he is overweight. He will also admit to easily 'losing his breath', often getting headaches and feeling 'flushed'.

In Frank's case a number of predisposing factors could have influenced his stroke. These might include stress, obesity, high alcohol consumption and cigarette smoking, which may have contributed to an increased risk of hypertension or heart disease.

Reduction in the incidence of stroke is a government *Health of the Nation* target (DH, 1992). Stroke preventive strategies include:
- discouraging smoking
- screening for and treating high blood pressure
- screening for abnormal lipids and treating as appropriate
- ensuring the optimal control of diabetes where appropriate (see also Chapter 25 on community care).

Success in the delivery of this strategy has led to a reduction in the mortality rate over the last decade (NAO, 2005).

Smoking

Cigarette smoking is a major cause of ill health and is implicated in a range of respiratory and circulatory disorders. Public health messages have been attempting to discourage people from starting smoking and encourage people to give up smoking for a number of years with only limited success. Frank describes himself as addicted, having tried to give up several times but failed. The addictive nature of smoking has been recognised in addition to the habitual element.

(a) Learning activity

Discuss the following in your learning group:
- Consider the smoking behaviour of people and reflect on antismoking campaigns.
- Consider strategies that could be deployed to reduce the number of people who smoke and the number of cigarettes that people smoke.
- Reflect on the use of nicotine replacement therapy as a method to reduce the number of people who smoke (see also Chapter 24 on care of the adult).

(S) Scenario continued

Frank suddenly collapses at home and loses consciousness. Joan accompanies him in the ambulance to the Accident and Emergency (A&E) department at the local general hospital. As Frank arrives he regains consciousness but is very confused and disorientated. Frank is seen immediately by the registrar and transferred to the admissions ward. It is strongly suspected that Frank has experienced a major stroke.

(a) Learning activity

What is a stroke and how does this differ from a TIA? (Consider what you may already know before reading on.)

Stroke

A stroke is defined as the rapid onset of neurological deficits that persist for at least 24 hours and are caused by either haemorrhage or partial or complete blockage of a blood vessel supplying or draining a part of the brain, leading to infarction of brain tissue.

Cerebrovascular accident is a term often used to refer to a stroke, frequently shortened to CVA. This term, while accurately describing the notion of damage to the part of the brain, the cerebrum, and that the cause is vascular, is now not commonly used. A stroke is a collective term for a syndrome. Additionally, a stroke is not an accident in the 'normal' meaning of this word.

Stroke is commonly caused by cerebral thrombosis or embolism, and less commonly by cerebral haemorrhage. The most common underlying pathology in these conditions is arterial damage, often associated with hypertension. The type of stroke often gives some indication of the prognosis and the onset of stroke can suggest the underlying type. For Frank Sargeant, it is important for investigations to be undertaken as a matter of urgency and this is discussed later.

> **a) Learning activity**
>
> If unsure, check out the meaning of the word 'syndrome'.

Types of stroke

The most common pattern of the onset and prognosis for stroke is set out in Table 28.1.

Table 28.1 Typical pattern of onset and prognosis according to type

Type	Onset	Prognosis
Thrombotic	Slow	
Embolic	Sudden	Variable: from good to very poor
Haemorrhagic	Sudden	Usually poor

Thrombosis refers to the formation of a blood clot within the blood vessels during life. Blood clotting within the body depends upon the same factors as in clotting outside the body, such as following a laceration. The rough edges of a wound or rough surface in the lining of a blood vessel will have similar effects, both trigger the blood clotting mechanism.

Therefore, an indirect cause of thrombosis is usually some damage to the smooth lining of the blood vessels brought about by inflammation or, most typically in stroke, the result of atheroma, a chronic disease of vessel walls.

Embolism refers to the plugging of a small blood vessel by material which has been carried through the larger vessels in the blood stream.

Haemorrhage means any escape of blood from the vessels which naturally contain it. It may occur from a wound on the skin, in which case it escapes externally, or into some internal cavity such as the stomach, or it may simply escape into the tissues surrounding the site of blood loss. In the case of cerebral haemorrhage the skull acts to contain all blood lost through haemorrhage, and hence any intracerebral haemorrhage not only irritates the neurological cells, but also acts to exert pressure on the brain.

> **a) Learning activity**
>
> Refer to a physiology textbook and study 'blood clotting mechanism'. You may wish to draw a diagram to show the cascade theory of blood clotting.

> **a) Learning activity**
>
> Reflect back on what you have already learnt about embolism in relation to TIAs. Research 'embolism' in more depth. Think about the different substances that form emboli and where emboli can lodge in relation to their origin.

Part

IV

Therefore, in summary, Frank Sargeant's stroke might have resulted from:

- **atheroma** (associated with cigarette smoking, high blood pressure, diabetes and hyperlipidaemia)
- **microaneurisms** (associated with high blood pressure)
- **emboli** (associated with a range of heart disorders)
- **thrombus** (associated with other conditions such as severe dehydration).

An understanding of the pathology of stroke gives some understanding on how to embark on prevention, including secondary prevention, and following a stroke, provides the basis for the range of investigations. As yet no specific treatment exists for stroke, but an understanding of the pathology provides the basis for considering treatment options.

How common are strokes?

A key resource is *Reducing Brain Damage: Faster access to better stroke care* (NAO, 2005).

(e) Evidence-based practice

Incidence of stroke – making use of statistics

Incidence refers to the number of new cases in a particular time frame, say one year, whereas *prevalence* is the number of existing cases. Stroke is a common problem, being the third most common cause of death in the United Kingdom; at any one time 25–35 patients with stroke will occupy beds in an average district general hospital (Wolfe, Rudd and Beech, 1996).

There are about 110,000 people who have their first strokes in any one year in the United Kingdom, and additionally, about a further 30,000 people have a recurrence or subsequent stroke in any one year (NAO, 2005). Hence at present between 174 and 216 cases of stroke are being seen per 100,000 members of the population (Mant et al, 2004). Stroke carries a high mortality, with around 80,000 people per year dying following a stroke. The consequence of these figures is that the prevalence of people with stroke is between 55,000 and 70,000 in the United Kingdom. It is noteworthy that men and women are equally affected, though a slight rise in the number of elderly women is noted, probably attributable to the greater proportion of elderly women than men in the older elderly sector of the population (Rudd et al, 1999). An average health district with a population of 250,000 can therefore expect to see about 500–650 new patients following a stroke per year. Many patients survive the initial stroke, but have a degree of residual disability. At a local level you could expect about 900–1200 people who have survived a stroke with some degree of disability (Wolfe et al, 1996).

(a) Learning activity

There are clear implications for stroke prevention. In your learning group, reflect back on the issues identified previously in relation to Frank's lifestyle and that of his family. How much at risk of stroke are Frank's children and grandchildren, and are they at any greater risk than the rest of the population?

Giving advice is an important role for all health practitioners. However, enabling individuals to understand and to concord with health advice is a key skill that all nurses have to develop.

(a) Learning activity

When you are next in a practice setting (in the community or elsewhere) try to observe a health education activity. Consider such issues as:

- Who takes the initiative in providing health education?
- How are health needs assessed?
- What format is used; for example, verbal information, leaflets, videos, one-to-one or

group activities?
- How is the activity evaluated?

You should also investigate what the Stroke Association's FAST campaign is all about.

You may like to begin to find out more about health education models and ascertain which model may be most effective in providing health advice for Frank, his wife, their children and grandchildren.

Nurses work as members of a multiprofessional team, which is essential in relation to the rehabilitation of patients following stroke, and to their family. Communication is key and nurses need to be able to not only converse with patients and relatives to enable clear understanding, but also to thoroughly understand the medical terminology.

Using key terms in relation to stroke

Stroke, which affects a major control system like the nervous system, gives rise to a number of clinical features, such as loss of consciousness, difficulty with mobility, difficulty with speech or swallowing, difficulty with understanding or perception. Many of these clinical features are described by the following terms:

- **Agnosia** is an inability to recognise sensory objects, as the sensory stimulus cannot be interpreted in spite of a normal sense organ.
- **Aphagia** refers to the loss of swallowing ability, and aphasia refers to the loss of speech, or the loss of power to understand the written or spoken word. The prefix 'a' meaning 'lacking' or 'loss of'.
- **Apraxia** refers to the inability to recognise common articles or perform correct movements because of a brain lesion, and not because of sensory impairment or loss of muscle power in the limbs.
- **Dysphagia** means difficulty in swallowing and **dysphasia** means difficulty in speaking. 'Dys' is used as a prefix meaning 'difficult'. Dysphasia may be receptive or expressive. Receptive dysphasia refers to difficulty in understanding. Expressive dysphasia means difficulty in speaking.
- **Hemiparesis** is a similar term, which refers to a partial paralysis of one side of the body.
- **Hemiplegia** refers to paralysis of one side of the body. It is due to cerebral disease. The lesion (damage to the brain) is in the side of the brain opposite to the side paralysed.

a Learning activity

Discuss the following questions in your learning group.

When Frank regained consciousness he was confused and disorientated. How would you be sure what you were doing was what Frank wanted? When his wife went home who would you ask? Would you always do what his wife requested?

What is the Mental Capacity Act 2005? How does it influence your actions?

S Scenario continued

Initial admission and assessment
Frank's wife had decided to go home to collect some nightclothes so did not accompany Frank to the ward. Once Frank was settled in bed on the emergency medical assessment ward, Staff Nurse Tatta had a brief discussion with the nurse responsible for Frank's care in the accident and emergency department. She then made an immediate assessment of his condition, decided on a number of priorities and instigated a plan of action. This she then handed quickly to a colleague, as she wanted to be off duty by 3 pm.

Part
IV

t⭐
Practice tip

Table 28.2 Care plan

Immediate Care Plan for: Mr Frank Sargeant Admitted to Ward: Aug 2nd, 14.30hrs
Named Nurse: Tatta Bose

ADL	Normal state	On admission	Actions
Breathing	SC	Semiconscious	GCS hourly TPR\BP hourly
Body temperature	SC	Semiconscious	Keep warm
Eating and drinking	SC	Semiconscious	Offer fluids
Elimination	SC	Semiconscious, incontinent of urine in casualty	Observe for incontinence. Offer bottle
Skin	INTACT	Semiconscious	Turn hourly
Mobility	SC	Semiconscious ? Rt hemiparesis	Bed rest
Rest and sleep	SC		
Communications	SC	Semiconscious? Some difficulty with speech	Answer patient's and relatives' questions
Sexuality			
Work and leisure	Retired		
Hygiene and grooming	SC		

Abbreviations

In Table 28.2 you will see several examples of abbreviations: ADL = activity of daily living; SC = self-caring; GCS = Glasgow Coma Scale. Many abbreviations are used in healthcare and especially in nursing and medical notes. It is a legal requirement that documentation is clearly written and understood by all, so it is very important that only accepted abbreviations are used. In your general reading, notice what accepted abbreviations are used and try to ascertain which are commonly accepted (such as TPR) and which are more doubtful (such as Rt). There is a need to avoid risk of confusion: for example, what does MI mean? Consider how such confusion might be avoided.

(a) Learning activity

(Key resource: Power et al, 2007.) Discuss the following questions in your learning group.

Put yourself in the shoes of healthcare professional Staff Nurse Tatta Bose. What might you have done differently over the first 24 hours and why? Consider the merits and shortcomings of Frank Sargeant's immediate plan of care with a colleague. How well does it:

- address Frank's immediate needs and those of his family?
- reflect on the function of an emergency assessment ward?

[S] Scenario continued

Frank is shortly due for transfer to the acute stroke unit, so try to find out about the purpose of such a unit. Consider its possible benefits and limitations.

(e) Evidence-based practice

The nature and purpose of stroke units
There have been a large number of randomised controlled trials comparing care provided in stroke units with that in acute medical and care of the elderly units. These trials demonstrate that patients who are cared for in a stroke unit have a lower rate of mortality and morbidity than those who are cared for in acute medical and care of the elderly units (SUTC, 1995). Hence, over the last ten years stroke units have opened in increasing numbers in many district general hospitals as required by the *National Service Framework for Older People* (DH, 2001).

(S) Scenario continued

Rehabilitation
The next day Frank is transferred to the hospital's acute stroke unit. His rehabilitation needs will have to be assessed by the multidisciplinary team.

(a) Learning activity

Work independently at first and then compare lists; validate your list in practice individually.

Many rehabilitation activities require specialist input from different members of the multidisciplinary team. Frank may well need a range of specialist interventions built into his plan of care. These might include compensatory training, managing cognitive and perceptual deficits, and managing speech and language disorders.

- Make a list of members of the multidisciplinary team: next time you are in practice seek them out and ask them what they have to offer a stoke patient.
- Try to arrange visits to rehabilitation areas and negotiate opportunities to work alongside members of the multidisciplinary team.

Working in a multidisciplinary team

Waters and Luker (1996) suggest that multidisciplinary teamwork is central to the policy and practice of care of the elderly, and further suggest that it is this notion of multidisciplinary teamwork that distinguishes care of the elderly from other medical specialities. Multiprofessional teamwork is recognised as the approach to complex problems where the services of more than one occupational group are necessary to improve patient outcomes. It has to be recognised, however, that each of the occupational groups have their own unique contribution to make in addition to the contribution to the team.

Recognising that the needs of a patient might be best met by the services of more than one professional group goes some way to encouraging the development of a multiprofessional team, and it follows that there must be some understanding of how that team will work together. It is evident, however, that tensions can exist between team members, and efforts have to be made by all parties to ensure that the work of the team is towards the common good.

The factors promoting interdisciplinary teams can be conceptualised as gains for the recipients of care and the organisation, that is third-party gains, rather than for the individual profession (first-party gains); hence the *raison d'être* of rehabilitation teams is to improve patient outcomes. An interdisciplinary approach requires, at least, that the members of the team collaborate with other colleagues and other professional groups with education being the key to interdisciplinary collaboration. Their exploration of the term 'collaborate' brings together two connotations: first, working together, especially in a joint intellectual effort; and

Part
IV

second, cooperating reasonably, as with an enemy occupying one's own country. The second interpretation of the word is interesting in that it raises issues of territory and domains of practice. This is of particular interest in the context of a rehabilitation team, where individual disciplines lay claim to specific areas of practice (territory), yet are requested to collaborate (work cooperatively) with other disciplines who may or may not have the same skills or knowledge.

(a) Learning activity

Research would suggest that there is much to gain from a multidisciplinary approach to rehabilitation, and yet the realities are that when any group gets together there are challenges that have to be addressed. Think of your own experiences of working in a group, or as a team. Can you relate to the commentary above? Identify the specific factors and behaviours that made it a comfortable and enabling experience, and think about how this could be applied in practice to promote holistic care and the achievement of agreed patient outcomes.

If you have worked in a team where there were tensions, how were these addressed and remedied?

(S) Scenario continued

Frank has arrived in the acute stroke unit accompanied by his wife Joan. He still has a right-sided hemiparesis and some difficulty with communication although he is now fully conscious and continent. Frank is feeling very depressed about the future.

Ongoing assessment

It is imperative to undertake a thorough assessment of the patient, initially to confirm the diagnosis of stroke, and second, to prescribe a patient management plan. The complex nature of stroke necessitates the use of numerous assessments, which are completed by appropriate members of the multiprofessional team. As we have acknowledged, each member of the team has a unique contribution to make in addition to the core aspects of care and patient management.

(c) Professional conversation

Jennifer Shepherd, nurse practitioner, discusses Frank's care with a physiotherapy student and a foundation degree student who are on placement: 'Although the initial assessment is undertaken on admission to hospital, I always see this as an ongoing process which informs the patient management plan. This in turn informs discharge planning and post in-patient care. In addition to the physical examination, which will be made by the doctor, assessments will be needed relating to Frank Sargeant's psychosocial status as well as detailed assessments of his functional ability. The multiprofessional nature of stroke care requires team work and we use single patient documentation (team notes) to facilitate this. It is working very well, as it avoids unnecessary duplication of records and everybody is kept updated on progress.'

The use of scales to assess progress by measurement offers a tangible way to monitor patient progress. A number of different assessment tools are available which are appropriate for assessing disability following stroke. These include, amongst others, the activity of daily living (ADL) scales, Barthel Index, Rivermead ADL Scale and the Nottingham 10-point ADL scale. In the acute stroke unit the team constantly review existing tools and seek out new developments. Some of these tools are discussed below.

t ☆
Practice tip

Measurement tools
Measurement tools have long been established to quantify aspects of patient care, and this is no less true for disabled people, including scales specifically designed for stroke patients. The battery of measurement tools includes those measuring impairment, the physiological consequences of pathology, disability, the functional consequences and handicap, and the social consequences. It is therefore important to consider what domain is to be assessed prior to employing an assessment tool.

a) Learning activity

Work independently to find some examples in practice of different assessment tools and consider what aspects of assessment are amenable to measurement. Think about the form of assessment tool that could be used as part of Frank Sargeant's rehabilitation in assessing progress in the biological, psychological and social domains. (Refer also to Chapters 10, 11 and 15 on nutrition, hydration and pain respectively.) Share your findings with your learning group.

A range of assessment tools

Activity of daily living scales are commonly used measurement scales, which are based on activities of daily living (ADLs). This concept will be reasonably familiar to most nurses, although it should not be confused with activities of living (ALs) as commonly associated with the activities of living model (Roper, Logan and Tierney 1985). ADLs have become the mainstay of disability measurement.

A number of these scales are general measures of disability which can be used for a range of client groups, whereas others have been specifically designed for the stroke patient. The commonly used scales include the **Barthel Index** (Mahoney and Barthel, 1965), which is a summed index (1–3 points per item), validated for assessing self-care, continence and mobility, and can be administered through formal testing, interview or informal assessment.

The **Rivermead ADL scale** (Whiting and Lincoln, 1980) was devised for use with stroke and head-injury patients and includes additional domestic items. It is a hierarchical scale and is administered as a formal assessment. It was revalidated for use with elderly stroke patients, which resulted in some re-ordering of items (Lincoln and Edmans, 1990).

The **Nottingham 10-point ADL scale** (Ebrahim, Nouri and Barer, 1985) was designed for use with stroke in-patients and, like the Rivermead scale, is hierarchical but does not include additional domestic items. The Nottingham 10-point scale can, however, be administered by observation, interview or by post.

Using tools would appear to be helpful to facilitate speed of assessment, ensuring that the same things are measured in the same way by each member of the multiprofessional team. They also facilitate effective communication. However, they need to have been proven to be effective before they are implemented in practice.

Accurate assessment tools

Assessment tools need to demonstrate *validity*; that is, they test what they are intended to test. They must also be *reliable*; that is, the same score is attained when applied to the same patient on two separate occasions unless a real change has occurred. The issue of *sensitivity* is closely related to reliability in that a measure of change is only useful if it can detect change relevant to the user. Tools used in clinical practice must be simple, but not at the expense of reliability or sensitivity. It is unlikely that a single tool will be developed that can usefully address all areas of disability.

Part
IV

Practitioners require tools that, in addition to their length, simplicity and sensitivity, can be used effectively and that facilitate communication between disciplines. The sensitivity of a tool may be compromised for the sake of simplicity. A single summary score which conveys the level of functional ability from one practitioner to another lends weight to the adoption of a hierarchical (Guttman) scale such as the Nottingham 10-point scale or Rivermead ADL scale. The Barthel Index, while it is recognised to be a good measure of physical disability and requires only a few minutes to complete, is not hierarchical and therefore does not provide a summated score which gives a clear indication of the level of disability. That is, the overall score can be gained by a variety of abilities. The completed assessment could, however, be communicated either verbally or in writing in a matter of seconds.

S Scenario continued

Frank has experienced quite severe depression following his stroke, symptoms which are distressing, but not unusual following such a devastating event. Assessment of mental state is of great importance, and assessment tools have been developed to assess anxiety, mood and other psychological traits. These tools are useful when used as an adjunct to clinical decision making; they can provide objective data on patient progress and give early warning of possible complications.

Investigations

These are required to confirm the diagnosis, to check for further pathology (for instance, has Frank also had a myocardial infarction?) and to establish baselines against which to measure change. In Frank's case the medical staff decided to request:

- full blood count
- erythrocyte sedimentation rate (ESR)
- carotid Doppler examination
- electrocardiogram (ECG)
- computerised tomography (CT) scan
- magnetic resonance imaging (MRI) scan
- cerebral angiography

with the following physiological parameters monitored and reviewed on an ongoing basis (as recommended by RCP 2004):

- blood pressure
- pulse/heart rhythm
- oxygen saturation
- temperature
- blood glucose
- hydration
- conscious level.

a Learning activity

In your learning group put yourself in the role of a healthcare professional caring for Frank Sargeant. How would you go about providing Frank and Joan with a clear explanation of the meaning and purpose of these investigations? What would the nurse's role be in preparing Frank for these investigations and caring for him during and after the investigation?

S Scenario continued

Following the initial multidisciplinary assessment of Frank on his admission to the stroke unit a plan of care was developed for the first 24 hours. The assessment was conducted by different members of the multidisciplinary team who communicated with each other to avoid duplication and repetition. The team now regularly meets together, involving Frank and his wife to review the care and treatment plan, check progress and adjust goals. Over the first 24 hours it was decided to:

- Monitor temperature, pulse, respiration and blood pressure.
- Continue with neurological assessment.
- Action swallowing assessment and request special diet if needed.
- Monitor continence and elimination.
- Carry out moving and handling assessment.

- Commence fluid balance recordings.
- Estimate tissue viability rating.
- Apply TED (thrombo-embolic deterrent) stockings.
- With Mr and Mrs Sargeant:
  - give introductory ward information
  - assess level of understanding of the situation
  - instigate initial planning regarding discharge.
- Set date for first interdisciplinary meeting with Mr and Mrs Sargeant.

In addition the medical staff included:

- Prescribe if required:
  - intravenous (IV) fluid
  - subcutaneous heparin

- dexamethazone
- thrombolysis.

These interventions were incorporated into Frank Sargeant's plan of care.

The evolving care plan

Assessment is ongoing and documentation is kept updated and the care plan amended as Frank's condition changes. Members of the multiprofessional team communicate changes in his condition, and consequent changes in care, to each other. This is effectively cascaded to others through written and verbal reports.

Ⓐ Learning activity

Reflect on the above action points. What information would you expect Mr and Mrs Sargeant to want regarding:

- the type of diet most suitable now and as the condition improves
- why IV fluids may be required
- the function of heparin and why this might help Frank.

What is thrombolysis, when is it undertaken and why?

One of the main concerns of the team is to avoid the potential of complications that follow stroke. A number of preventive strategies have therefore been introduced into the care plan. Stroke is a major illness which can kill at the time of onset. A large number of people do, however, survive the stroke, but are at risk of developing complications. Some of these are as a direct consequence of reduced mobility or bed rest. These include deep vein thrombosis (DVT), which can lead to pulmonary embolus, pneumonia/aspiration pneumonia, pressure ulcers, spasticity, urinary incontinence, contractures, malnutrition, anxiety and depression, neglect or inattention, poor coordination, visual loss, memory loss, sensory changes, speech problems, fatigue and sexual problems and shoulder pain or dislocation.

Ⓐ Learning activity

Before reading on you may like to consider what you know about each of these complications and the effects that they would have on Frank Sargeant. Find out why they occur and what actions might be taken to prevent them.

Depression

Depression is frequently seen following stroke and there is little doubt that stroke can give rise to considerable feelings of misery. Depression can act as a barrier to rehabilitation in that the patient lacks motivation to seek independence. Frank and his family will need time and space to grieve and adjust to the change in body image and any longer-term residual disability that there might be. Being listened to and acknowledged, involved and empowered to make decisions helps preserve self-esteem. The poor handling of the grieving process is therefore seen as the predominant cause of the common problem of post-stroke depression. (Kirkevold, 1997). The nurse's task therefore is to be instrumental in the reduction of the incidence of depression by the level of emotional support that they deliver (see Chapter 25 on care of the older adult, which explores the grieving process).

Part

IV

S Scenario continued

Frank has retained his cognitive and perceptual function and can engage in conversation. However, where there is significant cognitive and perceptual dysfunction it can be challenging to provide interventions which can lift mood. Company, the use of communication aids, and sensitive use of distraction through, for example, the radio or television, can all help to lift the mood. Medication in the form of antidepressants may sometimes be required.

a Learning activity

You may wish to check out how you can best recognise the characteristics of depression, especially in patients who have difficulty communicating. Review chapter 26 on mental health.

Care plan for depression:

- Frank and his family will need time and space to adjust to the change in body image and any longer term residual disability. Set aside time for listening to their needs and concerns, keeping them informed and involved in all decisions.
- Monitor mood through sleep pattern, appetite, activity and Frank's desire to communicate.

Deep vein thrombosis

Deep vein thrombosis refers to the development of a blood clot in one of the large veins, usually in the lower limb. This might go undetected as the patient may have a loss of sensation in the leg as a consequence of his stroke. Careful observation for signs associated with deep vein thrombosis need to be instigated. Preventive measures to reduce the likelihood of DVT include the use of elasticated stockings to reduce the risk of thrombus formation. These TED stockings should be carefully fitted as they work by exerting an external pressure on the legs, and subsequently the veins which force the blood back towards the heart. The stockings are designed to compensate for the loss of the 'muscle pump' which occurs in normal activity thereby assisting venous return. The one-way valves in the veins ensure that blood travels to the heart. Early mobilisation and regular and frequent passive limb exercises help to reduce the risk of developing deep vein thrombosis.

Care plan for DVT:

- Application of TED stockings.
- Observe for redness, tenderness/pain in calf.
- Early mobilisation and regular and frequent passive limb exercises.

Pneumonia

Pneumonia is a risk in all patients with reduced mobility and a particular problem in a person like Frank, following stroke, as a high proportion of patients have swallowing difficulties and lose their swallowing reflex. Saliva and aspirate fluid can more easily enter the lungs and create an environment rich for micro-organism growth and subsequent chest infection and pneumonia.

Care plan for pneumonia:

- Frequent positional change and chest physiotherapy to reduce the risk of pneumonia.
- Assess for swallowing deficit.
- Assist with choice of appropriate foods.
- Help to regain independence with feeding.

a Learning activity

Find out about swallowing deficit and the appropriate interventions used to maintain hydration and nutrition. Who can undertake a swallowing assessment?

Pressure ulcers

Pressure ulcers can result from inadequate perfusion of the tissues as a result of reduced mobility and loss of sensation, for example, by being confined to bed or chair. Risk increases due to a variety of factors including: debilitation, confusion, incontinence, poor diet and inadequate nutrition. Regular changes of position, the use of pressure-relieving aids, and interventions that address the risk factors will help to prevent pressure ulcers occurring (see Chapter 10 on Nutrition).

Care plan for pressure ulcers:
- Assess for pressure ulcer risk.
- Assist with frequent change of position (at least two-hourly).
- Assist with washing and choice of clothing to reduce accumulation of sweat.

Urinary tract infection

Urinary tract infection and incontinence can be distressing symptoms resulting from the stroke or its effects; thankfully, Frank Sargeant quickly regained continence following his stroke. Around 40 to 79 per cent of stroke patients experience alterations in their urinary continence to some degree in the acute stage (Patel et al, 2003) with 10–23 per cent having a longer-term problem (Patel et al, 2003). These alterations usually occur during the acute phase, and over the following subacute and rehabilitative phases; a significant number of these patients will recover their normal function with no interventions being required. Problems that might remain include urinary frequency, dysuria, urge incontinence and urinary retention.

Urinary tract infection is common in patients with reduced mobility, and particularly with those who are incontinent of urine. High standards of nursing care, paying particular attention to adequate hydration, positioning and hygiene, can help prevent urinary tract infection.

Care plan for urinary tract infection:
- Encourage fluids and initially monitor fluid intake and output.
- Monitor pattern of elimination for signs of urgency, dysuria and constipation.
- Discreetly place an urinal within easy reach, assess the patient's level of independence and assist if required.

Contractures

Contractures can be a distressing complication following stroke when the limbs contract towards the body, resulting in deformity and loss of functional ability. Contractures can be painful and once a limb is contracted, it is difficult to extend it again.

The positions outlined in Table 28.3 have been advocated following stroke in order to reduce the risk of spasticity and contractures.

These result from a consensus of opinion reached by Carr and Kenney (1992) taken from commonly used texts relating to recommended postures to be adopted following stroke. You may need to use a dictionary to identify the meaning of the anatomical terms used.

Strategic positioning will reduce the risk of contracture formation, while additionally ensuring the optimum functional position which will assist those who have the potential to make a full or near full recovery.

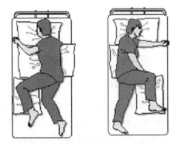

Figure 28.1 Sleep positions following stroke

© Clinical Skills Ltd.

Part

IV

Key positioning enables the patient to adopt a neutral or normal posture. The aim is to reduce spasticity and contractures by maintaining 'reflex inhibiting patterns of posture'.

Table 28.3 Consensus regarding positioning which maintains 'reflex inhibiting patterns'

Position	Lying on unaffected side	Lying on affected side	Supine-lying	Sitting-up in bed	Sitting in a chair
Part of body					
Head and neck	Neutral, symmetrical position.	Neutral, symmetrical position.	Support on pillow in 'slight' flexion.	Midline position.	Midline position.
Affected upper limb	Shoulder protracted and arm forward on pillow. Wrist in neutral position. Fingers extended. Thumb abducted.	Shoulder protracted to 90° of body if possible. Arm forward. Elbow extended. Forearm, hand supinated. Wrist neutral. Fingers extended. Thumb abducted.	Shoulder protracted and arm forward on pillow. Wrist in neutral position. Fingers extended. Thumb abducted. Thumb abducted.	Shoulder protracted and arm forward. Elbow flexed. Hand pronated. Wrist in neutral position. Fingers extended.	Shoulder protracted and arm forward. Hand pronated. Wrist in neutral position. Fingers extended. Thumb abducted.
Trunk	Straight.	Straight.	Straight.	Straight and supported by pillows.	Straight and supported.
Affected lower limb	Hip forward, flexed, supported. Knee forward, flexed supported.	Knee flexed.	Hip forward on pillow. Nothing against soles of feet.	Legs straight out in front.	Hips flexed at 90° to trunk. Knees flexed at 90° to hips. Equal weight through both hips. Feet flat on floor.
Unaffected lower limb(s)	Behind affected limb	Knee flexed? Supporting pillow.			

Source: Carr and Kenney (1992).

Care plan for contractures:

- Adhere to positioning guidelines which maintain reflex inhibiting patterns.

Shoulder pain

Shoulder pain is one consequence of the affected arm not being positioned or supported appropriately. The weight of the arm has the tendency to allow the head of the humerus to dislocate or 'subluxate' from the ball and socket joint formed with the scapula. Inappropriate moving and handling, such as repositioning the patient by using the arm as a lever, or raising the patient by gripping them either by the arm or under the arm, can cause or exacerbate the problem of shoulder pain and dislocation. Correct moving and handling techniques and correct positioning as described in the box above can help reduce the risk of these complications.

> **ⓐ Learning activity**
>
> Check the meaning of the word 'spasticity'.

Care plan for shoulder pain:
- Apply moving and handling strategies that minimise risk of shoulder injury.
- Particular care to be observed when assisting with bathing, dressing and walking practice.

a) Learning activity

Find out what is the latest local guidance for moving and handling, applied to the care of a person following stroke; and when in the practice setting, observe if these recommendations are followed. Discuss with colleagues the challenges of encouraging patient independence, while being responsible for their safety. Find out how each member of the multiprofessional team maintains their skill and keeps up to date with evidence-based practice in relation to moving and handling.

t☆ Practice tip

Throughout your healthcare career it is essential that you always keep up to date with the recommendations about moving and handling. Being appropriately assertive is an essential nursing skill, which will also enable you to ensure that those around you are also following recommendations which provide safe and effective practice in this area.

a) Learning activity

In your learning group you may like to consider how Mrs Sargeant and other family members can be directly involved to help prevent complications of stroke. Also, what about Frank's friends? What support might they need to be able to be involved? In practice observe whether relatives and friends are actively encouraged to play a part in rehabilitation. Consider the benefits and challenges.

s Scenario continued

Five days after his admission to hospital Frank is transferred to the stroke rehabilitation unit in a community hospital nearer his home, where his planned rehabilitation continues. Frank is making excellent progress, with sensation and power returning to his affected limbs. He is mobile, although he does require the use of a walking aid. He is eating well, generally caring for himself and much more optimistic about the future.

a) Learning activity

In your learning group take the opportunity to reflect back on the specific role of the nurse in Frank's rehabilitation. Look back at the different interventions that were included in his care plan. How many of these do you consider Frank's named nurse might be responsible for directly managing and evaluating?

The role of the healthcare professional in stroke rehabilitation

Research has identified specific roles for nurses and others within an increasing emphasis on interprofessional and multidisciplinary working. It is therefore essential that healthcare professionals are helped to clarify and develop a clear understanding of their specific contribution to the overall team.

Nolan and Nolan (1998a, 1998b, 1998c) found that while activities were clearly defined for the nurse in the acute setting, it is the acute-oriented physical activities that are more visibly being carried out, with the psychological, emotional and 'family' oriented aspects being less

Part
IV

well addressed. This was partly supported by O'Connor (1997) who identified that specific care in rehabilitation was care in which nurses believed that they had particular skills, above and beyond the remit of the 'average' nurse. Interventions required for caring for relatives, giving psychological care, continence care, and handling and positioning skills were areas in which they needed additional skills. However, in 1997 Kirkevold identified four specific nursing functions directly related to the nurses' role in rehabilitation, and these are set out below.

Rehabilitation nursing: four integrated nursing functions

- **Interpretative function** – Educating and supporting the patient and their carer through the delivery of the information required to understand, comprehend and make sense of the changes that have come about so suddenly as a result of their stroke. Information giving concerning stroke itself, its treatment and prognosis is seen as central to the nurse's role in this function.
- **Consoling function** – The support of the patient and their family through the emotional trauma of the stroke experience. The ability of the healthcare professional to facilitate the patients' and their carers' normal grieving process in the maintenance of hope and the prevention of depression is central to this function. People can be expected to grieve after the loss of the previously known self and loved one as a result of the stroke, and appropriate emotional care has to be planned.
- **Conserving function** – A dynamic delivery of essential care that prepares and maintains the patient in as fit a state as possible to fully partake in their rehabilitation programme. The patient can only fully partake in rehabilitation if they are as fit as possible to do so.
- **Integrative function** – Nurses and others translate the skills relearned in the therapy sessions, which usually take place in different distinct areas, to the everyday situations that patients experience. Hence patients and their carers rehearse skills in 'real' situations so that skills have a purpose; they become meaningful activities in that they can be related to the future lived experience and, if possible, integrated with a social focus (source: Kirkevold, 1997).

ⓐ Learning activity

When you have considered these empirical studies, discuss again in your learning group the role of the nurse and the other members of the caring team in stroke rehabilitation. Consider the relationship between the picture of stroke rehabilitation that you have, and that which would adequately describe rehabilitation in general.

Ⓢ Scenario continued

Frank is offered the opportunity to be assessed at home by the occupational therapist (OT), to see how he might cope and to see whether any specific equipment might need to be installed before it is safe for him to be discharged home. A convenient time is arranged with Frank's wife Joan and you (as the student) have an opportunity to go along.

ⓐ Learning activity

Discuss the following questions in your learning group:
- Consider the purpose of the home visit: what assessments may be undertaken, what recommendations made and outcomes achieved?
- Consider what anxieties the progress from hospital to home may create for Frank and his family: what services may be available to alleviate some if not all of these concerns?

- What is intermediate care, how relevant is this to Mr and Mrs Sargeant?
- What is a community rehabilitation team, what is its role in Mr and Mrs Sargeant's care at home?

Read the *National Service Framework for Older People* (DH, 2001, ch. 3), and debate its key messages.

S Scenario continued

Frank demonstrates his ability to be quite independent in most activities of living. He has, however, agreed to have his bed moved downstairs temporarily and a grab rail fitted in the downstairs shower and toilet. Luckily, there is level access to the property so no ramps or other alterations are required. Frank returns home and although he has been discharged from hospital, the policy of the stroke unit is to visit the patient and their family one month after discharge to see how things are going.

Both Frank's nurse and the OT arrange to meet Frank and his wife about a month after discharge. After the visit they record the following in Frank's notes:

20/10 4:30 p.m.
Mr Sargeant was very pleased to see us both and quickly commented that he missed the unit, especially the company of the other patients. While his wife was in the room he was cheerful and repeatedly said that things were going well. When his wife and Sarah (OT) went out to the kitchen, his mood changed and he was visibly upset. While he appreciated that his wife was doing her best, he complained that she did too much for him and that he felt that he had 'gone backwards' since he left the unit. He also mentioned that he thought his wife was tired and worried but would not say why.

Additional note by OT
In the kitchen Mrs Sargeant burst into tears and said that she did not know how much longer she would be able to cope. She had hurt her back lifting her husband out of his chair, even though she knew that he was quite capable of getting up himself. Also, she was dreadfully worried by the pressures on the rest of the family created by her having to care 24 hours a day for her husband.

Both the nurse and OT independently recorded Frank's Barthel Index as 18.

a Learning activity

Discuss the following in your learning group:
- List the problems that might have arisen since Frank's discharge.
- Reflect back on his care and think about how these problems might have been prevented.
- Consider the role of intermediate care services. Would this be an appropriate resource for Mr and Mrs Sargeant to access?

Your list may have included issues which relate to:
- caregiver burden
- caregiver burnout
- family overcompensation
- family role conflict.

a Learning activity

(Key resources: *No Secrets* (DH, 2000) and the policy on prevention of elder abuse in your local NHS Trust.)

Discuss the following in your learning group after you have answered the questions individually:
- What is elder abuse?
- How is it defined?
- What is your role in the protection of older people at risk?

S Scenario continued

The last six months have been difficult as Frank and his wife have adjusted to the fact that life has to be different. While Frank has continued with many of his interests, he finds the residual weakness in his arm and leg frustrating. Sometimes he vents his anger on the family, but they have all developed their own coping strategies. Joan has found particular support from the local branch of the Stroke Association, and although Frank is reluctant to attend she often helps out at the day centre. Frank has eventually given up smoking, which to him is a great achievement. They have also turned the downstairs dining-room into a proper bedroom; one of the things that the Sargeants were reluctant to talk about was their sexual needs. It transpired that one of the reasons for the initial lack of progress following discharge had been the need for Frank and his wife to sleep in separate rooms. They had always been sexually active and they are now happily reunited.

Within this chapter you have been introduced to a large number of concepts. Now that we have concluded our look at the experiences of Mr and Mrs Sargeant, in the final activity it is timely to invite you to reflect on the positive and negative impact that terminology has on client care.

> ## (a) Learning activity
>
> First, work individually and then discuss the following questions in your learning group.
>
>   Consider the two sets of WHO definitions below. Why might there have been a need to update these definitions between 1980 and 1999? Are there still shortcomings in the later definitions?
>
> **Rehabilitation and the World Health Organisation definitions (WHO, 1980):**
>
> **Impairment:** Any loss or abnormality of psychological, physiological or anatomical structure or function.
>
> **Disability:** Any restriction or lack (resulting from an impairment) of ability to perform an activity in the manner or within the range considered normal for a human being.
>
> **Handicap:** A disturbance for a given individual, resulting from an impairment or disability, that limits or prevents the fulfilment of a role that is normal (depending on age, sex, social and cultural factors) for that individual.
>
> **WHO International Committee on Impairment, Disability and Handicap (ICIDH) definitions (WHO, 1999)**
>
> **Impairment:** A loss or abnormality of body structure or of psychological function.
>
> **Activity:** The nature and extent of functioning at the level of the person. Activities may be limited in nature, duration and quality.
>
> **Participation:** The nature and extent of a person's involvement in life situations in relationship to impairments, activities, health conditions and contextual factors. Participation may be restricted in nature, duration and quality.
>
> **Disablement:** An umbrella term that covers all the negative dimensions (impairment, activity limitations and participation restrictions) either together or separately.

Conclusion

Through the scenario you will have experienced some of the challenges and identified some of the essential skills that nurses and other professionals use in the challenging field of rehabilitation following stroke. Many of these are to do with effective communication throughout assessment, the planning of care and its delivery. Ask any patient, or their family, what is most important to them and many will tell you that their needs are best met when professionals communicate with each other and actually work together. It will have been important to reflect on research about working in teams and how we can work together even more effectively (Davis and O'Connor, 1999).

Frank Sargeant and his family found it difficult to come to terms and adjust to the major changes to their routine following Frank's stroke. You will see the distress this caused not only in the early stages, but also later when everything seemed to be improving. This is a lesson for us all: the importance of long-term support which someone must arrange and be responsible for. It can be very convenient for planned care to just cease, and with it, all support to the client and their family. Thankfully, in Frank's case this did not happen.

We have posed many questions but by no means have we provided all the answers, for this was never the intention. Through the various activities and resources, you will have found an opportunity to explore and question the way that rehabilitation is provided and make comparisons with those services that you are familiar with.

Now reflect back on your experiences and try to answer one final question. Just what is meant by rehabilitation, and what more do you need to know?

Rererences

Baker, J. (1996) 'Shared record keeping in the multidisciplinary team', *Elderly Care* **10**(26), 39–41.

Borrie, M. J., Campbell, A. J. and Caradoc-Davies, T. H. (1986) 'Urinary incontinence after stroke: a prospective study', *Age and Ageing* **15**, 177.

Brunning, H. and Huffington, C. (1985) 'Altered images', *Nursing Times* **81**(31), 24–7.

Carr, E. K. and Kenney, F. D. (1992) 'Positioning of the stroke patient: a review of the literature', *International Journal of Nursing Studies* **29**(4), 355–69.

Davis, S. and O'Connor, S. E. (1999) *Rehabilitation Nursing: Foundations for practice*, London, Ballière Tindall.

Department of Health (DH) (1992) *The Health of the Nation*, London, HMSO.

DH (2000) *No Secrets: Guidance on developing and implementing multi-agency policies and procedures to protect vulnerable adults from abuse*, London, DH.

DH (2001) *National Service Framework for Older People*, London, TSO.

Donnan, G. A. (1992) 'Investigation of patients with stroke and transient ischaemic attacks', *The Lancet* **339**, 473–7.

Ebrahim, S., Nouri, F. and Barer, D. (1985) 'Measuring disability after stroke', *Journal of Epidemiology and Community Health* **39**, 86–9.

Forbes, E. J. and Fitzsimons, V. (1993) 'Education: the key for holistic interdisciplinary collaboration', *Holistic Nursing Practice* **7**(4), 1–10.

Fried, B. J. and Leatt, P. (1986) 'Role perception among occupational groups in an ambulatory care setting', *Human Relations* **39**(12), 1155–74.

Gibbon, B. (1991) 'Measuring stroke recovery', *Nursing Times* **87**(44), 32–4.

Gibbon, B. (1993) 'Implications for nurses in approaches to the management of stroke rehabilitation', *International Journal of Nursing Studies* **30**(2), 133–44.

Grenville, J. and Lyne, P. (1995) 'Patient-centred evaluation and rehabilitative care', *Journal of Advanced Nursing* **22**, 965–72.

Hamrin, E. (1982) 'Attitudes of nursing staff in general medical wards towards the activation of stroke patients', *Journal of Advanced Nursing* **7**, 33–42.

Kalra, L., Yu, G., Wilson, K. and Roots, P. (1995) 'Medical complications during stroke rehabilitation', *Stroke* **26**, 990–4.

Kirkevold, M. (1990) 'Caring for stroke patients: heavy or exciting?', *Journal of Nursing Scholarship* **22**(2), 79–83.

Kirkevold, M. (1997) 'The role of nursing in the rehabilitation of acute stroke patients: toward a unified theoretical perspective', *Advanced Nursing Science* **19**(4), 55–64.

Kratz, C. R. (1978) *Care of the Long-Term Sick in the Community: Particularly patients with stroke*, Edinburgh, Churchill Livingstone.

Lincoln, N. B. and Edmans, J. A. (1990) 'A re-evaluation of the Rivermead ADL Scale for elderly patients with stroke', *Age and Ageing* **19**, 19–24.

Mahoney, F. I. and Barthel, D. W. (1965) 'Functional evaluation: the Barthel Index', *Maryland State Medical Journal* **14**, 61–5.

Mant, J., Wade, D. T. and Winner, S. (2004) 'Health care needs assessment: stroke', in Stevens, A., Raftery, J., Mant, J. and Simpson, S. (eds), *Health Care Needs Assessment: The epidemiologically based needs assessment reviews*, 2nd edn, Oxford, Radcliffe Medical Press.

Mariano, C. (1989) 'The case for interdisciplinary collaboration', *Nursing Outlook* **37**(6), 285–8.

Marmot, M. G. and Poulter, N. R. (1992) 'Primary prevention in stroke', *The Lancet* **339**, 344–7.

McEwen, M. (1994) 'Promoting interdisciplinary collaboration', *Nursing and Health Care* **15**(6), 304–7.

Mullins, L. L., Keller, J. R. and Chaney, J. M. (1994) 'A systems and cognitive functioning approach to team functioning in physical rehabilitation settings', *Rehabilitation Psychology* **39**(3), 161–78.

Myco, F. (1984) 'Stroke and its rehabilitation: the perceived role', *Journal of Advanced Nursing* **9**, 437–9.

National Audit Office (NAO) (2005) *Reducing Brain Damage: Faster access to better stroke care*, London, TSO.

Nolan, M. and Nolan, J. (1998a) 'Stroke 1: a paradigm case in nursing rehabilitation', *British Journal of Nursing* **7**(6), 316–22.

Nolan, M. and Nolan, J. (1998b) 'Stroke 2: expanding the nurse's role in stroke rehabilitation', *British Journal of Nursing* **7**(7), 388–92.

Nolan, M. and Nolan, J. (1998c) 'Rehabilitation: scope for involvement in current practice', *British Journal of Nursing* **7**(9), 522–6.

O'Connor, S. E. (1993) 'Nursing and rehabilitation: the interventions of nurses in stroke patient care', *Journal of Clinical Nursing* **2**, 29–34.

O'Connor, S. E. (1997) 'An investigation to determine the nature of nursing in stroke units', unpublished PhD thesis, University of Southampton, Southampton.

Patel, M., Coshall, C., Rudd, A. G. and Wolfe, C. D. A. (2001) 'Natural history and effects on 2-year outcomes of urinary incontinence after stroke', *Stroke* **32**, 122–7.

Patrick, C. (1972) 'Forgotten patients on medical wards', *Canadian Nurse* **68**, 27–31.

Pearson, P. H. (1983) 'The interdisciplinary team process or the professional's Tower of Babel', *Developmental Medicine and Child Neurology* **25**(3), 390–5.

Power, M. L., Cross, S. P., Roberts, S. and Tyrrell, P. J. (2007) 'Evaluation of a service development to implement the top three process indicators for quality of stroke care', *Journal of Evaluation in Practice* **13**, 90–4.

Redfern, S. and Ross, M. (1999) *Nursing Older People*, 3rd edn, Edinburgh, Churchill Livingstone.

Roper, N., Logan, W. W. and Tierney, A. J. (1985) *The Elements of Nursing*, Edinburgh, Churchill Livingstone.

Royal College of Physicians (RCP) (2004) *National Clinical Guidelines for Stroke*, 2nd edn, London, RCP.

Rudd, A. G., Irwin, P., Rutledge, Z., Lowe, D., Morris, R. and Pearson, M. G. (1999) 'The national sentinel audit of stroke: a tool for raising standards of care', *Journal of the Royal College of Physicians* **30**, 460–4.

Smith, M. (1999) *Rehabilitation in Adult Nursing Practice*, Edinburgh, Churchill Livingstone.

Stockwell, F. (1972) *The Unpopular Patient*, London, Royal College of Nursing.

Strasser, D. C., Falconer, J. A. and Martino-Saltzmann, D. (1994) 'The rehabilitation team: staff perspectives of the hospital environment, and interprofessional relations', *Archives of Physical Medicine and Rehabilitation* **75**, 177–82.

Stroke Unit Trialists' Collaboration (SUTC) (1995) 'A systematic review of specialist multidisciplinary team (stroke unit) care for stroke inpatients', *The Cochrane Database of Systematic Reviews*, issue **1**.

Wade, D. T. (1988) 'Measurement in rehabilitation', *Age and Ageing* **17**, 289–92.

Waters, K. (1991) 'The role of the nurse in rehabilitation of elderly people in hospital', unpublished PhD thesis, University of Manchester, Manchester.

Waters, K. R. and Luker, K. A. (1996) 'Staff perspectives on the role of the nurse in rehabilitation wards for elderly people', *Journal of Clinical Nursing* **5**, 105–14.

Whiting, S. and Lincoln, N. (1980) 'An ADL assessment for stroke patients', *Occupational Therapy*, February, 44–6.

Wolfe, C., Rudd, A. and Beech, L. (eds) (1996) *Stroke Services and Research: An overview with recommendations for future research*, London, Stroke Association.

World Health Organisation (WHO) (1980) *International Classification of Impairments, Disabilities and Handicaps*, New York, WHO.

WHO (1999) *ICIDH-2 International Classification of Functioning and Disability: Beta 2 Draft*, New York, WHO.

Further reading

Anderson, R. (1992) *The Aftermath of Stroke*, Cambridge, Cambridge University Press. Stroke affects the personal, social, professional and family lives of patients and their carers. This book is based on a study in which 173 stroke patients and their family carers were followed from the time of the stroke for a period of 18 months. It tells of their experience of the illness and examines their patterns of coping, including physical, social, economic and emotional aspects. The book is written for all healthcare professionals involved with stroke patients and their carers, and directs attention to the practices which can improve the quality of life for people with chronic illness.

Barer, D. H. (1991) 'Stroke in Nottingham: Provision of nursing care and possible implications for the future', *Clinical Rehabilitation* **5**, 103–10. Report of a cross-sectional survey to measure the extent of the burden of stroke on health service resources. A total of 822 patients were surveyed out of a population of 700,000: 232 were in hospital (28 per cent) 221 were in nursing homes (27 per cent) and 369 at home with district nurse support (45 per cent). District nurses spend most time with the elderly, long-standing stroke patients. Increase in the proportion of elderly in the population and improvements in medical practice, which reduce fatalities in the early stages, are likely to increase the number of elderly disabled survivors.

Braithwaite, V. and McGown, A. (1993) 'Caregivers' emotional well-being and their capacity to learn about stroke', *Journal of Advanced Nursing* **18**, 195–202. Study examining the effect of distress on the capacity of informal care givers of stroke patients to absorb information about stroke and care giving. Care givers were given information at a seminar and were pre-and post-tested. Knowledge after the seminar was best predicted by age and pre-seminar knowledge. Emotional state did not affect how much they learnt, although emotional carers may be too shocked at the time. The data suggests that, given time to accept the care-giving role, emotional care givers are receptive to learning about stroke and stroke patients' needs.

Davies, S. M. (1994) 'An evaluation of nurse-led team care within a rehabilitation ward for elderly people', *Journal of Clinical Nursing* **3**, 25–33. Report of small quasi-experimental study considering the introduction of nurse-led team care against quality of care, job satisfaction, length of stay (LOS). Multimethod approach. Claims for nurse-led team care is based on time and presence with patient. Nurse-led team care improved quality, but had no effect on LOS or job satisfaction. It is still not clear how many members of a team can work effectively together nor what the mechanisms are for establishing appropriate team responsibilities and interprofessional boundaries.

Gibbon, B. (1993) 'Implications for nurses in approaches to the management of stroke rehabilitation: a review of the literature', *International Journal of Nursing Studies* **30**(2), 133–41. Literature review paper which contends that there is no generally agreed one best way to manage stroke patients. The three principle ways, that is, principles of SRU in GMW and peripatetic stroke service, are considered in the light of the implications for nurses. The author contends that understating and undervaluing nursing leads to underuse of essential resource. The findings of this paper have now been superseded by the systematic review conducted by the Stroke Unit Trialist's Collaboration.

Hamrin, E. K. F. and Lindmark, B. (1990) 'The effect of systematic care planning after acute stroke in general hospital medical wards', *Journal of Advanced Nursing* **15**, 1146–53. An experimental research project sought to determine the effect of systematic care planning on the functional outcome of stroke patients. While empirical evidence of greater satisfaction for both nurses and patients was reported, no statistically significant improvement could be found. It is noteworthy that the care plans were devised by a member of the research project group rather than the ward-based nurses.

McLean, J., Roper-Hall, A., Mayer, P. and Main, A. (1991) 'Service needs of stroke survivors and their informal carers: a pilot study', *Journal of Advanced Nursing* **16**, 559–64. Pilot study which sought to determine the needs of stroke patients and its survivors. Information was obtained about psychological, physical, social and service needs together with the feelings of stroke survivors and their informal carers. Methodology was by interview of patient and carers separately in their own homes. Research tools were refined and demonstrated several unmet needs in the psychosocial domain. Main finding was for more information about stroke and for counselling in relation to care problems arising out of the disability.

O'Connor, S. E. (1993) 'Nursing and rehabilitation: the interventions of nurses in stroke patient care', *Journal of Clinical Nursing* **2**, 29–34. This paper explores the therapeutic intervention of nurses given that it has been at the centre of debate for some time. It reviews existing (English-language) literature and concludes that the role of the nurse is still vague and that if nurses fail to define it, then others will.

Useful addresses

A cornucopia of rehabilitation information: www.codi.buffalo.edu.com
Archive of disability research: www.mailbox.ac.uk/lists-a-e/disability-research/archive.com
Association of Rehabilitation Nurses: www.rehabnurse.org/index.com
Essence of Care: patient-focused benchmarking for healthcare practitioners – www.doh.gov.uk/essenceofcare.htm
International Classification of Impairments, Activity and Participation (ICIAP): www.who.int/msa/mnh/ems/icidh/icidh.com
National Rehabilitation Information Centre: www.naric.com
National Service Framework for Older People: www.doh.gov.uk/nsf/olderpeople.htm

Stroke Forum: www.strokeforum.com
Stroke Association, CHSA House, Whitecross Street, London, EC1Y 8JJ. The Stroke Association is the only UK charitable organisation solely concerned with combating stroke. It was launched in November 1991 when the Chest, Heart and Stroke Association (CHSA) handed its work in chest and heart disease to other national charities, enabling it to concentrate on stroke. The Stroke Association sponsors programmes of research, health education and community services. The association produces a wide range of publications and cassettes in clear everyday language to help patients and carers to understand stroke and its effects.

Legislation

Mental Capacity Act 2005.

Chapter

29

Loss, grief, bereavement and palliative care

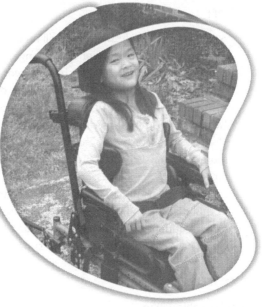

Lynda Rogers and
Pauline Turner

 Links to other chapters in *Foundation Studies for Caring*

2 Interprofessional learning
3 Evidence-based practice and
   research
5 Communication
6 Culture

9   Moving and handling
14 Pharmacology and medicines
15 Pain management
35 Complementary and alternative
    medicine

Links to other chapters in *Foundation Skills for Caring*

1   Fundamental concepts for skills
3   Communication
7   Breaking significant news
9   Patient hygiene
10 Pressure area care
12 Mouth care

28 Routes of medication
    administration
29 Patient-controlled analgesia
35 Oxygen therapy and suction
    therapy

W Don't forget to visit www.palgrave.com/glasper for additional
online resources relating to this chapter.

Part

IV

Introduction

As a healthcare professional you will meet and care for people who are experiencing loss and grief as a result of significant life changes. Colin Murray Parkes calls these 'dangerous life-change events' (1993: 91). The change might be because of a diagnosis of advanced, incurable illness; it might be because a loved one has died; it might be that someone has had to give up their home, their country or their independence; or a person might have suffered an injury (whether physical or psychological) which changes radically the way they see themselves. The way we adapt to any change throughout life can influence the way we deal with future, more substantial changes, and can also influence the way we develop our views and coping mechanisms.

This chapter defines and explores key concepts that are essential for practice when working in this challenging field. Having an understanding of some of the underpinning theory will help practitioners feel more confident and knowledgeable about providing care in situations which have the potential to be distressing and stressful.

Learning outcomes

The chapter should enable you to:

- identify how loss may affect individuals and families
- recognise the importance of self-awareness and how it may help you develop as a healthcare practitioner
- understand the principles of effective communication with the client/patient, their family and members of the healthcare team

- identify the principles of palliative and end of life care, which is about the care of people with advanced disease and who are approaching death
- consider how reflection may help us to learn and develop in our care of people at the end of their lives.

Concepts

- Palliative and end of life care
- Loss, bereavement and grief
- Self-awareness

- Reflection
- Working with families

- Communication
- Spirituality and whole person care

Health carers have contact with patients, clients and service users and their families in a variety of settings, for example in hospital, in the community, in outpatient departments and health clinics. Increasingly, they care for people with life-limiting illnesses and at the end of their lives. One of the arguments put forward by a number of researchers such as Kitson (1993) and Rogers (1992, 2002) is that students of healthcare, working with people across the lifespan who have physical, social or mental health needs, should have insight into loss and grief. This is so that they can not only provide good care, but are in some way prepared for the demands on them. They also need to know that loss and illness can affect the whole family. (In this context family does not just refer to biological family, but also to life partners, friends and significant others.)

Students of healthcare have identified feelings of stress when they feel unprepared in challenging practice situations:

> It's awful being left short of information about a patient's diagnosis.
> (a first-year healthcare student, cited in Rogers, 2002)

> When a child dies ... it's both ugly and obscene ... especially when you don't know your role in the team.
> (a nursing student, cited by Rogers, 2002)

Experiences of loss

One of the most stressful experiences a person can have is the loss of a significant person through death (Stroebe, Schut and Stroebe, 2007). However it is important to remember that people also experience major losses in ways other than by death. For example a person might lose their home or their country as a result of war or political instability. One person's adjustment to loss may be very different from another's, and is often influenced by a person's social and cultural background, the impact that the loss has on their life and the ways in which they are supported through the grieving experience (Payne, Seymour and Ingleton, 2004). It can be helpful to see loss as having two components. First, something or someone is missing – and grief, the emotional reaction to loss, is experienced (Stroebe et al, 2007); and second, changes have taken place because of the loss and a process of adjustment is needed.

The experience of loss usually affects every part of a person's life, and its effects will often be seen in some or all of their emotions, their cognitive abilities (the way they understand things), their behaviour, their physical health and well-being, their social interactions and relationships, and their spiritual and philosophical beliefs. It can also change the way a person sees the world – previously taken-for-granted views may no longer hold (Parkes, 1993). For this reason, Rogers (1992, 2002) suggests that knowing how different people may react to loss can help students and healthcare professionals to put patients', clients' and service users' (in this chapter, referred to as clients) needs as well as their own into perspective.

> Loss and grief are not signs of weakness or indulgence ... but more a sign of human need .... By developing insight into peoples' needs we can not only help the client/patient but also ourselves.
>
> (Rogers, 2002)

How loss and grief is expressed is something that is often influenced by social learning, culture, religious belief and the context in which we find ourselves. A person who is late for a bus because they cannot find the shoes they want to wear may feel a number of emotions – frustration, because they cannot find what they are looking for, and anger and perhaps blame because the shoes are not where they thought they were. Resolution may come when they decide that they have to wear another pair of shoes. If we transfer this pattern to healthcare experience, we can see how different situations may change our emotions and behaviour.

If as a healthcare professional you are with a client, for example, when they are given a life-changing diagnosis. you could feel uncomfortable or not know what to say if they turn to you for help and support. You might feel helpless or distressed, and 'at a loss for words'. You might feel angry because you feel you should not have been left to deal with this situation, or guilty because you simply do not have enough knowledge and experience to deal confidently with it. Being in a practice situation where someone appears to be looking to us for help, your actions (that is, your behaviour) might be very different from what you might do if you lost your shoes. Of course you will try to behave 'professionally', but that does not mean you will be immune from the stressful effects that such a situation brings.

Two students made these comments when confronted with situations in which they felt they did not know what to do:

> I need to know how to help people coping with bad news ... not just dying. How do I demonstrate understanding and professional caring when someone is told something they are not expecting and I just want to cry, but now I can't because John* and his family are the ones receiving the bad news, not me.
>
> (a learning disability student nurse, cited in Rogers, 1992)

> I felt awful this client was being told they had a problem and needed treatment as they had a serious mental illness .... I was angry and frightened all in one .... I thought, am I to

---

As elsewhere in this book, pseudonyms have been used to ensure confidentiality as required by the NMC *Code of Professional Conduct* (2008) and the DH *Confidentiality Code of Practice* (2003).

show sympathy, cry or not? How do I look professional when I am as scared as Simon ... and his mate?

(a first-year mental health student nurse, cited in Rogers, 2002)

A number of events can influence how we deal with a situation and express our grief. These can be classified as:

- antecedents
- concurrent social perspectives
- subsequent effects.

Antecedents

Things that have happened in the past may influence the way we deal with situations in the present:

- **Childhood experiences**. One of the earliest theorists about grief, Sigmund Freud, suggested that our childhood experiences influence our adult life (cited in Gross, 2001). If we have negative experiences during childhood, these incidents can negatively impact on the way we cope with similar issues in later life. Bowlby (1973, cited in Gross, 2001) argues that the loss of a mother during a child's early life can negatively influence the way the child copes and develops in later life. Although these theories have been disputed in a number of contemporary studies, it is still recognised that disruption of access to significant carers can still negatively affect a child's psychosocial development.
- **Previous history**. A number of studies support the idea that if a person has had a previous mental illness, loss can negatively affect the person's current mental well-being. Likewise, a person's social and cultural experience can affect the way they perceive and cope with loss and grief. A person who has a strong social network of friends and relatives may have greater opportunity to access support. Someone who does not have a strong social network might feel more isolated and withdraw further. A person's belief about their ability to talk with friends and family and be supported will also be influenced by past experiences.
- **Life crises.** Our experience of how we have dealt with crises in the past or been supported through them may influence how we adapt to change in the present.
- **Lifestyle**. Whether we have social and financial support to enable us to articulate our needs and access help will make a difference.
- **The timing of an event**. Whether it was expected or unexpected.

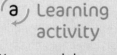

Learning activity

You can read about specific mental health illness in this context in a text such as Thomas, Hardy and Cuttings (1997).

Concurrent social perspectives

Sociologists such as Giddens (2006) argue that certain social and cultural norms can greatly influence the way a person deals with life issues. With regard to health it is suggested by Greenglass et al (cited in Sarafino, 2006) that culture and family influences as well as gender can influence the way a person deals with situations.

Therefore when considering how a person might cope with loss, a social perspective should also be taken into consideration. The following aspects may need to be considered:

- **Age.** Some people do not have to deal with their own or others' ill-health until they are well into middle age, whereas other people are familiar with life crises and family ill-health from an early age. It is recognised that over 15 per cent of primary carers (the person most likely to look after another person in their home) in the United Kingdom are children under the age of 12 (ONS, 2001).
- **Gender**. Giddens (2006) and Greenglass et al (1996, cited in Sarafino, 2006) found that men and women react differently to situations of loss. For example women, while more stoical in dealing with health issues, also express their emotions more freely. Men were found to be less willing to admit their emotions. However, each person is an individual and their needs must be viewed in relation to what else is happening in their life. It is not about generalising or stereotyping responses.

- **Personality.** Psychology theorists have been arguing about what personality is for many years. Malim and Birch (1998) suggest that personality encompasses aspects of the individual which make up the whole person. What is often referred to as 'personality' can include thinking skills, motivation, strategies adopted by the individual, the way they present their feelings, and the way they behave in a given situation. With reference to loss and grief, it is reasonable to suggest that some people present with a more extrovert or introvert personality than others. Some are open and articulate about what they are doing and how they are coping, while others may wish to say little and seek minimal or no support. Some feel that it is a good thing to seek support, while others feel that if they ask for support they will be seen as 'not coping' or 'weak'. Healthcarers should acknowledge that personality (including their own) may well influence the way a situation is managed, or how some people appear to cope and others do not.
- **Socioeconomic status.** Giddens (2006) argues that financial and social status can influence the way a person copes with a situation. For example a person may have fewer problems if they have enough money to support themselves and others during illness. Conversely, if a family is already living on social benefits the added burden of a reduced income will put a strain on the person who is ill as well as on their carers.

e Evidence-based practice

A study by Murray et al (2003) demonstrates how socioeconomic status can affect people's perspectives on priorities for healthcare. It looked at two groups of people who were terminally ill and needed healthcare intervention, one in Kenya and the other in Scotland. The study found that those from the richer socioeconomic background (in Scotland) were more focused on the psychological needs of their family and themselves, while the Kenyan patients, who generally have to pay for all their healthcare, were much more concerned with physical pain and financial issues. (A hospital stay in Kenya can cost as much as seven months of family income.)

- **Nationality and culture.** Mitchell (2002, cited in Payne, Seymour and Ingleton, 2004) argues that health carers need to understand that nationality and culture usually influence the way people respond to ill health and loss. Saunders (2000) argues that we should see some issues as being 'culturally common' and others as 'culturally specific'. If we adopt Saunders' view, we must acknowledge that all aspects of a person's culture are important to them, and seek to understand the cultural needs of each individual client. This will mean checking whether there are any specific requirements relating to cultural norms so that respect can be demonstrated and maintained in our healthcare practices.

Subsequent effects

The antecedents and concurrent social perspectives related to loss and grief can create subsequent effects. These are often manifest in:

- **Feelings of isolation.** Saunders (1960, cited in Open University, 2002) highlighted the fact that many clients feel very much alone. A person may have a lot of support and care from both professional and lay carers as well as their family and friends, but their journey can only be travelled by them, whether it involves moving from their longstanding home to a nursing home or receiving a diagnosis of a terminal disease.

Glaser and Strauss (1967) coined the phrase 'illness trajectory', when explaining the phenomena of an individual moving through the stages of well-being to ill health, and in some cases leading to palliative care and death. They wanted health carers to understand that clients have many different individual paths along this journey, and we as practitioners need to recognise the loneliness, possible stress and sometimes fear that people may experience.

Part

IV

S Scenario: Introducing Imran

Imran is 41 years old and has lived in the United Kingdom all his life. He currently lives with his elderly mother, who is his main carer. He has been having regular respite care at a social services care home in the community, about eight miles from his home, every eight weeks since his mother's health started to deteriorate six months ago.

Imran has limited cognitive ability coupled with very limited mobility, which means that he needs help to get out of bed and also with hygiene and dressing. Although he can feed himself he cannot buy his own food or cook it.

Imran's mother and her eldest son (who lives and works over 60 miles away) came with him to a multidisciplinary case conference regarding how best to support the family. Imran's mother wants him to remain at home but recognises that she can no longer give him the care he needs, so it is not possible for both of them to have a reasonable quality of life while he does so.

The professionals suggested that Imran should move to a special home in the community where both his health and his social needs can be addressed. He was assured that his mother and family would have regular contact with him.

a Learning activity

In your interprofessional learning group, discuss what Imran and his mother might be experiencing in relation to loss and grief. How would you feel if you were a member of the multidisciplinary team supporting them?

Theories and models of loss and grief

Theories and models can act as a framework to help practitioners understand what people who are undergoing loss and grief are experiencing. Here we introduce you to three of the many theories and models related to aspects of loss, grief and bereavement: 'stage' or 'phase' models (examples are Kubler-Ross, 1969, and Worden, 2003), a 'dual process' model (Stroebe and Schut, 1999), and a model based on a biographical approach.

Stage or phase models

Elizabeth Kubler-Ross developed one of the most frequently quoted models of loss and grief. She had had a great deal of experience as a young doctor working for the Red Cross towards the end of the Second World War. Her experiences during this conflict led her to undertake further studies in the United States, and she first published her findings in the late 1960s and early 1970s.

Kubler-Ross identified five stages of loss, outlined in Table 29.1.

Table 29.1 Kubler-Ross's stages of loss

Stage	Comments
Denial and isolation	The individual does not believe or accept the information given and often feels very alone and unsupported.
Anger	People often feel angry and frustrated at the situation. Common feelings and reactions are 'Why me?', 'What have I done to deserve this?' and 'It's not fair.'
Bargaining	Some people try to work through an illness or treatment option by attempting to make a pact with themselves or those who are caring for them, for example, 'If I do everything exactly as the professionals tell me, I'll get better.' It is important that healthcare practitioners recognise the need for some people to 'bargain' as a coping strategy but do not collude with it.

Stage	Comments
Depression	Practitioners need to understand the difference between 'feeling a bit down' and experiencing clinical depression. The latter needs to be recognised and treated. However, feeling low and 'depressed' may be part of a normal process for people facing loss.
Acceptance	Kubler-Ross originally suggested that in time a client will come to terms with their illness or loss and will learn to accept and adjust to their illness or deficit. However she revised her model some years later, having conducted further studies, arguing that some people may not achieve acceptance of their illness or its social, physical and psychological consequences.

Worden (2003) also presented a stage or phase model. He suggests that there are 'tasks' which help people to move on in their grief. If these tasks are completed successfully, healing can take place. If they are not completed, the healing may be incomplete. Healthcare professionals and counsellors who have insight into these 'tasks of grieving' will be able to facilitate people's journey through the grieving process.

Table 29.2 Worden's 'tasks of grieving'

Tasks of mourning	Description
1 Accept the reality of loss	Intellectual and emotional acceptance of loss
2 Work through the pain of grief	Experience of painful feelings
3 Adjust to the environment without the deceased (or body change)	Adjustments to change in circumstances/role(s)
4 Emotionally relocate loss and move on	Find a place for the deceased within. Letting go of feelings. Invest in future.

Source: Worden (2003).

Some people argue that the stage/phase models of loss and grief contain an assumption that distress and depression is always likely, when this is clearly not always the case. Many people deal with grief in their own individual, unique way. They argue that the idea of people grieving in 'stages' is fundamentally flawed from a research perspective because it is almost impossible to measure human responses to situations of loss. However, qualitative researchers could argue that responses can be measured by using a research approach that involves discussion or narrative about people's experiences and feelings.

The dual process model

It is important to compare models and theories of loss and grief in the context of our practice. The dual process model developed by Stroebe and Schut (1999) has an interesting approach. This model suggests that people do not experience loss and grief in a linear or phased way, but some have 'loss-oriented' coping strategies and others have more 'restoration-oriented' ones. Loss orientation will involve activities that have traditionally been associated with the 'tasks of grieving' concept: for example, going over events, crying, and getting in touch with a whole range of emotions. A restoration-oriented approach suggests that coping with grief does not occupy all of a bereaved person's time. It is embedded in everyday life experience which involves taking time off from grieving. Activities will involve focusing on what needs to be dealt with and how: for example, 'getting back to normal', returning to work and so on. Most people oscillate between the two methods of coping: at times they will be confronted by their loss and at other times they will avoid memories and seek distraction (Stroebe and Schut, 1999).

Part

IV

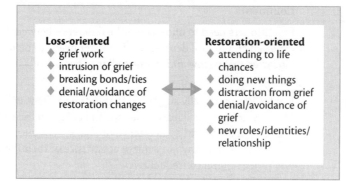

Loss-oriented
♦ grief work
♦ intrusion of grief
♦ breaking bonds/ties
♦ denial/avoidance of restoration changes

Restoration-oriented
♦ attending to life chances
♦ doing new things
♦ distraction from grief
♦ denial/avoidance of grief
♦ new roles/identities/relationship

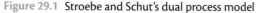

Figure 29.1 Stroebe and Schut's dual process model

Source: Stroebe and Schut (1999).

You may find that in your own experience you have perceived people grieving differently. Some people will want to return to 'normal' life as quickly as possible, and may resist others' efforts to engage them in conversations about the loss. Others will need to spend much more time talking through the circumstances that surrounded the loss and expressing emotion. Our intention is to make you aware of different theories of loss and grief, and enable you to consider how people, including yourself, react to different situations.

Learning activity

There is further reading related to the Stroebe and Schut model in Walker et al (2004).

The biographical model

Tony Walters' biographical model (1996) takes an entirely different approach to supporting people experiencing loss and grief. His work suggests that a person needs opportunities to explore the story of a deceased person's life. By doing this the sense of who that person was will increase and grow richer, with an accompanying diminution of the sense of loss.

Key features of Walters' thesis are that:
- telling the story provides an opportunity for the person to communicate their feelings
- using prompts enables the person to reconstruct the situation, for example how they felt when they received their diagnosis, the emotions experienced regarding a lost body part, or change to body function or image
- giving the person an opportunity to build up a 'bigger picture' of the situation, or a person who has died, enables them to begin to see the major issues and opportunities for change
- this construction, deconstruction and reconstruction can enable the person to explore the issue and go forward having found an 'end', or having decided where that experience or person will be in their memories.

Many people with advanced incurable disease experience huge loss, as do their families. The principles of palliative care, both as a specialty and as part of general clinical care, are hugely important for providing quality care for people who are approaching the end of their lives.

Palliative care

Palliative care as we know it today developed from the modern hospice movement, which was pioneered among others by Cicely Saunders, who wrote some of the earliest articles about care of the dying (Clark, 1997). In the 1980s palliative nursing became a specialty, and in 1985 the Association of Palliative Medicine for Great Britain was formed (Gamlin, 2001). Since then it has developed rapidly as a global concern, and presents some challenging issues particularly for developing countries (Gamlin, 2001).

> ### (a) Learning activity   W
>
> As part of your interprofessional learning group visit the International Observatory on End of Life Care website for information about the programmes and projects in palliative care that are being undertaken in different parts of the world: http://www. eolc-observatory.net

According to the World Health Organization (WHO, cited in Sepulveda et al, 2002), palliative care is:

> an approach that improves the quality of life of patients and their families facing the problems associated with life-threatening illness, through the prevention and relief of suffering by means of early identification and impeccable assessment and treatment of pain and other problems, physical, psychosocial and spiritual.

In other words, it is about providing care that means a person is able to get the most out of life from the time that they are diagnosed with a life-threatening illness until their death. It will involve looking at the needs of those closest to the patient – family and carers– and providing care in the place of choice where possible. The key principles of palliative care include:

- emphasis on quality of life, including good symptom control
- respect for patient autonomy and choice
- a holistic approach
- care of the dying person and those who matter to that person
- open and sensitive communication with patients, their informal carers and professional colleagues
- support for patient and family through the dying process and subsequent bereavement (adapted from NCPC, 2007).

All healthcare professionals need to subscribe to the philosophy of palliative care, and embrace it as part of their everyday practice with people who are approaching the end of their lives (Gamlin, 2001). Some people, however, will need referral to specialist palliative care services, which are for people with moderate to high complexity of need. These include in-patient units (hospices or palliative care units), hospital palliative care teams, community palliative care teams and palliative care day units. Most teams provide care for cancer patients and other people suffering with advanced illness, such as motor neurone disease and end-of-life cardiac and respiratory diseases (NCPC, 2007).

> ### (a) Learning activity   W
>
> In your interprofessional learning group, find out whether there is a specialist palliative care team in the area where you work. What is the role of individual members of the team? How is the team contacted?
>
> You may find it very useful to negotiate to spend some time with individuals in the team.
>
> For more information and definitions on palliative care visit the National Council for Palliative Care's website: http://www.ncpc.org.uk/palliaitve_care.html, and the NHS website on end-of-life care: http://endoflifecare.nhs.uk

Palliative care in the acute setting

Most people are cared for at the end of their lives in a hospital or other acute setting, although they may have spent a good part of the last year of their life at home or in another care setting. Studies by Skilbeck, Small and Ahmedzai (1999) and Gott, Ahmedzai and Wood (2001) suggest that a relatively high number of patients in the hospital setting will have palliative care needs. This presents a challenge for professionals on many fronts, and some of the studies that have looked at patient and family experiences in hospital have highlighted deficiencies in care (Rogers, Karlsen and Addington-Hall, 2000; Dunne and Sullivan, 2000).

Part

IV

It is possible that you will experience some negative experiences when caring for dying people. Here is an incident taken from a reflective account by a student, which illustrates how the reality of practice may be much less desirable than expected. This is what Johns (2000) calls the 'conflict of contradiction' through which the nurse may sometimes have to work to achieve 'desirable work':

> Alf was alone, MRSA positive, in a side room, and dying of cancer. There were no beds at the local hospice and he had no nearby relatives. When I came on night duty he was struggling to breathe and obviously distressed. The ward was quiet so I went and sat by him and held his hand. He linked his hand with mine.
>
> The night nurse came around and called me out of the side room and said, 'You shouldn't sit with him like that; you have to be careful because it makes people more frightened.' I felt hurt and angry that I was being told off for performing what I considered to be a nursing duty of care. I knew I wouldn't want to die alone in the night in a hospital side room.
>
> I have concluded that the night nurse wasn't good at handling patient deaths. I still to this day cannot see where I went wrong; after all, the ward was quiet and nothing else needed doing at that point in time. The others were sitting chatting and eating Pringles at the nursing station. The patient seemed comforted by my presence and I wasn't getting emotionally involved.
>
> If this situation arose again I would question the reason why what I was doing was wrong, and argue diplomatically that I believe sitting with someone whilst alone and dying is a duty of care and compassion. Both of these components are basic nursing principles.

By reflecting on the incident and thinking through her own values and beliefs, and her commitment to good care, and by also reflecting on what might have been influencing the other nurse, this student came to a position of more confidence about her own stance. She felt that if the situation arose again she would be more confident in standing by what she believed was good care.

Palliative care at home

Most people if given the choice would probably prefer to die at home, and so the support of family care givers becomes paramount. Although death is arguably becoming less of a taboo subject, many people will not have seen a death before, and need information and support about what to expect during the last stage of living. Many people are also cared for in residential and nursing homes, and the support and education of their staff is vital (Sidell, Katz and Komaromy, 2000; Katz, Komaromy and Sidell, 2000).

W

The Gold Standards Framework (GSF) (www.goldstandardsframework.nhs.uk) is a systematic evidence-based approach to optimising the care of people nearing the end of their lives in the community. It is concerned with helping people to live well until the end of life, and includes care in the final year of life for people with any end-stage illness in the community (GSF, 2005).

Working with the whole family

The diagnosis of a life-threatening illness will undoubtedly impact the family in many ways, not least in the family's ability to function normally. Writing about cancer, Colin Murray-Parkes suggests that it 'can affect a family in much the same way as it affects a body, causing

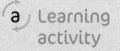

Learning activity

In your own field of practice learning group, think of what some of the challenges are in meeting the needs of the whole person in busy, acute settings.

Read Vanessa Taylor's chapter, 'Acute hospital care', in Payne et al (2004).

deterioration if left untreated' (cited in Monroe and Sheldon, 2004: 405). Working with the whole family is an essential component of preventive healthcare, and this involves helping the family think about what resources they already have and where they may need support, as well as giving information which enables them to make decisions, and helps them regain control where possible (Monroe and Sheldon, 2004).

(e) Evidence-based practice

A diagnosis of cancer not only impacts upon the identity of the patient but also affects the identities of their families and close social contacts (Lugton, 1997). Research suggests that family functioning helps to determine the outcome: that family dysfunction leads to increased rates of psychosocial morbidity in the bereaved (Kissane et al, 1997). Relatives' greatest support comes from seeing the patient being well cared for, with their symptoms adequately controlled (McIntyre, 2002).

The importance of assessment

All patients, but especially patients with advanced disease, benefit from a holistic assessment of needs. This should take into account the whole person, and develop an understanding of their needs, wishes and views, linking these to what can be offered and the skills available (Oliviere, Hargreaves and Monroe, 1998). Monroe and Sheldon (2004) suggest that assessment needs to focus on the individual, the family and those close to the individual, the physical resources available and the social resources, including cultural and spiritual aspects. There is evidence that what happens to the dying person affects the family and vice versa, and so good care must include an assessment of how the family is functioning (Monroe and Sheldon, 2004). Payne and colleagues (2004) make the point that people who are experiencing loss and change usually have families and friends, and so care needs to start from this socially embedded standpoint. In other words the patient should never be seen in isolation, but always within the context of their family and/or social network.

(s) Scenario: Introducing Harry

Harry is a 30-year-old adult with a severe learning disability. He was diagnosed with a degenerative neurological disorder some years ago, and had a percutaneous endoscopic gastrostomy (PEG) inserted recently because of his swallowing difficulties. He has recently been admitted to a medical unit, having pulled the PEG out. Some of the nurses on the unit think he did this deliberately because he no longer wants to live. Following a team discussion the medical staff decide that the tube will not be reinserted, as Harry's condition has deteriorated substantially and his quality of life appears to be poor. However, some of his family are very upset by this decision, and feel that he should be given 'every chance' to survive.

(a) Learning activity

In your field of practice learning group, discuss:
- How are end of life decisions made in practice?
- Who should be involved?
- What key areas need to be covered when assessing Harry and his family's needs?

t Practice tip

The assessment of Harry and his family should include enquiry about the following areas:
- Harry's physical needs: his symptoms, comfort, quality of life, the progression of his disease, its possible treatment and prognosis.
- Both Harry's and his family's psychological and emotional needs.
- Harry's spiritual needs.
- Support within the family.

Part

IV

Care of people's spiritual needs

When someone becomes ill, and especially at the end of life, they may need to explore ultimate questions about meaning and purpose, life and death, and relationships, both with the transcendent – something or someone beyond themselves (God or a Higher Being) – and with other people. When someone is approaching death they need to be cared for in an environment which acknowledges the spiritual aspects of a person's existence, acknowledges what is important to them and takes into account their religious and spiritual needs. The International Council of Nurses' *Code of Ethics* (2000) and the revised *Patient's Charter* (DH, 2001) put spirituality firmly in the realm of professional practice. It is thus very important that healthcare professionals understand what constitutes spiritual care and how it can be provided.

Lugton and Kindlen (1999) suggest that important questions which many see as fundamental to spirituality are 'Who am I?' and 'What am I?' These questions are dynamic throughout a person's life, and are contextualised within their culture, beliefs, relationships, identity and their overall understanding of what it means to be human.

Wright's study (2002) attempted to clarify and define spirituality. From his data five key domains emerged as follows:

- personhood: values, beliefs, achievements
- relationships: with self, others, the universe, a 'life force' or God
- religion: prayer, vocation, commitment and worship
- search for meaning: the 'big questions' of life and death, mortality
- transcendence: something beyond/something within.

Participants in his study included representatives of major world faiths and those of no faith, but what was clear was that the concept of spirituality was meaningful to all, whether they had a religious belief or not. This would confirm the importance of taking spirituality into account in care. At the end of their lives, people may need opportunities to explore these questions and reassess their beliefs (Hardwig, 2000).

Whatever people's beliefs, an important part of spiritual care is to spend time with someone in a way that strengthens and comforts them. Robinson, Kendrick and Brown (2003: 20) describe the experience of a seriously ill patient in intensive care who was unable to 'connect' with the nurse who was attending her at a crucial moment when terror had overtaken her on waking from a nightmare. The nurse's main concern, as perceived by the patient, was with monitoring the machines and supplying medicines – 'doing to' rather than 'being with.' The patient's recovery was significantly aided the next day, however, by the arrival of the hospital chaplain, who took her hand and spent time with her. The value of the ability to 'be present' with another in time of stress or difficulty cannot be overestimated (Nouwen, 1979), but it requires courage and self-awareness.

Healthcare professionals need to understand that for many people religious belief and ritual plays a very important part of their lives. You might or might not have any particular religion or belief system yourself, however it is very important that you recognise the role of religion and make every effort to gain insight and knowledge into the major religions of the world. You do not necessarily have to agree with the belief systems of your clients, but you do need to demonstrate respect and understanding of their needs, and the demands that their religion makes of them and their family. Our role is to provide for the religious requirements of people we are caring for within realistic boundaries.

Effective communication

One of the key skills in working with patients and families, as well as with other healthcare team members, is effective communication. Being able to reflect on the way you communicate with patients and families will help to highlight where communication enhances or hinders patient support.

Much has been written about the importance of good communication when caring for patients with cancer and their families. The challenge is to enter into open and honest dialogue in a way that enables them to express their anxieties and fears. This requires the development of good communication skills, which means paying attention to your nonverbal messages (body language), and the use of verbal skills such as active listening, open questioning and reflecting back to the patient an understanding of what they have said.

Effective communication requires courage, sensitivity, and a high level of self-awareness. Maguire (1999) suggests that there are barriers to effective communication. Some of these are 'patient-led' in that the patient does not wish to disclose their concerns, for any of a variety of reasons. Others are 'professional-led', and include behaviours like avoidance of emotionally focused questions, fear of releasing strong emotion or staying with uncertainty, lack of communication skills and lack of support.

(a) Learning activity

In your interprofessional learning group think about `avoidance' in communication. Consider any ways in which you have personally avoided certain responses from patients, and the reasons you have done so.

(c) Professional conversation

Callum and Geeta, two students, reflect on communication with a patient after reading Maguire's paper (1999).

Callum comments, 'I know I've avoided effective communication with a patient. I asked a patient how he was feeling yesterday and he replied, "Rough." Without thinking I continued, "But that pain in your leg is a lot better today, isn't it?" He muttered his agreement and went back to reading his paper. I was doing something else at the time and was relieved not to have to continue the conversation with him. But later when I thought about this incident I realised that I had switched the focus from an emotional one (how he was feeling) to a physical one (his pain), and had effectively avoided further conversation with him on this matter.'

Geeta says, 'I know what you mean. I was talking to a patient who was waiting to have a fairly unpleasant procedure performed. She told me she was feeling very anxious about it, and I said something to the effect that it was "fairly normal to feel like that". When I read Maguire's paper I realised that I had not wanted to hear how she was really feeling, in case her anxiety increased. By reassuring the patient that it was normal for her to feel like that, but without hearing her out and finding out what her anxieties really were, I'd practised avoidance. I hope that by reflecting on incidents like this I'll be more aware of my own communication with patients, and will listen more attentively to what they're saying.'

t☆ Practice tip

It is important that not only family and friends of the client, but also all members of the healthcare team, are able to express their thoughts and feelings.

Conclusion

While working through this chapter, many issues will have arisen for you about caring for people who are experiencing loss and/or a life-threatening illness. All have particular nursing needs, and the same principles of holistic care must be considered whether the person is in hospital, in a hospice, or is being nursed at home, to ensure that the best quality of life is attained for each individual.

Loss and grief raise professional and personal issues for all members of the healthcare team, who need to support each other as well as the patient and family. Perhaps you have been able to relate to the practice examples given in this chapter, and have reflected on your experiences to date of caring for people experiencing a great loss, for example loss of a limb or coping with terminal illness. You may wish to consider your own deficits in knowledge and understanding, and plan how you can access both information and support. Using a reflective tool may help you to review your own practice and highlight possible areas to further develop self-awareness, so you can care for people as effectively as possible in such challenging situations.

References

Clark, D. (1997) 'Someone to watch over me', *Nursing Times* **93**(34), 50–2.

Department of Health (DH) (1991, rev. 1995) *The Patients' Charter and You: A charter for England*, London, DH.

DH (2003) *Confidentiality Code of Practice* [online] www.dh.gov.uk/ipu/confident/protect/ (accessed 23 January 2009).

Dunne, K. and Sullivan, K. (2000) 'Family experiences of palliative care in the acute setting', *International Journal of Palliative Nursing* **6**(4), 170–8.

Fallowfield, L. (2004) 'Communication and palliative medicine', in Doyle et al (eds), *Oxford Textbook of Palliative Medicine*, 3rd edn, Oxford, Oxford University Press.

Gamlin, R. (2001) 'Palliative nursing: past, present and future', pp. 3–12 in Kinghorn, S. and Gamlin, R. (eds), *Pallative Nursing: Bringing comfort and hope*, London, Baillière Tindall.

Giddens, A. (2006) *Sociology*, Cambridge, Polity Press.

Glaser, B. G. and Strauss, A. L. (1967) *Time for Dying*, Chicago, Ill., Aldine Press.

Gott, C. M., Ahmedzai, S. H. and Wood, C. (2001) 'How many inpatients at an acute hospital have palliative care needs? Comparing the perspectives of medical and nursing staff', *Palliative Medicine* 15, 451–60.

Gross, R. (2001) *Psychology: The science of mind and behaviour*, 4th edn, London, Hodder & Stoughton.

Gold Standards Framework (GSF) (2005) reference to follow

Hardwig, J. (2000) 'Spiritual issues at the end of life: a call for discussion', *Hastings Center Report* **30**(2), 28–30.

International Council of Nurses (ICN) (2000) *Code of Ethics for Nurses*, Geneva, ICN.

Jarret, N. and Maslin-Prothero, S. (2004) 'Communication, the patient and the palliative care team', in Payne, S., Seymour, J. and Ingleton, C. (eds), *Palliative Care Nursing: Principles and evidence for practice*, Milton Keynes, Open University Press.

Johns, C. (2000) *Becoming a Reflective Practitioner*, Oxford, Blackwell.

Katz, J. T., Komaromy, C. and Sidell, M. (2000) 'Death in homes: bereavement needs of residents, relatives and staff', *International Journal of Palliative Nursing* **6**(6), 274–9.

Kinghorn, S. and Gamlin R. (2001) 'Promoting hope through meaningful communication', pp.115–96 in *Palliative Nursing: Bringing comfort and hope*, London, Baillière Tindall.

Kissane, D. W., Bloch, S., McKenzie, M., McDowall, A. C. and Nitzan, R. (1998) 'Family grief therapy: a preliminary account of a new model to promote healthy family functioning during palliative care and bereavement'. *Psycho-oncology* 7, 14–25.

Kitson, A. (1993) *Nursing: Art and science*, London, Chapman Hall.

Kubler Ross, E. (1969) *On Death and Dying*, New York, Macmillan.

Lugton, J. (1997) 'The nature of social support as experienced by women treated for breast cancer', *Journal of Advanced Nursing* 25, 1184–91.

Lugton, J., Frost, D. and Scavizzi, S. (2005) 'Communication and support in palliative care', in Lugton, J. and McIntyre, R. (eds), *Palliative Care: The nursing role*, 2nd edn, Edinburgh, Elsevier Churchill Livingstone.

Lugton, J. and Kindlen, M. (**1999**) *Palliative Care: The nursing role*, Edinburgh, Churchill Livingstone.

Maguire, P. (1999) 'Improving communication with cancer patients', *European Journal of Cancer* **35**(10),1415–22.

Malim, T. and Birch, A. (1998) *Introductory Psychology*, Basingstoke, Macmillan.

McIntyre, R. (2002) *Nursing Support for Families of Dying Patients*, London, Whurr.

Mitchell, K.(2002) *Medical Decisions at the End of Life that Hasten Death*, Ph.D. thesis, University of Auckland.

Monroe, B. and Sheldon, F. (2004) ''Psychosocial dimensions of care', in Sykes, N., Edmonds P. and Wiles, J. (eds), *Management of Advanced Disease*, 4th edn, London, Arnold.

Murray Parkes, C. (1993) 'Bereavement as a psychosocial transition: processes of adaptation to change', in Stroebe, M., Stroebe, W. and Hansson, R. (eds), *Handbook of Bereavement: Theory, research and intervention*, Cambridge, Cambridge University Press.

Murray, S. A., Grant, E., Grant, A. and Kendal, A.(2003) 'Dying from cancer in developed and developing countries: lessons from two qualitative interview studies of patients and their carers', *British Medical Journal* 7385, 326–68.

National Council for Palliative Care (2007) General information [online] http://www.ncpc.org.uk (accessed 8 January 2009).

Nouwen, H. (1979) *The Wounded Healer*, New York, Image Books.

Nursing and Midwifery Council (2008) *The Code: standards of conduct, performance and ethics for nurses and midwives*, London, NMC.

Office for National Statistics (2001) Census data for 2001 [online] http://www.statistics.gov.uk/census2001/access_results.asp (accessed 3 October 2008).

Oliviere D., Hargreaves R. and Monroe B. (1998) (2000) *Good Practices in Palliative Care: A psychosocial perspective*, place?, Ashgate Arena.

Open University Course Team (2002) *Health and Disease*, Book 5, Milton Keynes, Open University Press.

Parkes, C. M. (1993) 'Bereavement as a psychosocial transition: processes of adaptation to change', in Stroebe, M., Schut, H. and Stroebe, W. (eds), *Handbook of Bereavement: Theory, research and intervention*, New York, Cambridge University Press.

Pattison, R. (2001) 'Dumbing down the spirit' in Orchard, H. (ed.), *Spirituality in Health Care Contexts*, London, Jessica Kingsley.

Payne, S., Seymour, J. and Ingleton, C. (eds) (2004) *Palliative Care Nursing: Principles and evidence for practice*, Milton Keynes, Open University Press.

Robinson, S., Kendrick, K. and Brown, A. (2003) *Spirituality and the Practice of Healthcare*, Basingstoke, Palgrave Macmillan.

Rogers, A., Karlsen, S. and Addington-Hall, J. M. (2000) '''All the services were excellent. It was when the human element comes in that things go wrong'': dissatisfaction with hospital care in the last year of life', *Journal of Advanced Nursing* **31**(4), 768–74.

Rogers, L. (1992) *Dying Needs*, unpublished research Masters dissertation, University of Portsmouth

Rogers, L. (2002) *Actioning Curriculum Change: A collaboration with student nurses in developing an introductory programme regarding aspects of loss grief and bereavement with students*, unpublished

Ph.D. thesis, University of Southampton.

Sarafino, E. P. (2006) *Health Care Psychology: Bio-psychosocial interactions*, 5th edn, New York, John Wiley.

Saunders, C. (2000) 'The evolution of palliative care', *Patient Education and Counselling* 41, 7–13.

Sepulveda, C., Marlin, A., Yoshida, T. and Ullrich, A. (2002) 'Palliative care: the World Health Organisation's global perspective', *Journal of Pain and Symptom Management* 24(2), 91–6.

Sheldon, F. (1997) *Psychosocial Palliative Care*, London, Stanley Thornes.

Sheldon, F. (2004) 'Communication', in Sykes, N., Edmonds P. and Wiles, J. (eds), *Management of Advanced Disease*, 4th edn, London, Arnold.

Sidell, M., Katz, J. T. and Komaromy, C. (2000) 'The case for palliative care in residential and nursing homes', in Dickenson, S., Johnson, M. and Katz, J. S. (eds), *Death, Dying and Bereavement*, London. Sage.

Skilbeck, J., Small, N. and Ahmedzai, S. H. (1999) 'Nurses' perceptions of specialist palliative care in an acute hospital', *International Journal of Palliative Nursing* 5(3), 110–15.

Stroebe M. S. and Schut, H. (1998) 'Culture and grief', *Bereavement Care* 17(1), 7–10.

Stroebe, M. and Schut, H. (1999) 'The dual process model of coping with bereavement: rationale and description', *Death Studies* 23, 197–224.

Stroebe, M., Schut, H. and Stroebe, W. (2007) 'Health outcomes of bereavement', *The Lancet* 370(8 December), 9603–73.

Stuart, G. W and Sundeen, F. J. (1997) *Mental Health for Nursing: Principles and practice*, Washington, CV Mosby.

Thomas, B., Hardy, S. and Cuttings, P. (eds) (1997) *Stuart and Sundeen's Mental Health for Nursing*, London, Mosby Press.

Wakefield, ? (1993) 'Spirituality', in Payne, S., Seymour, J. and Ingleton, C. (eds), (2004) *Palliative Care Nursing: Principles and evidence for practice, Milton Keynes*, Open University Press.

Walker, J., Payne, S., Smith, P. and Jarrett, N. (2004) *Psychology for Nursing and the Caring Professions*, 2nd edn, Milton Keynes, Open University Press.

Walters, T. (1996) 'A new model of grief: bereavement and biography', *Mortality* 1(1), 7–25.

Worden, J. W. (2003) *Grief Counselling and Grief Therapy*, 3rd edn, London, Routledge.

Wortman, C. B. and Silver, R. C. (1989) 'The myths of coping with loss', *Journal of Consulting and Clinical Psychology* 57(3), 349–57.

Wright, M. C. (2002) 'The essence of spiritual care: a phenomenological enquiry', *Palliative Medicine* 16: 125–32.

Chapter

30

Emergency care and interventions

Jessica Knight and Rachel Palmer

Links to other chapters in *Foundation Studies for Caring*

3	Evidence-based practice and research	14	Pharmacology and medicines
5	Communication	31	Child emergency care and resuscitation
6	Culture	32	Adult emergency care and resuscitation
9	Moving and handling		

Links to other chapters in *Foundation Skills for Caring*

1	Fundamental concepts for skills	20	Neurological assessment
7	Breaking significant news	28	Routes of medication administration
9	Patient hygiene		
16	Vital signs	36	Basic life support: child
17	Blood pressure	37	Basic life support: adult
18	Pulse oximetry		

W Don't forget to visit www.palgrave.com/glasper for additional online resources relating to this chapter.

Introduction

This chapter focuses on the nursing care and interventions for a patient following a minor head injury. The scenario describes the typical emergency care and interventions for a person in this situation. Evidence-based practice (EBP) is the key to clinical effectiveness (Le May, 1999), and should be used by all health professionals. Guidelines such as NICE (2007) offer a concise insight into the assessment and management of head injury across the age span. Other documents and publications can always be used for a deeper knowledge base. EBP and sequential management are explored at each stage of the patient journey. The chapter covers initial assessment strategies through to discharge planning, incorporating health education to promote a return to a normal lifestyle. A sound underpinning knowledge of anatomy and physiology is fundamental to the chapter; you need to understand the normal physiology in order to appreciate the abnormalities caused by trauma or disease processes.

Learning outcomes

This chapter will enable you to:

- develop an understanding of how the underpinning knowledge relates to the components of neurological assessment
- consider the evidence base surrounding patient management
- explore aspects of decision making in relation to the neurological patient, such as frequency of observations, investigations, admission and discharge criteria

- develop an understanding of the signs and symptoms of raised intracranial pressure and other secondary complications which might impact on neurological function
- develop an understanding of the structure and function of the nervous system.

Concepts

- Initial assessment and observation
- Altered consciousness
- Defining head injury and NICE guidelines
- Concussion
- Point of injury assessment and decision making

- Assessment: Glasgow Coma Scale and AVPU
- Consciousness and altered levels
- Neurological assessment procedures
- Recognition of neurological deterioration and secondary complications

- Health education on cycle helmets
- Discharge advice
- Neurological anatomy and physiology

S   Scenario: Introducing Tom

Tom Hardy is a 19-year-old man who currently lives at home with his parents. He is about to leave home to start his university studies, where he will be living in a hall of residence. Tom is the only child of Helen and Ian Hardy, who are in their 50s and work full-time running the family business, a cycle shop.

During his gap year Tom took a part-time job at a local nature reserve where he was able to learn more about the environment, which will be the focus of his studies, and use his bicycle to get around. When the other rangers were cycling back to the rangers' hut for the regular morning meeting, they noticed that Tom was not with them.

This was very unusual as Tom was always punctual. They attempted to call him on his mobile but there was no reply. After five minutes there was still no sign of him, so a ranger, Kristof, went to check the route he would have taken.

Kristof found Tom sitting on the ground, rubbing the side of his head with his hand. Blood was trickling done the side of his face. Kristof immediately made contact with the base and warned them that Tom appeared dazed. An ambulance was called. Kristof sat down next to Tom to wait for further support and the ambulance crew.

The ambulance arrived quickly and the crew asked Tom what had happened to him, and whether he thought he

Part

IV

had lost consciousness. 'I was distracted by something in the trees,' Tom said, 'and I hit a rock. I remember coming over the handlebars and hitting the ground. I'm not sure how long ago it happened, but it wasn't long, maybe ten minutes.' The bicycle and Tom's helmet were nearby. Kristof checked them and found that the front wheel was buckled and his helmet was scratched and appeared cracked on the front.

The ambulance crew were concerned that Tom might have had a loss of consciousness, so they completed a neurological assessment.

Initial observations

The term 'neurological assessment' refers to a series of physical observations, comprising the Glasgow Coma Scale (GCS), vital signs (temperature, blood pressure, pulse and respiratory rate), pupil size and reaction to light; limb strength (power)/movement and sensation if required.

Altered consciousness refers to a transient period of time, ranging from seconds or minutes to hours, where the patient is unresponsive to sensory stimuli including auditory, visual, tactile and olfactory stimuli. They appear to be in a sleeplike, relaxed state but cannot be woken or roused. A person who is asleep can by contrast be roused by stimuli.

> ### ⓐ Learning activity
>
> Discuss with your peers, colleagues and other members of your multidisciplinary team what phrases or terminology they have heard or used to describe a loss of consciousness. Put the terms they come up with into an internet/database search engine and see what information comes up.

> ### ⒮ Scenario continued
>
> On arrival at the hospital Accident and Emergency department (A&E), the ambulance crew report that:
> - Tom has sustained a laceration to the left side of his head above his eye, and bruising and grazes to the left side of his body.
> - His GCS score at the scene was noted to be 13/15.
> - There was no witness to his accident: query loss of consciousness.
> - The ranger at the scene believed Tom had been 'knocked out' after talking to Tom about the accident.
>
> On initial assessment, following admission to hospital, Tom still has a GCS of 13/15. He complains of a headache, nausea and some dizziness. His vital signs are BP 105/70; pulse 65 bpm; respiratory rate 16 bpm; O$_2$ saturations 99 per cent on air; temperature 36.3 °C. A bloodstained gauze dressing is noted to be in place over his left temporal region. He has minor cuts and abrasions on his hands and forearms, and his shirt is ripped over his left shoulder.

> ### ⒞ Professional conversation
>
> Student nurse Lahti comments, 'I read the ambulance crew's report and noted that the ranger was concerned that Tom might have been "knocked out". My mentor explained to me that although lay people use terms like "knocked out" or "passed out", as healthcare professionals we refer to a loss or altered level of consciousness (LOC). This is potentially a serious medical condition which requires detailed and continuing assessment for a given period of time, so that's why following a minor head injury patients require hospitalisation or supervision at home.'

A large number of people have head injuries each year. Trauma is the leading cause of death in the first four decades of life, and head injury accounts for at least 50 per cent of these (Hutchinson and Kirkpatrick, 2002). 'Head injury' (HI) is defined as any trauma to the head, other than superficial injuries to the face (NICE, 2007). The most common reasons for these injuries are falls, road traffic accidents (RTAs), assaults such as fights (NICE, 2007) and occupational accidents. In the elderly, falls are a more common cause, and in younger patients RTAs (Evans, 2007). Alcohol is detectable in up to 60 per cent of patients hospitalised following HI, especially in younger people (Greenwood, 2002). From a gender perspective males are more likely to suffer from a mild HI, with a two to one ratio over females, and approximately half of all patients with mild HI are between 15 and 34 years old (Evans, 2007). A mild HI refers to someone with a GCS of 13–15 post trauma (see Table 30.1). A lower socio-economic status is a recognised risk factor for head injury (Evans, 2007).

Table 30.1 The Glasgow Coma Scale

Head Injury Grading	
Mild HI	GCS 13–15
Moderate	GCS 9–12
Severe	GCS 3–8

Sources: Greenwood (2002), Hickey (2003).

The scalp and skull absorb much of the impact when the head is hit, making a severe injury to the brain unusual. Less than one in a hundred of all head injuries involves a severe injury to the brain, and around 90 per cent are mild or minor head injuries (NICE, 2007). Hutchinson and Kirkpatrick (2002) highlight that annually in the United Kingdom 1500 per 100,000 of the population (a total of 1 million people) attend A&E departments with a head injury. Approximately 300 per 100,000 of the population require admission to hospital each year following a head injury, and of these 20–40 per cent will stay for no more than 48 hours (Greenwood, 2002). Fifteen per 100,000 per year are admitted to neurosurgical units, and nine of these people will die (Hutchinson and Kirkpatrick, 2002; Lasserson, Gabriel and Sharrack, 2000). The majority of those admitted are discharged within 48 hours (NICE, 2007). However mild head injuries can result in long-term problems, such as headaches occurring persistently or difficulty concentrating.

(a) Learning activity

Connect to the NICE website, and search for and read the short version of *Head Injury Triage, Assessment, Investigation and Early Management of Head Injury in Infants, Children and Adults* (NICE, 2007).

(e) Evidence-based practice

The management of head injury focuses on prevention, pre-hospital care, immediate, acute hospital care and rehabilitation if required. NICE (2007) is an essential piece of the evidence base for directing the management of individuals with a head injury.

Concussion literally means a violent shaking (Hickey, 2003). In concussions the symptoms are mild and short lived, as the brain injury is slight and resolves spontaneously. Those suffering from concussion may complain of feeling dizzy, seeing 'stars', headaches associated with nausea, just not feeling 'quite right' or 'out of sorts', and may appear confused and/or vacant. There may be amnesia of the actual trauma and events leading up to it. There is often little or no apparent permanent neurological deficit (Marieb and Hoehn, 2007). This reflects functional disturbance of the neurological system rather than structural injury, and is normally not associated with abnormal radiological imaging (Evans, 2007). Concussion can be induced by a blow to the head, face, neck or anywhere else in the body that transfers a force to the head (Evans, 2007).

People with concussion have often been 'knocked out' or suffered a LOC; however a mild concussion may not always be associated with an LOC. Concussion associated with contact sports such as rugby often goes unrecognised, as frequently there is no LOC and there may be risk of a repetitive brain injury. Repeated concussions or minor head injuries can have a cumulative effect, leading to problems such as the 'punch drunk syndrome' seen in boxers or those who have had frequent blows to the head (Lasserson et al, 2000). It can be associated with amnesia, loss of memory of events occurring immediately before the head injury (retrograde) or after it (antegrade).

Part
IV

Point of injury assessment and decision making

Following a head injury people should attend A&E if they have any of the following signs and symptoms (NICE, 2007):

- a high-energy head injury caused by an RTA, for example a pedestrian struck by a motor vehicle, or a fall from a height of greater than 1 metre or more than five stairs
- loss of consciousness or a reduced consciousness level: for example problems keeping eyes open; irritability or altered behaviour
- GCS score of less than 15 at any time since injury
- any episodes of vomiting since the injury
- any seizure activity since the injury
- any focal neurological deficit since the injury, which could include a limb weakness, speech deficits (slurring, expressive or receptive dysphasia or aphasia), loss of balance or problems walking, and visual disturbance or pupil irregularity
- amnesia of events before or after the injury
- persistent headache since the injury
- current drug or alcohol intoxication.

⌐S⌐ Scenario continued

When Lahti starts to admit and assess Tom, she notices that Tom is irritable and a little agitated. Tom is also being mildly uncooperative. Lahti has no concerns with Tom's admission vital signs (ABC components) but when assessing 'disability' he is responding to voice only (AVPU).

His GCS is 13/15 (E=3, V=4, M=6). As a result Tom will require further investigations and will be in the A&E department for a while longer. Lahti reports all this information to the qualified member of staff immediately.

Table 30.2 Glasgow Coma Scale chart

Glasgow Coma Scale	Eyes open	Spontaneously	4															C – eyes closed due to swelling	
		To speech	3																
		To pain	2																
		None	1																
	Best verbal response	Orientated	5															T – tracheostomy or endotracheal tube	
		Disorientated	4																
		Monosyllabic	3																
		Incomprehensible sounds	2																
		None	1																
	Best motor response	Obey commands	6															usually record best arm F – fit	
		Localise pain	5																
		Withdrawal to pain	4																
		Abnormal tension pain	3																
		Extension to pain	2																
		None	1																

⚠ **Professional alert!**

Patients presenting to A&E with impaired consciousness (GCS less than 15) should be assessed immediately by a trained member of staff (for example, a triage nurse) (NICE, 2007).

Assessment

Assessment normally follows a standard format, the ABCDE approach (American College of
Surgeons, 1993; Resuscitation Council (UK), 2006). See Table 30.3.

Table 30.3 Means of assessment

ABCDE	Disability includes
A = airway B = breathing and ventilation C = circulation D = disability: neurological status E = exposure	Conscious level assessment tools → AVPU → GCS Pupil assessment → Size → Reaction Blood glucose

A variety of assessment tools are used in clinical practice. The two most common tools
used are AVPU and the GCS.

AVPU (**a**lert, responds to **v**oice, **p**ain or **u**nresponsive) has a simple structure which is easy
to apply and has been incorporated into the **e**arly **w**arning **s**core (EWS), as many acutely ill
patients who deteriorate in general wards have an altered conscious level in the preceding 24
hours (Goldhill, White and Sumner, 1999; Goldhill, 2001; Schein et al, 1990; NICE, 2007).

Table 30.4 AVPU assessment

A – Alert	Responds spontaneously
V – Verbal	Responds to voice
P – Pain	Responds to pain
U – Unresponsive	No response to verbal or painful stimuli

GCS is the 'gold standard' tool used internationally by health professionals to make
repeated, effective, rapid evaluations of the conscious level (Harrahill, 1996). The three
components are eye opening (E), best verbal (V) and motor response (M) (Palmer and Knight,
2006).

E   Arousal or wakefulness: in other words, eye opening.

V   Alertness and awareness, that is, orientation and verbal communication.

M   Motor activity, an aspect of arousal, as in obeying commands.

> ### C) Professional conversation
>
> Lahti asks her mentor Mike how to score a patient who is asleep. Does the waking-up aspect alter the GCS scoring? 'A normal GCS in an awake individual is 15/15, falling to 14/15 if they are asleep,' Mike says. 'But they should be easily roused.
>
> 'Experienced observers might identify more subtle changes, which might not alter the GCS score at the point of assessment. At this point you should increase the frequency of assessments and involve the wider multidisciplinary team.'

The purpose of the GCS tool is to systematically assess the neurological function of the patient and provide a common language for communication between multidisciplinary groups (Aird and McIntosh, 2004; Fischer and Mathieson, 2001; Jennett, 1986). The 15-point GCS (revised from an earlier 14-point GCS) is the accepted version that has been commonly used for the last 30 years (Jennett and Teasdale, 1977; Wiese, 2003; NICE, 2007). GCS is applicable for adolescents as well as adults, and has been adapted for use in paediatrics.

It is essential that appropriate observations are instigated, whether this is AVPU or GCS, in order to assess neurological trends which will inform clinical decisions. Practitioners must recognise when to escalate assessment from AVPU to GCS. Neurological observations should only be conducted by healthcare practitioners who have been trained and deemed competent (NICE, 2007) to ensure appropriate use and consistency. The acquisition and maintenance of observation and recording skills requires dedicated education and training, and this should be available to all relevant staff. Specific training is required for the observation of infants and young children.

In order to competently assess neurological function, healthcare practitioners need to have some knowledge of the related anatomy and physiology (Palmer and Knight, 2006). Misinterpretation of neurological assessments could put your patient at risk of developing increasing and/or permanent neurological deficit or possibly even death.

Consciousness

There are many levels of consciousness, which range from being alert and responsive (generally considered normal) to a deep coma (abnormal). People with a head injury can fall anywhere in this range, depending on the extent of injury sustained and associated secondary complications. Alcohol and drug intoxication can make it more difficult to assess the conscious level accurately, and patients may not be compliant.

Many health professionals do not have a good understanding of the underlying mechanisms that produce altered levels of consciousness (Waterhouse, 2005; Shah, 1999; Addison and Crawford, 1999). Underpinning anatomical and physiological knowledge is required to competently interpret an assessment of level of consciousness.

> ### a) Learning activity
>
> You will hear and read many different terms used to define the continuum from consciousness to coma, including confusion, rousable, inattentiveness, delirium, clouding of consciousness, drowsiness, stupor, unrousable, flat, unconsciousness, obtundation, vegetative state or coma (Hickey, 2003; Goetz, 2003; Victor, and Ropper 2001). Look up and note down some definitions of these.

Consciousness is the most sensitive indicator of neurological change, and a reduced conscious level is usually the first sign to be observed. The conscious level can fluctuate, and assessments only reflect conscious level at the time the observations are made. Changes in conscious level can occur rapidly – in seconds, minutes or hours, for instance following a subarachnoid haemorrhage or head injury – or very slowly, over a period of days, weeks, months and years, as happens with a slow-growing tumour.

Arousal and awareness are the two distinct components of consciousness (Hickey, 2003).

- **Arousal** is a state or appearance of being awake. It demonstrates interaction between the reticular formation (RF) and cerebral hemispheres, as in motor response and speech (Palmer and Knight, 2006). Dysfunction is manifest in an altered level of consciousness and reflected in the GCS score.
- **Awareness** refers to the content of consciousness. This includes cognitive functions, and reflects the activity of the cerebral cortex. Dysfunction is manifest in altered mental and intellectual functions (Goetz, 2003; Hickey, 2003; Barker, 2002). There has to be interaction between the cerebral cortex and the RF for the individual to be aware (Palmer and Knight, 2006).

During sleep there is a reduced level of consciousness because of the inhibition of direct perception of sensory stimuli, but you can differentiate sleep from coma by the fact that you can wake a sleeping person. This is because cerebral uptake does not decrease during sleep as it does in coma (Barker, 2002).

Patients in any clinical setting may require assessment of conscious level for a number of reasons. Alteration of conscious level may result from intra or extracranial causes (see Table 30.5). Hypoxia, hypoglycaemia and sedative drug overdose are the most common metabolic causes of altered LOC seen in hospitalised patients (Hickey, 2003). An impaired conscious level may compound many other medical conditions: for instance, a patient may not be able to follow simple instructions to breathe deeply/cough to aid their respiratory care.

Table 30.5 Causes of altered conscious levels

Intracranial	**Extracranial**
Direct destruction of the anatomical structures by a disease or insult → space-occupying lesions – literally taking up intracranial space, such as a tumour or haematoma → head injury (falls, assaults, RTAs) → cerebrovascular accident (CVA) → seizures/epilepsy → raised intracranial pressure (ICP) → Infections	Metabolic causes → Hypoglycaemia/hyperglycaemia → Fluid/electrolyte imbalance Hypoxia (respiratory compromise) Hypotension/hypertension (cardiovascular instability) Shock Pharmacological agents e.g. → anaesthetics, sedatives and paralysing agents → opiate analgesics → anticonvulsants → antidepressants → recreational drugs and alcohol Sepsis Liver, renal and endocrine dysfunction

Sources: Teasdale and Jennett (1974), Jennett and Teasdale (1977), Fielding and Rowley (1990), Edwards (2001), Barker (2002), Hickey (2003), McLeod (2004), Lewis (2005).

> **S** Scenario continued
>
> It is decided that Tom has sustained a mild head injury but requires further review and investigations before a decision can be made on his discharge. Tom will require frequent assessment of his condition, which will include GCS and vital sign observations.
>
> Lahti asks Tom whether there is anyone he would like the hospital to contact. Tom is reluctant to call his parents until a further review has been completed. Lahti documents his wishes and next of kin contact details.

Part

IV

Based on the mechanism of injury the patient will be inspected for signs of bruising, lacerations and fractures of the head and neck, as associated injuries can occur. A general visual inspection of the patient is fundamental in the assessment process. Important information can be detected such as warning signs of a fractured base of skull, such as classic bruising behind the back of the ear (Battle's sign) and around the eyes (panda or racoon eyes) (Hutchinson and Kirkpatrick, 2002). These may take several hours to develop.

ⓔ Evidence-based practice

If there is any suspicion of a base of skull fracture the patient should not have a nasopharyngeal airway inserted or any nasopharyngeal suctioning or a nasogastric tube inserted.

The base of the skull sits behind the nose and above the roof of the mouth. This region of the skull is more fragile, and fractures can be transmitted to this area from trauma to the side of the skull. If the meninges are also breached the brain protection is compromised.

It is at this point in the patient's journey, as the scenario update has suggested, that there is a potential for Tom's condition to deteriorate. A summary of how to complete a GCS assessment now follows. You are also advised to review the associated anatomy and physiology of the neurological system at this stage. There is an overview later in this chapter.

Procedure for completing a neurological assessment

The AVPU and the GCS assessment tools provide a common language to improve communication in reporting neurological findings between all healthcare professionals (Aird and McIntosh, 2004; Fischer and Mathieson, 2001). Your observations begin as you approach the patient. Consider what information you can gather relating to their condition, for instance whether the patient is awake or appears asleep, their behaviour, position in bed and breathing patterns. Introduce yourself to your patient, indicating your name, role and what you intend to do whatever their conscious level. Gain the patient's verbal consent if they are conscious. Implied consent is assumed in the unconscious patient. To obtain the GCS score you add together the scores for each component. A minimum score is 3 (3/15) and a maximum score is 15 (15/15).

Table 30.6 **Best eye opening**

4	Spontaneously	As you approach the patient note whether there are eyes are open or closed. If open this is classed as open spontaneous and they score 4.
3	To speech	If they do not open their eyes spontaneously, speak to the patient in a normal tone, raising your voice if necessary. If their eyes open to voice this scores 3.
2	To pain	If they have still not opened their eyes, touch your patient on the arm or shoulder with a gentle shake, while speaking to them (for instance calling their name, or asking 'Can you open your eyes?'). If there is no response to this, apply a deeper stimulus such as pain (see pages 620–1). If they respond they score 2.
1	None	If there is no eye opening despite trying all the above, the patient scores 1.

Some patients respond to better to a familiar relative or friend's voice, or the lower pitch of a male voice. If a patient has severe orbital swelling it is normal to document closed eyes (noted as C on the chart) and not score this component.

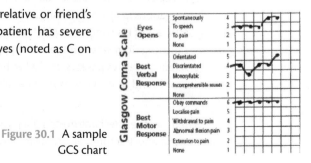

Figure 30.1 A sample GCS chart

Table 30.7 **Best verbal response**

5	Oriented	Talk to your patient. Start by asking them to tell you their name. This establishes that they are oriented to person if they can answer correctly. To establish if they are oriented to time ask whether they know the date or the day. Some patients may only be aware of the month, season or year. The final component is to assess orientation to place, so ask the patient to identify where they are (for instance the ward name, hospital or city). If they can answer all these components correctly, and are oriented to time, place and person, they score 5.
4	Confused conversation	If they have one or more of these elements wrong they are classed as disorientated/ confused and score 4.
3	Inappropriate words	If the patient can only answer in monosyllables or words, as opposed to sentences, which are out of context with the questions, they score 3.
2	Incomprehensible sounds	The patient scores a 2 if they are unable to format words and are only able to produce incomprehensible sounds such as moans or groans. This may be in response to verbal or pain/noxious stimuli.
1	None	If there is no verbal response despite trying all the above, the patient scores 1.

Remember this is a test of best verbal response. Even if they can write or communicate via other methods, they still score 1 if there are no verbal sounds. In paediatrics you may need to assess using appropriate developmental milestone questions, such as 'How old are you?' and 'What is your favourite toy's name?'

Table 30.8 **Best motor response**

6	Obeys	The best motor response is to be able to obey simple commands convincingly. This is a test of the best response in a single limb as opposed to all limbs. Ask the patient to squeeze and release their hands, or place a finger on their nose. Ensure that what you ask the patient to do is within their range of movements and physical ability. The patient scores 6 if able to obey commands.
5	Localises	If the patient localises to pain they will score 5. In order to localise you must observe the patient to move their hand to the stimulus and attempt to remove it. This is a purposeful movement.
4	Withdraws	The patient scores 4 if they withdraw (normal flexion) from the pain/noxious stimuli. The limbs will flex (bend at the elbows or knees).
3	Abnormal flexion	The patient scores 3 if they demonstrate abnormal flexion. Abnormal flexion is easiest to recognise in the arms. The arm flexes at the elbow, wrist and fingers, hands adducted into the body. The thumbs may be pushed through the curled fingers. This is also known as decorticate posturing.
2	Extends	The patient scores 2 if they exhibit extension. In extension the arms and legs are stretched (stiffly) downwards. The forearm pronates (turned away from the body) and the upper arm is held close to the body (adduction). The toes point down (planter flex) and foot may be rolled outwards.
1	None	If there is no motor response despite trying all the above, the patient scores 1.

Procedure for pupil assessment

Pupil assessment is composed of two aspects, pupil size and response to light.

Pupil size

Ask the patient to open both their eyes (if they are able), and assess the size of both pupils before testing light reflex. Compare this with the size charts that are commonly included on neurological assessment charts. The diameter across is measured in millimeters. Document the size of the pupils, both right and left, before testing for light reaction.

If the patient is unable to open their eyes, unless they are swollen tightly shut, you can gently open them and assess the pupil size and response to light. If possible try to assess the size of the pupils with both eyes open and before the light response is tested.

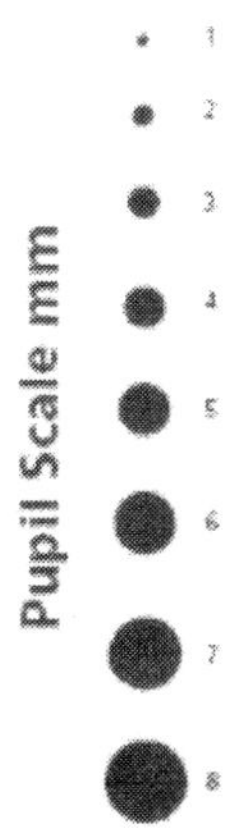

Pupil Scale mm

1
2
3
4
5
6
7
8

Part
IV

Figure 30.2 **Pupil scale measurement**

Pupil reaction to light

The pen torch should be shone onto the eye from the side of the face and not from directly in front. As you shine the light into the eye observe the pupil reaction: is there pupil constriction? If a reaction is not seen immediately, hold the light in position to check for a sluggish reaction or to establish no response. Document the reaction to light on the observation chart. It is common practice to document a positive reaction using a + sign, no response using a – sign, and sluggish response as SL.

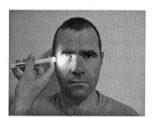

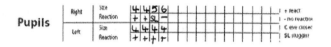

Figure 30.3 Position for testing light reaction   Figure 30.4 Pupil reaction chart

Unequal pupils, sluggish reaction or no response can be an indicator of raised intracranial pressure (ICP). Photophobia, irritability to light, is another. Pupil size can also be affected by some medications: for example constricted and pinpoint pupils are seen with the use of opiates, and pupils are dilated following the administration of mydriatic eye drops, which are often used in cases of eye casualty.

A hotly debated issue is the application of painful stimuli to a patient.

Painful stimuli

During neurological assessment, if a verbal or tactile stimulus does not elicit a response from the patient, then there is a need to apply noxious or painful stimuli. A peripheral stimulus is interpreted via the peripheral nervous system (spinal nerves) and communicates with the central nervous system via the spinal cord to the brain.

Trapezius muscle squeeze/twist is recognised as best practice (Palmer and Knight, 2006; Woodward, 1997; Addison and Crawford, 1999; Shah, 1999). Trapezius squeeze may be more difficult to perform on large or obese patients (Barker, 2002). When a noxious or painful stimulus is applied to a patient who subsequently responds, the patient is not comatose, as this demonstrates a degree of cortical function.

Position for trapezius squeeze

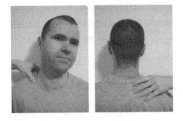

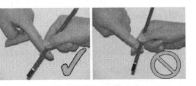

Position for peripheral pain stimuli

Pressure to edge of finger (just below the nail, below the interphalangeal joint)

Figure 30.5 Common painful stimuli

(e) Evidence-based practice

Sternal rub should be considered with caution because this soft tissue area bruises easily. Commonly this stimulus is applied with the knuckles, and trauma can be lessened by using a flat open hand (Barker, 2002). Teasdale (1975, 2004) advocates that nail bed stimuli (peripheral stimuli) are less painful than sternal rub (central stimuli); yet direct pressure over the nail bed can cause damage to the capillary network under the nail bed, resulting in bruising and potential loss of the nail. You are recommended to use the edge of the finger as opposed to the nail bed.

Vital signs

Vital signs offer a lot of information relating to the functioning of the central nervous system. Respiratory rate, rhythm and depth, pulse and blood pressure are regulated by control centres located within the brain stem. Temperature is regulated by the hypothalamus. These parameters may become altered indicating neurological deficit, for example in raised ICP. The blood pressure increases, the pulse rate slows to bradycardia and abnormal respiratory patterns may be observed in very late stages.

Muscle strength/power

Movement includes all the activities of the muscular system, supported by the bony framework of the skeleton, and activation of the muscles is via the central and peripheral nervous system (Marieb and Hoehn, 2007). Muscle strength and power is tested with resisted movements.

When interacting with your patient also observe their limbs, considering aspects such as symmetry of shape, size and strength. Note any atrophy, contractures, and involuntary movement such as tics, twitches, jerks or tremors. Consider the tone of their limbs, which can be described as the resting tension in muscles and can be affected in some neurological conditions. It can result in increased tone leading to spasticity or rigidity, as seen in Parkinson's disease, or reduced tone such as flaccid limbs, as seen in strokes.

Observe your patient's balance, coordination

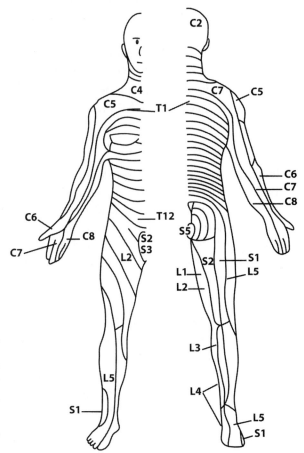

Figure 30.6 Dermatone map

Part

IV

and gait, as a variety of problems such as unsteadiness, loss of balance, widened stance, dragging of feet, shuffling or staggering can result from neurological problems.

Sensory impairment can occur when there are problems associated with either the parietal lobe or the spinothalamic tract within the spinal cord. Patients will need to be assessed for any diminished or abnormal sensation across all dermatones. Dermatones are the areas of skin innervated by the cutaneous branches of a single spinal nerve.

Some patients may also experience altered proprioception, which refers to our sense of position and body movement.

Patients who have suffered a minor head injury or are suspected to have a concussion may need to be admitted to a hospital for observation and monitoring post injury. A set of criteria has been created to ensure that a standardised approach can be applied.

> **(a) Learning activity**
>
> Practice power strength testing, vital signs and painful stimuli on a willing volunteer. Cross-reference the material contained in this chapter with the skills chapters in the companion volume to make sure you have all the correct procedures and protocols.

Criteria for admission following a head injury for 24-hour observation

Clients should be admitted for observation if (adapted from NICE, 2007):

- there is no responsible adult available to supervise them at home during the immediate 24–48 hours following discharge
- they have not returned to a GCS of 15/15
- they have signs and symptoms that give cause for concern following a head injury, such as irritability, drowsy, headaches and/or nausea and vomiting
- there are associated other injuries, haemodynamic instability (shock), cerebrospinal fluid leak, or other medical conditions which might exacerbate or be exacerbated by the HI (such as diabetes or cardiac history), or it is a nonaccidental injury
- a CT scan identifies something significant
- drugs or alcohol have made, or might make, assessment difficult.

When to make the neurological assessments and their frequency have been standardised and categorised by NICE (2007).

> **S Scenario continued**
>
> Tom has also sustained an injury to his forehead. He has an obvious haematoma developing and a laceration above his left eye. He will require very frequent neurological observations to monitor for any evolving signs and symptoms of neurological problems associated with frontal lobe trauma, such as: irritability, behavioural changes, memory/concentration problems or limb weakness.
>
> Tom at this point complains of a pounding headache and feels sick. He thinks he would be better off going home to sleep off his headache, as the A&E department is very bright and noisy. He is also extremely worried about how much damage has been done to his bicycle and helmet. He now reckons it would be a good idea to call his parents for some support and a lift home.

Frequency of observations

Observations should be performed and recorded on a half-hourly basis until GCS equal to 15 has been achieved. The minimum frequency of observation for a patient with GCS equal to 15 yet having a known history of a minor head injury should be:

- half-hourly for two hours
- then hourly for four hours
- then two-hourly thereafter.

Senior staff must review patient management when other signs and symptoms become progressively worse, such as nausea, vomiting, headache, agitation or inappropriate behaviour, unequal pupils, sluggish or no response to light, or abnormal or unexplained vital sign changes. Following a HI almost any focal neurological deficit can result, and reflects the site(s) of damage (Greenwood, 2002). Anosmia (loss of sense of smell) or disturbance of the sense of smell and/or taste is well recognised following injury to the brain, especially in the frontal or occipital regions (Greenwood, 2002). Various visual problems can occur and should be inquired about by nursing staff making an assessment of the patient.

A series of radiological imaging/diagnostic tests can be used with patients following a HI. The three most common are x-rays, computerised tomography (CT) and magnetic resonance imaging (MRI).

X-ray

This will be the first line of diagnostic imaging if a skull, facial or spinal fracture is suspected. Two-dimensional bony images of the area can be obtained quickly and efficiently in all major hospital facilities that have a 24-hour emergency care department. It is a painless and quick procedure that sends focused high-energy radiation through the affected area. In low doses x-rays are used to diagnose fractures by capturing images, often in digital form.

CT and MRI can provide greater detail. Both are painless procedures which require the patient to remain completely still. Some patients may require sedation to ensure they remain motionless for the duration of the scan. Body position may be maintained using plastic frames/moulds and Velcro strapping.

Computerised tomography

This is a specialized form of x-ray (radiation) that uses a computer to build up a layer of images based upon attenuation of exiting radiation from multidirectional simultaneous x-ray beams (Hickey, 2003), which can be reconstructed to produce three-dimensional computerised images. The patient is carefully positioned and immobilised, if unable to remain still, on a table which moves in and out of the scanner. CT scans can be completed in a matter of minutes if the patient is compliant. It is a painless procedure. CT is useful for the demonstration of the skull and vertebral bones and can detect haemorrhage, aneurysms and space-occupying lesions such as a tumour or abscess, hydrocephalus and the effects of raised intracranial pressure in the brain. Brain tissue appears in various shades of grey depending upon density. Fluid such as CSF will be black and bone will be white (Hickey, 2003). Based on known normal brain imagery, any differences or abnormalities in the patient's brain tissue and structures can be interpreted by the radiologist.

Part

IV

Radiological protocols

A CT scan of the head will normally be performed if there has been:

- a GCS score of 13 or 14/15 at two hours after the injury (where the person has not recovered full consciousness by the time of assessment)
- any sign of a fracture to the base of the skull or a penetrating injury
- seizures
- focal neurological deficit
- noted neurological deterioration.

Ⓐ Learning activity

Using an internet search engine that facilitates selection of images/pictures, find examples of skull fractures and haematomas.

Magnetic resonance imaging

MRI is a diagnostic tool commonly used in neuroscience patients to provide exquisitely detailed, cross-section images of the anatomical structures through the body (Hickey, 2003; British Brain and Spine Foundation). There is no radiation used in this procedure. This technology gives excellent pictures of soft tissue changes as they are not obscured by bone (Hickey, 2003). This is a painless procedure that uses strong magnetic fields to create cross-sectional images of tissue structures. All metal objects are restricted from the scanning area. Some patients may find the enclosed environment of the MRI scanner claustrophobic. As a rule, the patient is alone in the room during scanning.

Ⓒ Professional conversation

Lahti asks Mike, 'Is there anything else I should observe for in patients who have sustained a head injury?' 'There are plenty of other problems that crop up following head injuries,' Mike says. 'They could be associated with secondary injury, seizures, raised ICP, a CSF leak or haematomas. So you need to be aware of these possibilities, and of the signs to watch out for.'

Recognition of neurological deterioration

The potential for a patient to deteriorate post HI is ever present. Mike identified the key factors in the professional conversation.

Fundamental processes occur at a cellular level following brain injury, which can ultimately lead to cell death. Following any traumatic brain injury (TBI) (such as HI, or a subarachnoid haemorrhage) swelling of the parenchyma (brain tissue) can occur. The skull contains a confined rigid space called the cranium which contains the soft malleable brain tissue, cerebral spinal fluid and blood. Swelling of the brain parenchyma can result in an increase in ICP, since the space available for the brain cannot expand.

It is essential to promptly recognise and manage hypoxia (oxygen saturation < 95 per cent) and hypotension (systolic blood pressure < 90 mm Hg) following TBI, as these factors can contribute to an unfavourable outcome (Hutchinson and Kirkpatrick, 2002), which at the worst could be permanent neurological deficit or death. Patient management focuses on minimising the secondary injuries that can occur following TBI, with a focus on maintaining adequate oxygen saturations, respiratory care and fluid hydration to haemodynamic stability. Following a TBI delayed complications can be divided into vascular, infective, epileptic, cranial nerve palsies, and psychological/cognitive problems (Hutchinson and Kirkpatrick, 2002).

If there are signs of deterioration it may require referral to a neurosurgical team. Patients are referred based upon neurological assessment and diagnostic results such as x-rays and CT scans, which might demonstrate things such as a depressed skull fracture or an extradural haematoma, as these will require neurosurgical intervention.

(e) Evidence-based practice

Patients are also referred to the neurological team if they have any of the following (NICE, 2007):

- unexplained confusion which persists for more than four hours
- continued deterioration in GCS score after admission; greater attention should be paid to motor response deterioration
- progressive focal neurological signs such as arm weakness, speech or visual disturbance
- seizures
- penetrating skull injury
- cerebrospinal fluid leak (CSF).

If there is a persistently reduced GCS despite haemodynamic resuscitation, many trauma guidelines recommend airway protection: that is, intubation, and ventilation with a GCS below 8/15. 'Patients who do not follow commands, speak or open their eyes, with a GCS score of 8 or less, are by definition in coma' (Greenwood, 2002: i10).

Intracranial haemorrhage (bleeding inside the skull) usually occurs within the first few hours after the injury. The bleeding puts pressure on the brain, leading to raised ICP, and can be very serious if it is not recognised and treated promptly.

A subdural haematoma (an accumulation of blood below the dura, a protective layer over the brain) can be acute or chronic. When this happens it is usually within several days or weeks after a minor HI. The increasing intracranial pressure leads to progressive development of some or all of the following signs and symptoms: headaches, drowsiness, confusion, speech deficits or limb deficits.

(S) Scenario

Tom's headache and nausea have eased following simple analgesia and anti-emetics administered an hour ago. Tom is awaiting a CT scan and further medical review. Tom's mother has become very distressed about his need for a CT scan. She is now worried that he might develop epilepsy; as her friend had seizures and died prematurely.

Seizures and epilepsy

Epilepsy is a common neurological disorder (Brodie, Schachter and Kwan, 2005), characterised by recurrent spontaneous seizures (Lawal, 2005; Bahra and Cikurel, 1999). A seizure is a transient symptom and/or sign characterised by sudden, abnormal electrical activity within the brain (Bader and Littlejohns, 2004; Lawal, 2005), more specifically an abnormal electrical discharge from cerebral neurons (Bahra and Cikurel, 1999). A seizure will result in a temporary alteration of cerebral function (Hickey, 2003), depending on the region of the brain involved, and can cause an intermittent stereotyped disturbance of consciousness, behaviour, emotion, motor function and/or sensation. (You should refer to a textbook on anatomy and physiology if you need to be reminded of the functions of different regions of the brain.) Status epilepticus occurs when a seizure is continuous or there is no return to consciousness between recurrent seizures, and should be viewed as a medical emergency (Bahra and Cikurel, 1999). A seizure can occur in any individual, not just those with epilepsy, but susceptibility and thresholds vary with individuals, who might incur a seizure following head injury, an excessive volume of alcohol, alcohol withdrawal or illicit drug use (Hickey, 2003).

Seizures are classified according to a scale drawn by the International League Against Epilepsy (ILAE) and characterised as two broad groups, of partial and generalised seizures (see Table 30.9).

During a seizure the healthcare practitioner needs to remain calm and protect the person from injury (Hayes, 2004). During a convulsive seizure this may

(a) Learning activity

In a small group consider all of the components of care required by an individual who is having a seizure. Consider immediate and post-ictal management. You should explore the evidence base to establish best practice.

Part
IV

mean loosening tight clothing, cushioning the head and calling for help. It is important that someone stays with the person in case airway protection is required and to observe the nature of the seizure. As the seizure subsides the individual must be placed in the recovery position (Hayes, 2004). The healthcare practitioner should talk and reassure the patient during all seizures and subsequently document the event. Seizure charts act as a template to guide appropriate documentation. You should be able to describe a seizure you have observed, noting the time, duration and what the patient was doing prior to its commencement and during it. Consider what alerted you to the patient. Did they complain of a funny taste or smell, or did you notice any change in mood or behaviour? Key aspects to observe during a seizure are level of consciousness, eye movements, noises (groans or grunts), body and limb movements (tone, jerks or tongue biting), automatisms, continence and any respiratory changes.

Following a seizure, during the post-ictal period, the person may sleep, have slurred speech or dysphasia and/or complain of a headache. It is useful to ask the patient whether they had any warning, how they feel and what they can remember. Following a seizure all patients should be medically reviewed to establish the type of seizure (NICE, 2004) and instigate appropriate treatment if required. The history leading up to the seizure and description of

Table 30.9 International League Against Epilepsy classification of seizures

Partial (focal, local) seizures	Generalised seizures (convulsive or nonconvulsive)
Partial seizures are caused by epileptic activity in part of the brain. **Simple partial seizures (consciousness is not impaired):** The electrical activity is confined to one small part of the brain and the symptom will relate to the specific region, e.g. strong sense of déja vu or unpleasant smell/taste if the temporal region is involved; or a motor response such as a stiff arm or head drawn to one side of the body if the frontal region is involved. The parietal lobe will result in sensory symptoms and the occipital lobe in visual. **Complex partial seizures (with impairment of consciousness):** consciousness is altered and the individual will not remember the seizure. Lip smacking, chewing and swallowing, repeatedly scratching the head or searching for an object can occur and is referred to as an automatism. The person can still continue relatively complex actions such as walking, and to onlookers it may seem that the person is fully aware of what they are doing. Most commonly they originate in the temporal lobe. **Partial seizures evolving to secondary generalised seizures**: both simple partial and complex partial seizures can spread to the whole brain and result in a secondary generalised tonic-clonic seizure.	Generalised seizures involve epileptic activity in all or most of the brain. **Absence seizures**: a brief seizure where the person is 'absent' for a couple of seconds, going blank and staring. This can be very subtle and may be confused with daydreaming; usually only lasting a few seconds but can occur repeatedly. It usually involves both sides of the brain but not the entire brain. **Myoclonic seizures:** muscle jerk(s), sometimes violent, usually the arm or leg. **Clonic seizures:** the muscles contract and relax continuously, causing the person having the seizure to twitch and jerk repeatedly. **Tonic seizures:** all the muscles in the limbs and trunk suddenly stiffen and the person will fall. **Tonic-clonic seizures:** the person loses consciousness, the body stiffens, and then they fall to the ground. This is followed by jerking movements. Consciousness usually returns within a couple of minutes. There may be irregular breathing, cyanosis of lips, incontinence of urine or tongue biting. It is the most common form of generalised seizures. The person will have no memory of the seizure and recovery time varies from minutes for some to hours for others. **Atonic seizures:** all the muscles in the body suddenly go flaccid, sudden loss of tone, and they will fall.

Sources: adapted from Epilepsy Action (2007), National Society for Epilepsy (2007) and Hayes (2004).

the event are important diagnostic information. It is more important to be able to describe accurately what occurred rather than name the seizure type (Hayes, 2004). A diagnosis of epilepsy should be made by an epilepsy specialist or neurologist (SIGN, 2003), as it has important psychological and potential lifestyle implications.

Some people experience a sensation called an aura before a seizure starts. This may occur far enough in advance to give the person time to lie down and prevent injury from falling. The type of aura experienced varies from person to person, as auras are in fact a simple partial seizure: for example a change in body temperature, a feeling of tension or anxiety, a strange taste or smell, even musical sounds or visual disturbance. Some report a sense of heaviness, depression or general feeling of 'not being quite right' in themselves before a seizure. It can happen for hours or days before they have a seizure, and is referred to as a prodrome.

> **S** **Scenario continued**
>
> Tom's CT scan is normal and his GCS has returned to 15/15 for the last four hours. He is now able to be discharged to his parents' care.

Health education

At the point of discharge the patient's GCS should have returned to their normal level: that is, GCS 15/15, or the normal level for those people with an altered GCS level as their normal state (people with dementia or Alzheimer's disease). On discharge patients and carers should receive post-head-injury advice, both verbally and written. Multilingual communication and other formats of information should be made available. This advice should cover what to do if certain signs and symptoms arise, and be reiterated on a head injury advice card with emergency contact details. Every patient who has been admitted to hospital (treatment beyond the emergency department) following a head injury should be referred to their GP for a follow-up, as routine, within a week after discharge.

Table 30.10 gives the standard do's and don'ts for people who have had a head injury and have been discharged from hospital:

Table 30.10 Do's and don'ts after discharge following a head injury

Do	Don't
Do make sure a carer/responsible adult is with you for the first 48 hours after leaving hospital. **Do** make sure you stay within easy reach of a telephone and medical help. **Do** check whether or not you are able to take your regular medications, especially sleeping pills, sedatives or tranquillisers as these may mask signs or symptoms of further complications following your head injury. **Do** have plenty of rest and avoid stressful situations.	**Don't** stay at home alone for the first 48 hours after leaving hospital. **Don't** take any alcohol or recreational drugs. **Don't** play any contact sport (such as rugby or football) for at least three weeks without talking to your doctor first. **Don't** return to your normal school, college or work activity until you feel you have completely recovered. **Don't** drive a car, ride a motorbike or bicycle or operate machinery unless you feel you have completely recovered. **Don't** watch television or use computers for long periods.

> **a** **Learning activity**
>
> Tom needs to be made aware of the do's and don'ts following his head injury. Have a look in your clinical areas at the range of information available to support patients discharged following head injury. Consider the issues related to patient information such as language, literacy skills and visual impairment.

Part

IV

Potential problems after leaving hospital

In the initial phase after a head injury and discharge from hospital, some people may experience other symptoms which should disappear in the following two weeks after injury. These include a mild headache, feeling sick (without vomiting), dizziness, irritability or bad temper, problems concentrating, problems with memory, tiredness, lack of appetite or problems sleeping. If the problems do not appear to be resolving and reducing, patients should seek advice or be reviewed by their GP.

If a person who has had a head injury gets the symptoms listed above and they remain unresolved or appear to be getting worse (as noted below), they should seek advice immediately. Sudden onset of any of the following symptoms requires immediate medical assistance from a GP or emergency department (adapted from NICE, 2007):

- unconsciousness, or lack of full consciousness or difficulty in rousing (problems keeping their eyes open)
- any confusion (not knowing where they are, getting things muddled up)
- any drowsiness (feeling sleepy) that goes on for longer than one hour when they would normally be wide awake
- loss of consciousness for a short time followed by an apparent return to normality.
- any problems understanding conversation or difficulty with speech
- any loss of balance or problems walking, weakness in limbs
- very painful headache that won't go away.
- any nausea with vomiting
- seizures
- fluid (clear and thin) coming out of the ear or nose
- visual disturbances.

Thus the patient in the weeks and months following their head injury should return to their normal lifestyle. If there are late-onset neurological deficits these could be associated with hydrocephalus or a chronic subdural haematoma, and would be identified via a CT scan (Hutchinson and Kirkpatrick, 2002).

Support for families and carers

Early support in the form of verbal or written information can help the injured person's family or carer prepare for the effects on a person with a HI. The patient's family members often find themselves overwhelmed in a hospital, and dealing with different members of staff can cause additional stress. Hospital staff caring for the injured person, should introduce themselves to family members or carers, and briefly explain what they are doing. The person recovering consciousness can easily be confused by strange faces and the unfamiliar environment, so it is reassuring to have relatives and friends present. Headway, a charitable organisation, offers support for both patients and their families from within the hospital environment, and plays a major role in integrating people back into the community (Hutchinson and Kirkpatrick, 2002).

Long-term problems

Most people recover quickly and experience no long-term problems. However, a small number of people will have had a serious injury and are likely to have problems (cognitive and/or physical) which require rehabilitation and ongoing treatment (NICE, 2007).

Post-concussion syndrome can cause problems for months, even after a mild HI (Marieb and Hoehn, 2007; Hickey, 2003). Some people develop problems immediately, others after a few weeks, months or more. Problems associated with post-concussion syndrome include headaches, dizziness, poor concentration, memory loss, speech or hearing deficits, emotional and behavioural problems (Greenwood, 2002). In some cases the person's personality might be affected; for others problems are not obvious until they have returned to study or work (NICE, 2007). Life can be very difficult for patients and their families in these circumstances, and depression is not uncommon. In these situations there is a need for dedicated multidisciplinary neurorehabilitation units to maximise recovery following TBI. Minor head-injured patients have previously been neglected in this process, but there is now increased recognition of the benefits of neuropsychology within this patient group (Hutchinson and Kirkpatrick, 2002).

(a) Learning activity

Tom was wearing a cycle helmet but many people still do not. Explore the statistics regarding road traffic accidents to cyclists, the impact of wearing a cycle helmet and the extent of injury. Also consider when a helmet should be replaced.

As Tom's GCS has returned to his normal of 15/15 there is an opportunity to aid Tom in aspects of health education to avoid future risk of injury. According to the Nursing Midwifery Council (NMC, 2007), it is the nurse's responsibility to promote the health and well-being of those in their care, and a cycle helmet is evidence-based care as a possible preventive measure of reducing the head injury at point of impact.

Most people learn to ride a bike as children. Many adults choose this method of transportation as it is cheap, and often helps in beating traffic queues, while also providing healthy exercise. Cyclists as road users are more vulnerable than drivers of other vehicles. They have little protection from injury if they become involved in an accident (Headway). In a typical cycle accident the rider is knocked to the ground, suffering a blow to the head. Often the head bounces to a second or third impact. When an unprotected head strikes the edge of the pavement the skull will be deformed. The job of a helmet should be to absorb the impact rather than transferring it to the head. The force of the blow should be spread evenly within the helmet rather than on one concentrated spot. Headway (2007) has published the following statistics relating to UK injuries involving cycling:

- Each year approximately 200,000 people are injured through cycling accidents and receive hospital treatment.
- 70 per cent of all pedal cycle fatalities are caused by head injuries.
- Standard Approved cycle helmets are proven to be effective in reducing head injuries in cycle-related accidents by 85 per cent.
- The wearing of approved helmets by cyclists has been made compulsory in several states in Australia (1990), in the United States and more recently in New Zealand (1994).
- However the use of cycle helmets remains low in Britain, with only 18 per cent of young cyclists wearing them.

Awareness of general traffic noise and other road users is an essential way to interact and initiate appropriate measures whilst cycling on the road. If the cyclist is sensorily depriving themself of traffic and external environment sounds (by listening to an MP3 player for example) they will be slower to respond to the ever-changing roads conditions. They will not hear a car horn beeping or the sound of an approaching vehicle from behind.

[S] Scenario continued

Tom has made a full recovery and he always wears a cycle helmet but will be replacing it following his accident.

Anatomy and physiology of the neurological system

We have reviewed the clinical aspects of assessing conscious level and managing head injury, but if you are to become competent in this area you must also have a comprehensive understanding of the underpinning anatomy and physiology of the nervous system. This section provides an overview of this, which you will need if you are to make informed and accurate neurological assessments based on the principles of evidence-based care.

Part
IV

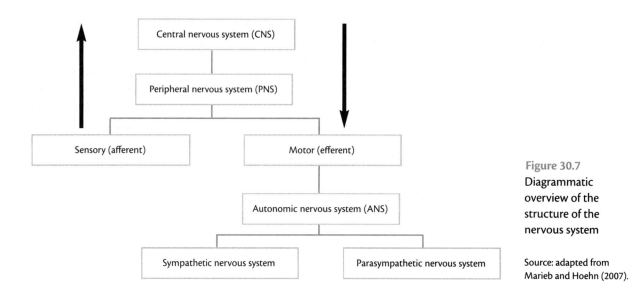

Figure 30.7
Diagrammatic overview of the structure of the nervous system

Source: adapted from Marieb and Hoehn (2007).

The nervous system can be seen as consisting of a number of functional areas that integrate sensory and motor function, as shown in Figure 30.7.

The central nervous system (CNS)

The CNS consists of the brain and the spinal cord, and has been compared to a supercomputer or a telephone switchboard. The brain is one-fiftieth of the total body weight, and consists of about two good fistfuls of quivering, pinkish-grey tissue with the consistency of porridge. It is wrinkled like a walnut to increase the surface area. The adult male brain weighs approximately 1600 grams (Marieb and Hoehn, 2007). The CNS interprets incoming sensory information and dictates motor responses based on past experiences, reflexes and current conditions.

CNS protection

The skull (fused bones) provides the outer protection for the brain, and the vertebrae does so for the spinal cord. The brain and spinal cord are completely covered by three protective membranes known as the meninges, which lay between the skull and brain or vertebra and spinal cord. The three layers are called the:

- dura mater, is the thickest and outer layer, closest to the skull
- arachnoid mater, where cerebrospinal fluid (CSF) flows between this layer and the pia mater in the subarachnoid space
- pia mater; a fine membrane intimately adherent to the brain (Marieb and Hoehn, 2007).

CSF is found in and around the brain and spinal cord, forming a liquid cushion that gives buoyancy to the CNS organs. It protects against blows or trauma and helps to nourish the brain. CSF circulates through the ventricles (fluid-filled spaces) of the brain, around the subarachnoid space and down the central canal around the spinal cord.

Blood supply

The blood supply to the brain is derived from the internal carotid arteries which supply the anterior territory, and is the vertebral arteries which supply the posterior. These arteries form an anastomosis at the base of the brain which is referred to as the Circle of Willis, which gives rise to the specific arteries which provide the fine network supplying the brain. Blood transports oxygen and other nutrients necessary for the health of neurons, so a constant flow of blood to the brain must be maintained. The brain is dependent on a constant internal environment. This is supported by the blood brain barrier (BBB). It is a selective barrier rather than an absolute one, allowing the transfer of nutrients across the tightly packed capillary membranes. Some drugs and alcohol can pass through the BBB.

Cerebral hemispheres

The brain is comprised of two cerebral hemispheres. Each hemisphere has four lobes, the frontal, parietal, temporal and occipital. Injury to these areas results in signs and symptoms on the opposite side of the body, which is referred to as a *contralateral deficit*. The left hemisphere is dominant in over 90 per cent of right-handed people and 60 per cent of left-handed people (Bahra and Cikurel, 1999). The speech centres of the brain are predominantly located in the frontal and temporal lobes of the left hemisphere of the brain (in right-handers).

The cerebral cortex is the outer layer of the cerebrum, also called the grey matter. Nerve cell bodies are mostly found in the grey matter. The four lobes of the brain each have specific functions.

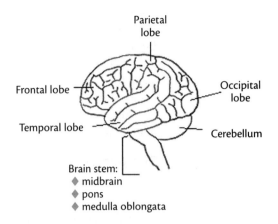

Figure 30.8 Lobes of the brain

The **frontal lobe** regulates behaviour and emotions. The motor cortex (homunculus) and Broca's area (relates to the motor function of speech) are located in the frontal lobe in the dominant hemisphere. Damage to the frontal lobe can result in personality change, inappropriate social behaviour, poor judgment, lack of concentration, difficulty in problem solving and expressive dysphasia. Broca's expressive dysphasia comprises non-fluent, hesitant speech or production of the wrong word, but with intact comprehension of spoken word (Bahra and Cikurel, 1999). Lesions of the frontal lobe because of their proximity are often associated with disturbance of the olfactory (sense of smell) and visual pathways (Bahra and Cikurel, 1999).

The **parietal lobe** interprets sensory information in conjunction with other lobes, and controls the ability to recognise and respond to touch, pressure and body position (Hickey, 2003). There is a sensory cortex (homunculus) mapped across this lobe. If this lobe is damaged then apraxia and neglect may occur. A person may have difficulty distinguishing between left and right and/or skills that involve numeracy.

The **temporal lobe** is the primary auditory area, and contains Wernicke's area. If this area is damaged the patient may experience problems comprehending spoken and written language; this is referred to as receptive dysphasia (Bahra and Cikurel, 1999). Damage to this lobe affects the ability to hear and interpret sound (auditory capabilities), smell and taste. Irritability and hallucinations can also occur.

The **occipital lobe** is responsible for visual perception and involuntary eye movements. It is the primary visual area and if it is damaged, hemianopia (loss of vision to half of the visual field) and other visual problems can occur (Marieb and Hoehn, 2007).

Other regions of the brain

The **hypothalamus** controls temperature, sleep, emotions, autonomic activity and the pituitary gland. The thalamus is the main relay station for incoming sensory pathways.

The **pituitary gland** has two lobes. The anterior lobe secretes six major hormones that relate to metabolic functions. The posterior lobe produces a hormone that controls the water content of the body (anti-diurectic hormone, ADH) (Hickey, 2003).

The **cerebellum** and its connections are responsible for rapid, coordinated and dextrous movements, posture and gait (Bahra and Cikurel, 1999; Lasserson et al, 2000).

The **brain stem** is made up of three areas: the **midbrain**,

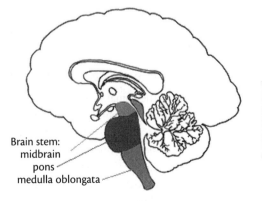

Figure 30.9 Regions of the brain

pons and **medulla oblongata**. The respiratory and cardiac centres are located within the pons and medulla oblongata, and control vital functions such as rate, rhythm and depth of breathing, pulse and blood pressure.

The **reticular formation** is a complex network (of nuclei and nerve fibres) in the brain stem (midbrain, pons and medulla oblongata), which passes through the thalamus and communicates with the cerebral cortex. It has an important role in automatic and reflex activities. The reticular activating system (RAS) provides the link between the cortex and the brain stem in relation to consciousness.

The peripheral nervous system (PNS)

The PNS is outside the CNS and consists mainly of the nerves that extend from the brain and spinal cord:

- 12 pairs of cranial nerves
- 31 pairs of spinal nerves.

There are two functional divisions of the PNS:

- sensory (afferent), which carries information from your skin and organs to the brain via the brain stem
- motor (efferent), which carries information from various sites in the brain to your skin, organs and muscles.

The first two cranial nerves originate from the functional areas associated with their names. The other cranial nerves originate from the brain stem.

Table 30.11 Cranial function

Cranial nerve		Function
I	Olfactory	Sense of smell
II	Optic	Vision (visual fields and acuity)
III	Oculomotor	Movement of eyes, pupil constriction and accommodation
IV	Trochlear	Movement of eyes
V	Trigeminal	General sensation of face and scalp and opening and of closing of mouth, chewing
VI	Abducens	Movement of eyes
VII	Facial	Facial movement, taste, salivation and lacrimation
VIII	Vestibulocochlear (or acoustic)	Vestibular sensation (balance) and auditory (hearing)
IX	Glossopharyngeal	Gag and swallow, sensation in oral cavity, taste, and salivation
X	Vagus	Swallowing, innervation of glands and viscera, speech and control of cardiovascular system, respiratory and gastrointestinal tracts
XI	(Spinal) Accessory	Movement of head and shoulders
XII	Hypoglossal	Movement and strength of the tongue

The spinal cord and column

The spinal cord runs through a hollow canal (formed by the spinal foramina) in the centre of the vertebral column, and is a cylindrical, pliable structure. It is suspended in the vertebral canal and surrounded by the meninges and cerebrospinal fluid. It is continuous with the medulla oblongata and extends to the lower border of L1-2 vertebrae (Marieb and Hoehn, 2007). The spinal cord terminates in a tapered cone shape called the conus medullaris, and divides into the cauda aquina. The spinal cord is approximately 45 cm long in an adult and is about as thick as an adult female's little finger (Marieb and Hoehn, 2007).

The spinal/vertebral column consists of 24 movable bones grouped into regions called the cervical, thoracic and lumbar vertebrae. The sacral area consists of five fused bones and finally the coccyx which consists of four fused bones. The spinal nerves exit the cord at segmental levels of the spinal column, and are numbered in relation to the level from which they exit.

Spinal tracts

During assessments sensory and motor functions are tested. Ascending (sensory/afferent) and descending (motor/efferent) nerve fibre tracts link the brain, via the brain stem and spinal cord, with the whole of the body, such as the skin, viscera and effector muscles. Figure 30.10 gives an overview of five key spinal tracts and their function. It is common practice for motor and sensory function to be colour-coded red and blue respectively.

Motor	Motor tracts			Sensory			Sensory
	Extra-pyramidal	**Cortico-spinal-pyramidal**	**Cortico-bulbar**	**Spinothalamic**		**Posterior dorsal column**	
	Regulates muscle movement: posture, tone	Control voluntary motor: trunk, limbs	Control motor: head, neck	Anterior Crude touch	Lateral Pain Temperature	Position Vibration Fine touch	

Figure 30.10 Key spinal tracts and their functions

Conclusion

If you have not yet done so, you should now complete the learning activities suggested in the chapter. Then revisit the learning outcomes and consider how this has contributed to your evolving knowledge base. This will ensure that you develop understanding of the underpinning knowledge base in relation to assessment and management of patients following a head injury.

Your knowledge base will expand and develop through exploration of the wider literature and discussion with peers, colleagues, mentors and academic advisors. With the application of the knowledge, the evidence base can be imbedded in clinical practice, promoting safe, quality patient care.

References

Addison, C. and Crawford, B. (1999) 'Not bad, just misunderstood', *Nursing Times* **95**(43), 52–3.

Aird, T. and McIntosh, M. (2004) 'Nursing tools and strategies to assess cognition and confusion', *British Journal of Nursing* **13**(10), 621–6.

American College of Surgeons (1993) *ATLS Advanced Trauma Life Support Program for Physicians: 1993 instructor manual*, 5th edn, Chicago, American College of Surgeons.

Bader, M. K. and Littlejohns, L. R. (eds) (2004) *AANN Core Curriculum for Neuroscience Nursing*, 4th edn, St Louis, Mo., Saunders.

Bahra, A. and Cikurel, K. (1999) *Mosby's Crash Course: Neurology*, London, Mosby.

Barker, E. (2002) *Neuroscience Nursing: A spectrum of care*, 2nd edn, St Louis, Mo., Mosby.

British National Formulary (BNF) (2005) *British National Formulary 49*, March, London, BMJ Publishing.

Brodie, M. J., Schachter, S. C. and Kwan, P. (2005) *Fast Facts: Epilepsy*, 3rd edn, Oxford, Health Press.

Crossman, A. R. and Neary, D. (2000) *Neuroanatomy: An illustrated colour text*, 2nd edn, Edinburgh, Churchill Livingstone.

Edwards, S. L. (2001) 'Using the Glasgow Coma Scale: analysis and limitations', *British Journal of Nursing* **10**(2), 92–101.

Epilepsy Action (2007) *Epilepsy Information: Seizure types* [online] http://www.epilepsy.org.uk/info/classifications.html (accessed 29 August 2007).

Evans, R. W. (2007) *UpToDate: Concussion and mild traumatic brain injury*, version 15.2 [online] Available at: http://utdol.com/utd/content/topic.do?topicKey=medneuro/5455&view=print (accessed 9 July 2007).

Fielding, K. and Rowley, G. (1990) 'Reliability of assessments by skilled observers using the Glasgow Coma Scale', *Australian Journal of Advanced Nursing* **7**(4), 13–17.

Fischer, J. and Mathieson, C. (2001) 'The history of the Glasgow Coma Scale: implications for practice', *Critical Care Nursing Quarterly* **23**(4), 52–8.

FitzGerald, M. J. T. and Folan-Curran, J. (2002) *Clinical Neuroanatomy and Related Neuroscience*, 4th edn, Edinburgh, W.B. Saunders.

Goetz, C. G. (2003) *Textbook of Clinical Neurology*, 2nd edn, Philadelphia, Pa., Saunders.

Goldhill, D. R. (2001) 'The critically ill: following your MEWS' (editorial), *Quarterly Journal of Medicine* 94, 507–10.

Goldhill, D. R., White, S. A. and Sumner, A. (1999) 'Physiological values and procedures in the 24h before ICU admission from the ward', *Anaesthesia* 54, 529–34.

Greenwood, R. (2002) 'Head injury for neurologists', *Journal of Neurology, Neurosurgery and Psychiatry* 73 (supp. I), i8–i16.

Harrahill, M. (1996) 'Glasgow Coma Scale: a quick review', *Journal of Emergency Nursing* (February), 81–3.

Hayes, C. (2004) 'Clinical skills: practical guide for managing adults with epilepsy', *British Journal of Nursing* 13(7), 380–7.

Hickey, J. V. (2003) *The Clinical Practice of Neurological and Neurosurgical Nursing*, 5th edn, Philadelphia, Pa., Lippincott.

Hutchinson, P. J. and Kirkpatrick, P. J. (2002) 'Acute head injury for the neurologist', *Journal of Neurology, Neurosurgery and Psychiatry* 73(Supp. I), i3–i7.

Jennett, B. (1986) 'Altered consciousness and coma', pp. 117–26 in Crockard, A., Hatward, R. and Hoff, J. T (eds), *Neurosurgery: The scientific basis of clinical practice*, Oxford, Blackwell Science.

Jennett, B. and Teasdale, G. (1977) 'Aspects of coma after severe head injury', *The Lancet* (23 April), 878–81.

Lasserson, D., Gabriel, C. and Sharrack, B. (2000) *Mosby's Crash Course: Nervous system and special senses*, Edinburgh, Mosby.

Lawal, M. (2005) 'Management and treatment options for epilepsy', *British Journal of Nursing* 14(16), 854–8.

Le May, A. (1999) *Evidence-Based Practice*, Nursing Times Monographs 1, London, NT Books.

Marieb, E. N. and Hoehn, K. (2007) *Human Anatomy and Physiology*, 7th edn, San Francisco, Calif., Pearson Benjamin Cummings.

McLeod, A. (2004) 'Intra and extracranial causes of alteration in level of consciousness', *British Journal of Nursing* 13(7), 354–61.

National Institute for Clinical Excellence (NICE) (2004) *The Epilepsies: The diagnosis and management of the epilepsies in adults and children in primary and secondary care*, Clinical Guideline 20, London, NICE.

NICE (2007) *Head Injury: Triage, Assessment, Investigation and Early Management of Head Injury in Infants, Children and Adults* (partial update of Clinical Guideline 4), London, NICE.

National Society for Epilepsy (2007) 'Information on epilepsy: back to basics – seizure classification' [online] http://www.epilepsynse.org.uk/pages/info/leaflets/b2bseizuresclass.cfm (accessed 29 August 2007).

Nursing and Midwifery Council (NMC) (2007) *Code of Professional Conduct* [online] http://www.nmc-uk.org/aFrameDisplay.aspx?DocumentID=606 (accessed 13 July 2007).

Palmer, R. and Knight, J. (2006) 'Assessment of altered conscious level in clinical practice', *British Journal of Nursing* 15(22), 1255–9.

Resuscitation Council (UK) (2006) *Advanced Life Support*, 5th edn, London, Resuscitation Council (UK).

Schein, R. M., Hazday, N., Pena, M., Ruben, B. H. and Sprung, C. L. (1990) 'Clinical antecedents to in-hospital cardiopulmonary arrest', *Chest* **98**(6), 1388–92.

Scottish Intercollegiate Guidelines Network (SIGN) (2003) *Diagnosis and Management of Epilepsy in Adults: A clinical guideline* (no. 70), Edinburgh, SIGN.

Shah, S. (1999) 'Neurological assessment', *Nursing Standard* 13(22), 49–56.

Teasdale, G. (1975) 'Acute impairment of brain function – 1: assessing 'conscious level', *Nursing Times* (12 June), 914–17.

Teasdale, G. M. (2004) 'The Glasgow Coma Scale – 30 years on', Leeds, Neurotrauma Symposium.

Teasdale, G. M. and Jennett, B. (1974) 'Assessment of the coma and impaired consciousness: a practical scale', *The Lancet* 2(7872), 81–4.

Victor, M. and Ropper, A. H. (2001) *Adams and Victor's Principles of Neurology*, New York, McGraw-Hill.

Waterhouse, C. (2005) 'The Glasgow Coma Scale and other neurological observations', *Nursing Standard* 19(33), 56–64.

Wiese, M. F. (2003) 'Different versions of the Glasgow Coma Scale: telephone survey', *British Medical Journal* 327, 782–3.

Woodward, S. (1997) 'Practical procedures for nurses no. 5.1: neurological observations 1, Glasgow Coma Scale'. *Nursing Times* **93**(supp. 45), 1–2.

Websites

British Brain and Spine Foundation: http://www.brainandspine.org.uk
Headway: http://www.headway.org.uk

Chapter

31

Child emergency care and resuscitation

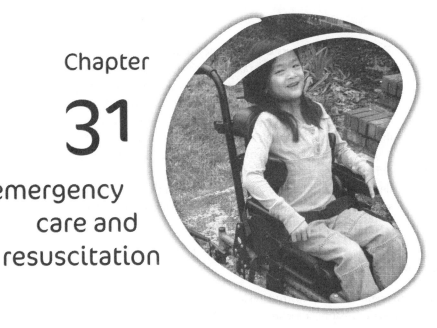

Janet Kelsey and Gill McEwing

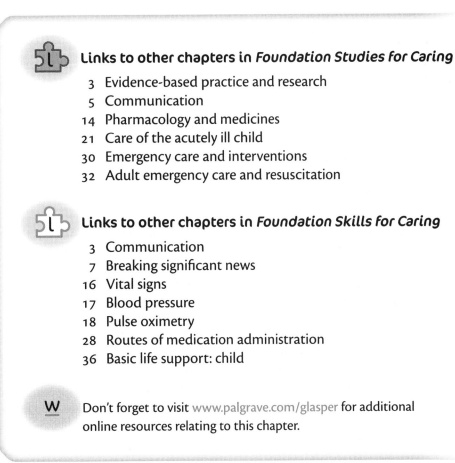

Links to other chapters in *Foundation Studies for Caring*

Links to other chapters in *Foundation Skills for Caring*

W   Don't forget to visit www.palgrave.com/glasper for additional online resources relating to this chapter.

Part

IV

Introduction

This chapter considers the emergency response to a child presenting with an acute incident in a community setting. It takes you through the stages of recognising and responding to a critical situation using the structured approach to care management. It discusses the relevant anatomical and physiological differences that need to be considered when caring for infants and children in an emergency situation. Communication, team work and support of the individuals involved in this situation are considered.

Babies and children are different from adults anatomically and physiologically as well as differing in the types of illnesses and injuries they sustain. The management of these may vary depending upon the age of the child. When they are involved in a life-threatening situation some of the anatomical differences must be taken into consideration.

Learning outcomes

This chapter will enable you to:

- recognise the signs of airway obstruction in a child
- provide emergency treatment for an infant or child with airway obstruction
- provide recovery care if the obstruction is relieved
- be aware of the anatomical and physiological differences of the respiratory and cardiovascular systems of babies and children.

- recognise when a cardiac arrest occurs in a child
- identify the keys stages in delivering basic life support for an infant and a child
- consider how to support parents witnessing their child in an emergency situation.

Concepts

- Emergency care
- Communication
- Assessment

- Decision making
- Safety

- Team working
- Family support

[S] Scenario: Introducing Sarah

Sarah is 3 years old; she is with her parents at the local fete. She is having a great time with her friends on the bouncy castle when she suddenly begins to cough, then she collapses.

Choking because of obstruction of the airway by an aspirated foreign body is a common problem in pre-school children. The foreign bodies could be objects such as a small toy, a marble, a coin or more commonly food such as sweets (Wayne, 2007). Infants and young children have few or no teeth, which reduces the probability of them masticating their food properly and increases the likelihood of their attempting to swallow larger pieces of food. Young children have also not developed the ability to coordinate chewing and swallowing in time with breathing. The consequence of this is that when objects are placed in the child's mouth there is a possibility that they will be inhaled, resulting in either partial or total occlusion of the airway.

[a] Learning activity

How many teeth will a child of 3 have? At what age would you expect Sarah's deciduous teeth to begin to fall out?

Inhalation of foreign bodies is a risk to young children. Visit your nearest health promotion unit and find the information available to parents and carers on this topic. Ask the manager of the unit how this information usually reaches parents.

A history of events is very important in helping establish whether the airway is obstructed by a foreign body or whether it is due to underlying pathology such as an allergic reaction or infection. Wayne (2007) suggests that the kind of questions you need to ask the parent/carer include:

- Were you or anyone else with the child at the time?
- Did you see what they playing with?
- Did you see the child put anything in their mouth? If so what?
- Have you a similar object with you?
- Has the child been ill with a recent respiratory illness?
- Have they had any recent difficulty in swallowing?
- Do they have any known allergies?
- Was the child eating? Could they have eaten anything that they are allergic to?

It is necessary to establish whether the airway is partially or totally obstructed. If the child is able to cry or talk then the trachea is only partly obstructed. If the child is coughing or wheezing and becoming cyanosed it is more likely that a total obstruction of the airway has been caused. It needs to be remembered that children do not go 'blue' but become pale with blue tinges to their lips, mucous membranes and nails (Wayne, 2007). If the child is unresponsive, with no spontaneous breathing and the history suggests aspiration, they may have totally occluded their airway and should be managed within the choking algorithm and cardiopulmonary resuscitation commenced (RCUK, 2005).

Most choking events in children occur during play or while eating (RCUK, 2005).The majority of deaths from foreign body aspiration occur in pre-school children (APLS, 2004; Cleaver and Webb, 2007). The foreign body obstruction sequence should only be used in children when there is a definite history of aspiration of a foreign body, when the onset of symptoms has been very sudden and there are no other signs of illness (RCUK, 2005; Cleaver and Webb, 2007).

The child's ability to cough effectively is the most important characteristic influencing how to manage the situation (Cleaver and Webb, 2007). The factors involved in determining whether the child can cough effectively are:

- crying or able to speak
- can take a breath before coughing
- is able to cough loudly
- is fully responsive/not losing consciousness.

In this situation help should be summoned, the child should be reassured, encouraged to cough and watched closely for any signs of deterioration in their condition. If the child's coughing either is or becomes ineffective help should be summoned and their conscious level reassessed.

> **S Scenario continued**
>
> Sarah's 6-year-old friend was on the bouncy castle. She is very upset, and tells her mother that she gave Sarah one of her chewy sweets.
>
> Given this information, you conclude that is highly possible Sarah has inhaled the sweet.

> **a Learning activity**
>
> How would you know whether Sarah's coughing is effective?

> **S Scenario continued**
>
> It is probable that Sarah has inhaled the sweet; she is no longer coughing or wheezing and has become very pale. The first aid officer is called to come and assist.

> **a Learning activity**
>
> How would you explain your actions to the parents of Sarah?

Physical methods (back blows, chest thrusts) of clearing the airway should be performed if there is clear evidence of an inhaled foreign body and the infant/child has increasing dyspnoea or becomes apnoeic with ineffective coughing. Only when a foreign body is easily visible and at the front of the mouth should an attempt at its removal be made by grasping the object firmly before removing (Wayne, 2007). A blind finger sweep must not be performed as this may push the foreign body further down and may cause trauma to the soft palate. If the child is conscious, allow the child to adopt the best position to maintain their airway and encourage coughing.

The management of choking in infants and children differs slightly. For the purposes of resuscitation and management of choking, the Resuscitation Council UK Guidelines (RCUK, 2005) define an infant as under 1 year of age, and a child as between 1 year and puberty.

In any situation where a child is choking it is important to ensure that you are not putting yourself in danger, to consider the safest way to manage the child and to summon assistance/call for help (RCUK, 2005).

Conscious child with airway obstruction

1 If the child is still conscious but has absent or ineffective coughing, give back blows.
2 If back blows do not relieve the foreign body obstruction, give chest thrusts to infants or abdominal thrusts to children. These manoeuvres create an 'artificial cough' to increase intrathoracic pressure and dislodge the foreign body.

Management of an infant with airway obstruction

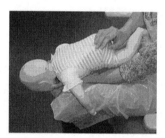

Figure 31.1 Position for managing an infant with airway obstruction

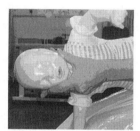

Figure 31.2 Supporting the head

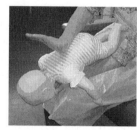

Figure 31.3 Performing back blows

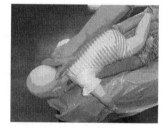

Figure 31.4 Turning to the supine position

1 Position the infant with their head down in prone position, along your thigh or knee for support. This will use gravity to assist removal of the foreign body. (See Figure 31.1.)
2 Support the head by placing your thumb at the angle of the lower jaw, and place one or two fingers of the same hand in a similar position on the other side of the jaw. (See Figure 31.2.)
3 Take care not to further obstruct the airway by compressing the soft tissues under the infant's jaw.
4 Perform five firm back blows, in

the middle of the back between shoulder blades, using the heel of one hand. (See Figure 31.3.)
5 Check the mouth after each back blow.
6 If there is a successful removal of foreign body cease the back blows.
7 If the infant remains obstructed and is still conscious, turn the infant over to the supine position remaining head down. The safest way to do this is to place the free arm along the infant's spine and hold the back of the infant's head in your hand. Remember to

support the head and neck when turning the infant. (See Figure 31.4.)
8 Support your arm by placing it down or across your thigh. (See Figure 31.5.)

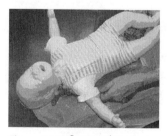

Figure 31.5 Supporting your arm for chest thrusts

9   Now perform five chest thrusts. Abdominal thrusts must not be used in infants because of the risk of intra-abdominal injury (Hoskins and Chandler, 2007).

10 Locate the lower sternum, approximately a finger's breadth above the xiphisternum.

11 Use the same fingers as for chest compressions and deliver chest compressions in an upward thrusting movement. This is similar to chest compressions but sharper in nature and performed at a slightly slower rate. (See Figure 31.6.)

12 Repeat five times checking for expulsion of the foreign body between thrusts.

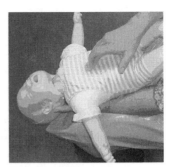

Figure 31.6 Chest thrusts

Management of a child with airway obstruction

1   Commence with five back blows, placing the child with their head lower than their chest.

2   Either sit the child on your knee, lean them forward, or place child over your knee, head down. (See Figure 31.7.)

3   Check the mouth after each blow.

4   If it is still obstructed, perform five abdominal thrusts. Stand or kneel behind the child. By placing your arms under the child's arms encircle the torso. Clench the fist of one hand and place it between the child's umbilicus and

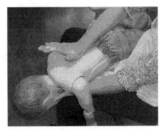

Figure 31.7 Position for managing a child with airway obstruction

xiphisternum. Grasp your fist with your other hand and pull sharply inwards and upwards. Avoid the xiphoid process and the lower rib

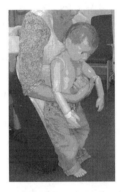

Figure 31.8 Abdominal thrusts

cage as this can cause abdominal trauma. (See Figure 31.8.)

S   Scenario continued

Sarah's condition does not improve. A crowd is gathering and asking what is happening.

---

a   Learning activity

How would you manage the scenario situation?

Reassessing the infant or child

If the airway is still obstructed and the patient is still conscious, continue with the sequence of back blows and chest (infant) or abdominal (child) thrusts.

Try to ensure that help has been summoned. If you are alone, call out, but do not leave the child/infant.

If the object has been expelled

Assess the child's condition. A piece of the object may still be present in the child's respiratory tract. Also physical methods to remove a foreign body may cause internal injuries, therefore it is important to continue to seek medical assistance.

If the infant or child becomes unconscious

1   Place the infant or child on a flat surface.

Part

IV

2 Ensure help has been summoned but do not leave the infant/child.

3 Open the mouth and look for the foreign body. If it is visible, attempt to remove it with one single finger sweep. Only perform a finger sweep if the object is clearly visible, and only attempt this once as repeated sweeps can impact the object more deeply, causing greater obstruction or damage.

If the infant or child is not breathing whether the object has been removed or not

1 Open the airway by using a chin lift/jaw thrust.

2 Attempt five rescue breaths.

3 If there is no response, proceed immediately to chest compressions and cardio pulmonary resuscitation, and follow the sequence for a single rescuer for one minute before summoning help. When the airway is opened for rescue breaths, check if the foreign body can be seen and removed with a single finger sweep.

If the obstruction is relieved

1 Open and check the airway.

2 If the infant/child is not breathing perform five rescue breaths.

3 If the infant/child regains consciousness and is able to breathe effectively, place them in a side lying recovery position, and monitor their breathing and level of consciousness until medical help arrives.

Positioning an infant or child to aid recovery

A number of recovery positions are currently advocated. No single one can be endorsed (Black, 2007). A suitable position should:

- be stable
- as near to a lateral position as possible, enabling free drainage of fluid from the mouth
- maintain a patent airway
- maintain a stable cervical spine
- avoid application of pressure on the chest that restricts breathing
- minimise the risk of aspiration
- limit pressure on bony prominences and peripheral nerves
- enable visualisation of the child's breathing and colour
- allow access to the child for interventions
- be easy and safe to achieve (including repositioning if required).

> **(a) Learning activity**
>
> Practise putting somebody into an effective recovery position.

An unconscious infant, breathing spontaneously can be held in the rescuer's arms. Ideally the infant should be face down with the head lower than the body. This position will help keep the airway open, allow fluids to drain from the mouth and keep the neck and spine in alignment (Black, 2007).

An unconscious child, breathing spontaneously needs to be positioned lying on their side (see Figure 31.9). In order to do this safely the following steps can be used.

1 Remove any bulky items either in the child's clothing or on the child (such as bags) and clear the immediate area of objects.

2 While kneeling next to the child, straighten the child's legs, and place the nearest arm at right angles to the body, elbow bent and palm up.

3 Bring the child's arm farthest away from you across the child's chest. Hold the hand palm outwards against the child's nearside cheek.

4 Using your other hand bend the knee of the far leg so that the foot is flat on the ground.

5 While supporting the child's hand against their cheek, use your other hand to pull the bent knee of the far leg. This will roll the child's towards you. With the child on their side, position the upper leg, bending both the hip and knee at right angles. This will prevent the child from rolling forward.

6 Tilt the child's head back slightly and adjust the child's hand position to maintain the airway and assist in the drainage of fluids from the mouth.

7 The child's position should be changed from side to side every 30 minutes unless the child's injuries prevent this.

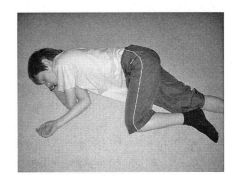

Figure 31.9 The recovery position for a child

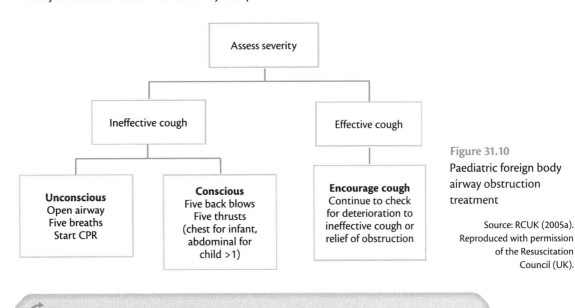

Figure 31.10

Paediatric foreign body airway obstruction treatment

Source: RCUK (2005a). Reproduced with permission of the Resuscitation Council (UK).

(a) Learning activity

Do you think Sarah is at risk of primary or secondary cardiorespiratory arrest?

Reasons that infants and children experience cardiorespiratory arrest

The underlying cause of cardiorespiratory arrest in infants and children is different from that of adults. The pathologies that affect children usually cause a secondary cardiorespiratory arrest as a result of respiratory and/or circulatory failure. Adults tend to experience primary cardiorespiratory arrest caused by cardiac dysfunction or arrhythmia.

Primary cardiorespiratory arrest

This is uncommon in children but can be seen when a child has existing cardiac disease or following cardiac surgery. It can also occur following hypothermia or poisoning. The cardiorespiratory arrest results from cardiac arrhythmias, usually ventricular fibrillation or pulseless ventricular tachycardia. The onset is sudden and immediate defibrillation is required. Any delay reduces the chance of a return to circulation by 10 per cent every minute (Kelly, 2007).

Secondary cardiorespiratory arrest

This sequence is more commonly seen in children, and is the result of the body's inability to

Part

IV

cope with the underlying illness or injury. The preterminal rhythm is bradycardia, which leads to asystole or pulseless electrical activity (Kelly, 2007). This can be preceded by either:

- Respiratory failure leading to inadequate oxygenation, hypoxia and hypercapnia causing acidosis. This then causes cell damage and cell death, leading to cardiac arrest.
- Circulatory failure when organs are deprived of essential nutrients and oxygen, plus the inability to remove waste products causes hypoxia and acidosis. Inadequate circulation will cause vital organs to be under perfused and cell damage will result.

Respiratory and circulatory failure can occur separately or together, but as the condition becomes worse, both will occur (Kelly, 2007).

It is broadly accepted that cardiopulmonary resuscitation including compressions and/or ventilations should be undertaken in children who have arrested. Although there are few systematic reviews, most clinicians regard bystander cardiopulmonary resuscitation to be an important intervention in out of hospital cardiopulmonary arrest. The 2006 International Liaison Committee on Resuscitation's consensus on science treatment recommendation encourages 'trained rescuers to provide both ventilations and chest compressions. The consensus recommendation goes on to encourage those rescuers who are reluctant or unable to perform ventilations to institute and continue chest compressions without interruption' (American Heart Organization, 2005).

> **S** Scenario continued
>
> Sarah's condition has not improved. The lack of oxygen entering her respiratory system has led to hypoxia and hypercapnia, and this has become so severe that she experiences a respiratory arrest and has become bradycardic.
>
> The ambulance has arrived and the paramedics take over the care of Sarah from the first aid officer. Basic life support is commenced.

When a child's body suffers respiratory problems, compensatory mechanisms will be utilised to try to provide oxygen to the vital organs. This will include tachycardia, tachypnoea and increased vascular resistance (Hoskins and Chandler, 2007). Increased secretion of antidiuretic hormone will compensate for fluid loss by reducing urine output and conserving water. Eventually the compensatory mechanisms fail and the child develops decompensatory shock, becoming bradycardic, leading to tissue hypoxia, myocardial dysfunction and eventually asystole (Hoskins and Chandler, 2007).

The anatomy and physiology of the respiratory and cardiovascular systems of babies and children differ from those of adults. These need to be considered when assessing and managing ill or injured children.

Table 31.1 The anatomy and physiology of respiratory and cardiovascular systems in babies and children

Anatomical factor	Practical considerations
Airway	
Large head, short neck, inability to support head.	Assistance required to maintain position of comfort. Can cause neck to flex in the unconscious child and contribute to airway obstruction.
Large tongue.	Airway is easily obstructed by tongue; proper positioning is often all that is necessary to open the airway.
The floor of the mouth is easily compressible.	Care is required in positioning of the fingers when holding the jaw.
Infants less than 6 months old are obligate nose breathers.	Obstruction of the nasal passages by mucus can compromise the infant's airway.
Smaller diameter of all airways (in a 1-year-old child, the tracheal diameter is less than the child's little finger).	Small amounts of mucus or swelling easily obstruct the airways. The child normally has increased airway resistance.

Anatomical factor	Practical considerations
The epiglottis is quite floppy and horseshoe shaped and projects posteriorly at 45 degrees. The larynx is high and anterior.	Tracheal intubation can be more difficult, it can be hard to visualise the cords. A straight blade laryngoscope is used and cricoid pressure may be necessary to facilitate intubation.
The tonsils and adenoids may be enlarged in children aged 3–8 years.	Can cause airway obstruction in the unconscious child (Hoskins and Chandler, 2007).
The trachea is short and soft. The cricoid cartilage is the narrowest portion of the neck.	The airway of an infant can be compressed if the neck is flexed or hyperextended. Tube displacement is more likely. It provides a natural seal for an endotracheal tube.
The cricoid ring is lined by pseudostratifed ciliated epithelium loosely bound to areolar tissue.	Particularly susceptible to oedema. Uncuffed tubes may be preferred in pre-pubertal children.
Breathing	
Infants rely mainly on diaphragmatic breathing. The ribs lie more horizontally in infants and contribute less to chest expansion.	Children are more prone to respiratory failure. Anything that impedes diaphragm contraction or movement, such as abdominal distension, can contribute to the development of respiratory failure.
The muscles have fewer type 1 fibres than adults.	Their muscles are more likely to fatigue than adults'.
The sternum and ribs are cartilaginous; the chest wall is soft; intercostal muscles are poorly developed.	An infant's chest wall may move inwards instead of outwards during inspiration (retractions) when lung compliance is decreased; greater intrathoracic pressure is generated during inspiration. The compliant chest wall may allow serious parenchymal injuries to occur without rib fracture.
Increased metabolic rate (about twice that of an adult); increased respiratory demand for oxygen consumption and carbon dioxide elimination.	Respiratory distress increases oxygen demand, as does any condition that increases metabolic rate, such as fever.
Lung compliance and high chest wall compliance in the neonate.	Respiratory function is inefficient during episodes of respiratory distress.
Smaller amount of elastic and collagen tissue in the paediatric lung.	May contribute to the increased incidence of pulmonary oedema, pneumomediastinum and pneumothorax in infants.
Circulation	
A child's circulating blood volume is larger per unit of body weight (70–80ml/kg) but absolute volume is relatively small; 70–80 per cent of newborn's body weight is water, compared with 50–60 per cent of an adult body weight; about half of this volume is extracellular.	Blood loss considered minor in an adult may lead to shock in a child; decreased fluid intake or increased fluid loss quickly leads to dehydration.
Stroke volume is small and relatively fixed in infants. Cardiac output is directly related to heart rate. By the age of 2 years the myocardial function and response to fluid are similar to that of an adult.	Stroke volume cannot increase to improve cardiac output. Response to volume therapy is therefore blunted. Tachycardia is the child's most efficient method of increasing cardiac output. However ventricular rates > 180–220 beats/min compromise diastolic filling time and coronary artery perfusion.
Systemic vascular resistance rises after birth and continues to do so until adulthood.	Children's normal values for blood pressure increase with age.
Short neck.	Can make it difficult to feel a carotid pulse or see jugular veins.

Basic life support

The basic principles of paediatric basic life support are the same as for adults, but there are some specific differences in technique for different sizes of children which are essential if the optimum support is to be given.

Part

IV

The major differences in technique for an infant

1 To open the airway the head and chin should be tilted to the 'sniffing position'. This is achieved by placing one hand on the forehead and tilting the head back into a neutral position, avoiding excessive neck extension and taking care not to press on the soft issues under the chin. A jaw thrust may be used if cervical spine injury is suspected. (See Figure 31.11.)

2 Deliver five rescue breaths. When delivering rescue breaths, cover the mouth and nose with your mouth, ensuring you have a good seal, and blow steadily into the mouth and nose over 1–1.5 seconds. (See Figure 31.12.)

3 If you are trained and experienced, check the circulation. The brachial pulse is easiest to feel on the inner aspect of the upper arm between the elbow and the shoulder. Gently press with your index and middle fingers until you feel the pulse. (See Figure 31.13.)

4 If the pulse rate is less than 60 beats per minute, that is less than 1 per second, external chest compressions should begin without delay. (See Figure 31.14.)

5 If you are alone, perform chest compressions by using two fingers of one hand to compress the lower third of the sternum. This is one finger's breadth above the xiphisternum. The xiphisternum is the angle where the lowest ribs join in the middle. If there are two rescuers use the encircling technique, place your thumbs flat side by side, on the lower third of the sternum with the tips pointing towards the infant's head. Spread the rest of both hands, with fingers together, encircling the lower part of the infants ribcage with the tips of the fingers supporting the infant's back. Depress the lower sternum with your thumbs to approximately one-third of the depth of the infant's chest (RCUK, 2005a).

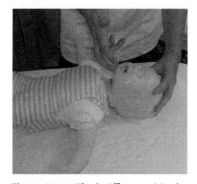
Figure 31.11   The 'sniffing position'

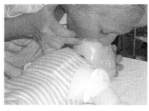
Figure 31.12   Rescue breaths

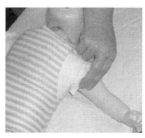
Figure 31.13   Checking the brachial pulse

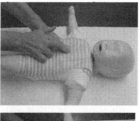
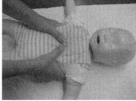
Figure 31.14   External chest compressions

The major differences in technique for a child

1 To open the airway place one hand on the forehead and tilt the head back into a neutral or slightly extended position. Lift the lower jaw with the tips of two fingers of the other hand. Avoid excessive neck extension and take care not to press on the soft issues under the chin. A jaw thrust may be used if cervical spine injury is suspected. (See Figure 31.15.)

2 To deliver rescue breaths make a mouth-to-mouth seal and pinch the soft part of the child's nose tightly with the thumb and index finger of the hand, maintaining head tilt. (See Figure 31.16.)

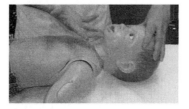
Figure 31.15   Resuscitation position for a child

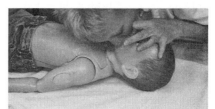
Figure 31.16   Rescue breaths for a child

3 If you are trained and experienced check the circulation. In children the carotid pulse should be palpated.

4 If the pulse is absent, then external chest compressions should begin without delay. (See Figure 31.17.)

5 In children the heel of one hand is used to compress the lower third of the sternum, which is one finger's breadth above the xiphisternum, ensuring that the fingers are lifted to prevent pressure being applied over the child's ribs. Position yourself vertically above the child's chest, with your arms straight. Compress the sternum one-third of the depth of the child's chest (RCUK, 2005a).

6 In larger children or when the rescuer is small it may be better to use both hands. Locate the lower half of the sternum and place the heel of one hand in position, then place the other hand directly on top of the first hand and interlock fingers. Raise the fingers off the chest to ensure that pressure is not applied to the child's ribs.

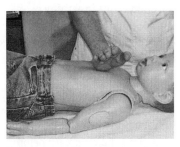

Figure 31.17 Chest compressions for a child

Basic life support in infants and children follows the airway, breathing and circulation sequence. They are the same in principle but utilise the different techniques relevant to the child's age as described earlier:

1 **Ensure safety of the rescuer and child.** It is essential that the rescuer does not become a victim and the child is removed from further danger as quickly as possible. This should precede all further actions.

2 **Assess the child's responsiveness.** Gently stimulate the child by speaking loudly and asking, 'Are you all right?' Shake by the shoulders or pinch gently. Do not shake children with suspected cervical spine injuries. A young child is unlikely to respond in a meaningful way, but may make some sound or open their eyes.

3 **If the child responds but is struggling to breathe,** leave them in the position in which you find them unless they are in further danger. Children with respiratory distress often position themselves to maintain patency of a partially obstructed airway. Attempts to improve a partially maintained airway, without advanced support being available, are potentially dangerous as total occlusion may occur. Check their condition regularly and get help if needed.

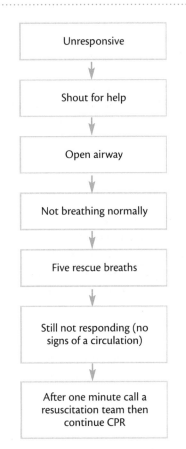

Figure 31.18 Paediatric basic life support

Reproduced with permission of the Resuscitation Council (UK).

If the child does not respond, the rescuer should shout for help and then provide basic life-support for one minute before going for assistance. It may be possible to take a small child or infant with you while summoning help. Check first

to see whether there is evidence of trauma. The likelihood of injury may be evident from the child's location or position: for example, a child found at the foot of a tree is more likely to have suffered trauma than a child found in bed. If more than one rescuer is present, then one should go for help whilst the other commences resuscitation.

After shouting for help, open the child's airway. Use the appropriate technique for the age of the child. Try to do this with the child in the position in which you find them. If this is not possible, then carefully turn the child onto their back and open the airway. Again if trauma is suspected, turn the child with head and neck firmly supported. Do not allow the head to twist, roll or tilt. Avoid head tilt if cervical spine injury is suspected.

4 **Keep the airway open and check breathing.** Look for chest and abdominal movement. Listen at the mouth and nose for breath sounds. Feel for expired air movement on your cheek.

Look, listen and feel for up to 10 seconds before deciding that breathing is absent. If the child is breathing, place them in the recovery position and continue to assess them.

Part

IV

The flow diagram in Figure 31.18 shows:
- Unresponsive
- Shout for help
- Open airway
- Not breathing normally
- Five rescue breaths
- Still not responding (no signs of a circulation)
- After one minute call a resuscitation team then continue CPR

5 **If the child is not breathing** or there is ineffective, gasping or obstructed breathing, carefully check for and remove any obvious airway obstruction, but do not perform a blind finger sweep.

Give up to five rescue breaths. With each breath, the child's chest should move. Take a breath before each rescue breath to optimise the amount of oxygen delivered to the child. Breath slowly and steadily for between 1 and 1.5 seconds. This minimises the risk of gastric distension, which can reduce the effectiveness of rescue breathing by pushing up the diaphragm and reducing lung volume. If the chest either does not rise or is inadequate, then the airway may be obstructed. Recheck the child's mouth for obvious obstruction. Readjust the airway position. Five attempts should be made to achieve two effective breaths. If you are still unsuccessful, then consider foreign body obstruction and move on to the airway obstruction sequence.

6 **Assess the child's circulation**. Take no more than 10 seconds to check the pulse using the correct technique for the age of the child (Infants; brachial or femoral, child; carotid). At the same time look for signs of life such as any movement including swallowing or breathing.

If you can detect signs of circulation within the 10 seconds but no breathing, then continue rescue breathing for one minute before going for help. If somebody else has gone for help, continue rescue breathing until the child starts breathing effectively on their own. If at this point the child remains unconscious, then turn them on to their side into the recovery position.

7 **If there is no palpable pulse**, or in infants, it is less than one beat per second, or you are not sure then start chest compressions using an age-appropriate technique and combine the chest compressions with rescue breathing.

Remember the ratio of compressions to breaths for infants and children is 30:2 for lay rescuers but for two or more rescuers with a duty to respond it is 15:2. The recommended rate of compressions is the same for all: 100 times per minute. However, this is the rate and not the number of compressions to be given in a minute, as there will be interruptions for ventilation.

8 You should continue to resuscitate until the child demonstrates spontaneous respiration and pulse, or help arrives, or you become exhausted.

(a) Learning activity   W

Once you are confident that you have achieved a good degree of knowledge about basic life support, you should practise these skills using a resuscitation mannequin in the clinical skills laboratory or on a practice placement. It is important that all nurses working with children practise these skills regularly so that they can quickly instigate resuscitation procedures on the rare occasions when they are required.

How much of this information do you think you would retain after practising on a mannequin?

Read the article by H. West (2000) on basic infant life-support. The guidelines for basic life support in children can be accessed on the internet at http://www.resus.org.uk/pages/pbls.pdf.

S   Scenario continued

Sarah's parents are very distressed. Her father becomes upset and doesn't want to watch the procedures, and he encourages his wife to come with him and sit down a short distance away. Sarah's mother becomes more distressed and does not want to leave Sarah.

Parents experience great distress when their child requires emergency treatment or resuscitation. This distress is not exacerbated if they choose to be present, and being with their child is sometimes more reassuring than not being present, which can intensify the anguish (Maxton, 2007). Parents usually have an inherent need to be with their child during periods of crisis. They should never be prevented from being with their child. However not every parent will wish to be present, and their wishes must also be respected without pressure to stay (Maxton, 2005).

Care of parents during the emergency

- Parents may exhibit a variety of behaviour responses. Crying does not necessarily mean the parent is not coping, and in some cases the parent who appears to be in control of their emotions may be nearer to crisis.

- If possible make sure you tell the parents what you are doing in terms that they can understand.
- Parents may feel comforted by the opportunity to touch their child's hand or foot. This should be offered when practically possible.
- If the parent is alone at the scene, where possible an appropriate adult should offer to give them support.
- The opportunity to make the decision to stay or leave the scene must be offered to parents at regular intervals, as their decisions may alter during the event. They should be given the opportunity to leave and return as they wish (Maxton, 2007).
- If the parent/parents decide not to stay at the scene, ensure that someone takes responsibility for keeping them informed.

S Scenario continued

The paramedics explain that Sarah is very ill and needs to go to hospital for emergency care. Sarah is transferred to hospital.

---

a Learning activity

What do you think is the likely outcome of this scenario?
  What advice would you give to a member of the public who approaches you after the ambulance has left and asks how they could be trained in basic life support?

It is important to remember that often being present comforts parents because they are able to provide comfort and love for their child irrespective of their own anguish.

Conclusion

Choking on a foreign body is a common occurrence in pre-school children. However if it is responded to swiftly, recovery is rapid. Few children progress to requiring basic life support. Advice on preventing choking should be readily available for all parents and carers of young children. The healthcare professional should be aware of this potential risk, and be competent to act promptly and effectively in situations such as those outlined in this chapter. This requires knowledge and practice in both the choking and resuscitation sequences for infants and children.

References

Advanced Paediatric Life Support group (APLS) (2004) *Advanced Paediatric Life Support: The practical approach*, 4th edn, London, BMJ Publishing.

American Heart Organisation (2005) *2005 International Consensus on CPR and ECC Science with Treatment Recommendations* [online] http://www.americanheart.org (accessed 4 February 2009).

Black, J. (2007) 'Recovery position in children and young people', in Glasper, E., McEwing, G. and Richardson, J. (eds), *Oxford Handbook of Children's and Young People's Nursing*, Oxford, Oxford University Press.

Cleaver, K. and Webb, J. (2007) *Emergency Care of Children and Young People*, Oxford, Blackwell.

Hoskins, R. and Chandler, K. (2007) 'Paediatric resuscitation', in Cleaver, K. and Webb, J. (eds), *Emergency Care of Children and Young People*, Oxford, Blackwell.

International Liaison Committee on Resuscitation (2006) The International Liaison Committee on Resuscitation (ILCOR) Consensus on science with treatment recommendations for pediatric and neonatal patients: pediatric basic and advanced life support', *Pediatrics* 117, e955–e977.

Kelly, M. (2007) 'Reasons why children arrest', in Glasper, E., McEwing,

G. and Richardson, J. (eds), *Oxford Handbook of Children's and Young People's Nursing*, Oxford, Oxford University Press.

Maxton, F. (2005) *Sharing and Surviving the Resuscitation: Parental presence during resuscitation of a child in PICU: the experiences of parents and nurses*, unpublished PhD thesis, University of Western Sydney, Australia.

Maxton, F. (2007) 'Parents witnessing arrest procedures', in Glasper, E., McEwing, G. and Richardson, J. (eds), *Oxford Handbook of Children's and Young People's Nursing*, Oxford, Oxford University Press.

Resuscitation Council (UK) (2005a) Paediatric basic life support [online] http://www.resus.org.uk/pages/pbls.pdf (accessed 23 December 2008).

RCUK (2005b) *Resuscitation Guidelines*, 2005, London, RCUK.

St John Ambulance (2002) *St Andrew's Ambulance Association and the British Red Cross Society First Aid Manual*, London, Dorling Kindersley.

Wayne, L. (2007) 'The choking infant and child', in Glasper, E., McEwing, G. and Richardson, J. (eds), *Oxford Handbook of Children's and Young People's Nursing*, Oxford, Oxford University Press.

West, H. (2000) 'Basic infant life support: retention of knowledge and skill', *Paediatric Nursing* 12(1) (February), 34–7 [online] http://www.ncbi.nlm.nih.gov/pubmed/11221327 (accessed 23 December 2008).

Part

IV

Chapter

32

Adult emergency care and resuscitation

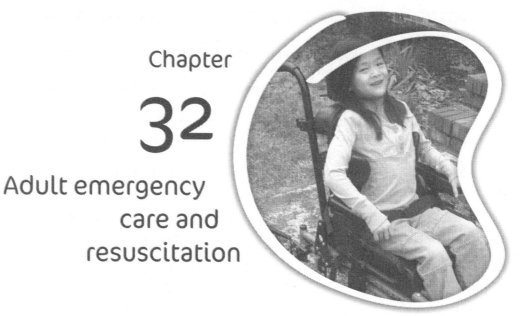

Jan Heath

Links to other chapters in *Foundation Studies for Caring*

Links to other chapters in *Foundation Skills for Caring*

W Don't forget to visit www.palgrave.com/glasper for additional online resources relating to this chapter.

Introduction

A bee or wasp sting is a common occurrence in late summer for most people. This is an uncomfortable experience but not life-threatening. However some people are allergic to the venom and can have a severe reaction. This chapter addresses the recognition of an anaphylactic reaction in a community setting. You are taken through the progression of events. The treatment of anaphylaxis and cardiac arrest is presented and discussed, and the dilemmas faced in such an emergency are considered.

Learning outcomes

This chapter will enable you to:

- define anaphylaxis
- describe the signs and symptoms of anaphylaxis
- recognise a cardiac arrest
- identify the key stages in delivering basic life support

- consider how to support relatives and friends witnessing a medical emergency

- think about the management of a community emergency when transferred to the emergency department.

Concepts

- Emergency care
- Responding to critical incidents
- Assessment

- Prioritising
- Decision making

- Communication
- Care of relatives

[S] Scenario: Introducing Simon

Simon is a 30-year-old plumber who was at the village Strawberry Fayre with his family. While watching a cookery demonstration he moved a waste bin to allow him to get a better view. This disturbed some wasps, which he felt sting his neck.

Simon immediately felt a sharp pain, and he flicked the wasps away and dashed away from where he had been standing. His neck was so sore that he went to the beer tent to ask for ice, which he applied wrapped in a cloth. The site of the sting was now swollen even though it was only a few minutes since he had been stung.

Simon asked for a glass of water and told the person behind the bar that he felt really odd.

A women at the bar described how she had been stung in the past and had investigations afterwards in hospital, and that she had been told to look for a number of symptoms which seemed similar to Simon's condition.

People in the bar sat Simon on the floor in a clear space where he could lean forward with his arms around his knees for support. The site of the sting was still very sore and swollen. Someone held ice to the site of the sting.

Simon was very restless by now, wanting to sit up as he was finding it difficult to breathe, but was complaining of

feeling very dizzy. He was increasingly anxious about his family who did not know where he was.

After about five minutes the people in the beer tent suggested Simon went to the first aid tent. As Simon tried to get up to go to the first aid tent he complained of having

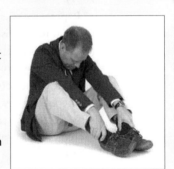

Figure 32.1 Simon seated after the sting

terrible abdominal cramps and felt sick. Other people were now aware of the problem as Simon's breathing was sounding increasingly noisy and he was quite distressed. He was helped to a chair and someone offered to go to get a first aider.

Simon was by now on his knees leaning on a chair, and gasping for breath.

It was now about 10 minutes since the initial sting. Simon's wife Donna then appeared as she been looking for him. She realised her husband's condition was serious, and asked someone to phone 999.

Anaphylaxis

Anaphylaxis is rare but severe, potentially fatal, hypersensitivity type 1 allergic reaction. There is not a conclusive definition for anaphylaxis but it should be considered when all of the following are identified.

● sudden onset of felling unwell
● mucosa or skin changes, for example swelling, itching or redness
● airway and/or breathing and/or circulation problems.

It is easier to confirm the problem when there is a history of exposure to a potential allergen. Other features are usually present:

● erythema
● generalised pruritis
● urticaria
● angio-odema
● wheeze
● rhinitis
● conjunctivitis
● itching of palate/external auditory meatus
● nausea, vomiting, abdominal pain
● palpitations
● sense of impending doom.

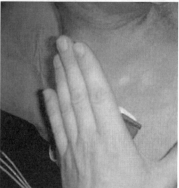

Figure 32.2 Simon with erythema

What happens during anaphylaxis

An anaphylactic reaction occurs following exposure to an allergen to which a person has been sensitised. People who have asthma and allergies are at high risk of anaphylaxis (Greenberger, 2007).

Repeated exposure results in specific IgE antibodies recognising the allergen and creating a reaction to it. This encourages mast cells to release inflammatory mediators, which cause an anaphylactic reaction. It consists of the rapid release of large quantities of mediators, which cause leakage of capillaries, and mucosal oedema, which in turn causes cardiovascular and respiratory shock (Greenberger, 2007).

There are many possible causes, most commonly:

● food especially seafood, peanuts, sesame and dairy products
● drugs such as aspirin or antibiotics
● latex
● stinging insects such as bees and wasps.

When dealing with patients presenting with difficulty with breathing, severe rashes or circulatory problems following exposure to elements that can cause anaphylaxis, urgent action is required.

There are approximately 20 deaths reported each year in the United Kingdom from anaphylaxis. However there may be many more that are not recorded (RCUK, 2008). The factors causing these reactions include the following (in numbers of suspected triggers or fatal anaphylactic reactions in the United Kingdom several years) (Pumphrey, 2004):

● 29 from wasp stings
● 4 from bee stings
● 10 from peanut
● 11 from contract medium
● 11 from penicillin
● 1 from banana
● 1 from snails.

In up to 40 per cent of cases of anaphylaxis there is no clear cause. This is called idiopathic anaphylaxis (Greenberger, 2007).

Fatal anaphylaxis occurs soon after exposure to the factor causing the reaction. It is shown that death from medicines can occur five minutes after they are administered, a reaction from a sting results in circulatory collapse 10–15 minutes after the event, while respiratory arrest happens 30–35 minutes after ingestion of food. Death will occur within six hours of exposure to the allergen. If the patient survives for this time the reaction is unlikely to be fatal (RCUK, 2008).

> ## ⒜ Learning activity   W̲
>
> Explore the statistics regarding anaphylaxis. More information can be found at www.resus.org.uk/pages/anadraft.htm

The treatment of an anaphylactic reaction

For severe anaphylaxis there is one immediate course of action that must be taken: administer adrenaline by the intramuscular route: for adults give 500 mcg of adrenaline 1:1000.

In the event of an anaphylactic reaction:

1 Act immediately.
2 Call for an ambulance.
3 Remove the item causing the event if possible: for instance, stop giving antibiotics.
4 If it is caused by an insect sting, immediately scrape away any insect parts at the site of the sting. Avoid squeezing.
5 Following ingestion of an allergen do not make the patient vomit.
6 Put the victim in a position where they are able to breathe more easily if possible. The victim might feel very faint or look very pale. If so, lie the victim down.
7 Loosen tight clothing and take a history from the victim or anyone who was present at the time.
8 Give 100 per cent oxygen if possible.
9 An experienced anaesthetist is mandatory if in hospital.

Medication for anaphylaxis in adults

- Intramuscular adrenaline 0.5 ml 1:1000 solution (500 mcg).
- If there is no improvement after five minutes repeat the dose.
- Fluids given intravenously are usually necessary.
- Salbutamol 5 mg given by nebuliser can be used to relieve bronchospasm.

Adrenaline (Epinepherine) facts

Adrenaline has a number of preparations including 1:10,000 and 1:1000. Adrenaline IM dose for adults = 0.5 mg IM which is 500 micrograms = 0.5 mL of 1:1000.

It is an alpha receptor antagonist and reverses peripheral vasodilation. It also reverses bronchodilation with its beta receptor activity. Intramuscular (IM) is the best route for most individuals to treat an anaphylactic reaction as it is safer, does not require cannulation of a vein and is easier to teach.

Specialists who are experienced in giving adrenaline intravenously in titrated doses may choose to use the intravenous route. These will be anaesthetists, intensive care doctors and experienced medical staff in the emergency department (Brown et al, 2004).

Bee and wasp stings

It is not pleasant being stung by an insect but it will happen to most people at some time. For most of us this is an incident that causes only temporary pain and discomfort. A few people however (between one and four in 1000) are allergic or hypersensitive to wasp or bee stings (Brown et al, 2004).

The sting is a modified egg-laying apparatus, hence only the female of the species will sting.

Part
IV

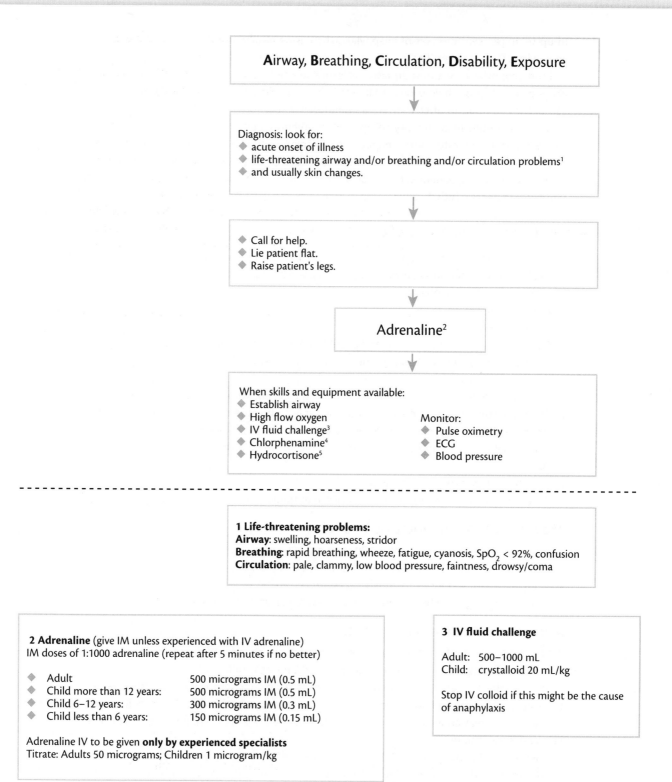

Airway, Breathing, Circulation, Disability, Exposure

Diagnosis: look for:
- acute onset of illness
- life-threatening airway and/or breathing and/or circulation problems[1]
- and usually skin changes.

- Call for help.
- Lie patient flat.
- Raise patient's legs.

Adrenaline[2]

When skills and equipment available:
- Establish airway
- High flow oxygen
- IV fluid challenge[3]
- Chlorphenamine[4]
- Hydrocortisone[5]

Monitor:
- Pulse oximetry
- ECG
- Blood pressure

---

1 Life-threatening problems:
Airway: swelling, hoarseness, stridor
Breathing: rapid breathing, wheeze, fatigue, cyanosis, SpO_2 < 92%, confusion
Circulation: pale, clammy, low blood pressure, faintness, drowsy/coma

2 Adrenaline (give IM unless experienced with IV adrenaline)
IM doses of 1:1000 adrenaline (repeat after 5 minutes if no better)

- Adult   500 micrograms IM (0.5 mL)
- Child more than 12 years: 500 micrograms IM (0.5 mL)
- Child 6–12 years: 300 micrograms IM (0.3 mL)
- Child less than 6 years: 150 micrograms IM (0.15 mL)

Adrenaline IV to be given **only by experienced specialists**
Titrate: Adults 50 micrograms; Children 1 microgram/kg

3 IV fluid challenge

Adult: 500–1000 mL
Child: crystalloid 20 mL/kg

Stop IV colloid if this might be the cause of anaphylaxis

Figure 32.3

Anaphylaxis algorithm

Source: RCUK (2008). Reproduced with permission of the Resuscitation Council (UK).

	4 Chlorphenamine (IM or slow IV)	**5 Hydrocortisone** (IM or slow IV)
Adult or child more than 12 years	10 mg	200 mg
Child 6–12 years	5 mg	100 mg
Child 6 months to 6 years	2.5 mg	50 mg
Child less than 6 months	250 micrograms/kg	25 mg

They will rarely sting when collecting pollen and nectar from flowers, but if provoked they will sting in defence. Often if caught in grass or hair they will panic and their barb will get caught, releasing the venom. It is this release of venom that causes pain when injected into the skin. The sharp pain lasts a few minutes, moving on to be a dull ache. This tenderness can last a few days.

When someone is stung their blood releases fluid to try to flush the venom from the tissue, causing swelling and redness of the area. The body's immune system will recognise the venom if the individual has been stung before, and the flushing mechanism will be more pronounced, causing greater swelling. This swelling and inflammation will be quite itchy, for which antihistamines taken either orally or applied topically may help (Brown et al, 2004).

When a honey bee stings the stinger is barbed and cannot be withdrawn by the bee. The stinger will be left in the skin, continues to pulsate, and releases venom for 45–60 seconds after impact. If it is removed during the first 15 seconds the sting is much less severe. Remove the stinger by scraping it out of the skin (do not pull it). After the stinger is removed, wash the wound and treat with a simple cold compress. There are numerous over-the-counter preparations together with many old wives' tales about how best to treat a sting. The key treatment is to cool the wound, elevate if swollen and observe (Brown et al, 2004). If the sting is in the mouth or eye, seek medical assistance. Stings in the mouth are not unusual as the insect may be in a drink or on food when someone is eating outdoors, while the eyes are vulnerable when people are tending bees. For this reason it is important that a veil is always worn when tending beehives.

> **S** Scenario continued
>
> Simon becomes unconscious and slumps to the ground. While waiting for the ambulance, bystanders put him into the recovery position. The first aid crew arrive and assess the situation. At this time Simon has no signs of respiration, palpable pulse or signs of life.

Application of theory to Simon's case history

If Simon had an anaphylactic reaction to the wasp sting he might complain of some of the following:

- itching
- blotchy skin
- urticaria
- swelling of the upper airways
- difficulty with breathing
- feeling faint
- wheezing
- runny nose
- itchy eyes
- discomfort of his mouth with swollen lips
- nausea, vomiting, abdominal pain
- palpitations.

> **t**☆ Practice tip
>
> An estimated 1 per cent of the population can perform basic life support effectively. However if that percentage was increased to 15–20 the mortality from out-of-hospital cardiac arrests would be significantly lower (RCUK, 2005).

> **a** Learning activity
>
> Revise your basic life support knowledge. If you have not had the opportunity to practise this for a while, make arrangements to go to the clinical skills practice area to practise on a mannequin.
>
> Explore how many of your friends and family have ever received any training in basic life support. Investigate where they could be directed to access such training.

Part
IV

Basic life support

Basic life support follows simple steps that can be most effective if applied promptly at the time of collapse. It may be performed by a single rescuer with no equipment.

It is important that little time is lost in calling for help, and that there are a minimum of pauses in the procedure. The recommendations in the 2005 guidelines (RCUK, 2005) placed the emphasis on looking for signs of life rather than spending time trying to assess for the presence of a carotid pulse, which was shown to be unreliable. This continues to be important, as does the absence of normal breathing. Too often patients who have irregular gasping breathing patterns are assessed to be breathing where they are actually having an end-stage respiratory pattern (agonal breathing), and as a result intervention is delayed. Forty per cent of victims of cardiac arrest have agonal respirations. Collapsed individuals who are unresponsive with irregular gasping breathing should have life support intervention (RCUK, 2005).

Basic life support is exhausting both physically and mentally, therefore help must be called for promptly. If you are alone with the victim, shout for help. If this is unlikely to raise assistance, then go to fetch help.

We can all imagine desperate situations where we could be alone with a collapsed individual with no prospect of help. In reality these are rare events, and the more likely scenario is that there will be access to a phone or other people can be alerted to the emergency.

Clear, sensible communication is essential in these circumstances. On the phone, dial an appropriate number (now 2222 in all hospitals). Tell the person what the emergency is and what help is required.

Steps to follow to deliver basic life support

1 Check that the person is unresponsive.
2 Shout for help.
3 Open the person's airway.
4 Check whether the person is now breathing normally.
5 If not, call for help.
6 Perform chest compressions.
7 Perform rescue breathing.

In more detail, this is the procedure:

1 Check: is it safe to approach the victim?
2 Approach carefully and ask clearly, 'Are you all right?'
3 If the victim responds, try to identify the problem and get help. Leave the victim in the position you found them, making sure you and the victim are not in danger.
4 If there is no response, call for help. Then with the victim on their back perform the airway opening manoeuvre by tilting the head back with one hand on their forehead and the fingertips of your other hand under the point of their chin, and lift the chin to attempt to open the airway.
5 Keeping the airway open assess for signs of normal breathing by:
   • **looking** for chest movements
   • **feeling** for air movement from the victim's mouth and nose
   • **listening** for any sounds of breathing.
6 If after no more than 10 seconds you are sure there are no normal respirations, get help by either going yourself or asking someone else to raise the emergency services.
7 Then begin to resuscitate the victim by performing chest compressions.

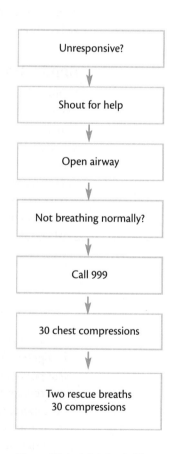

Figure 32.4 Adult basic life support

Reproduced with permission of the Resuscitation Council (UK).

Initially patients who have collapsed suddenly with no previous respiratory problems will have reasonable oxygen concentrations in their blood, which makes chest compressions more important than ventilation.

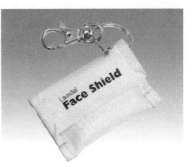

Figure 32.5 A face shield

To perform chest compressions you should:

1 Kneel by the side of the victim's chest, and place the heel of one hand in the centre of the chest, in line with the armpits. Place your other hand on top of the first. Interlock your fingers, keeping the heel of your hand only on the chest.

2 With elbows straight and your shoulders over the chest, deliver 30 compressions, pressing down enough to compress the chest by 4–5 cm.

3 You should aim to deliver 100 compressions over a minute, taking as long to release the pressure as you take to compress.

4 After each 30 compressions return to the airway and repeat the airway-opening manoeuvre. After taking a normal breath yourself, make a seal around the victim's mouth with your mouth and blow your expired air into the victim, enough to see their chest rise.

5 After two breaths return to the chest and deliver 30 compressions.

6 Continue without interruptions until help arrives to take over, the victim starts to respond (shown by movement or breathing) or you become too tired to continue.

7 In the event that you have some assistance, either perform two minutes of CPR alone then change over with your assistant, or work together with one person delivering compressions and the other giving the breaths. The breaths should be given after the 30 compressions while no chest compressions are being performed, because when delivering breaths there is an unprotected airway that is at risk of gastric regurgitation if the chest is being compressed during the inflation breaths.

Rescue breaths are not pleasant to perform, but they are essential to get breath into the victim. There are many devices available to provide a barrier between you and the victim, such as the face shield shown in Figure 32.5.

There is no evidence to suggest transmission of HIV during cardiopulmonary resuscitation (CPR), and there have been only isolated incidents of transmission of tuberculosis or severe acute respiratory distress syndrome (SARS).

Recovery position

There are a variety of guidelines to assist you in putting an individual in the recovery position (see Figure 32.6). The recommendation from the Resuscitation Council (2005) is as follows.

1 Remove the victim's spectacles, if any.

2 Kneel beside the victim and make sure that both their legs are straight.

3 Place the arm nearest to you out at right angles to their body, elbow bent, with the hand palm uppermost.

If at the initial assessment the victim is not responding to you but is breathing and has a pulse, call for assistance but make sure the victim is safe, away from danger and with a clear airway. Do not move the victim if there is a suspicion of trauma. If it is safe to do so, put the victim in the recovery position.

If the rescuer is unable or unwilling to perform mouth-to-mouth ventilation, compression-only resuscitation may be performed for a limited time, certainly no more than five minutes. This is not advised as a standard practice.

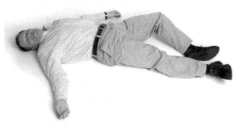

Figure 32.6 Preparing to put the victim in the recovery position

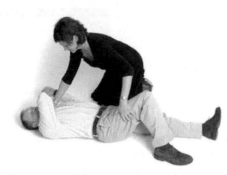

Figure 32.7 Pulling up the leg

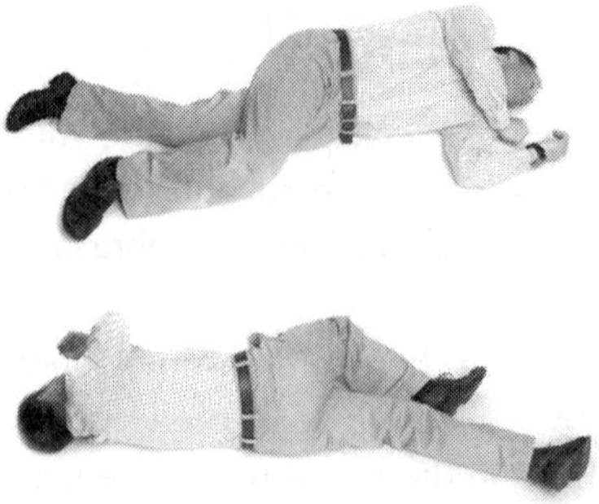

Figure 32.8 The recovery position

3 Bring the far arm across the chest, and hold the back of the hand against the victim's cheek nearest to you.
4 With your other hand, grasp the far leg just above the knee and pull it up, keeping the foot on the ground. (See Figure 32.7.)
5 Keeping the hand pressed against their cheek, pull on the far leg to roll the victim towards you onto their side.
6 Adjust the upper leg so that both the hip and knee are bent at right angles.
7 Tilt the head back to make sure the airway remains open.
8 Adjust the hand under the cheek if necessary, to keep the head tilted.
9 Check breathing regularly.

Issues to consider in Simon's case are that:
- there was a delay in recognising the intensity of the reaction
- the call for emergency services was delayed
- when Simon became unconscious he was put into the recovery position but his airway, breathing and circulation were not assessed
- Simon's wife was present from the time he became unconscious. It is never easy dealing with family friends who are present at an emergency. They may react in a variety of ways, some understandable, others more surprising.

> **t** ⭐
> ## Practice tip
> These guidelines should be practised and can be rehearsed using appropriate training manikins under the supervision of an experienced life support trainer, to help you feel comfortable in delivering these psychomotor skills (RCUK, 2004).

> **a**   **Learning activity**
>
> In your learning group discuss:
> - Should Simon have been given adrenaline immediately by the first aid crew?
> - When should the 999 call have been made?

> **S**   Scenario continued
>
> After 10 minutes of basic life support the ambulance could be heard, but in reality it took another 5 minutes for the ambulance to get into the arena to where Simon was being resuscitated. Simon had now been in cardiac arrest for 15 minutes.

> **a**   **Learning activity**
>
> Consider what has happened so far in the scenario, and think about why adults might collapse.

Intervention

The degree of intervention depends on many factors, including:

- the cause of collapse
- the location
- the help available
- the circumstances contributing to the collapse
- the ability of the persons attending.

Any intervention by healthcare professionals should be in accordance with the Resuscitation Council Guidelines based on the 2005 International Consensus on Cardiopulmonary Resuscitation.

t☆

Practice tip

The interventions should be practised on a regular basis in skills laboratories using appropriate training mannequin under the supervision of resuscitation officers or trained instructors. Up-to-date information is available from the Resuscitation Council website, www.resus.org

W

S Scenario continued

The ambulance crew arrived and reassessed the situation. The paramedics took over basic life support, delivering chest compressions and ventilation using a bag valve mask device with supplementary oxygen.

They acknowledged that Simon had suffered a cardiac arrest, probably secondary to respiratory distress brought on by an anaphylactic reaction. The situation is then managed as a cardiac arrest.

The important delivery of intramuscular adrenaline as first-line treatment for anaphylaxis had been missed. Ventilation was difficult because of upper airway swelling. The paramedic crew were trained in tracheal intubation, and using a size 6 mm endotracheal tube managed to intubate the trachea on the first attempt, secure the tube and inflate the chest using a self-inflating bag.

It would be appropriate to intubate an adult male with a 8–9 mm endotracheal tube. Simon had significant upper airway swelling. This would necessitate a smaller tube to secure his airway.

Basic life support was performed on Simon, with 100 chest compressions delivered over a minute and respirations at a rate of 10 breaths a minute.

Venous access was attempted three times without success. Adrenaline was then given via the endotracheal tube. At this point the adrenaline is being given in response to the cardiac arrest and not the anaphylaxis. The dose of adrenaline via this route is 3 mg diluted with a minimum of 10 ml of sterile water.

The ECG monitor was attached using hands-free defibrillation/monitor pads. The rhythm shown was sinus bradycardia with no corresponding pulse. The treatment algorithm to follow was therefore pulseless electrical activity (PEA).

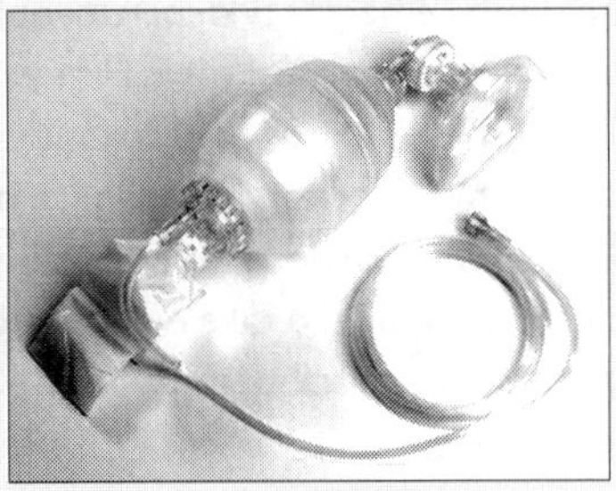

Figure 32.9 Mask and self-inflating bag with oxygen reservoir

---

PEA is the presence of electrical complexes with no palpable pulse. This might have a number of causes.

Management of PEA

The procedure for this is:

1 Maintain CPR 30:2.
2 As soon as intravenous (IV) access is successful, administer adrenaline 1 mg of 1:10,000. If this is not possible because of difficulty gaining IV access, the drug may be given via the endotracheal tube .The recommendation is to triple the dose when using this route.
3 Continue with CPR for at least two minutes. If there is no change in the rhythm and no pulse is palpated, continue with CPR.
4 If there is a change in rhythm and a pulse is palpable, stop and reassess the patient.

a Learning activity

Revise your knowledge of PEA, the four Hs and four Ts.

Part

IV

By this time Simon had no palpable pulse, his trachea was intubated and ventilation was performed by the use of a self-inflating bag with supplemental oxygen.

Chest compressions were being performed at a rate of 100 compressions a minute.

After a further two minutes Simon's condition was reassessed. He was found to have a fine weak pulse. Chest compressions were stopped and noted to correspond with the complexes on the ECG monitor.

Simon still had no signs of spontaneous respirations, for which ventilation continued using the self-inflating bag. A further attempt to insert an intravenous cannula was successful, and 1 litre of normal saline was infused rapidly.

Now that Simon was stable he was transferred to the ambulance, and the journey to hospital commenced.

It is normal practice for an ambulance crew to get a message to the receiving hospital to alert them to the state of the patient they are bringing in. The receiving team should reassess the patient and make decisions regarding the treatment required to continue from that given by the ambulance crew. This includes

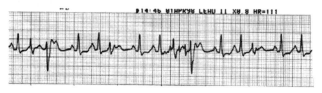

Figure 32.10 ECG monitor reading

assessing venous access and drugs administered, and a definitive airway, which in Simon's case would be a more appropriately sized endotracheal tube, probably 8 mm, and elective ventilation depending on his level of alertness.

After 20 minutes in the emergency department Simon was coughing on the endotracheal tube. His vital signs were BP 120/60, heart rate 100, oxygen saturations 97 per cent. His chest x-ray was clear and the rash had diminished considerably. The decision was made by the intensive care team attending to take out his endotracheal tube and give him nebulised salbutamol.

At this point Simon's airway was reassessed. After 10 minutes Simon was maintaining his own airway and maintained oxygen saturations of 97 per cent. He was cardiovascularly stable. The decision was made to transfer him to a high-dependency unit for observations.

In-hospital resuscitation

The resuscitation team

Each organisation will have its own action plan to attend individuals who collapse. There should be a team that responds to victims of cardiac arrest. The composition of the team will vary between organisations, but it should have a minimum of two doctors trained to deal with such emergencies.

The team should collectively have the skills to deal with

- airway interventions
- routes for drug administration
- monitoring and defibrillation
- knowledge of drugs and fluids
- post resuscitation management
- team leader skills

a   Learning activity

Anaphylaxis is a very familiar term given the number of people who are considered to be allergic to a vast range of substances. Consider people you have come across and how they cope. What do they avoid? How does it affect their lifestyle? Many individuals carry adrenaline. Think about the practicalities of carrying adrenaline, and who has received instruction and the opportunity to use the devices prescribed to deliver adrenaline in an emergency. Visit the websites relating to these devices.

Investigations

After the reaction has been treated, bloods should be taken for measurement of mast cell tryptase to assist with diagnosis of the anaphylaxis after the event:

- immediately
- after 6 hours
- after 24 hours.

Misdiagnosis of anaphylaxis

While there is a lot of publicity regarding anaphylaxis, actual observation of the event is rare. Hence it is not unreasonable to be concerned about making the wrong diagnosis, and indeed the symptoms can be confused with asthma, fainting and panic attacks.

The general opinion is that if you are unsure, you should treat for anaphylaxis, since it is a life-threatening event which can be treated by giving adrenaline early. If it is not anaphylaxis, the patient has nevertheless demonstrated quite severe symptoms, and will require close observation and monitoring.

Should the event turn out to not be an anaphylactic episode, appropriate guidance is to monitor the ECG and measurement troponic levels 10 hours after the adrenaline was given.

Conclusion

This chapter has demonstrated that life-threatening emergencies can happen anywhere in the community, and sometimes in unexpected situations. Intervention by people with key skills can make all the difference. The outcome from cardiac arrests could be so much better if more people knew what to do and had the confidence to deliver basic life support. Recognising an emergency situation, having the knowledge and confidence to act swiftly, call for help and perform basic life support skills will help save someone's life.

References

Axelsson, A., Zettergren, M. Axelsson, C. (2005) 'Good and bad experiences of family presence during acute care and resuscitation. what makes the difference?' *European Journal of Cardiovascular Nursing* 4, 161–9.

Bahr, J., Klingler, H., Panzer, W., Rode, H. and Kettler, D. (1997) 'Skills of lay people in checking the carotid pulse', *Resuscitation* 35, 23–6.

Brown, S. G., Blackman, K. E., Stenlake, V. and Heddle, R. J. (2004) 'Insect sting anaphylaxis; prospective evaluation of treatment with intravenous adrenaline and volume resuscitation', *Emergency Medical Journal* **21**(2),149–54.

Connolly, M., Toner, P., Connolly, D. and McCluskey, D. (2007) 'The ABC for life programme: teaching basic life support in schools', *Resuscitation* 72, 270–9.

European Resuscitation Council (2005) 'European Resuscitation Council Guidelines for Resuscitation 2005', *Resuscitation* 67(supp.1), S1–S190.

Greenberger, P. A. (2007) 'Idiopathic anaphylaxis', *Immunology Allergy Clinic of North America* **27**(2), 273–93, vii–viii.

Handley, A. J. (2002) 'Teaching hand placement for chest compression: a simpler technique', *Resuscitation* 53, 29–36.

Pumphrey, R. S. (2004) 'Fatal anaphylaxis in the UK,1992–2001', *Novartis Found Symptoms* 257, 116–28 (discussion 128–32, 157–60, 276–85.

Resuscitation Council UK (RCUK) (2004) *Cardiopulmonary Resuscitation: Standards for clinical practice and training*, London, RCUK.

RCUK (2005) *Resuscitation Guidelines 2005*, London, RCUK.

RCUK (2008) *Emergency Treatment of Anaphylactic Reactions*, London, RCUK.

Websites

Advanced Life Support Group: www.alsg.org.uk
Information on the Epipen: www.epipen.co.uk
Resuscitation Council UK: www.resus.org.uk
The Anaphylaxis Campaign: www.anaphylaxis.org.uk

Part

IV

Chapter

33

HIV and infectious disease management

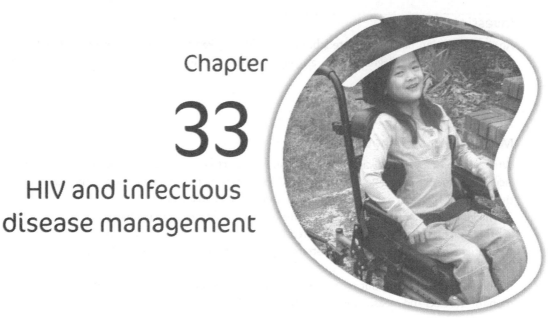

Vidar Melby

 Links to other chapters in *Foundation Studies for Caring*

 Links to other chapters in *Foundation Skills for Caring*

W Don't forget to visit www.palgrave.com/glasper for additional online resources relating to this chapter.

Introduction

The principal aim of this chapter is to introduce you to some of the fundamental challenges that face people living with the human immunodeficiency virus (PLH). This means you need to understand issues that relate to stigma and discrimination, pathophysiology of the human immunodeficiency virus (HIV), and gain an appreciation of a range of issues associated with care and treatment of PLH. The issues are presented through a case study of a 35-year-old gay man who has lived with HIV for eight years.

Learning outcomes

This chapter will enable you to:

- outline the range of issues facing people with HIV infection
- understand the concept of stigma in relation to certain illnesses and the impact of this
- describe the impact of enduring or chronic illness on adult patients

- understand how to generalise the ideas discussed here to the situation of others with severe nonacute infectious diseases requiring long-term treatment such as drug-resistant tuberculosis
- indicate how multidisciplinary action can help to satisfy the needs of those with complex physical, social and psychological needs.

Concepts

- Chronic infectious disorders and their impacts
- Human immunodeficiency virus and HIV infection

- Stigmatising illness
- Enduring and chronic health needs

[S] Scenario: Introducing John

John is a 35-year-old man who was diagnosed eight years previously with HIV. The infection was detected through normal testing at the nearest genito-urinary medicine (GUM) clinic, which John attended following an isolated experience of unprotected sexual intercourse.

Since diagnosis John has experienced a range of physical and emotional disturbances, and has attended the HIV clinic regularly. He has been on antiviral treatment for the past two years, which he finds difficult to cope with due to the many side-effects and the complicated treatment regime.

John is a trained teacher, but because of the physical and emotional strain associated with his HIV illness, he has been unable to teach in the last three months. He has experienced increasing hostility and discrimination from colleagues at the school where he works, and has made a decision to quit his teacher employment.

John lives with his male partner Cesare, who is not infected with HIV, in a jointly owned bungalow on the outskirts of Manchester. John knows that ending his employment will result in financial hardship, and he is very worried about this.

Terminology

The HIV literature is full of specialist terminology, and you need to understand some of the most common terms. The Centers for Disease Control and Prevention (CDC) (2001) provided a 1993 revised classification system for HIV infection and expanded surveillance case definition for AIDS among adolescents (aged over 13) and adults. In this classification, the CDC referred to the role of CD4+ t-lymphocytes, which denotes the number of uninfected t-lymphocytes that HIV loves to attach itself to. CD4+ t-lymphocytes are measured in terms of number of cells per microlitre (μL). With recent developments in diagnostics, the term viral load (VL) is increasingly common. Smith and Stein (2002) claimed that VL has emerged as an important biomarker for monitoring HIV disease and antiretroviral therapy (ART), and suggested that both baseline VL and changes in VL over time predicted HIV disease progression and death.

Viral load refers to the measurement of plasma HIV ribonucleic acid levels (RNA) levels, and is presented as HIV RNA, $\log_{10}$ copies/ml (Chan and Revicki, 1998). As a general reference point, no detectable virus is declared when there are fewer than 50 copies/ml. HIV disease progression (experienced through the presentation of symptoms) normally occurs when VL exceeds 10,000 copies/ml, and stage 3 HIV illness (that is, a diagnosis of AIDS) and death primarily occur in people with VL over 10,000 copies/ml.

Since the introduction of highly active antiretroviral therapy (HAART) in 1996, fewer PLH progress to stage 3 HIV illness with advanced clinical features such as pneumocystis carinii pneumonia (PCP), HIV-related dementia and life-threatening body wasting. HIV disease is thus better conceptualised as an infection on a continuum from asymptomatic to symptomatic, where symptoms can present in a variety of types and severity. An AIDS diagnosis serves no purpose to the patient or the physician from a treatment perspective, and this diagnosis has thus become redundant, so we shall not use this term here, and instead use simply PLH.

> **ⓐ Learning activity**
>
> How do you think John's life might be affected by an AIDS diagnosis as opposed to an HIV diagnosis?
>
> In your deliberations, think of what experiences people associate with the term AIDS.

Immunology

In a crude explanation, HIV attaches itself to lymphocytes that subsequently become neutralised, rendering the immune system ineffective. As a result, PLH become vulnerable to infections and other diseases (including some tumours) that are mediated by the immune system. There are several types, groups and subtypes of HIV, reflecting a virus that mutates very easily. The two main types are HIV-1 and HIV-2. Both are transmitted by sexual contact, through blood and from mother to child, and produce very similar clinical presentations. However, it seems that HIV-2 is less easily transmitted, and the period between initial infection and illness is longer than with HIV-1. Worldwide, the predominant virus is HIV-1.

The strains of HIV-1 can be classified into three groups: the Major (M) group, the Outlier (O) group and the New (N) group, with subtypes identified within each one. More than 90 per cent of HIV-1 infections belong to HIV-1 group M. To date subtype B has been the most common subtype in Europe, the Americas, Japan and Australia, although other subtypes have become more frequent, and in 2005 accounted for at least 25 per cent of new infections in Europe.

Daar (1998) claimed that primary (acute) human HIV-1 infection is accompanied by an acute illness termed the acute retroviral syndrome (ARS). ARS presents with fever, myalgia, rash, sore throat and lymphadenopathy, and diagnosis is confirmed by the presence of high levels of HIV viraemia along with an undetectable or evolving humoral immune response. There is considerable variation in how quickly this ARS emerges following infection, and it is possible that in due course we shall learn that not all PLH will develop ARS. The reasons for such human variation are as yet not clearly understood. Avert, a recognised HIV charity, provides simple and straightforward explanations of HIV on http://www.avert.org/

W

Epidemiology

We shall briefly outline the worldwide HIV epidemiology. It is particularly worth noting that sub-Saharan Africa, which includes countries such as Uganda, Malawi and Tanzania, accounts for about 70 per cent of all world HIV diagnoses (or estimations), and has considerably higher incidence rates for adults and children than other regions (Avert, 2007). In the United States, the United Kingdom and most developed countries, most infections have occurred through men having sex with men (MSM), while in developing countries the main transmission factor is heterosexual contact. It is also worth noting that there are major epidemiological differences between various ethnic or cultural subgroups in developed countries, in that epidemiological data confirms that HIV hits people from the black community harder than any other ethnic group. Across Europe there are considerable differences in prevalence and incidence rates across countries, with a frightening explosion of HIV in many Eastern European countries. While the numbers of people diagnosed with HIV are relatively modest in the United Kingdom compared with many other countries, it is likely that a considerable number of people are infected but have not yet been diagnosed. In an anonymous health survey of gay men in Northern Ireland (Carroll et al, 2002), it was intimated that while the number of diagnosed PLH in Northern Ireland was rather small, there could be as many as five times this number of undiagnosed PLH. It is likely that a similar pattern exists in all developed countries.

HIV diagnostics, pathology and treatment

CDC's revised classification system and definitions (2001) emphasised the clinical importance of the CD4+ T-lymphocyte count in the categorization of HIV-related clinical conditions. Testing for HIV is quite a simple process, which can be carried out sensitively but accurately in all GUM settings.

HIV illness has become associated with a range of conditions, and has the capability to affect all body systems and present with a variety of symptoms and clinical features. As HAART has reduced HIV mortality rates significantly, more PLH now live with HIV as a chronic illness and will endure a range of HIV-associated illness. Some of the most common physiological complaints are pain (Breitbart, 1998), body wasting (Earthman et al, 2002), cutaneous disorders (Myskowski and Ahkami, 1996), and oral manifestations (Cherry-Peppers et al, 2003). Neurological conditions are also common, including HIV encephalitis and neuropathy (Davies et al, 1997; Rao and Thomas, 2005), as are psychiatric disorders such as depression, dysthymia and generalised anxiety disorder (Perretta et al, 1996; Cruess et al, 2003). From the perspective of the PLH, this sudden change from a prognosis of certain death to long-term survival with a chronic illness has been referred to by some authors as the 'Lazarus phenomenon' (Brashers et al, 1999; Thompson, 2003).

W

Excellent overviews of HIV therapy are provided by Avert (http://www.avert.org). Principally there are four groups of drugs used to treat HIV, grouped and named according to how they interfere with the HIV replication process. Since 1996 it has become apparent that drugs from different groups work most effectively in combination, thus HAART is often referred to as *combination therapy*. The four groups of drugs commonly in use are the nucleoside/nucleotide reverse transcriptase inhibitors (NRTIs), which include drugs such as zidovudine (AZT) and didanosine, the non-nucleoside reverse transcriptase inhibitors (NNRTIs) (efavirenz and nevirapine), the protease inhibitors (PIs) (ritonavir and indinavir), and fusion inhibitors (FIs) (enfuvirtide). While HAART has resulted in reduced mortality and morbidity, and has changed the perception and classification of HIV disease from a terminal to a chronic disorder, the drugs are associated with a range of benign complications such as lipodystrophy (Burgoyne et al, 2004; Keiser et al, 2005) and more malevolent side-effects such as hyperlipidaemia and other cardiac disease (Fantoni, Autore and del Borgo, 2001; Steinhart and Emons, 2004).

While the development of ART drugs has progressed immensely since 1996, there remain numerous difficulties associated with ART such as drug resistance (Martinez-Picado et al, 2003) and adherence (Chesney et al, 2000; Siegel, Scrimshaw and Raveis, 2000; Brook et al, 2001; Adam, Maticka-Tyndale and Cohen, 2003). It is also not clear yet when ART should be commenced. PLH could remain symptom-free for years without ART, and the evidence on the benefits of early initiation of HAART to symptom-free individuals is not consistent. Thus in conclusion, from medical, immunological and pharmacological perspectives, it is evident that the quest must go on for new ART drugs that are safe, produce fewer side-effects and allow for a simplification of daily drug schedules (Marks and Gulick, 2004; Stanic and Schneider, 2005). In the meantime there appears to be no justification for withholding ART because of side-effects (Schackman et al, 2002).

Part

IV

a   Learning activity

In what circumstances should you encourage a person to undertake an HIV test? What are the main risk factors you would want to consider?

Living with HIV: the impact on individuals

Physical functioning

Pain

Symptomatic PLH present with a range of symptoms of variable and unpredictable severity and distress (Wachtel et al, 1992), Pain is a common presentation in HIV (Martinez-Picado et al, 2003), often strong enough to interfere with daily activities of living and sleep (Harrison et al, 1999), and is associated with a lower level of functioning in all aspects of life, in particular psychosocial distress (Rosenfeld et al, 1996). Martinez-Picado and colleagues (2003) suggested that interventions aimed at developing adaptive coping strategies and improving pain management could improve functional aspects for PLH. Evans and colleagues (1998) found that pain was widespread in PLH (25 per cent) and associated with considerable psychological and functional impairment, and reported additionally that PLH who experienced pain reported significantly more advanced disease with more physical and psychological symptoms. Sleep has an important function in human beings in restoring physical and mental functioning, and PLH experience considerable sleep disturbances, resulting from the effects of HIV-associated illness, pharmacological effects and social distress (Dreher, 2003).

Anaemia

Many authors have reviewed the impact of anaemia on PLH (Volberding, 2002; Siegel, Brown Bradley and Lekas, 2004a). These authors reported anaemia as the most common HIV-associated haematological abnormality, occurring with increasing frequency as HIV infection advances. The authors claimed that despite the high prevalence of anaemia in PLH, the symptoms were often overlooked or misinterpreted. Fatigue, for instance, which is the cardinal presentation of anaemia but also a principal presentation in HIV disease, was associated with impaired physical functioning. PLH whose haemoglobin levels had been raised to normal levels through the use of, amongst other, recombinant human erythropoietin (epoetin alfa), demonstrated significantly greater improvements in energy levels, and were better able to undertake their daily activities at home and at work.

Brain impairment

Stephenson and colleagues (2000) found brain impairment in PLH a disturbing expression of HIV disease, characterised by progressive cognitive impairment that might result in dementia or death. The authors noted that PLH with advanced brain involvement were clinically difficult to manage and that many needed residential care, although some PLH regained some functional ability. Benedict and colleagues (2000) reported considerable association between HIV infection and neuropsychological deficits, and found that cognitively impaired patients were more likely to be unemployed and fail cognitive tests such as medication management tasks. The authors concluded that their overall quality of life was poor, and that the cognitive deficiencies were serious as individuals were unable to manage their own medicines correctly and safely. Tozzi and colleagues (2003) reported that the presence of neurocognitive impairment was significantly associated with poorer daily functioning, in particular physical functioning (Crystal et al, 2000).

Diarrhoea

Henry and colleagues (1999) carried out a comparative study on the impact of diarrhoea on daily life, using a sample of 20 PLH with and 20 PLH without chronic diarrhoea. PLH without diarrhoea reported better self-reported health perceptions, and they also reported less fatigue, lower psychological distress and gastrointestinal discomfort. The intensity of chronic diarrhoea was reported as moderate to severe by 85 per cent of the sample. Snijders and colleagues (1998) claimed that diarrhoea in PLH was an important clinical problem, and that even people with mild diarrhoea could experience considerable limitations to social functioning, with the fear of faecal incontinence adding intolerable distress to actual incontinence. Diarrhoea can occur as a consequence of HAART, in particular if PI are used, or present as a clinical feature of opportunistic infections associated with HIV progression such as salmonella, cryptosporidium, isospora (protozoan parasite) and cytomegalovirus infections (CMV) (Tramarin et al, 2004).

> **S Scenario continued**
>
> John suffered for many weeks with diarrhoea, and during this time he felt isolated in his home and was afraid of going out socially as well as having friends visiting at home, because of his constant urge to go to the toilet.

> **a Learning activity**
>
> Outline a strategy for helping John to deal with this situation.
> Think about food and medications, but also how you can boost his self-confidence.

Fatigue

Fatigue is another common complaint in HIV (Breitbart et al, 1998; Rose et al, 1998). Breitbart and colleagues (1998) investigated the prevalence of fatigue in 427 ambulatory PLH in the United States. Fifty-four per cent of the participants reported fatigue, with women more likely to report fatigue than men, and gay people with HIV were less likely to report fatigue than those infected through injecting drug usage (IDU) or heterosexual contact. Fatigue was significantly associated with the number of HIV-related physical symptoms, current treatment for HIV-related medical disorders, anaemia and pain, and was consequently associated with poorer physical functioning.

The effects of diarrhoea, pain, anaemia, fatigue and associated loss of appetite contribute to body cell mass depletion in PLH, and this wasting syndrome has remained a considerable problem for PLH even following the introduction of HAART. Wagner, Ferrando and Rabkin (2000) found that 31 per cent of their sample of 187 PLH had significant body cell mass depletion at some point during the study, and that this was associated with significant increase in fatigue, emotional distress and depressive symptomatology, and reduced life satisfaction.

Opportunistic infections

A number of opportunistic infections are associated with HIV infection, in particular cytalomegalovirus retinitis and PCP, both common and severe infections that can lead to considerable limitations to life functioning.

HIV has been linked with many sexually transmitted infections (STIs) including herpes simplex virus (HSV), human papilloma virus and syphilis. Ormond and Mulcahy (1998) reported that many of these co-infections were characterised by nontraditional clinical features and therapeutic responses, because of the complex interaction between the STIs and HIV. The authors thus emphasised the potential for misdiagnosis and undertreatment, with a subsequent impact on people's lives. Hepatitis C (HCV) has also been linked with HIV disease, particularly in IDUs. While such co-infection does not appear to be related to any decline in immunological function and thus progression of HIV disease (Sulkowski et al, 2002), HCV has been associated with significant impairment in functioning, independent of the associated liver ailments of chronic hepatitis, hepatomegaly and carcinoma of the liver (Tillmann et al, 2004).

Part

IV

Depression

Mental health disturbances occur frequently in PLH (Koutsilieri et al. 2002), impair quality of life (Sherbourne et al. 2000), affect HIV prognosis, and impede treatment by compromising medication adherence. One of the most common HIV-associated mental health problems is depression, frequently unrecognised, underdiagnosed and undertreated (Tate et al. 2003; Valente 2003). In addition, people with mental illness are more likely to be involved in high-risk sexual and drug use behaviours (Kelly et al., 1993; Heller, 2004) and thus put themselves (and others) at increased risk of HIV infection (Checkley et al, 1996). Consequently, rates of HIV amongst people with mental illness is much higher than in the general population (Weiser, Wolfe and Bangsberg, 2004).

Suicide

Suicidal ideation has been reported in PLH who have concomitant mental illness (Haller and Miles, 2003), and is associated with the onset of symptoms and subsequent emergence of psychological distress which usually present during a high-risk period immediate post-diagnosis (Evangelisto, 1996; Kalichman et al, 2000). Such an acute stress disorder is commonly seen following the HIV diagnosis, and many PLH present with clinical features in which the acute stress reactions are significantly and positively related to prior traumatic life events that are indicators of post-traumatic stress disorder (Koopman et al, 2002).

The impact of injecting drug use on functioning was further demonstrated by other authors (Vogl et al, 1999; Knowlton et al, 2000; Valente, 2003). In Vogl and colleagues' (1999) study of 504 ambulatory PLH between 1992 and 1995 (pre-HAART), respondents who reported IDU as an HIV transmission factor reported more symptoms and higher overall physical symptom distress than those who reported homosexual or heterosexual contact as their transmission factor. Both the number of symptoms and symptom distress were highly associated with psychological distress and poorer functioning. In addition, co-infection with HCV has been associated with psychological states such as obsessive-compulsive disorder, phobic anxiety, paranoid ideation, and psychoticism (Grassi et al, 2002). Tate and colleagues (2003) suggested that both apathy and depression were more common in HIV positive than HIV negative participants.

The advent of HAART changed HIV from a terminal to a chronic disorder. As the association with death diminished and the hope for a future emerged, many psychological conditions remained and some new ones appeared (Catalan, Meadows and Douzenis, 2000). Nilsson Schönnesson (2002) maintained that medication could never totally remove the traumatic experiences of a HIV diagnosis, and reiterated that PLH still face the prospect of physical, social and sexual threats, stigma and discrimination associated with HIV.

Body image

Side-effects of HAART are numerous, some very harmful such as changes in serum lipid concentrations (increased triglyceride or cholesterol levels), and some less life-threatening such as alterations in body appearance (wasting, abdominal weight gain, buffalo hump). Corless and colleagues (2004) carried out a descriptive, correlational pilot study (23 men, 17 women) to ascertain the associations between these clinical features, body image and functioning. Better mental health functioning, vitality (energy/fatigue), and overall functioning correlated with weight gain towards normality; however these correlations did not occur in women. From her research, Chapman suggested there were three main spheres of influence on body image: physical, psychological and social, and that the way we think about the body in health and illness reflects the kind of society we live in (Chapman, 1998, 2002). People subsequently internalise representations towards them, such as perceived and received stigma. In addition to causing social isolation of PLH, the emotional problems triggered by the extreme changes in body shape may cause patients to discontinue or reduce their combination therapy (Shattuck, 2001).

S Scenario continued

John developed sunken cheeks and a buffalo hump as fat was redistributed around his body. He was very unhappy about this, saying, 'I don't mind having HIV, I don't mind being ill, I just don't want to LOOK ill!'

a Learning activity

Present a professional discussion in which you outline the principal arguments you would use to convince John that adhering to the medication regime is important to him. Consider the rationale for antiretroviral treatment – this must be sound! Weigh this up against the side-effects, some of which are benign.

Stigma

The association of stigma with HIV has been investigated by a number of authors (Cadwell, 1991; Sandelowski, Lambe and Barroso, 2004; Castro and Farmer, 2005; Herek, 2005), and the picture that emerged is confusing. It has been argued that stigma, perceived and received, is a barrier to accessing health and social care services. Other researchers have argued that it is in fact economic and behavioural factors (such as functioning) that are principal barriers to PLH accessing health and social care (Syme and Berkman, 2005).

Multiple stigmatisation

In an early paper prior to HAART, Cadwell (1991) claimed that PLH experience multiple stigmatisation because of associations with homosexuality, STIs, death and dying, and also with IDU (Peck and Secker, 1999; Burrage and Rocchiociolli, 2003). Crowther (1992) argued that as PLH face this stigmatisation in addition to the demands of their illness, this might result in a feeling of loss of control and might negatively impact their health and subsequent care. Herek and Capitanio (1993) studied public reactions to HIV in the United States with a general adult sample (n=1145), and most respondents showed at least some prejudice against PLH, with men more likely than women to support policies such as quarantine and stating a preference for avoiding PLH if they could. In a second paper based on the same sample (Herek and Capitanio, 1997), the authors reported that direct contact (versus vicarious contact) with PLH was associated with less support for coercive HIV policies, less blame towards PLH, and less avoidance of PLH.

Death and bereavement

Meyer (1995) reported that minority stressors, conceptualised as internalised homophobia and stigma, had significant independent associations with a variety of mental health measures. Slater and Bright (1995) broadened this to include isolation, rejection, breaches of confidentiality, guilt, anger, fear of infection and death, loss and bereavement. Range and Alliston (1995) examined stigma associated with suicide in PLH versus people living with cancer, and findings indicated that the person experienced more stigma when the diagnosis was HIV than with terminal cancer. Perceived or received stigma were also felt during bereavement, in which PLH who experienced bereavement reported a greater level of rejection from others and were more likely to conceal the cause of death from significant others, than people living with cancer (Kelly et al, 1996). This stigma extended to viewing the family as difficult to sympathise with, but not necessarily blameworthy. Courtesy stigma has also been reported, in which stigma is extended to include individuals related to, or in someway associated with, a PLH (Herek, 2005). This 'guilt by association' can happen to family members, children, parents, healthcare providers and caregivers (Powell-Cope and Brown, 1992).

a Learning activity

John was gay *and* he had HIV, thus he was at risk of double stigma. Discuss some of the arguments that might be levelled against him to justify such stigma. Is there a moral story?

Women and stigma

Research into women's experiences of stigma has reported multiple rejections by partners and children, friends, healthcare providers, employers, neighbours and church members (Carr and Gramling, 2004; Sandelowski et al, 2004). This rejection negatively impacted on their access to healthcare, medication adherence, social interaction and social support, and was sometimes expressed through direct violence. Sandelowski and colleagues (2004) noted a blurring between perceived and received stigma, and reported that women who were IDUs saw the diagnosis with HIV as a springboard to ending substance abuse and improving many aspects of their lives. Herek (2005) claimed that PLH were stigmatised throughout the world, and that this was expressed through social ostracism and personal rejection. The author argued that stigma varied from culture to culture and from country to country, and argued that the expectation and fear of stigma affected individuals' choices and decisions following diagnosis, in terms of testing and seeking help for their medical, social and psychological needs.

Disclosure

The fear of rejection from family, friends and other people in their social and occupational networks, and subsequent personal and social isolation, are often quoted as the reasons why PLH consider very carefully to whom they disclose their HIV status (Hays et al, 1993; Tewksbury and McGaughey, 1997), although disclosure has been associated with both positive and negative responses (Leask et al, 1997). HIV-positive gay men were found more likely to disclose their status to lovers and their closest gay friends than family members (Hays et al, 1993; Mansergh, Marks and Simoni, 1995), with asymptomatic men less likely than symptomatic men to disclose to relatives and colleagues. Disclosure to fathers was extremely low (Mansergh et al, 1995). Perry and colleagues (1994) reported that about one-third of the sexually active PLH did not disclose their HIV infection to any present sexual partner.

In a survey of 65 ethnically diverse women, Simoni and colleagues (1995) reported disclosure trends among women similar to those reported among men, with relatively low rates of disclosure of HIV status to extended family members, somewhat higher rates for immediate family members, and highest rates for lovers and friends, and that women considered carefully to whom they disclosed (Chandra et al, 2003). The authors also warned of cultural differences in disclosure.

Moneyham and colleagues (1996), using qualitative focus group interviews, examined the experiences of disclosure in 19 women infected with HIV, and found that participants expressed considerable concern about disclosing their HIV status because they expected and feared negative responses from others. Three main concerns were raised: discrimination, confidentiality, and the context of disclosure in relation to health care providers (HCP), sexual partners and their children. Chandra and colleagues (2003) emphasised the importance of awareness of cultural differences in disclosure. In their study based in India, 35 per cent of the participants reported disclosure without consent, mostly from HCP to immediate family members, but argued that such disclosure was not necessarily seen as ethically wrong, as the sharing of information to and within families is seen as a cultural norm in India.

Wiener and colleagues (1996) discussed issues surrounding disclosure to a child when a parent or close family member is HIV infected. They claimed that children were profoundly affected by the impact of HIV in this situation, although the initial reaction most adults have upon learning of their own, or a family member's, HIV diagnosis is that it must be kept a closely guarded secret. One reason frequently cited by parents and family members was their fear that the stigma of HIV would have a negative impact on their children (courtesy stigma). This delay in disclosure makes the children vulnerable to psychological distress (Roth, Siegel and Black, 1994).

Families

Miller and Murray (1999) discussed the impact of HIV on families, and claimed that HIV illness affects the whole family. Based on professional experience when working with HIV-infected families, but supported by research literature, the authors maintained that parental HIV illness placed stress on relationships between parents, between parents and children, and between parents and extended family members. While some relationships became closer, other became more distant, with suspicion and blame often proving central stressors. The authors further alleged that illness in one or both parents impeded their ability to care for their children, and that an inability to deal with the children's emotional and practical needs negatively influenced the children's developmental needs. Mok and Cooper (1997), in their study of PLH in Edinburgh, found that many families were fragmented and dysfunctional, and that 20 per cent of the children had cognitive and developmental disabilities, with a large proportion reported as presenting with disruptive and challenging behaviour.

When an HIV diagnosis has been made, people are faced with uncertainty which fluctuates over the course of the illness, and extends beyond that associated with medical diagnosis, treatment and recovery, to non-medical issues of identity, financial security, employment, and personal and social relationships. Identified sources of uncertainty, such as complex, ever-evolving treatments, ambiguous symptom patterns, and fear of stigma, have important implications on mental health and other aspects of daily functioning (Brashers et al, 1998, 2003). Brashers and colleagues (2003) further claimed that the uncertainty experienced by PLH was reduced over time, returned when illness recurred, and was highest during the period of diagnosis. Brashers, Neidig and Goldsmith (2004) considered how this uncertainty could be managed, and suggested that support from others helped PLH to manage uncertainty in different ways, including assisting with information seeking and providing instrumental support. In her qualitative study of PLH, Kendall (1996) reported an initial crisis associated with uncertainty, following which the individual sought help. Depending on the quality of interactions with family and friends in response to this help-seeking, PLH gained a new outlook on living with HIV.

Sexual functioning

Many authors have identified sexual functioning as an essential part of how people value their lives. Newshan, Taylor and Gold (1998) suggested it was important to understand sexual functioning and its relationship with HIV. They found that prevalence of sexual dysfunction increased with disease progression, and that those with sexual dysfunction reported poorer emotional functioning than those without sexual dysfunction. The authors concluded that low testosterone level (in men) as well as emotional distress and negative body image (in men and women) were significantly correlated with poor sexual functioning. Catalan and Meadows (2000), in their study of sexual dysfunction in PLH, reported primarily psychogenic causes in 44 per cent, primarily organic causes in 22 per cent and a mixed aetiology in 34 per cent of cases. Psychological and physical approaches to treatment, either separately or combined, resolved sexual dysfunction in 74 per cent of individuals.

Bova and Durante (2003), who focused on sexual activity in 101 women with HIV, claimed that additional issues became pertinent to women, such as transmissibility, partner disclosure, potential vertical transmission, and for some, problems associated with IDU. The study demonstrated that most women with HIV continued to be sexually active following the HIV diagnosis, that sexual functioning did not change as a result of HIV disease progression, and that few women reported that HIV itself caused worsening of their sexual functioning. Women who reported better quality of life had higher levels of sexual functioning.

Social and economic functioning

Martin and colleagues (2003), in a study of 1991 PLH, investigated perceived employment barriers and how these influenced individuals' decision to return to work after illness. The decision to return to work was dependent on considerations around discrimination, loss of benefit, the impact on health, and continued access to healthcare services. In general, the level

Part

IV

of acuity of HIV infection correlated positively with level of concern about return to work. Brooks and colleagues (2004) examined factors that influenced 757 PLH in the United States in their decision to return to work following illness. Concurring with the findings of Martin and colleagues (2003), the authors found that as many as 74 per cent of the participants were considering a return to employment. Blalock and colleagues (2002) investigated functioning amongst 200 employed and unemployed PLH, and found that employed participants reported significantly better functioning than unemployed PLH.

Vidrine and colleagues (2003) examined the impact of sociodemographic and behavioural variables on daily functioning among 385 multiethnic, economically disadvantaged PLH in the United States. Ethnic minorities reported significantly poorer physical functioning and work-role functioning, while participants with CD4+ counts > 500/mm^3, MSM HIV exposure, and education beyond secondary school, reported better physical functioning and work-role functioning. Overall quality of life and work-related functioning were significantly impaired amongst the economically disadvantaged ethnic minorities.

A pre-HAART study by Friedland, Renwick and McColl (1996) investigated how coping and social support affected daily functioning in 120 symptomatic and asymptomatic PLH. Respondents reported good levels of social support and used a variety of coping strategies, and regression analysis indicated that income, emotional social support, and problem-oriented and perception-oriented coping were positively related to good functioning. While respondents were generally happy with their support, they expressed a need for more emotional support. Unemployment was high despite participants being relatively healthy and well educated.

Diverse needs

Green and Smith (2004) reviewed psychosocial and health care needs of PLH in the United Kingdom, and outlined the evolution of diverse needs of different vulnerable groups of PLH such as migrants and asylum seekers, older people, women (particularly those who are pregnant), IDUs and prisoners. The authors confirmed that there had been a shift from acute mental health problems associated with dying to chronic mental health problems, and noted that stigma continued to concern PLH. The authors suggested that because of the optimism associated with HAART, a failure to respond to combination therapy might lead to a feeling of failure which could cause additional psychological distress. The authors cited poverty as a salient feature in the lives of the majority of PLH, and found that poverty was a serious barrier to accessing health and social care services. According to the authors, barriers to accessing services, such as difficulty in finding a general practitioner (GP) or dentist, linguistic problems, lack of cultural sensitivity or awareness by clinicians, mental health difficulties or disrupted social support, always hit marginalised groups unfairly hard.

> **a Learning activity**
>
> PLH do not form one homogenous population, but consist of several microcultures: smaller groups of people sharing a set of common ideals, values or standards. These include gay men, heterosexual men, women, drug users, haemophiliacs, older people, migrants, immigrants, asylum seekers and prisoners. How might an awareness of such microcultures enhance the quality of your care of PLH? Start with analysing your own culture – identifying your own values and beliefs.

Wachtel and colleagues (1992) and Campsmith, Nakashima and Davidson (2003), in their studies of 520 and 3778 PLH respectively during the period from 1992 to 1996 (pre/early HAART) in the United States, found that daily functioning was affected by older age, female sex, black or Hispanic ethnicity, IDU, lower education and income, no private health insurance, and lower CD4+ count. Other studies of women with HIV found that limitations to activities of living imposed by HIV additionally influenced relationships with partner, family and children, and led to a reduced sex life (Gray, 1999; O'Connell et al, 2003). Symptoms were perceived as a major stressor, as new symptoms were indicative of progression of HIV, and the uncertainty associated with stressors resulted in emotions of anger, depression and loneliness.

Age

Using effective combination therapy, more PLH reach old age than ever before (Stoff et al, 2004). In their comparative descriptive study of functioning in older (n = 73) versus younger (n = 640) PLH, Nokes and colleagues (2000) defined older age in PLH as 50, as prior to HAART very few PLH reached that age. There are many reasons that we might expect older people's experiences of living with HIV to be different from younger people's, and it is important to identify the underlying mechanisms that might account for such differences. As people grow older, they tend to develop chronic illnesses such as hypertension, arthritis and diabetes. According to Stoff and colleagues (2004), the neurocognitive and neuropsychiatric comorbidities are considered key factors for PLH because of their impact on daily functioning, in particular because of their likely impact on adherence to HAART and adjuvant medical treatment. Nokes and colleagues (2000) claimed that more needed to be known about the impact of pharmacodynamics in terms of drug–drug interactions in older PLH and whether these factors increase medication toxicities.

Several research studies have noted an association between HIV progression and age, and there is some evidence that the clinical conditions of older people deteriorate more quickly. Piette and colleagues (1995) reported that, in particular, physical functioning was more sensitive in older people to fluctuations in CD4+ counts. The authors found decreased physical and social functioning and health perception associated with advancing age. According to Nokes and colleagues (2000), this could be explained by immunological theory, which proposes that the immune system declines in older people as fewer T-cells reach the mature stage at which they become effective. Consequently, mortality rates are higher in older PLH. Compared with younger PLH, older PLH reported some advantages (O'Connell et al, 2003), such as possessing more wisdom, being more patient, and being more spiritual, while simultaneously reporting that they felt more socially isolated and that people in general afforded them less sympathy. More ominously, older PLH reported that doctors did not treat them with equal importance in terms of setting realistic and appropriate targets for treatment. It was also noted that older PLH tended to disclose their status to fewer people than younger PLH.

IDUs comprise a group of individuals that exist on the fringe of normal society in many ways, in terms of their sexual and drug behaviours, employment, criminal histories and health care usage. Wachtel and colleagues (1992) reported that IDUs present with poorer functioning in all domains, and that drug-using factors, in particular being in methadone treatment, significantly affected daily functioning (Carretero et al, 1996). In a qualitative study, Peck and Secker (1999) found that PLH who were IDUs saw their drug problems as more important than their HIV problems. Stigma associated with HIV was an important issue, as they feared being labelled and ostracised. IDUs also reported considerable abuse and trauma, and homelessness was a common feature in their lives.

The experience of health and social care

Wilson and colleagues (2002) noted in their study in the United States that there was limited information available on the experiences of PLH accessing health and social care services. The authors asked 1074 in-patients and 2204 outpatients to rate their visits to a healthcare facility, and found that more problems were associated with in-patient care than outpatient care, in particular in relation to communication between healthcare providers and PLH. Mental health was the only factor that was consistently related to problems associated with care.

Mouton and colleagues (1997) examined how people with serious illness communicated their care preferences to their physician. In an observational, cross-sectional survey of 1031 PLH, 861 individuals stated a treatment preference focused on comfort, even if it shortened life. Only 35.8 per cent had spoken to their physician about their preferred treatment. The main predicting factors were the emergence of symptoms and reduction in physical functioning. It was found that such discussions were less likely when the individuals had less education and lower income.

It has also been investigated whether access to community-based outpatient medical services would result in fewer hospitalisations of PLH (Cunningham et al, 1996, 1998). In this US-based study of 217 PLH, about 50 per cent of the respondents reported that medical services were readily accessible, and it was found that better reported access to services was significantly associated with not having been hospitalised over a defined time period. The authors found that access to services was particularly difficult for low-income people. Affordability, convenience and availability of medical care facilities were important factors identified by respondents, and the authors concluded that difficulty with access caused significant distress to individuals. Good physical and mental health was associated with fewer difficulties with access, and PLH reported significantly more difficulty with access than people with other chronic diseases. Masson and colleagues (2004) examined health service use amongst 190 PLH who also were IDUs, and found that over a two-year period, 71 per cent were treated in an emergency department, 64 per cent had been hospitalised, and the respondents averaged 12.9 outpatient visits. Homelessness was associated with higher use of emergency department and in-patient services, and drug use severity was associated with higher in-patient and outpatient service use.

The role of the healthcare professional

Schulman (1992) noted that stigma and the fear of virus acquisition were central reasons that dentists have refused to care for PLH in the United States. Robinson and Croucher (1993) undertook a survey of the dental experiences of 47 PLH in the United Kingdom. The authors noted that, despite regular attendance prior to HIV diagnosis, 60 per cent of the respondents had not visited a dentist since diagnosis, and as many as 25 per cent had been refused treatment. Gray (1999) noted that such lack of compassion and sensitivity by clinicians became reasons to terminate care or treatment, while Garcia and Cote (2003) suggested that a good relationship with clinicians was important to achieve adherence to ART.

Improving healthcare provision

Grimes and Cole (1996) examined dependence for help with daily living in a study of 83 PLH, and found that encouraging enabling skills would enhance self-help and subsequently enhance functioning. Holzemer and colleagues (1993) presented an instrument, the HIV-Quality Audit Marker (HIV-QAM), which was designed to measure changes in the status of hospitalised PLH brought about by nursing care. It captures the evaluation of the PLH based on vital signs assessment, personal interviews discussing previous and present health, and is concentrated on the areas of self-care, ambulation and psychological distress. Nicholas and colleagues (2003) further indicated that clinical interventions, including behavioural-medicine interventions, could enhance the lives of PLH. Pratt and Washer (1998) discussed care for PLH with HIV-related encephalopathy, and recommended a combination of intensive community support, residential care and respite care in preference to hospital care. They emphasised the importance of early neuropsychological assessment, the provision of a broad range of services with an appropriate skill mix of carers, and the need for staff education and support.

Meredith and colleagues (1997), who studied women's experiences of accessing healthcare, reported that getting a sense of personalised caring and respect was the most important, followed by having someone to talk to about problems, and being provided with honest

> **a) Learning activity**
>
> Melby (2007) found that many PLH had experienced negative communication and interactions with healthcare professionals. Can you think of some possible reasons for this? Do you think they include morality, fear, insecurity or lack of knowledge?

answers and education about their condition. Bride and Real (2003) noted that women in treatment for drug use reported more psychiatric symptoms, more depression and anxiety, lower self-esteem and higher rates of childhood sexual abuse than did men in treatment. The authors concluded that drug use in PLH had a negative effect on people's daily functioning, the use of health services and health outcomes. D'Souza and Garcia (2004) undertook a systematic review of services for pregnant women in the United Kingdom, and noted that while national service frameworks were set up to ensure high-quality services for all women, there were discernible differences in the quality of care provision, with the worst outcomes for women from minority ethnic groups, women experiencing domestic violence, women with mental illness and HIV-infected women.

How individuals respond to the challenges of HIV

Many authors (for example Derogatis,1986; Derogatis and Fleming,1996) have claimed that with advances in medicine and pharmacology and the resultant transformation of terminal diseases into chronic diseases, there has been an associated intensified interest in the concept of psychosocial adjustment in medicine. Many chronic disorders are disabling, and put heavy demands on individuals' coping skills, psychological integrity and social support networks. Appraising the psychosocial adjustment of PLH is thus essential, and should be viewed in terms of their behaviour at work, at home and during leisure time. Their psychosocial adjustment, good or poor, is reflected in their behaviours, and embraces interactions between individuals within the social and environmental context in which people live, and is much more than the consideration of purely intra-psychic processes. Home, work and leisure should be regarded as independent but correlated domains (Derogatis, 1986; Derogatis and Fleming, 1996). The authors also noted that the assessment of psychosocial adjustment was more applicable to people living with chronic conditions, as acute medical conditions and trauma were usually resolved comparatively quickly with immediate invasive and noninvasive treatment methods.

In a survey of 211 PLH, a statistically significant association between social support and psychosocial adjustment was found, with emotional support reported as enhancing subjective health status and social adjustment. According to these authors, coping strategies were not associated with psychosocial adjustment, and there was no evidence of the buffering theory of social support. As Wachtel and colleagues (1992) reported in the early 1990s, and as has been found repeatedly since then, the strongest single indicator of diminished daily functioning in PLH was the emergence of symptoms, particularly constitutional symptoms such as fever and weight loss (Testa and Lenderking, 1999). Discrimination against PLH has been demonstrated in employment, insurance, housing, medical and social care, and this has had observable effects on many areas of functioning. Some of the most severe impact of HIV extends beyond physical well-being to the psycho-social-spiritual and environmental areas of functioning, including social relationships, self-image and behaviour, with those who are homeless, have no education, or who are unemployed showing some of the poorest functioning (O'Connell et al, 2003; Conrad, 2005).

Suzman-Schwartz (2002) examined psychosocial factors that might be associated with reduced psychological distress and improved functioning in 104 HIV-infected men and women. A positive sense of meaning in life and fewer HIV-related symptoms were found to be the two predictors that uniquely contributed to reductions in psychological distress, and along with spirituality, also predicted better functioning. Farber and colleagues (2003) examined further the meaning of illness and psychological adjustment in 203 PLH. The authors claimed that psychologically traumatic events, including the diagnosis of life-threatening diseases, could challenge core personal assumptions and expectations, and reported that positive meaning was associated with enhanced psychological well-being and a reduction in depression. It was suggested by the authors that positive meaning formed a new coping strategy that they termed positive reappraisal.

Part

IV

Kylma, Vehvilainen-Julkunen and Lahdevirta (2001) investigated hope, despair and hopelessness in PLH, and noted that many PLH presented with psychosocial needs of loss, uncertainty, fear, difficulties in relationships and problems with care. When PLH reconstructed their lives, individuals reported gaining help through constructive life experiences, constructive relationships, finding meaning and zest for life, and caring for other people.

Krikorian, Kay and Liang (1995) examined emotional distress, coping and adjustment in 57 ambulatory PLH and 17 HIV seronegative controls. The authors suggested that suicidal ideation was present in many HIV-positive individuals and that it lasted about two months post-diagnosis. Self-reported symptoms were correlated with increased somatic concern, and disruptions in many aspects of daily living were noted, in the domestic, vocational, social and sexual domains. Pakenham and Rinaldis (2002), in their survey of 132 PLH, investigated the role of stress in adjustment to living with HIV. Higher levels of stress were correlated with more HIV symptoms, reliance on emotion-focused coping, lower social support and poorer levels of adjustment.

> **(a) Learning activity**
>
> Research by Melby (2007) suggested that following diagnosis PLH underwent a chaotic period in which a range of dependent behaviours were acted out, such as unprotected sexual intercourse and unsafe intravenous drug use. Major health promotion issues thus arise. Can you propose some ways of challenging such behaviour? How would you approach these people? What would you say? Who could you collaborate with?

The impact of gender

Studies have confirmed that psychosocial adjustment is more complex for women than for men, more complex for other vulnerable groups such as IDUs and ethnic minorities, and that adjustment is associated with more difficulty for PLH than for people suffering from other chronic diseases. Karus, Siegel and Raveis (1999), who investigated psychosocial adjustment in a multi-ethnic sample in New York, found that while there were ethnic differences, difficulties with sexual relationships were reported amongst all groups, and women in all ethnic groups reported difficulties in psychosocial adjustment relative to normative data for cancer patients.

Siegel, Karus and Dean (2004b) studied psychosocial characteristics of 74 New York City HIV-infected women before and after the advent of HAART, and found significant differences related to their domestic environment, with more difficulties reported by the participants receiving HAART. Thus there was no evidence that HAART, while improving immunological status and thus survival, significantly improved psychological health for women. Bova (2001) claimed that symptom experience was the major predictor of adjustment in women, and reported that social support, while not having a direct effect on adjustment, was mediated by personal appraisal of illness and symptom experience.

An investigation of well-educated women infected with HIV by Nannis, Patterson and Semple (1997) suggested that social support correlated with a positive coping strategy, and was additionally associated with less depression and reduced loneliness, while a helpless coping strategy was associated with less social support and more depression. Chung and Magraw (1992) claimed that the unique psychosocial problems of women with HIV infection were often overlooked, and economic, personal, and social resources to meet their needs were therefore often inadequate or inappropriate. According to the authors, women with HIV experienced social isolation, perceived and real stigma, shame, lost or changed roles as women, mothers and wives, and experienced anxiety and confusion about options for sexual activity. Shorposner and colleagues (2000) reported significant socioeconomic inequities between men and women who are IDUs and how this impacts psychosocial adjustment, with women significantly more likely to be homeless than men. Poorer psychosocial adjustment was also associated with less social support.

The impact of social support

Norbeck (1988) carried out a review of social support research in nursing, and confirmed that models proposed that social support buffers the effect of stress on health and that it also has direct effects on stress and health. Various authors saw as core issues the number of social support resources (who and how many in the social network), satisfaction with support, perceived social support, loss, frequency of support, and quality of support. Norbeck and Tilden (1988) further discussed the conceptual basis for assuming that social support is a universal phenomenon, and that the buffering effect applies to all cultures. The authors concluded that social support is a universal phenomenon, although certain manifestations of social support may be culture-specific. Hutchison (1999) claimed that while the positive effect of social support on health had been noted by several authors, the absence of a clear definition made it difficult to compare social support across studies, and maintained that the main conceptual components were emotional, instrumental, informational, appraisal assistance and social integration.

Sarason, Sarason and Pierce (1994) argued that an individual's interpretation of the quality of their social support (that is, their perceived support) was the most important factor in determining the effect on adjustment. They argued that perceived social support was related to health status but also influenced by the individual's personality, including self-image. The authors also pointed out that there were gender differences to take into consideration. In their interpretation, social support was dependent on disease-related issues, psychological distress and relationship issues. Perceived support involves a process in which the person rates their expectations of people in their social network.

Namir, Wolcott and Fawzy (1989) corroborated that the principal domains of social support were emotional, tangible (instrumental) and informational, and suggested that different types of support might be more useful at different stages of illness. The authors found that PLH were more likely to ask friends for help than their families, and that help was needed to gain information, deal with practical difficulties, and cope with emotions. Wilcox and Vernberg (1985) suggested that social support was a response-set to stressors in life, which create adaptational demands of varying amounts and intensity. They argued that social support is effective when there are sufficient social resources to make the necessary adaptations. In all stressful situations, individuals attempt to match the threat to them with the resources available to them, and respond according to the balance they perceive. However, some stressors may be viewed as so traumatic that all coping mechanisms, including social support, are ineffectual.

Barnes and Duck (1994) claimed that in a crisis, most people turn to those they have a continuous relationship with, most often their partner, and argued that normal conversation and interaction between partners are crucial components of social support. They saw this as involving six supportive functions, including giving and receiving information, early detection in changes in condition, and ventilation of emotions. In some situations clinicians are needed to provide additional specialist support. Kimberly and Serovich (1996) investigated perceived social support among 77 PLH, and noted that for gay PLH, friends are more important social support providers than family members primarily because of the stigma associated with HIV, with subsequent lack of disclosure to family members, friends and colleagues. These important members of the social support network are consequently unable to provide support.

Many researchers (Pakenham, Dadds and Terry, 1994; Friedland et al, 1996; Bor, du Plessis and Russel, 2004) have claimed that partners and close friends are most closely linked with satisfaction of support, and highlighted that emotional support is related to better subjective health status and illness-related adjustment. The authors could not find evidence for the direction of causality between social support and adjustment, so this gives little support to arguments about the buffering effect of social support. Rather, adjustment was seen as related to physical health variables such as the number of symptoms. Barroso (1997) carried out a

Part

IV

qualitative study of social support in people who had lived with HIV for a long time, and confirmed that social support had a positive effect on a person's health status, in particular emotional aspects, such as psychological adjustment, greater sense of coherence, higher self-esteem and decreased anxiety. When HIV symptoms appeared there was a decline in total support, possibly reflecting people withdrawing from the social network.

Green (1993) maintained that early research on social support in PLH was almost exclusively focused on gay, middle-class, white men in the United States, with little or no research into vulnerable groups such as ethnic minorities, women or IDUs. She argued that such research could indeed bring to light new issues in the relationship between social support and health in PLH. Barroso (1997), in her in-depth interview study of 14 men and six women, found that partner support was seen as crucial, but pointed out that men and women sensed and used their social support differently, with women with children citing their children as the major reason to live. Pakenham, Dadds and Terry (1994), in their study of 96 gay men with HIV, found that having a partner was associated with poorer adjustment and an increase in physical symptoms, possibly indicating a partner dependency issue (a passive relationship). Gielen and colleagues (2001), in their study of 287 women with HIV, reported that women with larger social support networks reported better mental health and overall quality of life, with instrumental support strongly associated with better physical and mental health.

House, Lantz and Herd (2005) revealed that socially isolated people were unhealthier and died earlier than those who had good social relationships. Social relationships are the foundation of social support, and the nature and quality and thus perceptions of these relationships are influenced by age, gender, ethnicity and socioeconomic status. Fleishman and colleagues (2000) indicated that conflictual social interactions were strongly related to negative mood and coping behaviours such as social isolation, anger and wishful thinking. PLH who are IDUs experience heightened emotional distress, are often homeless and unemployed, and live in social isolation (Fleishman and Fogel, 1994), and improved drug behaviour has been associated with better social support in terms of having people to talk to, and a social network that excludes other IDUs (Zapka, Stoddard and McCusker, 1993).

While the benefits of social support have been clearly demonstrated, there is also evidence that social support for PLH may have negative consequences (Barroso, 1997; Vosvick et al, 2004). These studies have reported that social relationships can concurrently be a source of stress, and that actions intended to be supportive may instead be experienced as psychologically disturbing. Such negative interactions might have a poor effect on mental health. Some of the negative interactions noted by the respondents in this study were ineffective help, excessive help (treating the PLH as an invalid), and unwanted or unpleasant interactions. Goldsmith (1994) further explained that advice could be interpreted as negative, when people do not want to be told what to do.

Coping strategies

Coping appears as another factor in adjustment. Several researchers have presented data that suggests that active, cognitive coping strategies lower psychosocial distress and aid adjustment (Fleishman et al. 2000; Tuck, McCain and Elswick, 2001; Vosvick et al, 2002; Weaver et al, 2004). How each PLH responds to a diagnosis with HIV appears to be specific to that individual, but many find that social support has a positive effect on their psychosocial adjustment. According to Grummon and colleagues (1994), perceived social support from family correlated positively with psychological adjustment, although perceived social support from friends did not. Linn and colleagues (1994) suggested that PLH derive a greater sense of purpose in their life with good social support.

Barroso (1997) reported that helping other PLH was part of coping with adjustment, as was partaking in support groups (Leserman et al, 1994). Spiritual revival was common (Regan-Kubinski and Sharts-Hopko, 1995), but this was rarely religious, and was associated with enhanced daily functioning (Tuck et al, 2001; Weaver et al, 2004). Wayment, Silver and

Kemeny (1995) reported that 'survivors' guilt' was common in gay men with HIV, and noted that benefit was experienced from gay-related community group involvement. Another means of helping other PLH is volunteering in 'buddy' programmes, in which PLH provide a variety of support to other PLH. Burrage and Demi (2003), using a convenience sample of 46 PLH, found that PLH perceived adequate social support and assistance with this system, and there was very good satisfaction with client–volunteer relationships.

Complementary and alternative therapies (CAMs) are commonly used by PLH (Lutgendorf et al, 1994; Wootton and Sparber, 2001; Nicholas et al, 2003), in particular body therapies such as massage and aromatherapy, which have been found to be associated with better social functioning. The use of other CAMs, such as nutritional therapies, relaxation exercises and psychospiritual therapies, has been associated with better mental health and social support and subsequently enhanced adjustment.

Kirksey and colleagues (2002) investigated the use of CAMs in PLH in the United States. Using a convenience sample of 422 PLH, they found significant differences for gender and for ethnicity, with females and African-Americans using CAMs more frequently. Overall more than one-third of the participants used at least one CAM, and the authors suggested that CAM use might enhance the quality of people's lives through the cushioning or reduction of side-effects associated with HIV disease and HAART treatments. Ozsoy and Ernst (1999) carried out a systematic review of 14 studies covering herbal treatments (two studies), vitamins and other supplements (five), stress management (five), one massage therapy and one acupuncture. While the review concluded that few rigorous studies of the utilisation of CAM in PLH existed, CAMs appeared to enhance the quality of people's lives, with stress management found to be particularly effective. Pawluch, Cain and Gillett (2000) reported from their qualitative study that PLH used CAMs as a part of a health maintenance strategy, as a healing strategy, as an alternative to traditional medicine, and as a way of mitigating the side-effects of drug therapies, thus confirming the integration of CAMs into coping as a strategy to maximize daily functioning.

> **a** Learning activity
>
> Undertake a literature search and examine the evidence base for the use of complementary therapies in clinical practice. What does the evidence tell us?

Conclusion

This chapter has established the importance of examining how PLH function across a range of activities in their daily lives. In addition, we must take account of the impact of social support and the effects of perceived and received stigma experiences. Those PLH who are substance-dependent, come from an ethnic minority, or who are socioeconomically disadvantaged, appear to be more exposed to negative experiences in their daily lives and are less able to respond positively to psychosocial demands. A holistic examination of how people live with HIV should ideally incorporate all of these variables, as they all impact how PLH adjust to a HIV diagnosis and will shape the quality of life that individuals with HIV enjoy.

References

Adam, B. D., Maticka-Tyndale, E. and Cohen, J. J. (2003) 'Adherence practices among people living with HIV', *AIDS Care* **15**(2), 263–74.

Avert (2007) 'HIV and AIDS in countries and region' [online] http://www.avert.org/aids-countries.htm (accessed 14 June 2007).

Barnes, M. K. and Duck, S. (1994) 'Everyday communicative contexts for social support'. pp. 175–94 in Burleson, B. R., Albrecht, T. L. and Sarason, I. G. (eds), *Communication of Social Support: Messages, interactions, relationships and community*, Thousand Oaks, Calif., Sage.

Barroso, J. (1997) 'Social support and long-term survivors of AIDS',

Western Journal of Nursing Research **19**(5), 554–73.

Benedict, R. H. B., Mezhir, J. J., Walsh, K. and Hewitt, R. G. (2000) 'Impact of human immunodeficiency virus type-1-associated cognitive dysfunction on activities of daily living and quality of life', *Archives of Clinical Neuropsychology* **15**(6), 529–34.

Blalock, A. C., McDaniel, J. S. and Farber, E. W. (2002) 'Effect of employment on quality of life and psychological functioning in patients with HIV/AIDS', *Psychosomatics* **43**(5), 400–4.

Bor, R., du Plessis, P. and Russell, M. (2004) 'The impact of disclosure of HIV on the index patient's self-defined family', *Journal of Family*

Therapy **26**(2), 167–92.

Bova, C. (2001) 'Adjustment to chronic illness among HIV-infected women', *Journal of Nursing Scholarship* **33**(3), 217–23.

Bova, C. and Durante, A. (2003) 'Sexual functioning among HIV-infected women', *AIDS Patient Care and STDs* **17**(2), 75–83.

Brashers, D. E., Neidig, J. L., Cardillo, L. W., Dobbs, L. K. and Al, E. (1999) '"In an important way, I did die": uncertainty and revival in persons living with HIV or AIDS', *AIDS Care* **11**(2), 201–19.

Brashers, D. E., Neidig, J. L. and Goldsmith, D. J. (2004) 'Social support and the management of uncertainty for people living with HIV or AIDS', *Health Communication* **16**(3), 305–31.

Brashers, D. E., Neidig, J. L., Reynolds, N. R. and Haas, S. M. (1998) 'Uncertainty in illness across the HIV/AIDS trajectory', *Journal of the Association of Nurses in AIDS Care* **9**(1), 66–77.

Brashers, D. E., Neidig, J. L., Russell, J. A., Cardillo, L. W., Haas, S. M., Dobbs, L. K., Garland, M., McCartney, B. and Nemeth, S. (2003) 'The medical, personal, and social causes of uncertainty in HIV illness', *Issues in Mental Health Nursing* **24**(5), 497–522.

Breitbart, W. (1998) 'Pain in AIDS: an overview', *Pain Reviews* **5**(4), 247–72.

Breitbart, W., McDonald, M. V., Rosenfeld, B., Monkman, N. D. and Passik, S. (1998) 'Fatigue in ambulatory AIDS patients', *Journal of Pain and Symptom Management* **15**(3), 159–67.

Bride, B. E. and Real, E. (2003) 'Project assist: a modified therapeutic community for homeless women living with HIV/AIDS and chemical dependency' *Health and Social Work* **28**(2), 166.

Brook, M. G., Dale, A., Tomlinson, D., Waterworth, C. and Al, E. (2001) 'Adherence to highly active antiretroviral therapy in the real world: experience of twelve English HIV units' *AIDS Patient Care and STDs* **15**(9), 491–4.

Brooks, R. A., Martin, D. J., Ortiz, D. J. and Veniegas, R. C. (2004) 'Perceived barriers to employment among persons living with HIV/AIDS', *AIDS Care* **16**(6), 756–66.

Burgoyne, R. W., Rourke, S. B., Behrens, D. M. and Salit, I. E. (2004) 'Long-term quality-of-life outcomes among adults living with HIV in the HAART era: the interplay of changes in clinical factors and symptom profile', *AIDS and Behavior* **8**(2), 151–63.

Burrage, J. and Demi, A. (2003) 'Buddy programs for people infected with HIV', *Journal of the Association of Nurses in AIDS Care* **14**(1), 52–62.

Burrage, J. and Rocchiociolli, J. (2003) 'HIV related stigma: implications for multi-cultural nursing', *Journal of Multicultural Nursing and Health* **9**(1), 13–17.

Cadwell, S. (1991) 'Twice removed: the stigma suffered by gay men with AIDS', *Smith College Studies in Social Work* **61**(3), 236–46.

Campsmith, M. L., Nakashima, A. K. and Davidson, A. J. (2003) 'Self-reported health-related quality of life in persons with HIV infection: results from a multi-site interview project', *Health and Quality of Life Outcomes* **1**(12), 1–6.

Carr, R. L. and Gramling, L. F. (2004) 'Stigma: a health barrier for women with HIV/AIDS', *Journal of the Association of Nurses in AIDS Care* **15**(5), 30–9.

Carretero, M. D., Burgess, A. P., Soler, P., Soler, M. and Catalan, J. (1996) 'Reliability and validity of an HIV-specific health-related quality-of-life measure for use with injecting drug users', *AIDS* **10**(14), 1699–705.

Carroll, D., Foley, B., Hickson, F., O'Connor, J., Quinlan, M., Sheehan, B., Watters, R. and Weatherburn, P. (2002) *Vital Statistics Ireland: Findings from the All-Ireland Gay Men's Sex Survey*, Dublin, Gay Health Network.

Castro, A. and Farmer, P. (2005) 'Understanding and addressing AIDS-related stigma: from anthropological theory to clinical practice in Haiti', *American Journal of Public Health* **95**(1), 53–9.

Catalan, J. and Meadows, J. (2000) 'Sexual dysfunction in gay and bisexual men with HIV infection: evaluation, treatment and implications', *AIDS Care* **12**(3), 279–86.

Catalan, J., Meadows, J. and Douzenis, A. (2000) 'The changing pattern of mental health problems in HIV infection: The view from London, UK', *AIDS Care* **12**(3), 333–41.

Centers for Disease Control and Prevention (CDC) (2001) '1993 Revised classification system for HIV infection and expanded surveillance case definition for AIDS among adolescents and adults', *Mortality and Morbidity Weekly Reports* **41**(RR-17), 9 December 2005 [online] http://www.cdc.gov/mmwr/preview/mmwrhtml/00018871.htm (accessed 22 December 2008).

Chan, K. S. and Revicki, D. A. (1998) 'Changes in surrogate laboratory markers, clinical endpoints, and health-related quality of life in patients infected with the human immunodeficiency virus', *Evaluation and the Health Professions* **21**(2), 265–81.

Chandra, P. S., Deepthivarma, S., Jairam, K. R. and Thomas, T. (2003) 'Relationship of psychological morbidity and quality of life to illness-related disclosure among HIV-infected persons', *Journal of Psychosomatic Research* **54**(3), 199–203.

Chapman, E. (1998) 'Body image and HIV: implications for support and care', *AIDS Care* **10** (supp. 2), S179–S187.

Chapman, E. (2002) 'Patient impact of negative representations of HIV', *AIDS Patient Care and STDs* **16**(4), 173–7.

Checkley, G. E., Thompson, S. C., Crofts, N. and Mijch, A. M. (1996) 'HIV in the mentally ill', *Australian and New Zealand Journal of Psychiatry* **30**(2), 184–94.

Cherry-Peppers, G., Daniels, C. O., Meeks, V., Sanders, C. F. and Reznik, D. (2003) 'Oral manifestations in the era of HAART', *Journal of the National Medical Association* **95** (supp. 2), 21S–32S.

Chesney, M. A., Ickovics, J. R., Chambers, D. B., Gifford, A. L., Neidig, J., Zwickl, B. and Wu, A. W. (2000) 'Self-reported adherence to antiretroviral medications among participants in HIV clinical trials: the AACTG adherence instruments, Patient Care Committee and Adherence Working Group of the Outcomes Committee of the Adult AIDS Clinical Trials Group (AACTG)', *AIDS Care* **12**(3), 255–66.

Chung, J. Y. and Magraw, M. M. (1992) 'A group approach to psychosocial issues faced by HIV-positive women', *Hospital and Community Psychiatry* **43**(9), 891–4.

Conrad, P. (2005) 'The experience of illness', pp. 130–2 in P. Conrad (ed.), *The Sociology of Health and Illness: Critical perspectives*, 7th edn, New York, Worth.

Corless, I. B., Nicholas, P. K., McGibbon, C. A. and Wilson, C. (2004) 'Weight change, body image, and quality of life in HIV disease: a pilot study', *Applied Nursing Research* **17**(4), 292–6.

Crowther, M. (1992) '"I am a person, not a disease": Experiences of people living with HIV/AIDS', *Professional Nurse* **7**(6), 381–5.

Cruess, D. G., Evans, D. L., Repetto, M. J., Gettes, D., Douglas, S. D. and Petitto, J. M. (2003) 'Prevalence, diagnosis, and pharmacological treatment of mood disorders in HIV disease', *Biological Psychiatry* **54**(3), 307–16.

Crystal, S., Fleishman, J.A., Hays, R.D., Shapiro, M.F. and Bozzette, S.A. (2000) 'Physical and role functioning among persons with HIV: results from a nationally representative survey', *Medical Care* **38**(12), 1210–23.

Cunningham, W. E., Hays, R. D., Ettl, M. K., Dixon, W. J., Liu, R. C., Beck, C. K. and Shapiro, M. F. (1998) 'The prospective effect of access to medical care on health-related quality-of-life outcomes in patients with symptomatic HIV disease', *Medical Care* **36**(3), 295–306.

Cunningham, W. E., Mosen, D. M., Hays, R. D., Andersen, R. M. and Shapiro, M. F. (1996) 'Access to community-based medical services and number of hospitalizations among patients with HIV disease: are they related?' *Journal of Acquired Immune Deficiency Syndromes and Human Retrovirology* **13**(4), 327–35.

D'Souza, L. and Garcia, J. (2004) 'Improving services for disadvantaged childbearing women', *Child: Care, Health and Development* **30**(6), 599–611.

Daar, E. S. (1998) 'Virology and immunology of acute HIV type 1 infection', *AIDS Research and Human Retroviruses* **14** (Suppl 3), S229–S234.

Davies, J., Everall, I. P., Weich, S., McLaughlin, J., Scaravilli, F. and Lantos, P. L. (1997) 'HIV-associated brain pathology in the United Kingdom: an epidemiological study', *AIDS* **11**(9), 1145–50.

Derogatis, L.R. (1986) 'Psychosocial Adjustment to Illness Scale (PAIS)', *Journal of Psychosomatic Research* **30**(1), 77–91.

Derogatis, L. R. and Fleming, M. P. (1996) 'Psychological adjustment to illness scale: PAIS and PAIS-SR', pp. 287–99 in B. Spilker (ed.), *Quality of Life and Pharmacoeconomics in Clinical Trials*, 2nd edn, Philadelphia, Pa., Lippincott-Raven.

Dreher, H. M. (2003) 'Measuring health status in HIV disease: challenges from a sleep study', *Holistic Nursing Practice* **17**(2), 81–90.

Earthman, C. P., Reid, P. M., Harper, I. T., Ravussin, E. and Howell, W.H. (2002) 'Body cell mass repletion and improved quality of life in HIV-infected individuals receiving oxandrolone', *Journal of Parenteral and Enteral Nutrition* **26**(6), 357–65.

Evangelisto, M. (1996) 'Death with dignity: end-of-life issues for the HIV/AIDS patient', *Journal of Psychosocial Nursing and Mental Health Services* **34**(6), 45–7.

Evans, S., Ferrando, S., Sewell, M., Goggin, K., Fishman, B. and Rabkin, J. (1998) 'Pain and depression in HIV illness', *Psychosomatics* **39**(6), 528–35.

Fantoni, M., Autore, C. and Del Borgo, C. (2001) 'Drugs and cardiotoxicity in HIV and AIDS', *Annals of the New York Academy of Sciences* 946, 179–99.

Farber, E. W., Mirsalimi, H., Williams, K. A. and McDaniel, J. S. (2003) 'Meaning of illness and psychological adjustment to HIV/AIDS', *Psychosomatics* **44**(6), 485–91.

Fleishman, J. A., Sherbourne, C. D., Crystal, S., Collins, R. L., Marshall, G. N., Kelly, M., Bozzette, S. A., Shapiro, M. F. and Hays, R. D. (2000) 'Coping, conflictual social interactions, social support, and mood among HIV-infected persons, HCSUS Consortium', *American Journal of Community Psychology* **28**(4), 421–53.

Fleishman, J. A. and Fogel, B. (1994) 'Coping and depressive symptoms among young people with AIDS', *Health Psychology* **13**(2), 156–69.

Friedland, J., Renwick, R. and McColl, M. (1996) 'Coping and social support as determinants of quality of life in HIV/AIDS', *AIDS Care* **8**(1), 15–31.

Garcia, P. R. and Cote, J. K. (2003) 'Factors affecting adherence to antiretroviral therapy in people living with HIV/AIDS', *Journal of the Association of Nurses in AIDS Care* **14**(4), 37–45.

Gielen, A.C., McDonnell, K.A., Wu, A.W., O'Campo, P. and Faden, R. (2001) 'Quality of life among women living with HIV: the importance of violence, social support, and self care behaviors', *Social Science and Medicine* **52**(2), 315–22.

Goldsmith, D. J. (1994) 'The role of facework in supportive communication', pp. 29–49 in Burleson, B. R., Albrecht, T. L. and Sarason, I. G. (eds) *Communication of Social Support: Messages, interactions, relationships and community*, Thousand Oaks, Calif., Sage.

Grassi, L., Satriano, J., Serra, A., Biancosino, B., Zotos, S., Sighinolfi, L. and Ghinelli, F. (2002) 'Emotional stress, psychosocial variables and coping associated with hepatitis C virus and human immunodeficiency virus infections in intravenous drug users', *Psychotherapy and Psychosomatics* **71**(6), 342–9.

Gray, J. J. (1999) 'The difficulties of women living with HIV infection', *Journal of Psychosocial Nursing and Mental Health Services* **37**(5), 39–43.

Green, G. (1993) 'Social support and HIV', *AIDS Care* **5**(1), 87–104.

Green, G. and Smith, R. (2004) 'The psychosocial and health care needs of HIV-positive people in the United Kingdom: a review', *HIV Medicine* **5**(supp. 1), 5–46.

Grimes, D. E. and Cole, F. L. (1996) 'Self-help and life quality in persons with HIV disease', *AIDS Care* **8**(6), 691–9.

Grummon, K., Rigby, E. D., Orr, D., Procidano, M. and Reznikoff, M. (1994) 'Psychosocial variables that affect the psychological adjustment of IVDU patients with AIDS', *Journal of Clinical Psychology* **50**(4), 488–502.

Haller, D. L. and Miles, D. R. (2003) 'Suicidal ideation among psychiatric patients with HIV: psychiatric morbidity and quality of life', *AIDS and Behavior* **7**(2), 101–8.

Harrison, R. A., Soong, S., Weiss, H. L., Gnann, J. W. and Whitley, R. J. (1999) 'A mixed model for factors predictive of pain in AIDS patients with herpes zoster', *Journal of Pain and Symptom Management* **17**(6), 410–17.

Hays, R. B., McKusick, L., Pollack, L., Hilliard, R., Hoff, C. and Coates, T.J. (1993) 'Disclosing HIV seropositivity to significant others', *AIDS* **7**(3), 425–31.

Heller, S. (2004) 'The missing link: perceived stigma as a contributing variable to HIV high-risk behaviors among people with severe mental illness', *Dissertation Abstracts International Section A: Humanities and Social Sciences* 6412-A, pp. 4371.

Henry, S. B., Holzemer, W. L., Weaver, K. and Stotts, N. (1999) 'Quality of life and self-care management strategies of PLWAs with chronic diarrhea', *Journal of the Association of Nurses in AIDS Care* **10**(2), 46–54.

Herek, G. M. (2005) 'AIDS and stigma', pp. 121–9 in Conrad, P. (ed.), *The Sociology of Health and Illness: Critical perspectives*, 7th edn, New York: Worth.

Herek, G. M. and Capitanio, J. P. (1993) 'Public reactions to AIDS in the United States: a second decade of stigma', *American Journal of Public Health* **83**(4) 574–7.

Herek, G. M. and Capitanio, J. P. (1997) 'AIDS stigma and contact with persons with AIDS: effects of direct and vicarious contact', *Journal of Applied Social Psychology* **27**(1), 1–36.

Holzemer, W. L., Henry, S. B., Stewart, A. and Janson-Bjerklie, S. (1993) 'The HIV quality audit marker (HIV-QAM): an outcome measure for hospitalized AIDS patients', *Quality of Life Research* **2**(2), 99–107.

House, J.S., Lantz, P.M. and Herd, P. (2005) 'Continuity and change in the social stratification of aging and health over the life course: evidence from a nationally representative longitudinal study from 1986 to 2001/2002 (Americans' Changing Lives Study)', *Journals of Gerontology. Series B, Psychological Sciences and Social Sciences* **60**(Spec. no. 2), 15–26.

Hutchison, C. (1999) 'Social support: factors to consider when designing studies that measure social support', *Journal of Advanced Nursing* **29**(6), 1520–6.

Kalichman, S.C., Heckman, T., Kochman, A., Sikkema, K. and Bergholte, J. (2000) 'Depression and thoughts of suicide among middle-aged and older persons living with HIV-AIDS', *Psychiatric Services* **51**(7), 903–7.

Karus, D., Siegel, K. and Raveis, V. H. (1999) 'Psychosocial adjustment of women to living with HIV/AIDS', *AIDS and Behavior* 3(4), 277–87.

Keiser, P., Sension, M., Dejesus, E., Rodriguez, A., Olliffe, J., Williams, V., Wakeford, J., Snidow, J., Shachoy-Clark, A., Fleming, J., Pakes, G., Hernandez, J. and for the ESS40003 Study Team (2005) 'Substituting abacavir for hyperlipidemia-associated protease inhibitors in HAART regimens improves fasting lipid profiles, maintains virologic suppression, and simplifies treatment', *BMC Infectious Diseases* 5(1), 2.

Kelly, B., Raphael, B., Statham, D., Ross, M., Eastwood, H., McLean, S., O'Loughlin, B. and Brittain, K. (1996) 'A comparison of the psychosocial aspects of AIDS and cancer-related bereavement', *International Journal of Psychiatry in Medicine* 26(1), 35–49.

Kelly, J. A., Murphy, D. A., Bahr, G. R., Koob, J. J., Morgan, M. G., Kalichman, S. C., Stevenson, L.Y., Brasfield, T. L., Bernstein, B. M. and St Lawrence, J. S. (1993) 'Factors associated with severity of depression and high-risk sexual behavior among persons diagnosed with human immunodeficiency virus (HIV) infection', *Health Psychology* 12(3), 215–19.

Kendall, J. (1996) 'Human association as a factor influencing wellness in homosexual men with human immunodeficiency virus disease', *Applied Nursing Research* 9(4), 195–203.

Kimberly, J. A. and Serovich, J. M. (1996) 'Perceived social support among people living with HIV/AIDS' , *American Journal of Family Therapy* 24(1), 41–53.

Kirksey, K. M., Goodroad, B. K., Kemppainen, J. K., Holzemer, W. L., Bunch, E. H., Corless, I. B., Eller, L. S., Nicholas, P. K., Nokes, K. and Bain, C. (2002) 'Complementary therapy use in persons with HIV/AIDS', *Journal of Holistic Nursing* 20(3), 264–78.

Knowlton, A. R., Latkin, C. A., Chung, S., Hoover, D. R., Ensminger, M. and Celentano, D. D. (2000) 'HIV and depressive symptoms among low-income illicit drug users', *AIDS and Behavior* 4(4), 353–60.

Koopman, C., Gore-Felton, C., Azimi, N., O'Shea, K., Ashton, E., Power, R., de Maria, S., Israelski, D. and Spiegel, D. (2002) 'Acute stress reactions to recent life events among women and men living with HIV/AIDS', *International Journal of Psychiatry in Medicine* 32(4), 361–78.

Koutsilieri, E., Scheller, C., Sopper, S., Ter Meulen, V. and Riederer, P. (2002) 'Psychiatric complications in human immunodeficiency virus infection', *Journal of Neurovirology* 8(supp. 2), 129–33.

Krikorian, R., Kay, J. and Liang, W.M. (1995) 'Emotional distress, coping, and adjustment in human immunodeficiency virus infection and acquired immune deficiency syndrome', *Journal of Nervous and Mental Disease* 183 (5), 293–8.

Kylma, J., Vehvilainen-Julkunen, K. and Lahdevirta, J. (2001) 'Hope, despair and hopelessness in living with HIV/AIDS: a grounded theory study', *Journal of Advanced Nursing* 33(6), 764–75.

Leask, C., Elford, J., Bor, R. and Miller, R. (1997) 'Selective disclosure: a pilot investigation into changes in family relationships since HIV diagnosis', *Journal of Family Therapy* 19(1), 59-–69.

Leserman, J., Disantostefano, R., Perkins, D. O. and Evans, D. L. (1994) 'Gay identification and psychological health in HIV-positive and HIV-negative gay men', *Journal of Applied Social Psychology* 24(24), 2193–208.

Linn, J. G., Anema, M. G., Estrada, J. J., Cain, V. A. and Usoh, D. M. (1994) 'HIV illness and mental distress in female clients of AIDS care and referral centers', *AIDS Patient Care* 8(5), 254–9.

Lutgendorf, S., Antoni, M. H., Schneiderman, N. and Fletcher, M. A. (1994) 'Psychosocial counseling to improve quality of life in HIV infection', *Patient Education and Counseling* 24(3), 217–35.

Mansergh, G., Marks, G. and Simoni, J.M. (1995) 'Self-disclosure of HIV infection among men who vary in time since seropositive diagnosis and symptomatic status', *AIDS* 9(6), 639–44.

Marks, K. and Gulick, R. M. (2004) 'New antiretroviral agents for the treatment of HIV infection', *Current HIV/AIDS Reports* 1(2), 82–8.

Martin, D. J., Brooks, R. A., Ortiz, D. J. and Veniegas, R. C. (2003) 'Perceived employment barriers and their relation to workforce-entry intent among people with HIV/AIDS', *Journal of Occupational Health Psychology* 8 (3), 181–94.

Martinez-Picado, J., Negredo, E., Ruiz, L., Shintani, A., Fumaz, C. R., Zala, C., Domingo, P., Vilaro, J., Llibre, J. M., Viciana, P., Hertogs, K., Boucher, C., D'Aquila, R. T., Clotet, B. and Swatch Study, T. (2003) 'Alternation of antiretroviral drug regimens for HIV infection: a randomized, controlled trial', *Annals of Internal Medicine* 139(2), 81–9.

Masson, C. L., Sorensen, J. L., Phibbs, C. S. and Okin, R. L. (2004) 'Predictors of medical service utilization among individuals with co-occurring HIV infection and substance abuse disorders', *AIDS Care* 16(6), 744–55.

Melby, V. (2007) *Quality of Life of People Living with HIV in Ireland*, Ph.D. thesis, Coleraine, Northern Ireland, University of Ulster.

Meredith, K., Delaney, J., Horgan, M., Fisher, E., Jr and Fraser, V. (1997) 'A survey of women with HIV about their expectations for care', *AIDS Care* 9(5), 513–22.

Meyer, I. H. (1995) 'Minority stress and mental health in gay men', *Journal of Health and Social Behavior* 36(1), 38–56.

Miller, R. and Murray, D. (1999) 'The impact of HIV illness on parents and children, with particular reference to African families', *Journal of Family Therapy* 21(3), 284–302.

Mok, J. and Cooper, S. (1997) 'The needs of children whose mothers have HIV infection', *Archives of Disease in Childhood* 77(6), 483–7.

Moneyham, L., Seals, B., Demi, A., Sowell, R., Cohen, L. and Guillory, J. (1996) 'Experiences of disclosure in women infected with HIV', *Health Care for Women International* 17(3), 209–21.

Mouton, C., Teno, J. M., Mor, V. and Piette, J. (1997) 'Communication of preferences for care among human immunodeficiency virus-infected patients. Barriers to informed decisions?' *Archives of Family Medicine* 6(4), 342–7.

Myskowski, P. L. and Ahkami, R. (1996) 'Dermatologic complications of HIV infection', *Medical Clinics of North America* 80(6), 1415–35.

Namir, S., Wolcott, D. L. and Fawzy, F. I. (1989) 'Social support and HIV spectrum disease: clinical and research perspectives', *Psychiatric Medicine* 7(2), 97–105.

Nannis, E. D., Patterson, T. L. and Semple, S. J. (1997) 'Coping with HIV disease among seropositive women: psychosocial correlates', *Women and Health* 25(1), 1–22.

Newshan, G., Taylor, B. and Gold, R. (1998) 'Sexual functioning in ambulatory men with HIV/AIDS', *International Journal of STD and AIDS* 9(11), 672–6.

Nicholas, P. K., Corless, I. B., Webster, A., McGibbon, C. A. and Al, E. (2003) 'A behavioral-medicine program in HIV: Implications for quality of life', *Journal of Holistic Nursing* 21(2), 163–78.

Nilsson Schönnesson, L. (2002) 'Psychological and existential issues and quality of life in people living with HIV infection', *AIDS Care* 14(3), 399–404.

Nokes, K. M., Holzemer, W. L., Corless, I. B., Bakken, S., Brown, M., Powell-Cope, G. M., Inouye, J. and Turner, J. (2000) 'Health-related quality of life in persons younger and older than 50 who are living with HIV/AIDS', *Research on Aging* 22(3), 290–310.

Norbeck, J. S. (1988) 'Social support', *Annual Review of Nursing Research* 6, 85–109.

Norbeck, J. S. and Tilden, V. P. (1988) 'International nursing research in social support: theoretical and methodological issues', *Journal of Advanced Nursing* 13(2), 173–8.

O'Connell, K., Skevington, S., Saxena, S. and WHOQOL HIV Group (2003) 'Preliminary development of the World Health Organization's Quality of Life HIV instrument (WHOQOL-HIV): analysis of the pilot version', *Social Science and Medicine* **57**(7), 1259–75.

Ormond, P. and Mulcahy, F. (1998) 'Sexually transmitted diseases in HIV-positive patients', *Dermatologic Clinics* **16**(4), 853–7.

Ozsoy, M. and Ernst, E. (1999) 'How effective are complementary therapies for HIV and AIDS? – a systematic review', *International Journal of STD and AIDS* **10**(10), 629–35.

Pakenham, K. I., Dadds, M. R. and Terry, D. J. (1994) 'Relationships between adjustment to HIV and both social support and coping', *Journal of Consulting and Clinical Psychology* **62**(6), 1194–1203.

Pakenham, K.I. and Rinaldis, M. (2002) 'Development of the HIV/AIDS stress scale', *Psychology and Health* **17**(2), 203–19.

Pawluch, D., Cain, R. and Gillett, J. (2000) 'Lay constructions of HIV and complementary therapy use', *Social Science and Medicine* **51**(2), 251–64.

Peck, E. and Secker, J. (1999) 'Piths, pearls, and provocation. Quality criteria for qualitative research: does context make a difference?' *Qualitative Health Research* **9**(4), 552–8.

Perretta, P., Nisita, C., Zaccagnini, E., Lorenzetti, C., Nuccorini, A., Cassano, G. B. and Akiskal, H. S. (1996) 'Psychopathology in 90 consecutive human immunodeficiency virus-seropositive and acquired immune deficiency syndrome patients with mostly intravenous drug use history', *Comprehensive Psychiatry* **37**(4), 267–72.

Perry, S. W., Card, C. A., Moffatt, M. J. R., Ashman, T., Fishman, B. and Jacobsberg, L. B. (1994) 'Self-disclosure of HIV infection to sexual partners after repeated counseling', *AIDS Education and Prevention* **6**(5), 403–11.

Piette, J., Wachtel, T.J., Mor, V. and Mayer, K. (1995) 'The impact of age on the quality of life in persons with HIV infection', *Journal of Aging and Health* **7**(2), 163–78.

Powell-Cope, G.M. and Brown, M.A. (1992) 'Going public as an AIDS family caregiver', *Social Science and Medicine* **34**(5), 571–80.

Pratt, R. and Washer, P. (1998) 'HIV-related encephalopathy', *Nursing Standard* **13**(7), 38–40.

Range, L.M. and Alliston, J.R. (1995) 'Reacting to AIDS-related suicide: does time since diagnosis matter?' *Death Studies* **19**(3), 277–82.

Rao, V. K. and Thomas, F. P. (2005) 'Neurological complications of HIV/AIDS', *Beta Bulletin of Experimental Treatments for Aids* **17**(2), 37–46.

Regan-Kubinski, M.J. and Sharts-Hopko, N. (1995) 'Illness cognition of HIV-infected mothers', *Issues in Mental Health Nursing* **16**(4), 327–44.

Robinson, P.G. and Croucher, R. (1993) 'Access to dental care: experiences of men with HIV infection in the United Kingdom', *Community Dentistry and Oral Epidemiology* **21**(5), 306–8.

Rose, L., Pugh, L.C., Lears, K. and Gordon, D.L. (1998) 'The fatigue experience: persons with HIV infection', *Journal of Advanced Nursing* **28**(2), 295–304.

Rosenfeld, B, Breitbart, W, McDonald, M V, Passik, S. D., Thaler H. and Portenoy, R. K. (1996) 'Pain in ambulatory AIDS patients II: impact of pain on psychological functioning and quality of life', *Pain* **68**(2–3), 323–8.

Roth, J., Siegel, R. and Black, S. (1994) 'Identifying the mental health needs of children living in families with AIDS or HIV infection', *Community Mental Health Journal* **30**(6), 581–93.

Sandelowski, M., Lambe, C. and Barroso, J. (2004) 'Stigma in HIV-positive women', *Journal of Nursing Scholarship* **36**(2), 122–8.

Sarason, I. G., Sarason, B. R. and Pierce, G. R. (1994)

'Relationship-specific social support', pp. 91–112 in Burleson, B. R., Albrecht, T. L. and Sarason, I. G. (eds), *Communication of Social Support: Messages, interactions, relationships and community*, Thousand Oaks, Calif., Sage.

Schackman, B. R., Freedberg, K. A., Weinstein, M. C., Sax, P. E., Losina, E., Zhang, H. and Goldie, S. J. (2002) 'Cost-effectiveness implications of the timing of antiretroviral therapy in HIV-infected adults', *Archives of Internal Medicine* **162**(21), 2478–86.

Schulman, D. I. (1992) 'Stigma, risk, and the Florida AIDS dental cases: point of view', *AIDS Patient Care* **6** (1), 3–4.

Shattuck, D. (2001) 'Complexities beyond simple survival: challenges in providing care for HIV patients', *Journal of the American Dietetic Association* **101**(1), 13–15.

Sherbourne, C. D., Hays, R. D., Fleishman, J. A., Vitiello, B., Magruder, K. M., Bing, E. G., McCaffrey, D., Burnam, A., Longshore, D., Eggan, F., Bozzette, S. A. and Shapiro, M. F. (2000) 'Impact of psychiatric conditions on health-related quality of life in persons with HIV infection', *American Journal of Psychiatry* **157**(2), 248–54.

Shorposner, G., Lecusay, R., Miguezburbano, M. J., Quesada, J., Rodriguez, A., Ruiz, P., O'Mellan, S., Campa, A., Rincon, H., Wilkie, F., Page, J.B. and Baum, M.K. (2000) 'Quality of life measures in the Miami HIV-1 infected drug abusers cohort: relationship to gender and disease status', *Journal of Substance Abuse* **11**(4), 395–404.

Siegel, K., Karus, D. and Dean, L. (2004b) 'Psychosocial characteristics of New York City HIV-infected women before and after the advent of HAART', *American Journal of Public Health* **94**(7), 1127–32.

Siegel, K., Karus, D. and Schrimshaw, E.W. (2000) 'Racial differences in attitudes toward protease inhibitors among older HIV-infected men', *AIDS Care* **12**(4), 423–34.

Siegel, K., Brown Bradley, C.J. and Lekas, H. (2004a) 'Strategies for coping with fatigue among HIV-positive individuals fifty years and older', *AIDS Patient Care and STDs* **18**(5), 275–88.

Siegel, K., Schrimshaw, E.W. and Raveis, V.H. (2000) 'Accounts for non-adherence to antiviral combination therapies among older HIV-infected adults', *Psychology, Health and Medicine* **5**(1), 29–42.

Simoni, J. M., Mason, H. R., Marks, G., Ruiz, M. S., Reed, D. and Richardson, J. L. (1995) 'Women's self-disclosure of HIV infection: rates, reasons, and reactions', *Journal of Consulting and Clinical Psychology* **63**(3), 474–8.

Slater, C. and Bright, J. (1995) 'HIV: the story of a family', *Nursing Standard* **9**(41), 50–2.

Smith, C.L. and Stein, G.E. (2002) 'Viral load as a surrogate end point in HIV disease', *Annals of Pharmacotherapy* **36**(2), 280–7.

Snijders, F., De Boer, J. B., Steenbergen, B., Schouten, M., DAnner, S. A. and Van Dam, F. S. (1998) 'Impact of diarrhoea and faecal incontinence on the daily life of HIV-infected patients', *AIDS Care* **10**(5), 629–37.

Stanic, A. and Schneider, T.K. (2005) 'Overview of antiretroviral agents in 2005', *Journal of Pharmacy Practice* **18**(4), 228–46.

Steinhart, C. R. and Emons, M. F. (2004) 'Risks of cardiovascular disease in patients receiving antiretroviral therapy for HIV infection: implications for treatment', *AIDS Reader* **14**(2), 86–90.

Stephenson, J., Woods, S., Scott, B. and Meadway, J. (2000) 'HIV-related brain impairment from palliative care to rehabilitation', *International Journal of Palliative Nursing* **6**(1), 6–11.

Stoff, D. M., Khalsa, J. H., Monjan, A. and Portegies, P. (2004) 'Introduction: HIV/AIDS and aging', *AIDS* **18**(supp. 1), S1–S2.

Sulkowski, M. S., Moore, R. D., Mehta, S. H., Chaisson, R. E. and Thomas, D. L. (2002) 'Hepatitis C and progression of HIV disease', *Journal of the American Medical Association* **288**(2), 199–206.

Suzman-Schwartz, K. (2002) 'Predictors of adjustment to HIV/AIDS:

the role of personal meaning construction and spirituality in a stress and coping model', *Dissertation Abstracts International: Section B: The Sciences and Engineering* 628-B, pp. 3816.

Syme, S. L. and Berkman, L. F. (2005) 'Social relationships and health', pp. 24–30 in Conrad, P. (ed.), *The Sociology of Health and Illness: Critical perspectives*, 7th edn, New York, Worth.

Tate, D., Paul, R. H., Flanigan, T. P., Tashima, K., Nash, J., Adair, C., Boland, R. and Cohen, R. A. (2003) 'The impact of apathy and depression on quality of life in patients infected with HIV', *AIDS Patient Care and STDs* 17(3), 115–20.

Testa, M. A. and Lenderking, W. R. (1999) 'The impact of AIDS-associated wasting on quality of life: qualitative issues of measurement and evaluation', *Journal of Nutrition* 129(1S Suppl), 282S–289S.

Tewksbury, R. and McGaughey, D. (1997) 'Stigmatization of persons with HIV disease: perceptions, management, and consequences of AIDS', *Sociological Spectrum* 17(1), 49–70.

Thompson, B. (2003) 'Lazarus phenomena: an exploratory study of gay men living with HIV', *Social Work in Health Care* 37(1), 87–114.

Tillmann, H. L., Manns, M. P., Claes, C., Heiken, H., Schmidt, R. E. and Stoll, M. (2004) 'GB virus C infection and quality of life in HIV-positive patients', *AIDS Care* 16(6), 736–43.

Tozzi, V., Balestra, P., Galgani, S., Murri, R., Bellagamba, R., Narciso, P., Antinori, A., Giulianelli, M., Tosi, G., Costa, M., Sampaolesi, A., Fantoni, M., Noto, P., Ippolito, G. and Wu, A. W. (2003) 'Neurocognitive performance and quality of life in patients with HIV infection', *AIDS Research and Human Retroviruses* 19(8), 643–52.

Tramarin, A., Parise, N., Campostrini, S., Yin, D. D., Postma, M. J., Lyu, R., Grisetti, R., Capetti, A., Cattelan, A. M., Di Toro, M. T., Mastroianni, A., Pignattari, E., Mondardini, V., Calleri, G., Raise, E., Starace, F. and Palladio Study Group (2004) 'Association between diarrhea and quality of life in HIV-infected patients receiving highly active antiretroviral therapy', *Quality of Life Research* 13(1), 243–50.

Tuck, I., McCain, N. L. and Elswick, R. K., Jr (2001) 'Spirituality and psychosocial factors in persons living with HIV', *Journal of Advanced Nursing* 33(6), 776–83.

Valente, S. M. (2003) 'Depression and HIV disease', *Journal of the Association of Nurses in AIDS Care* 14(2), 41–51.

VIdrine, D. J., Amick, B. C. I. I. I., Gritz, E. R. and Arduino, R. C. (2003) 'Functional status and overall quality of life in a multiethnic HIV-positive population', *AIDS Patient Care and STDs* 17(4), 187–97.

Vogl, D., Rosenfeld, B., Breitbart, W., Thaler, H., Passik, S., McDonald, M. and Portenoy, R. K. (1999) 'Symptom prevalence, characteristics, and distress in AIDS outpatients', *Journal of Pain and Symptom Management* 18(4), 253–62.

Volberding, P. (2002) 'The impact of anemia on quality of life in human immunodeficiency virus-infected patients', *Journal of Infectious Diseases* 185(supp. 2), S110–S114.

Vosvick, M., Gore-Felton, C., Ashton, E., Koopman, C., Fluery, T., Israelski, D. and Spiegel, D. (2004) 'Sleep disturbances among HIV-positive adults: the role of pain, stress, and social support', *Journal of Psychosomatic Research* 57(5), 459–63.

Vosvick, M., Gore-felton, C., Koopman, C., Thoresen, C., Krumboltz, J. and Spiegel, D. (2002) 'Maladaptive coping strategies in relation to quality of life among HIV+ adults', *AIDS and Behavior* 6(1), 97–106.

Wachtel, T., Piette, J., Mor, V., Stein, M., Fleishman, J. and Carpenter, C. (1992) 'Quality of life in persons with human immunodeficiency virus infection: measurement by the Medical Outcomes Study instrument', *Annals of Internal Medicine* 116(2), 129–37.

Wagner, G. J., Ferrando, S. J. and Rabkin, J. G. (2000) 'Psychological and physical health correlates of body cell mass depletion among HIV+ men', *Journal of Psychosomatic Research* 49(1), 55–7.

Wayment, H. A., Silver, R. C. and Kemeny, M. E. (1995) 'Spared at random: survivor reactions in the gay community', *Journal of Applied Social Psychology* 25(3), 187–209.

Weaver, K. E., Antoni, M. H., Lechner, S. C., Duran, R. E. F., Penedo, F., Fernandez, M. I., Ironson, G. and Schneiderman, N. (2004) 'Perceived stress mediates the effects of coping on the quality of life of HIV-positive women on highly active antiretroviral therapy', *AIDS and Behavior* 8(2), 175–83.

Weiser, S. D., Wolfe, W. R. and Bangsberg, D. R. (2004) 'The HIV epidemic among individuals with mental illness in the United States', *Current HIV/AIDS Reports* 1(4), 186–92.

Wiener, L. S., Battles, H. B., Heilman, N., Sigelman, C. K. and Pizzo, P. A. (1996) 'Factors associated with disclosure of diagnosis to children with HIV/AIDS', *Pediatric AIDS and HIV Infection* 7(5), 310–24.

Wilcox, B. L. and Vernberg, E. M. (1985) 'Conceptual and theoretical dilemmas facing social support research', pp. 3–20 in Sarason, I. G. and Sarason, B. R. (eds), *Social Support: Theory, research and applications*, Dordrecht, Martinus Nijhoff.

Wilson, I. B., Ding, L., Hays, R. D., Shapiro, M. F., Bozzette, S. A. and Cleary, P. D. (2002) 'HIV patients' experiences with inpatient and outpatient care: results of a national survey', *Medical Care* 40(12), 1149–60.

Wootton, J. C. and Sparber, A. (2001) 'Surveys of complementary and alternative medicine: part III, use of alternative and complementary therapies for HIV/AIDS', *Journal of Alternative and Complementary Medicine* 7(4), 371–7.

Zapka, J. G., Stoddard, A. M. and McCusker, J. (1993) 'Social network, support and influence: relationships with drug use and protective AIDS behavior', *AIDS Education and Prevention* 5(4), 352–66.

Websites

For UK statistics: http://www.hpa.org.uk
For US statistics: http://www.cdc.gov/

Chapter

34

Primary care

Sian Maslin-Prothero,
Sue Ashby and Sarah Taylor

Links to other chapters in *Foundation Studies for Caring*

2 Interprofessional learning
3 Evidence-based practice and research
4 Ethical, legal and professional issues
6 Culture
7 Public health and health promotion
9 Moving and handling

10 Nutritional assessment and needs
14 Pharmacology and medicines
17 Safeguarding adults
25 Care of the older adult – community
35 Complementary and alternative medicine

Links to other chapters in *Foundation Skills for Caring*

1 Fundamental concepts for skills
3 Communication
9 Patient hygiene
10 Pressure area care
16 Vital signs
28 Routes of medication administration

31 Wound assessment
32 Aseptic technique and wound management
41 Specimen collection

W Don't forget to visit www.palgrave.com/glasper for additional online resources relating to this chapter.

Introduction

The government paper *Making a Difference* (DH, 1999) launched the challenge to redesign services around the needs of the patient. Since then there have been a number of key phrases, such as right person, right time, right place and person-centred care, which have challenged the more traditional ways in which health and social care has been delivered. As a result the roles of health and social care practitioners have developed in primary care to support the shift from hospital care to care being delivered in the home environment or closer to home. This makes use of existing resources such as community hospitals (DH, 2006). Care that had taken place in hospital settings is now being supported at home by the development of enhanced packages of care delivered by teams of health and social care professionals (DH, 2002, 2005a).

There has been an increasing emphasis on the proactive management of chronic disease, with reports from the National Health Service (NHS) advising that people with chronic conditions are significantly more likely to see their general practitioner (GP), accounting for up to 80 per cent of GP consultations (DH, 2004a, 2004b, 2004c). In addition 60 per cent of hospital bed days are for patients with chronic disease-related complications, and two-thirds of patients admitted as medical emergencies have a chronic disease or an exacerbation of one. Some people are highly intensive users of services, with 10 per cent of in-patients accounting for 55 per cent of in-patient days and 5 per cent of in-patients accounting for 40 per cent of in-patient days (NHS Modernisation Agency, 2004: 13).

This chapter explores primary care and how healthcare need is assessed and provided, adopting a whole systems approach. This is accomplished by the use of two scenarios illustrating the issues which can present when meeting the health needs of an individual in the community. The management of diabetes has been highlighted because it is recognised as a major and growing health problem that is increasingly managed in primary care (DH, 2008: Renders et al, 2001). The scenarios also demonstrate the interface between primary and secondary care in relation to the management of both type 1 and type 2 diabetes.

Learning outcomes

This chapter will enable you to:

- understand the primary care service in the United Kingdom using a whole systems approach
- using diabetes as a focus, examine how primary care and other agencies work collaboratively to plan and provide services for clients
- discuss key terms and concepts including whole systems, multidisciplinary, interdisciplinary and multi-agency working
- appreciate how care is planned and delivered for clients and their families in the community setting
- examine primary, secondary and tertiary care in the community using a whole systems approach.

Concepts

- Whole systems approach
- Primary care
- Diabetes
- Multidisciplinary
- Multi-agency
- Partnership
- Person-centred
- Interdisciplinary
- Quality and Outcomes Framework (QOF)

Living in a community

Communities present healthcare practitioners with an array of differing circumstances in which an individual might require professional advice or support. There are many aspects that influence an individual's health (see Chapter 25, Care of the older adult – community). Working within the community requires a level of understanding regarding the locality issues as well as the individual's presenting health need(s) (Robinson and Elkan, 1996). In the United Kingdom primary care trusts (PCTs) have responsibilities to ensure that they understand the needs of their community, and to work with surrounding authorities and other agencies that provide health and social care to make sure that their community's needs are effectively being met.

The PCTs develop local strategic partnerships supporting determinants of health, for example:

- promoting safer communities with less crime and fear of crime
- working with the local education authorities, ensuring equal access to good education, engaging the local community in planning and decision making
- working to make services, information and advice more accessible
- working with the local housing authority with the aim of providing affordable homes suited to need, and a high-quality environment available to everyone.

This partnership approach strives for equal opportunity and accessible resources with the aim of improving health, well-being and quality of life.

Local action plans need to be sensitive to locality need as well as guided by national targets directed by the Department of Health (DH). The strategic health authority (SHA) in which the PCT is situated will also fix targets determined by the national targets relevant to the area's specific circumstances. This guidance will be informed by existing knowledge about local health issues and the views of other NHS and social care organisations in these strategic partnerships.

a Learning activity

In your interprofessional learning group read through your local authority's latest census information and determine a demographic profile of the population of your local area. Identify issues that could impact upon an individual's health.

Compare this information with your local PCT's health delivery plan.

Establish which areas have been targeted for development.

How will this information impact on how health and social care professionals plan care in the community?

When we consider the local strategic partnerships in the community setting, it becomes apparent how many different professionals and organisations a healthcare practitioner might work with.

Definitions

You will encounter a number of terms in your practice as well as in this chapter, and you need to understand what is meant by them.

Primary care is the collective term for all services that are people's first point of contact with the NHS, for example the services provided by district nurses (DN) and midwives, GPs and dentists.

Secondary care is the collective term for those services to which a patient is referred by a consultant. Usually this refers to NHS hospitals offering specialised medical and surgical services, and care.

Intermediate care are those integrated services for people that promote faster recovery from illness, prevent unnecessary hospital admissions and maximise independent living.

A *whole systems approach* is concerned with all agencies working together in their localities, in partnership. This approach recognises that a wide range of factors such as demographic, social and economic factors, and available services, interact with agencies, for example clients and their families, professional health and social services. That is, nothing works independently of anything else. Therefore a problem or issue is not the responsibility of one factor, individual or team, but is about working together with the relevant agencies to find solutions. A whole systems approach acknowledges that systems can be complex and dynamic.

Partnership working is based on the appreciation that no one organisation, even one as large as the NHS, can meet all the needs of all the people who use it, all of the time. We need to move to an NHS that provides plurality of provision based on sound and genuine partnership working with the voluntary and community sector and others outside the NHS itself, providing real choices and services that are equitable and responsive to the diverse needs and preferences of the population. Each partner has to be open to ideas for developing how services are delivered, acknowledge potential barriers to involvement, and find joint solutions to the challenges. In addition, this requires people to work within financial constraints, and offer value for money as well as a high quality of care. An example of partnership working and collaboration is the Strategic Agreement between the Department of Health, the NHS and the voluntary and community sector (VCS), in which the NHS and VCS organisations work together to build effective partnerships and contribute together to provide a truly patient-centred health service (DH, 2004c). By agreeing a shared vision of improved services and by working strategically in partnership at every level, we can develop and expand the scope, versatility and capacity of all health services for the benefit of patients, carers and service users.

Voluntary and community sector organisations support service users and carers, act as advocates, provide a range of health and support services and are a conduit for information, particularly on health promotion. Local community groups with an interest or role in health and/or social care are an important source of expertise in their specialist areas: for example, care for older people, mental health, palliative care or learning disabilities. They also contribute to mainstream health service and social care delivery.

> ## (a) Learning activity
>
> In your interprofessional learning group explore your local community and list the professionals who work in your primary healthcare team. Then consider who are the members of the wider community team.
>
> Consider Figure 34.1. Had you realised that a community nurse had the potential to be working with so many other professionals and agencies?

Figure 34.1

Care in the community

Source: reproduced with permission from Johnson (2003).

Ambulance service
Chiropodist
Community psychiatric nurse (CPN)
Chronic disease management teams
Citizen's Advice Bureau
Community hospitals
Community midwife
Community matrons
Community Transport Council
Dietician
District nurse
Fire Service
GP
Home care assessor
Health visitor
Housing departments
Intermediate care team
Learning disabilities services
Meals on Wheels
Minor injuries unit

Wider community team

Primary health care team

Wider community team

Nurse practitioners
Nursing homes
NHS Direct
Occupational therapist
Orthoptist
Outpatient departments
Paediatric district nursing service
Physiotherapist
Police force
Primary care trusts
Practice nurses
Public health departments
Residential homes
Rehabilitation teams
School nurse
Social services
Social worker
Speech and language therapist
Voluntary services
Walk-in centre

Traditionally, primary healthcare teams have been represented by GPs, nurses and therapists working for the PCT, as they were predominantly the first point of professional contact for a person presenting with a health need. These roles have been developed in response to the presenting needs of the community (DH, 2000), resulting in roles such as nurse practitioners, community matrons and intermediate care coordinators. These professionals may work in a variety of settings as opposed to health centres or GP surgeries such as walk-in centres and minor injuries units. Some areas hold satellite clinics in supermarkets and community centres to promote accessibility. The wider community team (indicated in green in Figure 34.1) usually consists of members who work closely with healthcare professionals ensuring that the physical, social and environmental influences on the health of individuals, groups and communities are properly taken into account.

Partnership working

Health policy goes beyond the traditional reach of the NHS to include the wider social, environmental and economic determinants of health. The NHS has limited scope to address these wider determinants unless it works in partnership with other agencies in order to address the complex and interconnected issues affecting the health of individuals and communities. Effective partnership arrangements – with local government, the voluntary and private sectors – are considered essential for taking forward health policy and improving services. Services based on partnership and collaborative ways of working are referred to as integrated care: that is, joined-up working between agencies, leading to the effective integration of services for the benefit of service users and their carers. It could be argued that this is more pronounced in Scotland and Wales than in England (Woods, 2001; Wanless and HM Treasury, 2002; Integrated Care Network, 2003; NHS Scotland, 2003; Scottish Executive, 2003; Henk, 2006). Partnership is one of the NHS's ten core principles (DH, 2000), and is a central feature of health and social care policy. The 2004 *Choosing Health* white paper (DH, 2004c) identified working together to address all the factors that interact to determine health, as one of three core principles of a new approach to public health.

As mentioned earlier, PCT staff are required to form partnerships/alliances with local authorities, social services, housing, education, welfare, and other statutory and voluntary agencies in order to provide appropriate and relevant care. Service users and the general public are encouraged to take an active role in describing and identifying the health and care needs of their community.

Multi-agency working

The Health Act 1999 stated that NHS bodies had a statutory duty to cooperate with each other and with local authorities. The Act enabled the pooling of budgets and resources to facilitate joint working between health and social agencies, and it increased the arrangements for ensuring quality in service delivery.

The Health and Social Care Act 2001 gave the government powers to direct local authorities and healthcare organisations to pool their budgets, especially where services are failing, and reinforced the earlier commitment to interdisciplinary working and quality improvement. High-quality continuing care services depend fundamentally on the availability of an appropriately trained workforce able to perform its role effectively and efficiently. *The NHS Plan* (DH, 2000) acknowledged that changes were needed to deliver person-centred services, and that traditional patterns of professional practice were effectively holding back innovation. It expressed the intention for the new plans to 'shatter old demarcations which have held back staff and slowed down care' (DH, 2000: 9.5). The vision of a reconfigured workforce and the need to improve efficiency and cost effectiveness have provoked a re-evaluation of the manner in which services are delivered, and have led to an examination of skill mix and the development of new roles to fill some of the gaps in provision.

The two scenarios in this chapter illustrate how clients may present within the community, how needs are assessed and how support is offered from a person-centred approach using resources and expertise across the spectrum of health and social care provision, and spanning the interface of primary and secondary care. The relevant management of diabetes is explored as a recognised long-term condition (Renders et al, 2001), and applied to the individual's presenting circumstances.

S Scenario: Introducing Bill

Bill is recently widowed and lives at home with his dog Bess. Their home was once a working farm. Bill has a difficult relationship with his only son, Mark, who chose not to be a farmer, breaking with the family tradition. Bill has difficulty seeing clearly and his vision has become blurred; as a result he cannot read his daily paper. By his own admission he is also struggling to draw up and administer his insulin. He has a sore area on his heel, which his wife used to take care of. On a bereavement visit his GP asked Bill about the blood on his slipper; he also noticed an unpleasant smell. Bill responded, 'It's nothing, doctor. I manage, and it's not giving me any pain.' Throughout the doctor's visit Bess barked persistently. On returning to the surgery the GP asked one of the DNs, Arjuna, to visit Bill to assess him more fully.

a Learning activity

Bill has type 2 insulin-treated diabetes. What support mechanisms (involving the primary healthcare team or voluntary agencies) could be in place to help him manage his diabetes more effectively?

Prevalence of diabetes mellitus

In the United Kingdom 2.3 million people (3.5 per cent of the population) have been diagnosed with diabetes, and it is estimated that a further 500,000 remain undiagnosed (Diabetes UK, 2008). The World Health Organization (WHO) estimates that 180 million people worldwide have diabetes, and suggests that this is likely to double by 2030 (WHO, 2006). This global increase in diabetes will occur because of population ageing, growth, and increasing trends towards obesity, unhealthy diets and sedentary lifestyles (Wanless et al, 2007). Type 2 diabetes accounts for 85–95 per cent of all people with diabetes, and up to 50 per cent of people will already have complications at diagnosis.

- People with diabetes have a fivefold increased risk of cardiovascular disease (CVD) compared with those without diabetes.
- Diabetes is the leading cause of blindness in people of working age in the United Kingdom.
- Kidney disease develops very slowly and is most common in people who have had the condition for 20 years. One in three people with diabetes might go on to develop kidney disease (Diabetes UK, 2006a).
- About 5 per cent of the total NHS spend and up to 10 per cent of the hospital in-patient spend is used for the care of people with diabetes (DH, 2007a).

S Scenario: Introducing Lui

Lui is 18 years old. She has recently started university and is living in a hall of residence. In the last week she has become increasingly tired and lethargic, and has lost about 3 kg in weight. Initially, she attributed this to the stress of moving away from home and settling into university life. However, as she has felt increasingly unwell, and after speaking with her mother the previous evening she attends an appointment with the practice nurse at the university health practice.

The practice nurse takes a history from Lui and identifies that she has been very thirsty and has been passing urine much more frequently than normal.

Fortunately, the practice nurse has recently attended an update on diabetes mellitus and suspects that this might be the cause of Lui's symptoms. She tests Lui's urine and performs a finger-prick blood glucose measurement. (For further information on blood glucose and monitoring please refer to Chapter 19 in the accompanying Skills book.) The urinalysis shows large levels of both glucose and ketones, and the blood test reveals a blood glucose level of 17 mmol per litre. (See below for more detail on diagnostic criteria for diabetes.)

(a) Learning activity

Visit www.diabetes.org.uk/Guide-to-diabetes and look at the two main types of diabetes, and identify the major differences between the two types.

Once you have examined the different types of diabetes, can you say what type of diabetes Lui appears to have?

Diabetes recognition and management

This section will help you to define diabetes mellitus, identify methods and criteria for diagnosis, outline treatment plans and how the primary healthcare team work in partnership with secondary care to support prevention and management of this condition. This is centred on engagement with the individual and promoting self-management as far as possible (Nagelkerk, Reick and Meengs, 2006; Sturt, Whitlock and Hearnshaw, 2006). A potentially life-threatening complication of type 1 diabetes is ketoacidosis; this is identified and discussed in Lui's scenario, and guidelines are given for detection and management.

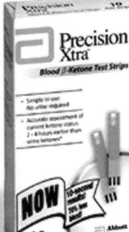

Diabetes mellitus is a chronic disease that presents when the amount of glucose (sugar) in the blood is too high, because the body is unable to utilise it properly. This is normally controlled by the hormone insulin, and diabetes occurs when insulin is not being produced by the pancreas, or there is insufficient insulin or insulin action for the body's needs (Williams and Pickup, 2004).

This common, chronic disease is increasingly managed in primary care (DH, 2008: Renders et al, 2000). The increasing prevalence of diabetes has been highlighted and the importance of controlling this progression has been acknowledged. In particular the *National Service Framework (NSF) for Diabetes* (DH, 2001a) began to address this, and the targets set in the *Quality and Outcomes Framework (QOF)* (DH, 2004d) helped to confirm this (Farooq, 2007). Ninety-three points have been allocated to diabetes management,. and 31 of these points are related to glycosylated haemoglobin (HbA1c) (DH, 2004d). HbA1c is the most important monitoring tool for glucose control, and measures the amount of glucose carried by the red blood cells over a period of two to three months. Glucose sticks to the haemoglobin and forms a 'glycosolated haemoglobin' molecule. A normal nondiabetic HbA1c is usually 3.5 to 5.5 per cent. There is clear evidence that achieving and maintaining good glycaemic control reduces the risk of complications (UKPDS,1998; DCCT, 1993), and the result of this should be a reduction in the burden of the disease to both individuals and the health service.

Figure 34.2 A blood ketone strip

Lifestyle, in particular diet and exercise, is an important factor in the management of this disease, and this can mean considerable life changes for some people. Also significant are the use of medication, and engaging people to manage their own diabetes and promote concordance. It should also be recognised that changes in routine and/or illness can alter outcomes. There can be differences in individuals' circumstances between being monitored within a hospital setting and being at home: for example, meal times may vary and there may be differing levels of activity. All of this requires consideration and acknowledgement when transferring care from different environments and with any subsequent care planning.

Part

IV

Methods and criteria for diagnosing diabetes mellitus

The WHO (1999) advises that if there are diabetes symptoms (that is, polyuria, polydipsia and unexplained weight loss), the investigation should be either a random venous plasma glucose concentration > 11.1 mmol/l or a fasting plasma glucose concentration >7.0 mmol/l; or a two-hour plasma glucose concentration > 11.1 mmol/l two hours after 75g anhydrous glucose load in an oral glucose tolerance test (OGTT).

With no symptoms, diagnosis should not be based on a single glucose determination but requires confirmatory plasma venous determination. At least one additional glucose test result on another day with a value in the diabetic range is essential, either fasting, from a random sample, or from the two-hour post glucose load. If the fasting or random values are not diagnostic the two-hour value should be used.

The main differences between type 1 and type 2 diabetes are:

- **Type 1** mainly occurs in childhood or early adult life, and accounts for 5–15 per cent of all people with diabetes. It is caused by autoimmune destruction of the beta (β) cells of the islets of Langerhans in the pancreas, and results in absolute insulin deficiency. The symptoms of type 1 diabetes usually develop quickly, over a period of a few days or weeks. People with type 1 diabetes require insulin to sustain life.
- **Type 2** is usually a disease of the middle-aged or elderly. However, it is now becoming a problem in children (Wanless et al, 2007). It is caused by both impaired insulin production and insulin resistance (the insulin produced does not work properly). In most cases, type 2 diabetes is linked to being overweight. People with type 2 diabetes can be treated with diet, oral medication and/or insulin.

The main aim of treatment is to achieve not only blood glucose levels as near to normal as possible, but also as near to normal as possible blood pressure and cholesterol levels. It is these, along with a healthy lifestyle, that will help to improve well-being and will protect against long-term damage to the eyes, kidneys, heart and the major arteries caused by atherosclerosis.

The healthcare team

In order to achieve the best possible diabetes care, people with diabetes need to work in partnership with multidisciplinary teams, in primary and secondary care, in order to provide the most effective and appropriate care for the individual (DH, 2007b). This may include a GP, practice nurse, DN, diabetic specialist nurse (DSN) (in the hospital and/or community), consultant physician, dietician, chiropodist, pharmacist, optometrist/opthalmologist, psychologist and other specialists.

Other agencies that can or may be involved include interpreters, and local and national support groups or charities, in particular Diabetes UK. Diabetes care can take place at a number of different levels, and the choice will depend on what care is available in a particular area and to some degree patient choice. The options are a GP clinic, hospital clinic, community clinic, primary care centre or home.

One important and quite recent feature of diabetes care has been life-long learning and structured education. Having diabetes involves a life-long learning process, and NHS guidelines (NICE, 2003) recommend that people with diabetes receive structured education and support to enable them to manage their diabetes (Diabetes UK, 2006c).

Another important aspect of diabetes care is an annual review (Diabetes UK, 2006b). This usually takes place at the GP surgery (refer to the QOF targets for detailed information). This will involve:

- Laboratory tests and investigations:
  - HbA1c
  - cholesterol
  - kidney function (checking for protein).

- Physical examination:
  - body mass index (BMI)
  - waist measurement (see Table 34.1)
  - examination of legs and feet (circulation and nerve supply for evidence of neuropathy)
  - blood pressure
  - examination of eyes (fundoscopy for evidence of retinopathy).
- Lifestyle:
  - treatment
  - control
  - coping mechanisms, managing challenges
  - other potential side-effects/issues: smoking, alcohol, stress, sexual problems, physical activity, healthy eating,

Table 34.1 shows how your waist measurement can affect your chance of getting health problems. The numbers given are for a measurement taken just above the top of the hips, roughly at the level of the umbilicus (BMJ, 2007).

Table 34.1 Waist measurement and the risk of health problems

Waist measurement	Slightly higher chance of health problems	Much higher chance of health problems
Men	94 cm (37 in)	102 cm (40 in)
Women	80 cm (31 in)	88 cm (35 in)

S Scenario continued: Bill

Communication between primary and secondary care

Arjuna, the DN, visits Bill but finds no one at home. She can see several newspapers pushed through the letterbox in the porch. The nurse looks through the front window and checks the back of the house. There is a dog barking in the garden which prevents further investigation. As Arjuna leaves the lane, a neighbour waves and stops her. She says that Bill's son rang for an ambulance that morning as he was concerned about his father.

On returning to the practice Arjuna checks with the hospital and is advised that Bill is in the medical assessment unit (MAU), presenting with elevated blood glucose levels and an infected foot ulcer. She explains that she had intended to see Bill at home and plan his care with him. The unit staff explain that he is very concerned about his dog and is not cooperating with the medical team. He is also very upset that his son called an ambulance.

Bill is understandably concerned about his dog, Bess, but does not appear to understand the implications and risks associated with his foot being infected and his diabetic condition. By first listening to Bill and acknowledging what is important to him, the health and social care professionals can support and empower him to make informed choices about his care. Bill in turn needs an understanding of the roles and responsibilities of the multidisciplinary team, and the expertise of agencies working alongside them. This should mean that Bill's needs are acknowledged, and he and the professionals are able to jointly plan his care (see NICE, 2004a).

a Learning activity

Recall the circumstances leading to Bill's arrival at the medical assessment unit. Bill is not presenting with an acute medical emergency, he has raised blood glucose and an infected foot ulcer. The primary care professionals are able to manage these conditions working as part of an integrated, multidisciplinary team.

Review the latest clinical guidelines for diabetic foot ulcer management and management of Type 2 diabetes (NICE, 2004a) and indicate the key issues regarding Bill's lifestyle and recent circumstances.

In the scenario, it seems that in Bill's current circumstances, Arjuna is the most appropriate professional to coordinate the multidisciplinary team in the primary care setting because she is the person in most frequent contact with Bill. Visits will be required to evaluate the healing of Bill's foot ulcer, redressing, and to observe Bill administering his insulin. Professionals trained in the management of diabetic foot conditions may also be involved in Bill's plan of care, and work interprofessionally to classify Bill's foot risk and manage care (NICE, 2004a). Other methods for administering insulin may be considered to maintain Bill's independence, such as pen devices. The DSN will be able to offer guidance and support to the primary care team on these issues.

(c) Professional conversation

Arjuna comments, 'On my return to the health centre, I telephoned the MAU explaining that I had attempted to visit Bill that morning, but it appeared that Mark, Bill's son, had called for an ambulance before my arrival. In preparation for my visit I had liaised with the practice nurse. I gave the hospital staff details of Bill's latest monitoring and annual diabetic review, which were within acceptable limits. I informed the staff of Bill's bereavement, and how it was early days and that he was still adjusting to the loss of his wife, living alone and managing his condition. I was able to tell the staff that Bill usually had a good understanding of his condition, but had relied on his wife to administer his insulin. He regularly attended appointments with the practice nurse, who monitored his foot ulcer (together with the chiropodist), giving instructions to his wife to re-dress it as required between appointments.

'Following this telephone conversation I forwarded to the MAU an electronic copy of the single assessment process (SAP) document, which included the specialist foot ulcer mapping, grading assessments and vascular reports. The impression Bill was giving to hospital staff was of noncompliance, which was quickly rectified. As I learned of Bill's concerns regarding his dog, I was able to relay information given by a neighbour that they had taken Bess for a walk and planned to look after her until Bill came home; the neighbour was aware that Bill would not settle until he knew Bess was being cared for.

'I checked my caseload and staffing levels for the next 48 hours, and advised the MAU that depending on Bill's time of discharge I could visit later that day or early the next morning. I gave my contact information and those of the out of hours district nursing team so that they could be recorded on Bill's MAU notes. This allowed staff to confirm Bill's discharge details with myself or colleagues, and provide Bill with a point of contact when he left hospital.'

Some district and practice nurses are experienced in managing long-term conditions such as diabetes. However the support of the specialist nurse ensures that the latest guidelines and protocols are followed and the latest devices/equipment used. The specialist nurse often has an extended role (DH, 2002), enabling the multidisciplinary team to access diagnostics, secondary care and manage medication in a timely way. Using a whole systems approach this makes best use of medics' time, allowing them to focus on situations requiring their specific expertise and skills.

Following the latest clinical guidelines Bill's foot will be risk assessed and the appropriate level of management involving the multidisciplinary team will be offered.

(a) Learning activity

The DSN can be either hospital or community based, and in some locations DSNs work across both settings.

Determine how the DSN works in your area, and how their role is interpreted across the interface of primary and secondary care. Locate the members of the 'foot protection team' (see NICE, 2004a) in your area.

Find out whether a care pathway has been developed in your locality. How would you refer clients in a timely way to the most appropriate professional (this will depend on their presenting condition and management of any associated risk)?

Planning care delivery

Depending on the presenting needs of the patient/client, the coordinator of the multidisciplinary team approach to care could be any member of the primary healthcare team. This is a dynamic role which changes to meet the requirements of the individual. For example for housebound clients the DN might take the lead role, while for ambulant clients the practice nurse might be the most appropriate person. Close monitoring is necessary to determine the necessity for home visits, even if the individual is ambulant, such as four-hourly treatments, observations/monitoring or specialist expertise (such as wound care). Using the nursing process ensures that the timely assessment, planning, implementation and evaluation of an individual's needs will use the most appropriate skills and resources (including the appropriate environment to deliver care, which could be home (including a long-stay care facility), a clinic or a community hospital). This maximises the individual's potential for rehabilitation, recovery, self-management and/or maintenance (Nagelkerk, Reick and Meengs, 2006; Sturt, Whitlock and Hearnshaw, 2006).

There are many aspects to consider when planning care in the community. The healthcare professional must consider whether the health and social care needs of the person can be met. The GP is responsible for the medical management, and needs to be in agreement with the multidisciplinary team in order that the right level of care is determined and provided. This is particularly significant when considering the development of specialist teams in the community who provide 'hospital at home' type provision where care – of a kind traditionally delivered in a hospital – is provided within the home setting (such as intravenous therapy). Medical cover must also be available to ensure robust management. Depending on the area this might be by the GP, medical officer employed within the enhanced team, or outreach by a designated hospital medic. Commissioning for differing types of service provision has been directed to local areas (DH, 1997), with PCTs, SHAs and hospital clinicians agreeing whether a service should be commissioned for the whole population across the health authority or more locally. 'Quality standards, service protocols and agreements should be clearly set by direct discussion between clinicians to ensure primary care and secondary care services are properly integrated and programmes of care are developed to reflect patient needs' (DH, 1997: 40).

Professionals working in a purpose-built facility such as a clinic or hospital have a degree of control over their environment, whereas the home environment changes with every client, and the team involved must consider both their and their clients' safety whilst delivering care in the home. This may also involve consideration of the level of care that can be delivered, such as 24-hour care, night sitting services, episodes of intense care delivery over two or three hours, or visits lasting 15–60 minutes. Joint visits are required where visiting alone could in itself be a risk, for example when there is a need for moving and handling assistance. Environmental hazards such as the presence of animals such as dogs might not be an issue for the client, but may need to be considered when delivering care.

Caring for clients and their families in the community setting

When nursing within the home, you must consider others who share the same accommodation, and the impact on family and carers, as well as their relationship with the person in receipt of care. The dynamics within this group can vary greatly. There might be a high level of family support and care; at the other extreme there is sometimes a possibility of aggression to the professional, or neglect of the person receiving care in the home. Consideration needs to be given to the effects on the family of the illness of a family member which could include admission to hospital or long-term care. For example, this person might have been the main wage earner, or the main carer for another family member.

You should also consider issues such as invasion of privacy and the space required for care purposes. The environment is not within your control, and you need to negotiate with all those involved to plan and provide care. It can be challenging to maintain confidentiality, privacy and dignity when sharing an environment with others.

S Scenario continued

Planning Bill's care

Bill was assessed by the MAU team, and directed to the vascular team as an outpatient, with management by the multidisciplinary team in the community. The MAU team had assessed Bill's social circumstances in anticipation of planning his care, using the SAP (DH, 2001b) documentation. Bill explained to the MAU nurse his concern for his dog, Bess, and emphasised that he was sure he could manage at home in spite of his son's fear for his well-being.

From this Arjuna began to build a picture of Bill's daily routine, and she identified some possible areas of vulnerability around his diet and meal preparation. On the MAU Bill has been encouraged to be self-caring, and was observed administering his insulin. On one occasion the staff noted that he had drawn an incorrect dose, and he was stopped from administering it.

On closer questioning the MAY staff learned that Bill had not visited an optician for five years and that he had not attended the chiropodist since his wife's death. Bill acknowledged that he was struggling with some of his activities of daily living, yet when given time he could show the MAY staff that he understood how to manage his diabetes. Arjuna encouraged Bill to identify what he felt he needed to meet his needs, and using this information explained what services were available to support him in his own home. Subsequently, Bill agreed to Arjuna visiting him at home to discuss and plan his care.

Bill's son Mark was concerned that his father had deteriorated since his mother's death, but now felt reassured that professionals would be monitoring his condition. He agreed to stay with his father for a couple of days, but made it clear that he could not maintain this indefinitely because of his work and other family commitments.

The unit team liaised with Arjuna, and advised her about the condition of Bill's ulcer and dressings applied. They negotiated a timed visit to coincide with Bill's discharge and insulin regime. On discharge the necessary documentation and a supply of dressings were to be sent home with Bill.

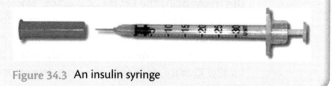

Figure 34.3 An insulin syringe

---

a Learning activity

In your interprofessional learning group briefly think about someone you have recently cared for in a hospital setting. During this episode of care, what was the impact on their care of the:

- general cleanliness of the location?
- space available?
- access to bathroom facilities?
- equipment used and maintenance of it?
- heat?
- lighting?
- skills required to provide care?
- timeliness of care delivery?
- carers/family members?

Now imagine you are responsible for discharging this person to their home environment for nursing care. Depending upon the type and intensity of care required these factors could determine whether the patient can be nursed safely within their own environment, whether other forms of support or care are needed, and whether they meet the requirements for discharge from an acute area of care.

How does this impact on appropriate use of acute care provision, patient choice, carers' rights, Health and Safety at Work regulations, and risk management?

Managing a caseload

Let's now look at the many factors that must be considered when planning care in the community setting from the perspective of a professional managing a primary care caseload. These individuals usually have responsibility for an area of care that is determined by an attachment to a GP practice: in other words they respond to the nursing need of patients registered with one or more named GPs. In some areas of the United Kingdom this arrangement has now been reviewed, and caseloads are instead divided up geographically, to minimise the time spent travelling.

a Learning activity

In your learning group, find out what the caseload is for your community nurses or another professional group in your GP practice. Do they have a designated geographical area, or an allocation by GP? What is the population size and type of area covered? Refer to local statistics based on census data.

What challenges do you think the community nurse or other key healthcare worker would face in responding in a timely manner to patient need and choice? Do certain times of the day present differing challenges? And if so, what are these? Think about the specific differences between urban and rural locations.

Community nurses might work in or manage a team (as happens in district nursing) or have sole management of a specific area, as school nurses and health visitors typically do. Increasingly, there have been moves to combine community nursing with specialities: individuals might be trained in two or more specific roles such as psychology. district nursing, health visiting or school nursing, and the recently developed public health role (NMC, 2004).

We have seen that someone of any discipline might appropriately manage a multi-disciplinary team. It is not unusual for a social work or allied health professional to manage a predominantly nursing team, and vice versa, for example in intermediate care teams and enablement teams. The team manager will respond to the needs of the presenting client and monitor their condition, and delegate aspects of their health or social care appropriately to other team members. This includes considering the management of care, appropriate skills in the team, types of care, time of visit, location and environmental circumstances.

Unlike a bed-based service there is no fixed caseload size. The number of clients varies, depending on many factors such as the type, frequency, time and location of visits. A professional in this role needs to continually assess the workload and resources available. If they are conscious of insufficient resources to manage the load safely, they will be required to present risk assessments, and look to negotiate further resources or redirection of care. It is important to be proactive in managing people's care. This ensures timely transfer to areas of least dependency, or self-care appropriate to the individual, and that skills are directed to the most appropriate professional or area of care (Sturt et al, 2006).

The professional will draw up a daily plan of care for all their patients/clients, taking all these issues into account, but there will also be unplanned visits to new referrals, or known clients who require an emergency response (for instance, if they have a blocked supra-pubic or urethral catheter). At times, too, some clients will have intensive needs, for example in terminal care. To manage these different situations calls for clinical expertise, an in-depth knowledge of the caseload and the ability to reorganise and delegate to ensure all needs are met in a safe and timely manner.

In addition to management within the team, the caseload holder will work in an interdisciplinary way across organisations and agencies whenever a client requires multidisciplinary expertise. The coordination of this in the community can become complex, and communication is key to ensure everyone concerned is aware of the situation, and safety is maintained for both clients and staff.

It has been acknowledged that changes in the management of long-term conditions and earlier discharges from the acute sector have resulted in increasing pressure on the community services workload (DH, 2005b; Baldwin, 2006; Queen's Nursing Institute, 2006). Health policy has directed investment in resources and development of nursing roles and multidisciplinary working to make best use of the skills and expertise in the workforce (DH, 2002); PCTs have responded to meet the needs of their population.

a Learning activity

In your interprofessional learning group, consider what the implications might be if documentation and records are not maintained or are inaccurate. Review the current documentation used by your community teams. How do they communicate within the multidisciplinary team?

Part
IV

Case management is 'the process of planning, coordinating, managing and reviewing the care of an individual' (Kings Fund, 2004). The roles of caseload holders are currently undergoing change, and case management is increasingly being undertaken by community matrons. This role varies in approach, and is influenced by models such as Kaisser (Feachem, Sekhr; and White, 2002) and Evercare (National Primary and Research Development Centre, 2005). These case management models help to inform the future development of services, but no model as yet has an evidence base demonstrating that it is superior to the others (Gill, 2004).

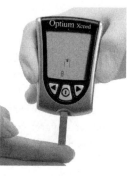

Figure 34.4   Example of a blood glucose meter

S Scenario continued

Bill's care in the primary care setting

Bill has an uneventful journey home from the hospital with his son Mark. Arjuna arrives at the house as planned, and introduces herself to Bill and Mark. Because detailed information about Bill's home circumstances and needs has been communicated between secondary and primary care she quickly gains Bill's and his son's confidence. She watches Bill monitor and record his blood glucose, and administer his insulin. She offers advice and provides relevant contact numbers. It has been a long and tiring day for Bill and Mark, so Arjuna agrees to visit again the next day so they can have a longer discussion and plan together what Bill needs to manage his own healthcare. She will visit at 09.00 to check Bill's blood glucose reading and observe his insulin administration, and again at 11.00 to assess his foot and agree on ongoing management. She asks that Bess be kept in another room for future visits, explaining that there could be a risk of introducing infection.

---

a Learning activity

How might Arjuna negotiate the time of her visits with Bill with reference to:

- the patient's circumstances?
- building relationship and trust?
- decision making?
- management of caseload?

S Scenario continued

Bill's plan of care

Arjuna visits as planned the following morning and observes Bill's routine. She returns later that day and assesses Bill using a single assessment with Mark. They discuss Bill's daily activities and Arjuna gives him some dietary advice. She suggests he could use some help with meal preparation, but Bill says no, he doesn't need that. When his wife was alive he was the one who prepared meals, it's just that it's not the same cooking only for one. Arjuna asks too about shopping, and Bill explains that he has an arrangement with a neighbour who visits weekly and does his shopping for him. Bill appears to appreciate and understand the importance of eating regular, nutritious meals, and what foods to avoid, and this shows an understanding too of the management of his diabetes.

Bill is still grieving for his wife and adjusting to living alone. His foot ulcer is superficial but requires close monitoring as it could deteriorate. He is able to take an accurate blood glucose checks, and explain the significance of both high and low blood glucose readings. His blood glucose readings are still elevated and the

HbA1c taken at the hospital was still high at 9 per cent. Because Bill has not been taking his insulin correctly for some time, and the impact of the infection, this would have caused his blood glucose levels to raise steadily, leading to an elevated Hba1c. On the basis of information from MAU staff and her own observation, Arjuna notices that Bill has a tendency to draw up less insulin than is prescribed. She asks about this, and Bill explains that he can't see the markings on the syringe clearly. He has blurred vision at times, so Arjuna helps him to urgently arrange an eye test.

Arjuna decides that until Bill's vision is sorted out, she will need to continue with twice-daily visits for support with his insulin administration, monitoring of dietary intake and blood glucose levels, and on alternate days dressings of his foot ulcer. The team will also look at alternative methods of insulin delivery, such as a pen device. She also requests an urgent chiropody appointment as Bill shows signs of peripheral vascular disease. Bill already has an outpatient vascular team appointment.

W

a Learning activity

Adopting the DN assessment, formulate a care plan for Bill, applying the latest clinical guidelines for management of type 2 diabetes and diabetic foot management.

- How would you plan the care for Bill?
- On which other professionals' skill and expertise do you think you would need to call as part of the multidisciplinary team managing Bill's condition?
- Demonstrate this involvement within your plan of care for Bill.

You might find it useful to check out the NICE website (http://www.nice.org.uk): the home page directs you to the latest clinical guidelines by topic. Remember that individual webpages may alter as the latest guidelines are released. Also look at the NHS National Diabetic Support Team website on http://www.diabetes.nhs.uk/ Information on diabetic foot care is available on http://www.diabetes.nhs.uk/downloads/NDST_Diabetic_Foot_Guide.pdf

S Scenario, continued: Lui's case

Communication between primary and secondary care

Lui is referred urgently to the assessment unit at the local hospital. She is diagnosed with type 1 diabetes and admitted to hospital because of diabetic ketoacidosis (DKA), a potentially life-threatening complication of diabetes.

People with type 1 diabetes are typically affected with DKA (see the scenario), but it can also be precipitated in people with type 2 diabetes during severe infections and other illnesses. Many factors can precipitate DKA in type 1 diabetes, such as new diagnosis, insulin errors, omissions, infections and noncompliance.

DKA is caused by an inadequate concentration of insulin in the blood. As a result cells in the body are unable to use glucose as an energy source and have to rely on the body's fat reserves. Blood glucose levels rise, and the byproducts of fat metabolism (that is, ketone bodies) cause the blood to become acidic. Insulin deficiency together with the presence of catabolic counter-regulatory 'stress' hormones leads to hepatic overproduction of glucose and ketones, which promotes lipolysis, a release of fatty acids from adipose tissue. In the liver these are oxidised to ketone bodies and acetoacetic acid.

DKA is a medical emergency, and requires treatment with insulin and intravenous fluids. It can carry a high fatality risk if it is suboptimally managed. In order to reduce this risk there are government recommendations, and guidance for protocols is in place (DH, 2001a; NICE, 2004b).

a Learning activity

Look at the recommendations for managing DKA (NICE, 2004b). Check with your local hospital/diabetes service: are guidelines in place, and if so, do they fulfil the requirements?

S Scenario continued: Lui

By the next day Lui is feeling much better. She manages to eat breakfast and is no longer dehydrated. She is seen by the DSN, who starts on education and information giving. This involves Lui being taught how to monitor her own blood glucose levels and how to inject herself with insulin. The DSN gives her appropriate literature, with the emphasis on Lui learning to monitor and manage her diabetes herself, with support from professionals where necessary. This is understandably quite an anxious time for Lui, and you should appreciate that people with newly diagnosed diabetes may not be able to fully take in all the information they are given.

C Professional conversation

Mairi, the diabetic specialist nurse (DSN), says, 'I met Lui on the second day of her hospital stay. She was no longer dehydrated and the intravenous infusion of fluid and insulin had recently been discontinued. She had received her first subcutaneous injection just before lunch and this had been administered by the staff nurse; during our conversation Lui informed me that she had been surprised as she had hardly felt the injection. I introduced myself and explained that I wanted to talk her, provide information, and answer any questions that she might have about diabetes.

Lui now knew that she had type 1 diabetes and it was clear that, although feeling physically better, she was still shocked and upset about her diagnosis. I did offer to come back the following day if she felt she was not ready for more information, but she said that she was keen to go home as soon as possible. A diagnosis of diabetes can be overwhelming, and I assured Lui that she would receive ongoing support and that I did not expect her to understand everything immediately. At this point her mum arrived on the ward and Lui visibly relaxed. Although Lui will ultimately take responsibility for her diabetes it was extremely useful to have her mum involved at this initial session. Considerable progress was made in explaining the condition, showing Lui how to test her blood glucose levels, learning how to inject the insulin and having some awareness of what to do if the blood glucose levels were too low or too high. With support from the district nurse this made sure that Lui had enough information to allow her to go home the following day. I provided Lui with the date of a follow-up session with the DSN and said I would phone her the day after discharge to see how she was getting on.'

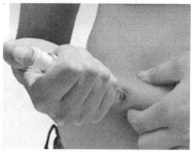

Figure 34.5 Subcutaneous injection using a pen driver

S Scenario continued

In order to ensure a safe and quick discharge from hospital Lui was referred to the DN, who was able to visit her at home for two days to ensure that she was competent at monitoring her glucose levels and injecting insulin. The GP and practice nurse (PN) were informed of Lui's diagnosis, and she was able to visit the PN to discuss her prescriptions and to learn more about any ongoing care that she might require. Lui is managed initially by both primary and secondary care to ensure that she has access to the appropriate level of support and education to enable her gain confidence in coping effectively with her diabetes.

There is currently no cure for diabetes, and although their needs will differ, both Bill and Lui will require ongoing input from the healthcare team.

a Learning activity   W

How would you feel if you or a relative were diagnosed with a chronic condition? What care and support do you think you might require?

Visit www.diabetes.org. uk to find out what care is recommended and the support networks available for people with diabetes.

Primary care

There has been a marked change in health services, with a shift from hospital to community; in the United Kingdom 86 per cent of all problems presenting to the NHS are managed through primary care services. (Devolution has created distinct differences between the health services of England, Scotland, Wales and Northern Ireland, particularly in their organisation and management. The broad aims for health services across the four countries are similar; to recognise the need to streamline the acute sector, provide more care in community settings and make more preventative interventions, particularly for individuals with long-term conditions. For further discussion see Maslin-Prothero, Masterson and Jones, 2008.) Children under 5 years old and people over 75 years average up to seven contacts a year with their GP (Pereira Gray, 2003). The increased availability and cost-effectiveness of medical technologies demonstrates the growth of the primary care-led health service (Toward and Maslin-Prothero, 2007), and increasing numbers of services are being delivered in primary care or outpatient settings, without the need for hospital admission, as illustrated through the scenarios in this chapter.

> ### (a) Learning activity
>
> Read through the chief nursing officer's 10 key roles for nurses set out in Chapter 9 of the *NHS Plan* (DH, 2000). Find out what new roles for nurses, midwives and health visitors have been developed in primary care settings.

In mental health, services have become increasingly community based with the development of assertive outreach teams, crisis resolution teams and early intervention teams (Chisholm and Ford, 2004). The growing emphasis on improved management of long-term, chronic conditions will further shift the emphasis to primary care (DH, 2004b). These developments, coupled with the European Working Time Directive reducing junior doctors' hours, are opening up a number of opportunities for nurses, midwives and health visitors to extend and expand their roles (CNO, 2003), for example through the creation of community matron posts.

At the macro level, organisational and budgetary arrangements for primary care reflect the direction in healthcare policy; PCTs control over 80 per cent of the NHS budget and have a key role in planning and commissioning primary and secondary care services on behalf of their patients (DH, 2005a). This development has affected referral decisions, and creates significant differences in the services available to patients both within individual PCTs and between them, such as the provision of Herceptin in one PCT but not another.

In Scotland commissioning and purchasing have been integrated, whereas in Wales the purchaser–provider split has been maintained with an emphasis on partnership. In Northern Ireland, there has been a reorganisation of Northern Ireland's Health and Social Services (HPSS) with the establishment of a Health and Social Services Authority (HSSA); this has created five integrated health and social service trusts (Woods, 2001; DHSSPS, 2006).

Key issues for nurse, midwives and health visitors arising from recent health policy developments

The NHS currently employs over 300,000 whole-time-equivalent nurses and midwives, and nursing is the largest of the health professions and the biggest staff group in the NHS workforce (DH, 1999; RCN, 2000). Nurses use significant resources in order to deliver or directly supervise the majority of direct care provided by the NHS. What nurses and midwives do and the way they perform directly influences quality and costs as well as the patient experience. Subsequently clinical effectiveness and cost efficiency are significantly affected by the way in which nurses are organised, deployed and practise (DH, 2000).

The Welsh Assembly government's health and social care strategy, *Designed For Life – Creating world class health and social care for Wales in the 21st century*, is a 10 year strategy for Wales (Welsh Assembly, 2005); the philosophy was to transform the NHS from an illness-based model to a health-based model. In *The NHS Plan* (DH, 2000), *Choosing Health* (DH, 2004c), and *Our Health, Our Care, Our Say: A new direction for community services* (DH, 2006), the government outlined its commitment to preventing as well as treating ill-health and reducing health inequalities in England. The Scottish plan for health, *Better Health, Better Care* (NHS Scotland, 2007) outlined the actions required to improve health, tackle health inequalities and enhance the quality of services, with an emphasis on creating an integrated health system, and developing care pathways that build on clinical networks between specialist acute services and primary care. Likewise, Northern Ireland is going through a process of reorganisation where health and personal social care is to become an integrated service; and like Wales and Scotland there is a focus on public health (DHSSPS, 2007).

Challenging the current inequitable access to health and healthcare resources, economic impoverishment and unsafe physical surroundings which threaten the health and well-being of countless people, requires an understanding of the interprofessional contribution – not only in terms of service delivery but also in shaping the policy process itself. Nursing and healthcare are clearly areas for political activity and debate, as scarce resources are allocated amongst competing and equally worthy groups and needs; for example healthcare policy and policy for health could be seen as representing competing causes when it comes to resource allocation (see Toward and Maslin-Prothero, 2007 for a more in-depth discussion). It is essential for nurses and other health and social care professionals to be accepted by the wider policy community and be thinking in a politically informed way if they are to have the issues they are concerned about taken seriously (Hart, 2004; Masterson and Maslin-Prothero, 2005).

Currently, healthcare professionals work in systems that still exclude or disadvantage large numbers of people needing care, and are confronted by health issues caused by sexism, racism, ageism and the inequitable distribution of resources. In the United Kingdom the statutory regulatory body, the NMC's *Code* states that you must 'work with others to protect and promote the health and wellbeing of those in your care, their families and carers, and the wider community' (NMC, 2008: 1).

Inequalities that may determine health status permeate healthcare structures and can constrain our ability to deliver healthcare, possibly because of the difficulty in presenting a united front (Masterson and Maslin-Prothero, 2005).

The former NHS chief executive, Sir Nigel Crisp (DH, 2004e), described nursing leadership as 'pivotal' to patient-centred care, leadership and influencing the future. He stated nursing leadership was key:

- in championing better health and services for local people
- within a reforming NHS
- professionally.

Interdisciplinary working

We have seen that interdisciplinary working – where professionals work towards shared client centred goals and team members cross traditional professional boundaries to meet client need – has led to the development of a range of new roles and the demise of some. For example, in rheumatology services, nurses, physiotherapists and occupational therapists in parts of the United Kingdom have developed their roles to become 'rheumatology practitioners' (Read et al, 2001), taking on a new autonomous role as the lead practitioner in the continuing care of rheumatology patients with chronic conditions.

However other nursing and health specialist roles, for example in learning disability services, have practically disappeared over the first decade of the twenty-first century. The white paper *Valuing People: A new strategy for learning disability for the 21st century* (DH, 2001c) set out the government's plans for improving the lives of people with learning disabilities. These plans were built around people with learning disabilities, their families, local councils, the health service and voluntary organisations working together. Joint investment planning was seen as a practical means for bringing together the wide range of organisations that support people with learning disabilities. Case management and coordination is now predominantly managed by social workers, and the majority of continuing care for people with learning disabilities now takes place in the community (Masterson and Maslin-Prothero, 2005).

The government's report on learning disability, *Valuing People: Moving forward together* (DH, 2004f), illustrates the different ways that the government has tried to move the concerns of people living with learning disabilities forward, and demonstrates new ways of working, and how people with learning disabilities are influencing key decisions and policy makers. It has been argued that people with learning disabilities and their carers were not given a choice about the transfer of services to social care (Manthorpe, 2003). Also there is a recognition that models of interdisciplinary working do not always meet the needs or priorities of clients, such as people with learning disabilities from black and ethnic minority communities (Healthcare Commission, 2004).

An outcome of the modernisation of the health and social care services in the United Kingdom has been the increased move towards interdisciplinary working in continuing care services (Miller, Freeman and Ross, 2001). Effective interdisciplinary working between health and social care professionals in such services is believed to promote improved client/ patient care (Borril et al, 2000, 2001; Freeth and Reeves, 2002). For teams to work effectively, traditional divisions between professions must be challenged, and ways of working differently and collaboratively explored. This requires health and social care professionals to become more flexible and develop a greater mutual understanding and respect for each other (Freeth and Reeves, 2002; Humphris and Hean, 2004); interdisciplinary education has been promoted as a means of achieving this.

Interdisciplinary education

Interdisciplinary education has been promoted as a means of implementing reforms in health and social care (Glen, 2004). Policy documents have emphasised the government's commitment to interprofessional education pre and post qualification (DH, 2000, 2001b, 2002), and interprofessional education is believed to enable health and social care practitioners to deliver more person-centred services and to be fundamental to successful joint working across health and social care. Davies (2000) suggests that when incorporating new models of collaboration it is not what people have in common, but their differences that make collaborative work more powerful than working separately. Through working together there needs to be an acknowledgment that all participants bring equally valid knowledge and expertise from their professional and personal experience (Beattie, 2003).

Conclusion

This chapter has highlighted current health policy and the drive to bring care closer to home, with the aim of ensuring acute hospital beds are used appropriately, with enhanced care provision being provided in the community setting. The examples of type 1 and 2 diabetes to illustrate the management of long-term conditions have showed the importance of empowering people to change and adapt lifestyles to improve their health and well-being, and the role of the primary healthcare team and other professionals in meeting their needs. The significance of working with a whole-system approach, recognising the roles and responsibilities of the many professions within health and social care and the important role of voluntary and charitable agencies, is a necessary requisite of interprofessional care today and the future.

References

Baldwin, M. (2006) 'The Warrington workload tool: determining its use in one trust', *British Journal of Community Nursing* **11**(9), 391–5.

Beattie, A. (2003) 'Journeys into third space: health alliances and the challenge of border crossing', pp. 146–57 in Leathard, A. (ed.), *Interprofessional Collaboration: From policy to practice in health and social care*, Hove, Brunner-Routledge.

Borrill, C., West, M., Dawson, J., Shapiro, D., Rees, A., Richards, A., Garrod, S., Carletta, J. and Carter, A. (2001) *Team Working and Effectiveness in Healthcare: Findings from the Healthcare Effectiveness Project*, Aston, University of Aston.

Borrill, C., West, M., Shapiro, D. and Rees, A. (2000) 'Team working and effectiveness in healthcare', *British Journal of Healthcare Management* 6, 364–71.

British Medical Journal (BMJ) (2007) Obesity: how do doctors diagnose obesity? [online] http://besttreatments.bmj.com/btuk/conditions/12939.html (accessed 16 September 2007).

Chief Nursing Officer (CNO) (2003) 'Rising to the challenge of the working time directive', *CNO Bulletin*, November [online] www.doh.gov.uk/cno/bulletindetail_nov.htm#topnews (accessed 12 December 2003).

Chisholm, A. and Ford, R. (2004) *Transforming Mental Healthcare*, London, Sainsbury Centre for Mental Health.

Davies, C. (2000) 'Getting health professionals to work together', *British Medical Journal* 320, 1021–2.

Department of Health (DH) (1997) *The New NHS: Modern, dependable*, London, DH.

DH (1999) *Making a Difference: Strengthening the nursing, midwifery and health visiting contribution to health and healthcare*, London, DH.

DH (2000) *The NHS Plan*, London, DH.

DH (2001a) *National Service Framework for Diabetes*, London, DH.

DH (2001b) *National Service Framework for the Older Person*, London, DH.

DH (2001c) *Valuing People: A new strategy for learning disability for the 21st century*, London, DH.

DH (2002) *Liberating the Talents: Helping primary care trusts and nurses to deliver the NHS Plan*, London, DH.

DH (2004a) *Chronic Disease Management. A compendium of information*, London, DH.

DH (2004b) *Making Partnership Work for Patients, Carers and Service Users: A strategic agreement between the Department of Health, the NHS and the Voluntary and Community Sector* [online] http://www.dh.gov.uk/en/Publicationsandstatistics/Publications/PublicationsPolicyAndGuidance/Browsable/DH_4095983 (accessed 16 September 2007).

DH (2004c) *Choosing Health: Making healthier choices easier*, Cm 6374, London, The Stationery Office [online] http://www.dh.gov.uk/en/Publicationsandstatistics/Publications/PublicationsPolicyAndGuidance/DH_4094550 (accessed 19 November 2007).

DH (2004d) *The Quality and Outcomes Framework* [online] www.ic.nhs.uk/services/qof (accessed 19 November 2007).

DH (2004e) Chief Nursing Officer's Conference 2004, Manchester, 3–5 November 2004 [online] http://www.dh.gov.uk/NewsHome/ConferenceAndEventReports/ConferenceReportsConferenceReportsArticle/fs/en?CONTENT_ID=4097515&chk=mdHshD (accessed 7 June 2006).

DH (2004f) *Valuing People: Moving forward together*, London, DH.

DH (2005a) *Independence, Well-being and Choice: Our vision for the future of social care for adults in England*, Social Care green paper, London, DH.

DH (2005b) *The National Service Framework for Long-Term Conditions*, March, London, DH.

DH (2005c) *Supporting People with Long Term Conditions: Liberating the talents of nurses who care for people with long term conditions*, London, DH.

DH (2006) *Our Health, Our Care, Our Say: Making it happen*, London, DH.

DH (2007a) 'About diabetes' [online] http://www.dh.gov.uk/Policy and guidance/health and social care topics (accessed 10 October 2007).

DH (2007b) *Working Together for Better Diabetes Care*, London, DH.

DH (2008) *Raising the Profile of Long Term Conditions*, London, DH.

Department of Health, Social Services and Public Safety. Northern Ireland (DHSSPS) (2006) *Review of Public Administration* [online] http://www.dhsspsni.gov.uk/index/hss/rpa-home.htm (accessed 16 September 2007).

DHSSPS (2007) *Health and Social Care* [online] http://www.dhsspsni.gov.uk/index/hss.htm (accessed 24 December 2007).

Diabetes Control and Complications Trial (DCCT) Research Group (1993) 'The effect of intensive treatment of diabetes on the development of long-term complications in insulin-dependent diabetes mellitus' *New England Journal of Medicine* **329**(14), 977–86.

Diabetes UK (2006a) *Complications* [online] www.diabetes.org.uk/Guide to diabetes (accessed 9 January 2009).

Diabetes UK (2006b) *At Your Annual Review* [online] www.diabetes.org.uk/Guide to diabetes/What care to expect (accessed 9 January 2009).

Diabetes UK (2006c) *Structured Education* [online] www.diabetes.org.uk/Guide to diabetes/Treatment and your health (accessed 9 January 2009).

Diabetes UK (2008) *What is Diabetes?* [online] www.diabetes.org.uk/Guide to diabetes/Introduction to diabetes (accessed 9 January 2009).

Farooq, A. (2007) 'Achieving Quality and Outcomes Framework glycaemia targets', *Prescriber* (19 April), 30–8 [online] www3.interscience.wiley.com/cgi-bin/fulltext/114294735/PDFSTART (accessed 9 January 2009).

Feacham, G. A., Sekhri, N. K. and White, K. L. (2002) 'Getting more for their dollar: a comparison of the NHS with California's Kaiser Permanente', *British Medical Journal* **3**(24), 135–43.

Freeth, D. and Reeves, S. (2002) 'Evaluation of an interprofessional training ward: pilot phase', pp. 116–138 in Leiba, T. and Glen, S. (eds), *Multi-Professional Learning for Nurses: Breaking the boundaries*, Basingstoke, Palgrave.

Gill, K. (2004) *Strategic Framework for Management Of Long Term Conditions*, Report prepared by Kate Gill to Essex Strategic Health Authority [online] http://www.essex.nhs.uk/documents/framework/longtermconditions.pdf (accessed 29 September 2007).

Glen, S. (2004) 'Interprofessional education: the policy context', pp. 1–15 in Glen, S. and Leiba, T. (eds), *Interprofessional Post-qualifying Education for Nurses: Working together in health and social care*, Basingstoke, Palgrave Macmillan.

Hart, C. (2004) *Nurses and Politics: The impact of power and practice*, Basingstoke, Palgrave Macmillan.

Healthcare Commission (2004) *State of Healthcare*, London, Healthcare Commission.

Henk, N. (2006) 'Managing effective partnerships in older people's services', *Health and Social Care in the Community* **14**(5), 391–9.

Humphris, D. and Hean, S. (2004) 'Educating the workforce: building the evidence about interprofessional learning', *Journal of Health Service Research and Policy* **9**(1), 24–7.

Integrated Care Network (2003) About Integrated Care. London [online] http://www.integratedcarenetwork.gov.uk/themes/integration.php (accessed 3 December 2004 – no longer available).

Kings Fund (2004) *Case Managing Long Term Conditions*, London, Kings Fund.

Manthorpe, J. (2003) 'The perspective of users and carers', pp. 238–48 in Leathard, A. (ed.), *Interprofessional Collaboration: From policy to practice in health and social care*, Hove, Brunner-Routledge.

Maslin-Prothero, S. E., Masterson, A. and Jones, K. (2008) 'Four parts or one whole: the National Health Service (NHS) post-devolution', *Journal of Nursing Management* 16, 662–672.

Masterson, A. and Maslin-Prothero, S. E. (2005) 'Interdisciplinary working and education in continuing care' , ch. 14 in Roe, B. and Beech, R. (eds), *Intermediate and Continuing Care: Policy and practice*, Oxford, Blackwell.

Miller, C., Freeman, M. and Ross, N. (2001) *Interprofessional Practice in Health and Social Care*, London, Arnold.

Nagelkerk, J., Reick, K. and Meengs, L. (2006) 'Perceived barriers and effective strategies to diabetes self-management', *Journal of Advanced Nursing* **54**(2), 151–8.

National Diabetes Support Team (2006) *Diabetic Foot Guide* [online] http://www.diabetes.nhs.uk/downloads/NDST_Diabetic_Foot_Guide.pdf (accessed 29 September 2007).

NHS Modernisation Agency (2004) *Learning Distillation of Chronic Disease Management Programmes in the UK*, Matrix Research Consultancy/Modernisation Agency, July.

NHS Scotland (2003) *Partnership for Care: Scotland's Health white paper* [online] http://www.show.scot.nhs.uk/sehd/publications/PartnershipforCareHWP.pdf (accessed 19 November 2007).

NHS Scotland (2007) *Better Health, Better Care* [online] http://www.scotland.gov.uk/Resource/Doc/206458/0054871.pdf (accessed 16 December 2007).

National Institute for Clinical Excellence (NICE) (2003) *TA60 Diabetes (type 1 and 2) Patient Education Models: Guidance*, London, NICE.

NICE (2004a) *Type 2 Diabetes: Prevention and management of foot problems*, Clinical Guideline 10, London, NICE.

NICE (2004b) *Diagnosis and Management if Type 1 Diabetes in Children, Young People and Adults*, Clinical Guideline 15, London, NICE.

National Primary and Research Development Centre (2005) *Evercare Evaluation Interim Report: Implications for supporting people with long-term conditions*, 19 January, University of Manchester/University of York.

Nursing and Midwifery Council (NMC) (2004) *Standards of Proficiency for Specialist Community Public Health Nurses*, London, NMC.

The Code: Standards of conduct, performance and ethics for nurses and midwives, London, NMC.

Pereira Gray, D. (2003) '2020 vision', *Health Service Journal* (2 October), 18–19.

Queen's Nursing Institute (QNI) (2006) *Vision and Values: A call for action on community nursing*, London, QNI.

Read, S., Doyal, L., Vaughan, B. Lloyd-Jones, M., Collins, K., McDonnell, A., Jones, R., Cameron, A., Masterson, A., Dowling, S., Furlong, S. and Scholes, J. (2001) *Exploring New Roles in Practice: Final report*, Sheffield, School of Health and Related Research, University of Sheffield.

Reeves, S. and Freeth, D. (2003) 'New forms of technology, new forms of collaboration' In Leathard A (ed) *Interprofessional Collaboration: From policy to practice in health and social care*, Hove, Brunner-Routledge, pp 79–92.

Renders, C. M., Valk, G. D., Griffin, S. J., Wagner, E. H., van Eijk, J. T. and Assendelft ,W. J. J. (2001) 'Interventions to improve the management of diabetes in primary care, outpatient, and community settings: a systematic review', *Diabetes Care* 24, 1821–33.

Robinson, J. and Elkan, R. (1996) *Health Needs Assessment: Theory and practice*, Edinburgh, Churchill Livingstone.

Royal College of Nursing (RCN) (2000) *Making Up the Difference: A review of the UK nursing labour market in 2000*, London, RCN.

Scottish Executive (2003) *Community Health Partnerships*, 18 July [online] http://www.scotland.gov.uk/consultations/health/comhealpart.pdf (accessed 19 November 2007).

Sturt, J., Whitlock, S. and Hearnshaw, H. (2006) 'Complex intervention development for diabetes self-management', *Journal of Advanced Nursing* **54**(3), 293–303.

Toward, S. and Maslin-Prothero, S. (2007) 'The impact of health and social policy on the planning and delivery of nursing care', pp. 113–134 in Brown, J. and Libberton, P. (eds), *Principles of Professional Studies in Nursing*, Basingstoke, Palgrave Macmillan.

UK Prospective Diabetes Study (UKPDS) Group (1998) 'Intensive blood-glucose control with sulphonylureas or insulin compared with conventional treatment and risk of complications in patients with type 2 diabetes', *The Lancet* **352**(9131), 837–53.

Wanless, D. and HM Treasury (2002) *Working Together: Effective partnership working on the ground*, London, HM Treasury.

Wanless, D., Appleby, J., Harrison, A. and Patel, D. (2007) *Our Future Health Secured? A review of NHS funding and performance*, London, King's Fund.

Welsh Assembly (2005) *Designed for Life: Creating world class health and social care for Wales in the 21st century* [online] http://www.wales.nhs.uk/documents/designed-for-life-e.pdf (accessed 24 December 2007).

Williams, G. and Pickup, J. C. (2004) *Handbook of Diabetes*, 3rd edn, Oxford, Blackwell.

Woods, K. J. (2001) 'The development of integrated healthcare models in Scotland', *International Journal of Integrated Care* 1(e41, Apr–June) [online] http://www.pubmedcentral.nih.gov/articlerender.fcgi?artid=1525338 (accessed 21 November 2007).

World Health Organization (WHO) (1999) *Part 1 Diagnosis and Classification of Diabetes Mellitus*, Geneva, WHO.

WHO (2006) Diabetes programme Factsheet 312 [online] www.who.int/diabetes/facts/en (accessed 9 January 2009).

Legislation

Health Act 1999

Health and Social Care Act 2001

Part

IV

Chapter

35

Complementary and alternative medicine

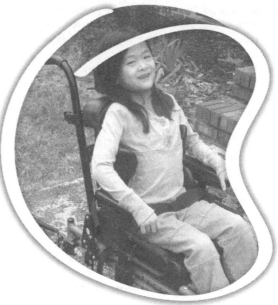

Alistair McConnon

 Links to other chapters in *Foundation Studies for Caring*

2 Interprofessional learning
3 Evidence-based practice and research
4 Ethical, legal and professional issues
5 Communication
6 Culture
7 Public health and health promotion
8 Healthcare governance
14 Pharmacology and medicines
28 Rehabilitation
34 Primary care

 Links to other chapters in *Foundation Skills for Caring*

1 Fundamental concepts for skills
3 Communication
28 Routes of medication administration

W Don't forget to visit www.palgrave.com/glasper for additional online resources relating to this chapter.

Introduction

This chapter aims to provide you with a basic introduction to the most commonly used forms of complementary and alternative medicine (CAM). The text and activities encourage you to investigate and discuss these therapies and their use, either individually or in groups. There is information on complementary and alternative therapies in relation to professional clinical practice at the end of this chapter. The chapter also introduces the main complementary and alternative professional bodies, so you can gain more information about the therapies and will know how to check whether a complementary or alternative practitioner belongs to a professional body.

CAM is currently undergoing a change of name, so although this is the name used in this chapter, you might find the new name 'integrated healthcare' in some journals. This name implies that there is, or will be in future, a close partnership between modern medicine and complementary medicine.

The areas addressed in this chapter are herbalism, traditional Chinese medicine, acupuncture, chiropractic, osteopathy, homeopathy, massage, aromatherapy, reflexology and healing. It also reviews the current status regarding training, and professional and legal aspects. Where there is a scientific basis to support the therapy, this is outlined. If you consider the use of complementary medicine it should not be seen in isolation from modern medicine, but rather used where appropriate in conjunction with modern medicine.

Learning outcomes

This chapter will enable you to:

- demonstrate a basic understanding of each of the therapies mentioned in this chapter
- discuss the position of the Nursing and Midwifery Council (NMC) regarding complementary therapies
- identify the need for more research into CAM in order to protect the public

- recognise the role, present and future, of CAM in healthcare
- demonstrate an awareness of the need for regulation of all CAM
- be aware of some of the ethical issues that those who practise a CAM therapy might face.

Concepts

- Complementary medicine
- Homeopathy
- Herbalism
- Traditional Chinese medicine
- Acupuncture
- Chiropody
- Osteopathy
- Massage
- Aromatherapy
- Reflexology
- Healing

Issues to consider when using complementary and alternative medicine

The House of Lords Science and Technology Committee's *Sixth Report* on CAM (2000) made recommendations for the regulation and training of CAM practitioners and therapists. These recommendations are resulting in the gradual organisation of training and regulation for CAM. The previous training is being improved upon and standards set. You must bear in mind that because of these developments, any information about training and regulation is liable to change, and you should consult the relevant organisations (many of which are named here) to find out the current position.

There is also an increasing quantity and quality of research into CAM therapies, but unfortunately this is from a very low base: much research to date lacks methodological rigour. Rigorous designs need to be applied to research studies that aim to investigate the efficacy of CAM therapies, and their results need to be tested for validity. It could be argued that many

Part

IV

of the claimed results of CAM studies are not readily quantifiable, and that the random controlled trials that are perceived as the gold standard of medical research are not the most appropriate way of researching them: if so, it is necessary to develop other methodologies in order that these less quantifiable aspects can be investigated and tested thoroughly.

Note too that while it is increasingly easy to buy for example homeopathic and herbal remedies over the counter in a variety of outlets, it is always wise to seek the advice of a qualified practitioner of the therapy. Making an appointment to see a herbalist or homeopath for example, and having a professional consultation, is by far the most reliable method of using these therapies.

CAM practitioners and therapists whose professional organisations have codes of conduct are usually required, if a person who approaches them for treatment is currently receiving conventional medical treatment, to liaise with, or seek permission to administer the therapy from, the medical staff under whose care they are. Thus the medical practitioner retains overall control of the individual's treatment, and can consider the appropriateness of the therapy and any contraindications for it. One problem that may arise is that not all medical practitioners know enough about the complementary therapies to make an informed judgement. To try to remedy this information deficit, the reputable training organisations and professional bodies relating to CAM have sent information regarding the main complementary therapies to primary care groups (DH, 2000).

A nurse or other healthcare professional who wishes to administer a form of complementary therapy themselves is required to have undertaken an approved course in that particular therapy, and have been appropriately accredited by the relevant examining body (NMC, 2008). The individual must be aware of contraindications to the use of any remedies, herbs or essential oils used in the therapy (NMC, 2008). They also need to discuss the appropriateness of the therapy with their multidisciplinary team (NMC, 2008). Employers may have local policies regarding complementary and alternative therapies, and you should make yourself aware of these and adhere to them. You will also need current personal insurance which covers any therapy you choose to use (NMC, 2008).

If you consider using some other practitioner or therapist of any complementary or alternative therapy, you should ask to see proof of training, qualifications, current membership of an organisation and current insurance. It is important to check that the practitioner or therapist has had recent updated sessions or courses in relation to their therapy, since this helps to ensure that they follow current best practice. It is also wise to verify the cost of the therapy, and to inform yourself about what is involved, including risks and possible side-effects. You may find a recommendation from a friend or colleague is also useful when choosing a practitioner/therapist.

Ernst (2000) supports the argument that no therapy can cure a disease, and even their strongest supporters are unlikely to disagree. However that does not mean CAM is necessarily without merit: research into the complementary therapies has shown that some therapies improve the relaxation response, reduce anxiety and generally improve the well-being of the individual, and these are worthwhile benefits. You should be aware yourself, and make sure that your patients/clients are aware, of what can realistically be expected if they use CAM.

Herbalism

Herbalism is also referred to as phytotherapy: *phyto* is the Greek word denoting a plant. Evidence of plants as a form of medicine has been found over the centuries in written

> **S** **Scenario: Introducing Paul and Sarah**
>
> Paul is a first-year physiotherapy student on placement in an orthopaedic ward. His mentor Sarah is an experienced physiotherapist who has been linked to orthopaedics for a number of years. Sarah is also a qualified acupuncturist, and occasionally uses this form of CAM with patients, particularly those with lower back pain.

texts from many different cultures. The writings of Greek physicians Hippocrates, Galen of Pergamon and Dioscorides of Anazarbus, Islamic physicians such as Hunayn ibn Ishaq, Sassanian (ancient Persian) texts (Portmann and Savage-Smith, 2007), Chinese medicine, Ayurvedic medicine, Native North American medicine (Mills and Bone, 2000), and also Western European physicians such as St Hildegarde of Bingen (Libster, 2002) all mention the use of herbs in a variety of medicinal forms.

The use of plants as medicine is often referred to as *simple* medicine, in as much as the plants can often be used in simple form such as tea. Plants, however, are naturally occurring complex chemicals. Therefore the practitioner of herbal medicine needs to possess a great deal of knowledge about the origin, varieties, appearance and chemical structure, evidence-based knowledge regarding uses, the most suitable remedy to use for each individual, and side-effects of the plants. Plant medicines provided by the herbalist contain the essence of the plant. Plant nutrients, chemical compounds and esoteric properties can stimulate and improve a person's own healing abilities, affecting them physically, emotionally, mentally and spiritually (Libster, 2002), thus restoring a state of health to the individual.

Herbs and modern drugs both have complex chemical compositions, and therefore they can work in similar ways. A difference between the two is that plants and herbs use a rather indirect route to the blood stream and target cells and organs, and their results are normally less dramatic and slower of onset than those of conventional pharmaceuticals (Kuhn, 1999). Most pharmacological actions of herbs are understood, but a good number of herbs possess pharmacological activities which are inharmonious with present-day pharmacological understanding (Mills and Bone, 2000: Libster, 2002). For example a herb given when the body's processes are in an overactive state to aid return controlled homeostasis, can also be given when the body's processes are in a state of underactivity (Libster, 2002; Kuhn, 1999). The toxicity of herbs is generally less than that of synthetic drugs, and herbs also, probably because of their natural and whole composition, act in a manner that treats the cause of the disharmony in the person's state of health (Kuhn, 1999; Mills and Bone, 2000). Manufactured drugs tend to be aimed at alleviating the symptoms of the disease and not the underpinning cause.

Herbalism is used to treat, and in the management of, a wide variety of complaints and illnesses. It is not possible to list them all here, but they include respiratory problems such as mild to moderate bronchitis, infectious conditions, moderate acute hepatitis, and cardiac problems including mild to moderate hypertension (Libster, 2002; Mills and Bone, 2000).

When using herbs there is a need to optimise safety, as the herbs can have interactions with conventional drugs that result in adverse effects for the patient. There is a growing body of sound, empirical evidence on all aspects relating to the uses of herbs. Therefore in order to maximise safety, only a qualified herbalist should prescribe herbs and herbal remedies. It is not advisable to purchase herbal remedies over the counter unless either a qualified herbalist has been consulted, or information regarding the herb has been gained from a reputable book on herbalism, such as that by Mills and Bone (2000).

> **(a) Learning activity**
>
> In your interprofessional learning group consider the use of St John's wort, which has received publicity over the last few years. Find out the proper name for this plant, and what conditions it might be used to treat. Find evidence to support your findings. Be sure to use proper scientific sources!

> **(a) Learning activity**
>
> In your learning group consider how herbalist medicine could be used in the treatment of patients alongside conventional medicine. What advantages and disadvantages might it have from the point of view of the patient?

Part
IV

Training to become a qualified herbalist takes between three and five years. The National Institute of Medical Herbalists, a professional body, has an Accreditation Board which accredits courses which meet the board's minimum standards (Kayne, 2002). One of the requirements is that each student must complete supervised practice of a minimum of 500 hours. Currently the European Herbal Practitioners Association is harmonising the standards of training across Europe.

Traditional Chinese medicine

The theories and philosophies of traditional Chinese medicine (TCM) are complex, simple and at the same time profound, and are also alien to Western thought. This last point in particular makes TCM very difficult for the western scholar to comprehend. However I shall attempt to provide an outline of the main conceptual basis, with apologies to practitioners and scholars for the limitations of my knowledge.

One aspect of the theoretical basis of main theoretical basis of TCM, the yin–yang concept, is according to Maciocia (1989) referred to in the *I Ching* or *Book of Changes*, which predates the Christian calendar by 700 years. European travellers to China in the seventeenth century found it being practised throughout China (Kuriyama, 2002), as indeed it is today.

The yin–yang concept is probably the best known concept of TCM in the west, as is its symbol, a circle divided by a reverse S-shaped line into two equal halves, one white, one black. The lighter half represents yang and the darker half represents yin. In each half, however, is a small circle of the opposing colour. The yin–yang concept is applied to everything in the universe, although nothing is totally one or the other (Maciocia, 1989; Kaptchuk, 2002). There is always a part of yin in yang and vice versa, as represented by the circles of opposite colour. While yin and yang are opposites they are also interdependent on each other, both requiring the other in order to exist (Maciocia, 1989).

A straight line dividing a circle tends to be perceived as static, whereas a reversed S-shaped divisional line may be suggestive of movement. This is the case with the yin–yang concept, which includes the idea that yin can become yang and yang can become yin (Maciocia, 1989). There must, however, be a balance of yin and yang in order to maintain health. An imbalance is described, according to Maciocia (1989), as an excess or a depletion of one or the other resulting in disharmony. This disharmony results in what we in the western world call disease. In Chinese medicine the body's state of harmony is said to be disturbed by influences which also disturb the balance of the whole energy system of the body. Therefore when it comes to treatment in Chinese medicine, one must never lose sight of the balanced whole.

TCM identifies six external factors that can influence the body's state of harmony: wind, cold, fire and heat, damp, dryness, and summer heat (Williams, 1995), which are intrinsic to the five elements of water, fire, wood, metal and earth. These five elements constitute a construction of a relationship, which in Chinese medicine exists amongst the body's internal viscera, and also between the organs and the different types of tissue, sense organs, smells, tastes, sounds and colours. Chinese medical philosophy weaves all those factors and elements into a complex and intricate form of medicine and treatment. Chinese medicine involves the main treatment modes of acupuncture (discussed on page 709), herbalism, meditation, nutrition and energy balancing, and development exercises such as Qigong and T'ia Chi (Kaptchuk, 2002; Williams, 1995; Maciocia, 1989).

a) Learning activity

For a learning group activity find a picture of the diagrammatic representation of the yin–yang concept. Give some examples of what might be yin and what might be yang. What might be the significance of these for patients who believe in this concept? It will also be useful for nursing students and other healthcare students to understand these ideas so that they can understand how some of their patients might be reacting to being ill.

Qi, pronounce 'chee', is the other main aspect of TCM, and is described in detail in the section on acupuncture.

> ## ⟲ⓐ Learning activity
>
> In your learning group choose two of the other treatment modes and find out whether they have any relevance in modern medicine. It will be especially useful to consider how believing in these systems might influence patients' reactions to having a health problem.

Research into TCM has been received with much criticism and doubt in the west. Most of the research involves acupuncture, which is used for a variety of conditions: one prominent condition for which it is often tried is back pain. You are encouraged to critically analyse research into TCM to help you decide on its validity, bearing in mind that the methods of research used by westerners may not be totally applicable to TCM.

Training for TCM is carried out at universities, the first British university to run a degree in TCM being Middlesex University. Those successfully completing the degree course are then eligible to progress to postgraduate studies. The Association of Traditional Chinese Medicine, which has amalgamated with the British Society of Chinese Medicine, is a professional organisation for practitioners of TCM. This organisation has a code of professional conduct and a code of practice, which promote safe and competent practice of TCM, and to which members are bound at all times.

> ## ⟲ⓐ Learning activity
>
> For a learning group presentation find out where your nearest practitioner of TCM is based, and find out about the Chinese approach to the whole person. Compare this with the holistic approach in western nursing. What lessons can you learn from this comparison?

This section has only superficially touched on the main aspects of the philosophy of TCM. Sources of further reading are provided at the end of the chapter.

Acupuncture

Acupuncture is an ancient method used in Chinese medicine, the first mention of which was in the *I Ching* (Mole, 1992). *Qi* (sometimes spelled ch'i and pronounced 'chee') forms the basis of Chinese medicine (Maciocia, 1989), and is a concept also found in other countries such as India, where it is known as *prana*. Common translations into English in order to make sense of this concept include 'vital force' and 'energy'. *Qi* can be seen as the thread which links everything from minerals to human beings, and indeed is present throughout the universe. It is effectively a form of energy, which is in state of constant motion and aggregation, emerging on both the physical and spiritual level at the same time (Maciocia, 1989). Meridians, which are each linked to organs of the body, are the pathways or channels (Kaptchuk, 2002), much like roads, along which the *qi* flows to every cell in the body. According to Kaptchuk (2002), the meridians in Chinese meridian theory are not visible to the naked eye but form an invisible web-like structure which serves as an information mesh.

The density of the *qi* varies within 'normal' boundaries. Should these boundaries be exceeded, lumps or clots of *qi* are formed. Thus the flow of *qi* is interrupted and a pathological condition ensues (Maciocia, 1989). Disease also occurs if the *qi* is weak or if it flows in a direction other that in that which it should.

Before acupuncture is used, a concrete diagnosis must be made. This can be achieved by questioning and by examination of the six pulses on each wrist, each pulse being related to a major organ (including the tongue and the skin). Depending on the diagnosis the acupuncturist inserts very fine, sterile needles into the relevant acupuncture points to stimulate the flow of *qi*. This unblocks the clot which is impairing flow of *qi*, allowing it to flow freely and thus return health to the affected part of the body. This may take several sessions with the acupuncturist, who must be highly knowledgeable and skilled.

(c) Professional conversation

Paul, the physiotherapy student, is angry to overhear another healthcare practitioner being critical of Sarah's use of acupuncture with a patient. He takes up his concerns with Sarah at a one-to-one meeting later in the shift. 'It doesn't trouble me particularly,' Sarah assures him. 'Most people who are sceptical of acupuncture are those who have never looked into it. Would you like to look through my folder? This is where I keep copies of published journal papers highlighting the evidence base for acupuncture.'

Paul takes up the offer, and returns to the conversation once he has read some of the articles. 'You're right, Sarah,' he says. 'I've tried to take a critical look at the research, but on the whole it does seem to be well founded. I feel comfortable now that there is after all a good provenance for this CAM therapy.'

Acupuncture can be used to treat a wide variety of medical conditions, and not just in the treatment of pain, although it is with this that acupuncture tends to be most commonly associated.

(a) Learning activity

In your learning group find out what other methods of treatment are incorporated in TCM. Choose one method and find out more about that method of treatment. How will this help you in working collaboratively with patients who believe in this method of treatment?

Training to become an acupuncturist varies (DH, 2008). Nonqualified acupuncturists, many of whom belong to the British Acupuncture Council, have undertaken a three-year programme in both traditional acupuncture and studies in western medicine at higher education institutes accredited by the British Acupuncture Accreditation Board. According to the British Medical Acupuncture Society, qualified doctors can take a short course in acupuncture which is generally part time. The acupuncture profession is continuing to develop both written standards for practice and guidelines for specialist areas in the clinical field (DH, 2008).

Practitioners claim that acupuncture, like other complementary therapies, can be used to maintain a healthy state.

(a) Learning activity

Within your learning group source and critically analyse two published journal papers on the effect of acupuncture on pain.

Chiropractic

The term 'chiropractic' has its origins in the Greek words *cheir*, meaning hand, and *praxis*, which means action, so its base meaning is 'done by hand' (Horowitz, 2007).

Daniel Palmer was the founder of the Palmer School of Chiropractic in 1897, in Iowa (Horowitz, 2007) after a claimed meeting with Andrew Sill, the founder of osteopathy (Vickers and Zollman, 1999). Chiropractics is a form of manipulative therapy which utilises both manual and physiological approaches to healing (Kuhn, 1999), with the underpinning belief that the body possesses an innate ability to self-heal (Horowitz, 2007).

The premise on which chiropractics is based is that mechanical dysfunction particularly of the spine, such as vertebral subluxation, the pelvis and distal articulations, can cause a disturbance in the associated nerves (Kuhn, 1999). Pain and in some instances ill health can result from this mechanical dysfunction. This forms the nucleus of chiropractic theory, while the focus of chiropractic practice is on ascertaining the dysfunction and reestablishing normal function. The chiropractic practitioner uses gentle manual manipulation of the spine and pelvis in order to resolve the mechanical dysfunction and thus help restore health. Palmer considered chiropractics to be a complete therapeutic system (Kuhn, 1999). Some of the common conditions that chiropractors are able to treat or improve are carpal tunnel syndrome, headaches, respiratory disorders, backache, sciatica and whiplash (Kuhn, 1999). Chiropractics can also be a means of health promotion by offering what might be termed a 'spinal service', helping to prevent problems or identifying potential problems early and establishing treatment.

> **(a) Learning activity**
>
> Revise the anatomy and physiology of the spinal cord and the spinal nerves. Establish the relevance of this knowledge to your understanding of therapies that involve spinal manipulation.

Treatment risks associated with chiropractics range from headaches, tiredness, local and radiating discomfort through to spinal injury (Sendstad, Leboeuf-Yole and Borchgreuint, 1996). Research shows mixed opinions on the effectiveness of chiropractics. Cherkin and colleagues (1998) both found short-term benefits of chiropractic treatment in the relief of chronic pain and functional abilities. A recent review of systematic reviews of spinal manipulation by Ernst and Calder (2006) concluded that there was no demonstrable evidence to suggest that chiropractics was of benefit in any condition, and that it should not be recommended as a treatment.

> **(a) Learning activity**
>
> As a learning group activity source four research articles on treating back pain with chiropractics, and consider the quality of the evidence for effectiveness of the treatment.

Chiropractic practitioners work in a variety of settings such as clinics with other complementary practitioners and/or health professionals, general practices, and clinics in their own homes (Vickers and Zollman, 1999). The majority of chiropractors work alone, although a few have contractual agreements with primary care trusts.

Chiropractors or chiropractic practitioners are governed by a professional organisation, the General Chiropractic Council, and by the Chiropractors Act 1994. This Act regulates registration, professional education, professional conduct and fitness to practice, appeals, offences, monopolies, competitive practice, and includes the powers of the Privy Council. All chiropractors must be registered with the General Chiropractic Council and cannot call themselves a chiropractor or practise as one unless they are registered. In order to register the applicant must hold a qualification in chiropractics, usually a four-year course at B.Sc. level, inclusive of a year of postgraduate training in an approved practice, which is recognised by the Chiropractors Act 1994.

Osteopathy

Osteopathy, like chiropractics, has its roots in the folk traditions of 'bone setting', a practice that can be traced back to the Ayurvedic texts on medicine (Pole, 2006) and the ancient Chinese texts (Veitch, 2002). In 1864 an American practitioner, Andrew Taylor Still, devised a new system of healing in which he formulated the fundamental principles of osteopathy (Howell, 1999). Eight years later Still founded the first osteopathic medical school in Kirksville, Missouri (Howell, 1999).

Osteopathy, a manual therapy, is said to be one of the oldest means of treating injured joints, muscles and ligaments, and is used in both the detection and treatment of damaged or injured muscles, ligaments, joints and nerves (General Osteopathic Council, 2008).

Part

IV

Defects or dysfunction of these parts of the body, according to osteopathic theory, influence the natural functioning of the internal organs. Osteopathy is said to help the body fulfil its natural capacity to restore health. The osteopath can use drugs, x-rays, surgery, nutrition and mechanical means, as well as manual treatment.

Osteopaths can treat a variety of conditions. These include changes in posture caused by pregnancy, sports training and work-related problems, as well as injuries to the muscles, ligaments, joints and nerves.

⟲ⓐ Learning activity

For a learning group activity presentation, revise the anatomy and physiology of the muscles, and prepare a flipchart poster that names on a diagram the major muscles of the chest, back, neck, abdomen, arms and legs.

Identify the most common muscles strained or pulled or ruptured in the field of sport. Find out the ways in which osteopathic practitioners claim to be able to treat these problems.

The training of an osteopath is over four to five years at BSc(Hons) level, and incorporates intensive clinical training. The training is governed by the General Osteopathic Council, which was a product of the Osteopathic Act 1993. This act covers the same topics as mentioned in the Chiropractors Act 1994. This allows osteopaths to diagnose and prescribe treatment as independent practitioners.

⟲ⓐ Learning activity

In your interprofessional learning group explain the differences between physiotherapy and osteopathy. In what ways do you consider these to be significant?

Risks from osteopathic treatment, although very slight (between 1:20,000 to 1 per million procedures), include spinal cord injuries after cervical manipulation, with a reduction in recent years as a result of increasing awareness and safer techniques (Vickers and Zollman, 1999).

Homeopathy

Samuel Hahnemann (1755–843), a German physician, read when translating a herbal text, with a high degree of disbelief, that cinchona bark (*China officalis*) was an effective cure for malaria. The argument for this was that it was bitter (Wayne et.al, 2003). Hahnemann ingested several doses of cinchona bark and found that he presented with symptoms similar to malaria. He concluded that like cured like. His discoveries led him to develop the therapeutic system of homeopathy. Homeopathy has three principles which differ from modern medicine (Millgrom, 2006): the principle of similars, the principle of potentisation and the principle of vital force.

The principle of similars is based on treating like with like. The argument is that a minute dose of a substance that in a larger dose would cause symptoms can cure the person of the symptoms (Kuhn, 1999). For example if a given substance from a plant, animal or mineral induces nausea in a person, this same substance in a minute dose can be used to treat people who suffer from the condition of nausea.

The principle of potentisation is perhaps the most difficult principle to understand and to accept. Homeopathic remedies undergo a process called succussion. This process involves a substance being serially diluted and then being agitated in a turbulent manner (Millgrom, 2006). The serial dilution of a substance reduces the toxicity of the substance. However, the degree of dilution can be so great that it results in no molecules of the original homeopathic remedy remaining in the water, or water-based solution, that is used for treatment (Coulter, 1981).

The absence of molecules of the homeopathic remedy in the solution has led to homeopathy being perceived as implausible in medical circles. Recent advances in science have, however, provided evidence that water has a 'memory'. This evidence is not conclusive but is very strong. Zhalko-Tytarenko, Lednyiczky and Topping (1998) state that information from the solute stored in the hydrogen bond network is transferred to the organism, where it is stored via resonance interactions. Succussion causes the molecules in solution to vibrate with great intensity, thus emitting the molecules' electromagnetic signature (Oschman, 2000). These signatures of the biologically active molecules are then transferred to the water (Oschman, 2000). The hydrogen bonds handcuff the water molecules to a helix-like structure in the water through which the current induced by the vibrating molecules flows. When the water containing the homeopathic remedy is further diluted, the signals from the current transfer to the new water molecules contained in the water used for dilution (Zhalko-Tytarenko et al, 1998). Thus the memory of the molecules' information is passed on. Potentisation stimulates the body's vital force to cure itself (Castro, 1992).

The principle of the vital force refers to the term that Hahnemann used to describe the energy behind the animation of all living beings, the energy that gives life (Castro, 1992). This vital force is perceived by homeopathy as being independent of any chemical or physical forces, and it is argued that it keeps the person healthy and balanced. The vital force can be equated to what modern medicine calls homeostasis, in as much as it is seen as self-regulating, and possessing an innate aptitude to preserve equilibrium and compensate for disruption to the norm (Castro, 1992; Millgrom, 2006). Disease, according to the belief of homeopaths, occurs when the vital force is weak. Homeopathic remedies are seen as a catalyst, which can activate the body's own energy and thus the body's self-healing ability.

> ### ⟲ⓐ Learning activity
>
> For a learning group activity prepare a brief presentation in which you identify the common name and use for *Calendula Officinalis*. What evidence is there for the efficacy of this plant?

Training for homeopathy is undergoing reform in order to bring parity across training institutions regarding the standards of the training of practitioners and safety of the public. This is in line with the recommendations of the report by the House of Lords Select Committee on Science and Technology (2000) on complementary and alternative medicine.

A government document entitled *Homeopathic Services* was distributed to directors of commissioning in the NHS early in 2007. While this document does not represent any policy on commissioning, it could be interpreted as indicating that homeopathy is being considered as a possible adjunct to treatments in the NHS.

> ### ⟲ⓐ Learning activity
>
> In your learning group source a range of articles on how homeopathy might be used in healthcare, and discuss the feasibility of this partnership. Can you suggest how such a strategy might improve patients' experience of care?

Massage

Massage has been used as a means of treating people for thousands of years. Chinese literature provides evidence that massage was recommended as part of treatment around 2600 BC (Van Why, 1992). The ancient Greeks and Romans also incorporated massage into their treatment repertoire (Bendick, 2002), as did the ancient Islamic doctors (Deuraseh, 2005). Frenchman Ambrose Pare recommended massage as a treatment for a variety of complaints in the sixteenth century, while some 300 years later Per Hendrik Ling, a Swedish doctor, developed a system of massage and in 1894 founded the Society of Trained Masseurs (Holey and Cook, 2003).

Many definitions of the term 'massage' can be found, each embroidering the main concept of manipulation of tissue. Holey and Cook define massage as 'the manipulation of the soft tissues of the body by a trained therapist as a component of a holistic therapeutic intervention' (2003: 6). Perhaps this definition would be more accurate were we to insert the words 'awareness and conscious' from Westland's (1993) definition before 'manipulation'.

Part

IV

Many nurses are showing considerable enthusiasm for the use of therapeutic massage, with a view to making the rather technologically focused experience of the patient more human and caring (Hill, 1995). Massage is one of the more popular complementary therapies in Britain (Ernst, 2000), and continues to increase in popularity.

Systemic reviews of massage for nonspecific lower back pain (Furlan et al, 2002; Cherkin, Sherman and Deyo, 2003) indicate that massage may be beneficial for people with this condition when combined with education and exercise, and for those with persistent back pain. The systemic reviews do, however, strongly suggest the need for more studies. There is also some (but by no means compelling) evidence that massage seems to improve anxiety, depression and self-esteem in people with multiple sclerosis (Huntley and Ernst, 2000).

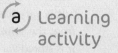 Learning activity

In your learning group consider uses for massage, by a qualified masseuse, in healthcare.

Learning activity

Complete this exercise as part of a learning group activity. It is to relax your eyes, neck and shoulders.

1 Sit upright in a chair with your back supported and your feet flat on the ground, or if you are able to, sit cross-legged on the floor. Whichever position you choose, make sure you are comfortable. Should you choose to sit on a chair, have a table in front of you.
2 Roll your shoulders simultaneously forward then backwards eight times.
3 Vigorously rub your hands together until they feel warm, then place the palms of your hands over your eyes, excluding the light.

4 Place your elbows on the table (if seated) or on your knees (if sitting cross-legged).
5 Breathing deeply, slowly inhale through the mouth and exhale through the mouth. Do this for two minutes.
6 Lower your hands slowly until your face is cupped in your hands.
7 Gently stroke along the line of your eyebrows to your temples with your fingers. Repeat this eight times.
8 Gently open your eyes and relax your arms into a comfortable position.

Note how you now feel and compare it with how you felt before this form of self-massage.

The main bodies for training people in massage such as the International Therapy Exam Council have been working, and continue to work, together to develop national vocational standards to both improve and standardise the training and safety of massage. This is in line with the recommendations by the House of Lords Science and Technology Committee (2000).

Aromatherapy

History shows that aromatherapy has been used for many centuries, particularly in far eastern countries such as Egypt as far back as 1500 BC, and in the Indian subcontinent from around 1000 BC. Aromatherapy involves massage using oils derived from plants, mixed with a base oil (Vickers and Zollman, 1999), such as grapeseed oil or soya oil, which acts as a lubricant. The oils extracted from plants are called 'essential oils' (Fowler and Wall, 1997) and are thought to have a broad range of therapeutic uses and benefits to the recipient of the aromatherapy massage (Vickers and Zollman, 1999).

There is however a need to consider a number of issues surrounding the safety of essential oils, which are in their own right complex chemicals (Fowler and Wall, 1997). The essential oils are used and administered by means of oil burners, vaporisers, inhalations and massage. The use of an oil burner in particular means that the spread of the smell of the oil cannot be controlled, and thus could prove harmful to other people in the vicinity. These complex

Learning activity

In your interprofessional learning group find out whether aromatherapy oils can be used in your clinical area, and if so, by whom and for what they are used. Find out what side-effects and cautions it will be important for you to be aware of when aromatherapy is used.

chemicals have many components, some of which cancel out any potential harmful effects of other components (Carson and Riley, 2001). There are, however, some prevalent components which dominate the pharmacological and toxicological effects of oils (Tisserand, 1996; Carson and Riley, 2001). The toxic effects of some oils can be minor, almost negligible, while the effects of others can prove more serious. For example peppermint, a stimulant, could cause minor cardiac reactions which might be dangerous to those who are being treated for cardiac conditions. Some essentials oils, for example tea tree oil, are governed by the Control of Substances Hazardous to Health Regulations (COSHH) 1994 (Fowler and Wall, 1997). These regulations require safety data sheets and identification of hazards of chemicals to be supplied by manufacturers and suppliers (HSC, 1994). Therefore each user, qualified aromatherapist or not, of essential oils should be aware of possible toxic effects before using the oils.

> ### ⟲ⓐ Learning activity
>
> Florence Nightingale used lavender to treat patients wounded in the Crimea War. Find research to support possible uses of lavender today. Suggest how it might be used in practice and what benefits for patients/clients might be expected.

Since they are complex chemical compounds there is a high risk that essential oils will react with the chemicals in orthodox drugs a patient might be taking, possibly enhancing or negating their effects. In view of the dearth of clinical trials on the reaction between the drugs and essential oils, aromatherapists are advised not to treat any client who is on prescribed medication. A nurse who is a qualified aromatherapist, and wishes to use essential oils in the treatment of their patients, needs to consult with the trust for which they work to find out their position on essential oils. Some trusts consider essential oils to be drugs.

The essential oils that aromatherapists use in their practices raise issues which need to be answered in order to protect the public who use aromatherapy. The essential oils are not licensed under the Medicine Act (1968), Section 12 (1), which means that the oils can be marketed without provision of evidence of their safety, efficacy or quality (Barnes, 2003). This lack of evidence could prove detrimental to the health and safety of the public.

The botanic origin of the plant from which the oil is derived can raise questions of safety, as plants often belong to a family or species, only one of which is the source of an oil, and it is not always guaranteed that the right species has been used. For example the Melaleuca species from which tea tree oil is derived includes M cajuputi, M quinquenervia and Malternifolia. Tea tree oil is only derived from the last of these.

Essential oils now come under the new European Community Regulation on the Registration, Evaluation, Authorisation and Restriction of Chemicals (REACH) which was adopted in 2006 and aims to improve the protection of human health. REACH should improve the safety of manufacture and use of the essential oils.

There have already been improvements to the training for aromatherapists have in response to the House of Lords Science and Technology *Sixth Report* (2000). The Aromatherapy Organisation Council – Education and Training, now the Aromatherapy Council (AC), published national vocational standards in 1998. Valid training courses must be mapped to these for those passing them to be licensed to practise as an aromatherapist. For example the course must now include a module on the chemistry of oils, which is a step towards increasing the safety of clients and practitioners alike.

Aromatherapists need to be aware of both the over-the-counter drugs and the prescribed medication a client is taking: they can identify the uses and side-effects through free access to the British National Formulary, which is now accessible online at www.bnf.org.uk. While the AC is raising awareness of the potential effects of interactions between drugs and essential oils, this does not appear to be research-based. Rigorous clinical trials need to be carried out to check on specific interactions, but there has been little or no progress as yet in this direction.

W

Research into aromatherapy indicates that there is disagreement over its benefits for people experiencing anxiety and relaxation. Cooke and Ernst (2000) made a systematic review of available research but stated that the evidence was probably of insufficient depth to justify any firm conclusion. A systematic review of the use of aromatherapy in the treatment of premenstrual tension resulted in a similar conclusion (Stevinson and Ernst, 2001). These results strongly suggests the need for more rigorous research into the uses of aromatherapy.

Reflexology

Hieroglyphic inscriptions showing physicians or practitioners working on the hands and feet of other people have been found on the walls of an ancient Egyptian physician's tomb at Saqqara. This suggests that a form of reflexology, which might be a direct forerunner of today's discipline, was used in ancient Egypt around 2300 BC.

Reflexology, a natural and holistic therapy, has its base in the claim that specific locations on a person's hands and feet relate to all human organs, structures and systems within the body (Pitman, 2002). This close relationship is called a 'reflex': a more specific use of the general term for application of a stimulus to one area resulting in a reaction in another area (Pitman, 2002). Reflexology involves the reflexologist applying pressure via their thumbs and fingertips, to stimulate pre-identified points on the hands and feet of the recipient. It is claimed that this can detect and resolve imbalances of energy in organs, tissues and systems, thus restoring balance and well-being (Pitman, 2002).

A search of systematic reviews involving reflexology has provided no firm evidence that reflexology is an effective treatment or adjunct to conventional treatment. A greater quantity of rigorous research on the use of reflexology in the treatment of medical conditions is required.

> ### ⟲ⓐ Learning activity
>
> Choose a common condition, perhaps from the clinical area in which you are working. Find two research articles which discuss the use of reflexology and your chosen topic, and assess their results.

Healing

The word 'healing' is derived from the Anglo-Saxon word 'haelan' which means whole, incorporating the physical, mental and spiritual aspects of the body (Furner, 2004). Healing. in the sense of the laying-on of hands, has been used for thousands of years in all cultures. There are many different forms depending on the local culture, but with the rise of modern scientifically based medicine this form of healing was reduced to folklore medicine (Porter, 1997). Healing has, however, had a revival of interest, through the developing use and interest in modern medicine and also through advances in scientific discoveries.

In today's world of medicine and science these nonscientific forms of healing are collectively referred to as 'energy healing'. (Here we use the terms 'healing' and 'healing energy' as necessary for clarity.)

The contemporary forms of hands-on healing that you might encounter include spiritual healing, including distant healing/prayer, Reiki, and therapeutic touch (Gerber, 1988, 2000). The basic thesis underpinning all these varieties of healing is that the therapist or healer can channel energy (from a source that corresponds with the therapists' and patients' belief system) into the recipient (Gerber, 1988). This healing energy then stimulates the person's ability to self-heal (Gerber, 1988).

Oschman claims that 'Healing energy, whether produced by a medical device or projected from the human body, is energy of a particular frequency that stimulates the repair of one or more tissues' (2006: 87). This concept of variation in signal frequencies had been noted in earlier research by Zimmerman (1990), who recorded signals from a healing practitioner's hands and found that there were variations between the signal frequencies. These ranged from 3 to 30 Hz, with a cluster around 7–8 Hz. Research has found that the healing effects of specific frequencies of healing energy differ (Sisken and Walker, 1995, cited in Oschman, 2000). While this does not answer the questions whether, and how, this form of healing works, it does offer an avenue for further research.

> ### a Learning activity
>
> Find out if any GP surgeries, hospitals or charities connected to hospitals in your area employ spiritual healers or Reiki practitioners, refer individuals to them, or offer either therapy to patients. If so, for which complaints is this considered?

The results of a systematic review of random controlled trials of spiritual healing (Astin et al, 2000) were inconclusive regarding whether or not this was an effective intervention. The authors recommended that many and more rigorous trials be carried out in future.

> ### a Learning activity
>
> Try this small experiment into healing techniques.
> 1 Sit facing a partner with your knees almost touching each other and your feet flat on the floor, shoulder width apart.
> 2 Ask your partner to rest their hands on their legs, with palms facing upwards, keeping the hands relaxed.
> 3 Sitting with your knees very close to your partner, place the palms of your hands over your partner's palms so that both sets of palms are gently touching. Your eyes can be open or closed.
> 4 Slowly raise your hands 2–3 inches above your partner's, keeping your palms directly above theirs, then hold this position for 1–2 minutes.
> 5 Repeat this deliberate raising of your hands four or five more times, pausing above your partner's hands each time for 1–2 minutes, then reverse the process until your hands are again gently touching your partner's hands.
> 6 Reverse the position of your hands so they are resting palms upwards on your knees. Your partner then performs the active role outlined above.
>
> Discuss the results of this exercise.

CAM and clinical healthcare practice

The increasing public use and acceptance of forms of CAM presents professional nurses and other healthcare professionals with new challenges. Whether you are preparing to introduce CAM into your own area of practice, need to respond to a patient's enquiry, or are considering suggesting that a client try an additional form of therapy, there are several issues you must take into consideration.

You must always remember that you are bound by your professional code of practice, for example the Nursing and Midwifery Council's *Code of Professional Practice* (NMC, 2008). It is integral to this code is that nurses must deliver a safe standard of care, and the code explicitly mentions that this care should be 'based on the best available evidence' (NMC, 2008). This chapter has shown, albeit briefly, that there is a lack of evidence based on rigorous scientific search for the outcomes of many therapies, particularly the ones most practised by nurses, such as massage and reflexology.

It is important that you do not either use, or provide information about and encourage clients to use, any therapy unless you have identified and familiarised yourself with the best of the research into it that is available. This requires study skills of the kind that you are likely to acquire in your professional course (see also Chapter 1).

Another essential is that you discover whether your employer has a policy on the use of CAM, and that you adhere to it at all times. If you find that there is no such policy, it would

Part
IV

be an useful protection for yourself as well as your clients to suggest that one be drawn up. If there is a policy (as should be the case if your employer is providing CAM to patients), there should be a clinical protocol in place. This will set boundaries for practice within which you must work.

Other areas for consideration include consultation with the other members of a multidisciplinary team that is responsible for the individual. All relevant individuals should be aware of the proposed use of a CAM, and should agree on this way forward before the therapy is practised. This will involve determining which if any therapy is appropriate for the individual, considering evidence on its risk, and identifying the accountability and responsibility of the staff delivering the therapy, as well as any other relevant issues. Patients must give consent to CAM treatment as they do to conventional treatment, and it might be necessary to draw up a specific consent form for this purpose, as the standard form might not be appropriate. Because of the possible legal implications your healthcare organisation will want to review and agree the consent process before any treatment is given.

Discussions with your employing organisation must also include the environment in which the therapy will be carried out. This is particularly important if aromatherapy oils are being used, as the aroma of the oils cannot be contained, and inhalation of the odour by another patient, visitor or member of staff might cause an allergic reaction or other unwanted effect.

Of course there are also financial implications, which include both staff time (or the time of brought-in practitioners) and resources. If a salaried professional is to provide the therapy as an adjunct to their normal duties, this might require an adjustment to their contract of employment. The question of insurance must also be addressed, and so must equal opportunity issues. Other issues to be considered include evaluation and auditing, to determine the effectiveness or otherwise of the therapy, and how many people have used the service.

As has been noted earlier, there are a number of organisations that regulate the provision of CAM, and any practitioner should be appropriately trained and become a member of the relevant professional body or bodies. This should also provide access to insurance and continuing professional development, issues that must be considered carefully. A nurse belonging to the Royal College of Nursing (RCN) and qualifying and practising in a field of CAM would, for example, continue to be covered by RCN indemnity insurance providing they remained appropriately qualified and/or registered, did not breach their employer's policies and protocols, and operated within the NMC Code of Conduct (2008).

Experience must be considered as well as training, as is indeed the case for any form of healthcare. Newly qualified practitioners should initially be supervised by the more experienced. This should prove easier in areas where CAM therapies have already been established. Should there be no local person with suitable experience in your own field of work, you might need to carry out research to locate an appropriate supervisor: perhaps an experienced practitioner in the therapy whose primary work is another clinical area.

The requirements are less stringent if you do not plan to practise a therapy yourself, but when you give any advice to individuals you should ensure that you are appropriately informed to do so.

> ### ⓐ Learning activity
>
> A district nurse visits a patient in the community to re-dress a leg wound which is not healing after two weeks of orthodox treatment. 'I've read an article in a magazine,' the patient says, 'that suggests Manuka honey is a good thing to use for wounds that aren't healing very well. You spread it on a cabbage leaf, and tie it on instead of the usual kind of dressing, apparently. I've bought the honey: here it is. Will you fix that for me please?'
>
> In your learning group, discuss how the nurse should respond to this request. What professional and ethical issues does it raise?

Conclusion

This chapter has provided a brief introduction to some of the CAM therapies you might encounter. You should now realise why it is necessary for all health practitioners to have at least a broad awareness of the therapies currently being used, and the evidence on their results. If you are considering including a CAM therapy in your clinical practice, you will want to research it in considerably more depth. A good resource to start you on continued research is the RCN publication *Complementary Therapies in Nursing, Midwifery and Health Visiting* (2003).

References

Angelo, J. (2002) *Spiritual Healing: A practical guide to hands-on healing*, London, Godsfield Press.

Astin, J. A., Harkness, E. and Ernst, E. (2000) 'The efficacy of "distant healing": a systematic review of randomized trials', *Annals of Internal Medicine* **132**(11), 903–10.

Barnes, J. (2003) 'Quality, efficacy and safety of complementary medicines: fashions, facts and the future, Part 1: Regulation and quality', *British Journal of Clinical Pharmacology* 55, 226–33.

Bendick, J. (2002) *Galen and the Gateway to Medicine*, San Francisco, Bethlehem Books/Ignatius Press,

Brennan, B. (1990) *Hands of Light: Guide to healing through the human energy field*, rev. edn, London, Bantam.

Carson, C. F. and Riley, T. V. (2001) 'Safety, efficacy and province of tea tree (Melaleuca Alternifolia)', *Contact Dermatitis* 45, 63–7.

Castro, M. (2003) *The Complete Homeopathy Handbook*, London, St. Martin Press.

Cherkin, D. C., Deyo, R. A., Battie, M., Street, J. and Bralow, W. (1998) 'A comparison of physical therapy, chiropractic manipulation and provision of an educational booklet for the treatment of patients with low back pain', *New England Journal of Medicine* **339**(15), 1021–9.

Cherkin, D. C., Sherman, K. J. and Deyo, P. G. (2003) 'A review of the evidence for the effectiveness, safety and cost of acupuncture, massage therapy and spinal manipulation for low back pain', *Annals of Internal Medicine* **138**(11) (3 June), 898–906.

Cooke, B and Ernst, E. (2000) 'Aromatherapy: a systematic review', *British Journal of General Practice* 50(455) (1 June), 493–6.

Coulter, 1981)

Deuraseh, N. (2005) 'Medical care during the middle ages', *Journal of the International Society for the History of Islamic Medicine* 4(8) (October), 1–21.

Department of Health (DH) (2000) *Complementary Medicine: Information for primary care clinicians*, June, London, DH.

DH (2008) *Report to Ministers for the Department of Health Steering Group on the Statutory Regulation of Practitioners of Acupuncture, Herbal Medicine, Traditional Chinese Medicine and Other Traditional Medicine Systems Practised in the UK*, London, DH.

Dougans, I. (2005) *Reflexology: The 5 elements and their meridians – a unique approach*, rev. edn, London, Thorsons.

Ernst, E. (2000) 'The role of complementary and alternative medicine', *British Medical Journal* 321 (4 November), 1133–5.

Ernst, E. and Calder, P. H. (2006) 'A systematic review of systematic reviews of spinal manipulation', *Journal of the Royal Society of Medicine* 99, 192–6.

Ernst, E., Pittler, B., Wilder, B. and Boddy, K. (2007) 'Massage therapy: is evidence-base getting stronger?' *Complementary Health Practice Review* 12, 178–83.

Fowler, P and Wall, M. (1997) 'COSHH and CHIPS: ensuring the safety of aromatherapy', *Complementary Therapies in Medicine* 15, 112–15.

Furlan, A. D., Brosseau, L., Imamura, M. and Irvin, E., (2003) 'Massage for low back pain', *Cochrane Database of Systematic Reviews* 2007, Issue 2.

Furner, J. (2004) 'Healing the mind and body as spirit fails', *Nursing* 34(4).50–1.

General Osteopathic Council (GOC) (2008) *Good Health in Good Hands: UK osteopathy today*, January, London, GOC.

Gerber, R. (1988) *Vibrational Medicine*, Santa Fe/New York. Bear.

Gerber, R. (2000) *Vibrational Medicine for the 21st Century*, London, Piatkus.

Gillanders, A. (1994) *Reflexology: The theory and practice*, Jenny Lee.

Health and Safety Commission (HSC) (1994) *The Control of Substances hazardous to Health Regulations*, London, HMSO.

Hicks, A. (2005) *The Acupuncture Handbook: How acupuncture works and how it can help you*, London, Piatkus.

Hill, F. (1995) 'Massage in intensive care nursing: a literature review', *Complementary Therapies in Medicine* **3**(2), 100–4.

Holey, E. and Cook, E. (2003) *Evidence-Based Therapeutic Massage: A practical guide for therapists*, Edinburgh, Churchill Livingstone/ Elsevier.

Horowitz, S. (2007) 'Evidence based application for chiropractic', *Alternative and Complementary Therapies* **13**(5), 248–53.

House of Lords Select Committee on Science and Technology (2000) *Complementary and Alternative Medicine: 6th Report (session 1999–2000)*, reprinted 2003 [online] http://www.parliament.the-stationery-office.co.uk/pa/ld199900/ldselect/ldsctech/123/12301. htm (accessed 18 December 2008).

Howell, J. D. (1999) 'The paradox of osteopathy', *New England Journal of Medicine* **341**(19), 1465–8.

Huan Ti (1995) *The Yellow Emperor's Classic of Internal Medicine*, trans. N. I. Maoshing, Boston, M.A., Shambala.

Huntley, A. and Ernst, E. (2000) 'Complementary and alternative therapies for treating multiple sclerosis symptoms: a systematic review', *Complementary Therapies in Medicine* **8**(2) (June), 97–105.

Kaptchuk, E. K. (2002) *The Web That Has No Weaver*, New York, Contemporary Books.

Kayne, S. B. (2002) *Alternative Medicine*, London, Pharmaceutical Press.

Kuhn, M. A. (1999) *Complementary Therapies for Healthcare Providers*, Baltimore, Md., Lippincott Williams & Wilkins.

Kuriyama, S., (2002) *The Eexpressiveness of the Body and the Divergence of Greek and Chinese Medicine*, New York, Zone.

Libster, M. (2002) *Delmar's Integrative Herb Guide for Nurses*, United States, Thomson Learning.

Lubeck, W., Petter F.A. and Brand W.L. (2001) *The Spirit of Reiki: The complete handbook of the Reiki System from tradition to the present*,

Twin Lakes, Wis., USA, Lotus Press.

Maciocia, G. (1989) *The Foundations of Chinese Medicine*, Edinburgh, Churchill Livingstone.

McIntyre, E. (2004) 'Therapeutic massage: an amazing modality', *Home Healthcare Management Practice* 14, 516–20.

McKone, W. L. (2001) *Osteopathic Medicine: Philosophy, principles and practice*, Oxford, Wiley Blackwell.

Millgrom, L. R. (2006) 'Is homeopathy possible?' *Journal of the Royal Society for the Promotion of Health* **126**(5) September, 211–18.

Mills, S. and Bone. K. (2000) *Principles of Phytotherapy: Modern herbal medicine*, Edinburgh, Elsevier.

Mole, P. E. (1992) *Acupuncture: Eenergy balancing for body, mind and spirit, health essentials*, Dorset, Element Books.

Nursing and Midwifery Council (NMC) (2008) *The Code: Standards of conduct, performance and ethics for nurses and midwives*, London, NMC.

Oschman, J. L. (2000) *Energy Medicine: The scientific basis*, Edinburgh, Churchill Livingstone.

Pitman, V. (2002) *Reflexology: A practical approach*, 2nd edn, Cheltenham, Nelson Thornes.

Pole, S. (2006) *Ayurvedic Medicine: The principles of traditional practice*, Edinburgh, Churchill Livingstone.

Porter, R. (1997) *The Greatest Benefit to Mankind: A medical history of humanity*, New York, Morton.

Portmann, P. E. and Savage-Smith, E. (2007) *Medieval Islamic Medicine: The new Islamic surveys*, Edinburgh, Edinburgh University Press,

Royal College of Nursing (RCN) (2003) *Complementary Therapies in Nursing, Midwifery and Health Visiting Practice*, London, RCN.

Sendstad, O., Leboeuf-Yde, C. and Borchgrevink, C. F. (1996) 'Side effects of chiropractic spinal manipulation: types frequency, discomfort and course', *Scandinavian Journal of Primary Healthcare*

14(1), 50–3.

Stevinson, C. and Ernst, E. (2001) 'Complementary/alternative therapies for premenstrual syndrome: a systematic review of randomized controlled trials', *American Journal of Obstetrics and Gynaecology* **165**(1), 227–95.

Stone, J. (2002) *An Ethical Framework for Complementary and Alternative Therapists*, London, Routledge.

Tisserand, R. (1996) 'Essential oil safety', *International Journal of Aromatherapy* vol. 7.

Van Why, R. P. (1992) *The History of Massage and its Relevance to Today's Practitioner*, New York, Wappingers Falls.

Veitch, I, (2002) *Yellow Emperor's Classic of Internal Medicine*, Berkeley, C.A., California University Press.

Vickers, A. and Zollman, C. (1999) 'ABC of complementary medicine: massage therapies', *British Medical Journal* 319, 1254–7.

Wayne, B., Jones, M. D., Kaptchuk, T. J. and Linde, K. (2003) 'A critical overview of homeopathy', *Annals of Internal Medicine* **138**(5), 393–9.

Westland, G. (1993) 'Massage as a therapeutic tool', *British Journal of Occupational Therapy* **56**(4), 129–34; 56(3), 177–80.

Williams, T. (1995) *Chinese Medicine: Acupuncture, herbal remedies, nutrition, qigong and meditation for total health*, Australia, Element Books.

Wisneski, L.A. and Anderson, L. (2005) *The Scientific Basis of Integrative Medicine*, New York, CRC Press.

Zhalko-Tytarenko, A., Lednyiczky, G. and Topping, S. (1998) 'Towards a biophysics of homeopathy, 1: conceptual approach', *Journal of Advancement in Medicine* **11**(1) (March), 27–33.

Zimmerman, J. (1990) 'Laying-on-of-hands healing and therapeutic touch: a testable theory, BEMI currents', *Journal of the Bio-electric Magnetics Institutes* 24, 8–17.

Journals

Today's Therapist: www.todaystherapist.com
Complementary Therapies in Nursing and Midwifery
International Journal of Aromatherapy.

Websites

British National Formulary: www.bnf.org.uk
British Acupuncture Council/Accreditation Board: www.acupuncture.org.uk
British Medical Acupuncture Society: www.medical-acupuncture.co.uk

Legislation

Control of Substances Hazardous to Health Regulations (COSHH) 1994
E C Regulation on the Registration, Evaluation, Authorisation and Restriction of Chemicals (REACH) 2006

Names index

Subject index